SECOND OPINION

SECOND OPINION
An Introduction to Health Sociology

FOURTH EDITION

Edited by **JOHN GERMOV**

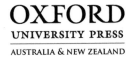

OXFORD
UNIVERSITY PRESS
AUSTRALIA & NEW ZEALAND

OXFORD
UNIVERSITY PRESS

Oxford University Press is a department of the University of Oxford.
It furthers the University's objective of excellence in research,
scholarship, and education by publishing worldwide. Oxford is a registered
trademark of Oxford University Press in the UK and in certain other
countries.

Published in Australia by
Oxford University Press
253 Normanby Road, South Melbourne, Victoria 3205, Australia

© John Germov 2009

The moral rights of the author have been asserted

First edition published 1998
Revised edition published 1999
Second edition published 2002
Third edition published 2005
Fourth edition published 2009
Reprinted 2009, 2010 (twice), 2011

National Library of Australia Cataloguing-in-Publication data

Germov, John
Second opinion : an introduction to health sociology / John Germov
4th ed.

ISBN 978 0 19 556281 1 (pbk)

Previous ed.: 2005.
Includes index.
Bibliography.

Social medicine—Australia.
Health—Social aspects—Australia.

306.4610994

Edited by Lisa Fraley
Cover illustration by Diana Platt
Text design by Mason Design
Typeset by Mason Design
Proofread by James Anderson
Indexed by Russell Brooks
Printed in Hong Kong by Sheck Wah Tong Printing Press Ltd

Contents

Expanded Contents

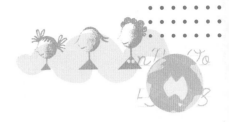

Preface to the Fourth Edition

It has been over a decade since the first edition of *Second Opinion*. This milestone marked an appropriate time to give the book its most significant revision to date. The fourth edition has new chapters, new authors, new pedagogic features, and a new format. That said, *Second Opinion* retains its accessible yet authoritative overview of key debates, research findings, and theories in the field of health sociology.

New to the fourth edition:

- **New chapters** on Global Public Health (Alex Broom & John Germov), Workplace Health (Toni Schofield), Rural Health (Clarissa Hughes), Mental Illness (Pauline Savy & Anne-Maree Sawyer), The Illness Experience (Daphne Habibis), and Media and Health (John Germov & Maria Freij)
- **New authors** for chapters on the Sociology of Nursing (Helen Keleher), the Sociology of Complementary and Alternative Medicine (Alex Broom), Ageing, Health and the Demographic Revolution (Marilyn Poole), plus an expanded Appendix on writing health sociology essays
- **A new reader-friendly dual-colour layout** with an expanded range of pedagogic features. Each chapter begins with a topical vignette to draw attention to relevant sociological issues. All chapters include highlighted 'doing health sociology' boxes that show the application of health sociology to real-life issues of health policy and practice. In addition, a list of recommended documentaries and films has been added to each chapter
- **Expanded book website:** the website now includes online access to chapter-relevant supplementary reading, access to chapters from the previous edition, topical case studies, and updated web links for all websites recommended in the book

Guide to the book

In addition to being a contemporary reader on the field of health sociology, the book is also designed to be used as a teaching text, with the following pedagogic features:

- **Overview:** each chapter opens with three main questions it seeks to address
- **Introductory vignettes** begin each chapter to grab the readers' interest and to encourage a sociologically reflexive approach to the topic
- **Key terms and concepts** are highlighted in bold in the text and defined in separate margin paragraphs and also appear in a **glossary** at the end of the book

- **Doing health sociology boxes** (new to this edition) highlight the insights of sociological research and theories for informing health care practice, health policy, and public understanding of the social origins of health and illness
- **Theory Links boxes** clearly cross-reference theoretical discussions in different chapters
- **Summary of main points**
- **Sociological reflection exercises** are self-directed or class-based exercises that help students apply their learning and highlight the relevance of sociological analysis
- **Discussion questions**
- **Further investigation** essay-style questions
- **Further reading**
- **Recommended chapter-specific web resources**
- **Recommended chapter-specific documentaries and films** (new to this edition)
- **Expanded appendix on essay writing** provides advice for students on the planning, writing, and referencing of health sociology essays, including tips on the critical use of web resources, how to reference the web, and how to reference chapters in this book
- **Expanded** *Second Opinion* **website** <www.oup.com.au/orc/germov/>:
    - **Online case studies** dealing with contemporary health issues for each chapter
    - **Links to all the web resources** recommended in the book
    - **Supplementary readings**
    - **Access to chapters from previous editions:** the Body, Medicine, and Society (Deborah Lupton), Ageing, Dying, and Death in the Twenty-first Century (Maureen Strazzari), Nursing and Sociology: An Uneasy Relationship (Deidre Wicks), Alternative Medicine (Gary Easthope), and Citizenship, Rights, and Health Care (Bryan Turner)
- Updated teaching resources for lecturers:
    - **Teaching Manual:** short tutorial exercises in the form of 'ice-breakers' for each chapter to facilitate student discussion
    - **Test Bank of Multiple-choice Questions:** over 200 questions and answers organised by chapter
    - **Downloadable PowerPoint slides** of all diagrams and tables in the book
      The Teaching Manual, Test Bank, and PowerPoint slides are available free of charge from the publisher for those using the book as a course text.

Suggestions, comments, and feedback

I am very interested in receiving feedback on the book and suggestions for future editions; many of the new features in this edition resulted from user feedback. Please contact me at: <John.Germov@newcastle.edu.au>

John Germov
The University of Newcastle, January 2009

Guided Tour

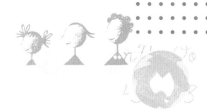

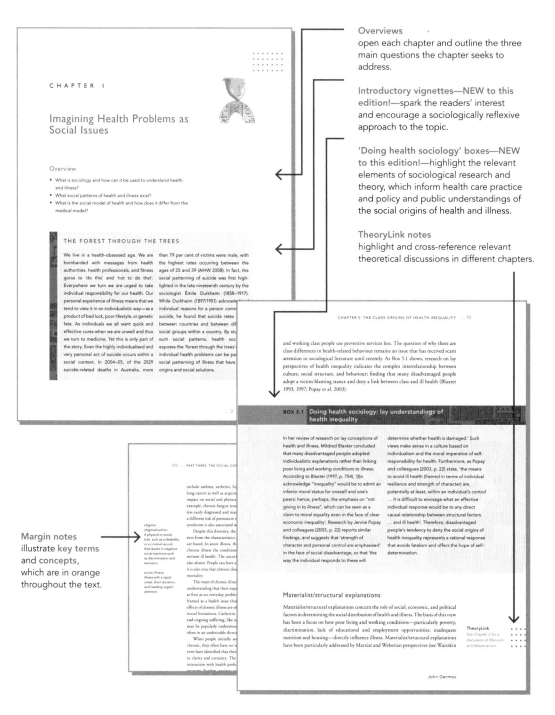

Overviews
open each chapter and outline the three main questions the chapter seeks to address.

Introductory vignettes—NEW to this edition!—spark the readers' interest and encourage a sociologically reflexive approach to the topic.

'Doing health sociology' boxes—NEW to this edition!—highlight the relevant elements of sociological research and theory, which inform health care practice and policy and public understandings of the social origins of health and illness.

TheoryLink notes
highlight and cross-reference relevant theoretical discussions in different chapters.

Margin notes
illustrate key terms and concepts, which are in orange throughout the text.

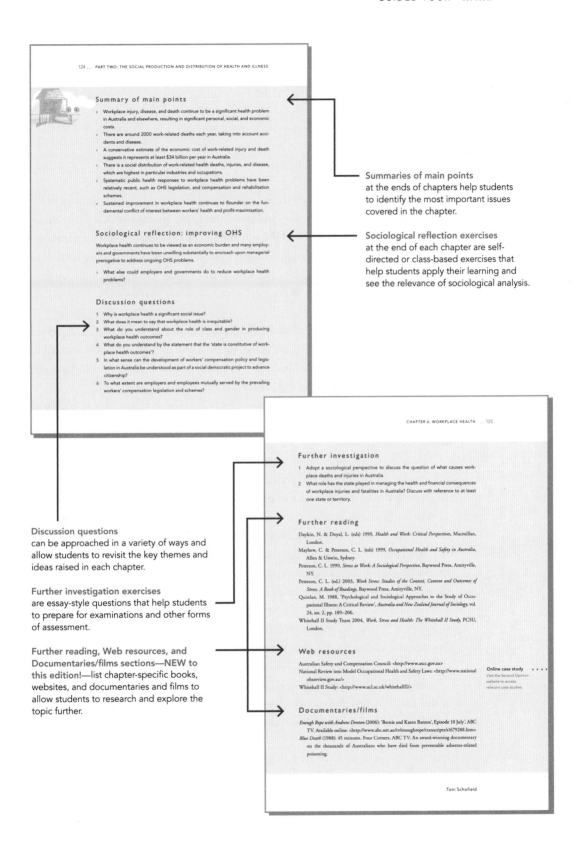

124 ... PART TWO: THE SOCIAL PRODUCTION AND DISTRIBUTION OF HEALTH AND ILLNESS

Summary of main points

- Workplace injury, disease, and death continue to be a significant health problem in Australia and elsewhere, resulting in significant personal, social, and economic costs.
- There are around 2000 work-related deaths each year, taking into account accidents and disease.
- A conservative estimate of the economic cost of work-related injury and death suggests it represents at least $34 billion per year in Australia.
- There is a social distribution of work-related health deaths, injuries, and disease, which are highest in particular industries and occupations.
- Systematic public health responses to workplace health problems have been relatively recent, such as OHS legislation, and compensation and rehabilitation schemes.
- Sustained improvement in workplace health continues to flounder on the fundamental conflict of interest between workers' health and profit-maximisation.

Sociological reflection: improving OHS

Workplace health continues to be viewed as an economic burden and many employers and governments have been unwilling substantially to encroach upon managerial prerogative to address ongoing OHS problems.

- What else could employers and governments do to reduce workplace health problems?

Discussion questions

1 Why is workplace health a significant social issue?
2 What does it mean to say that workplace health is inequitable?
3 What do you understand about the role of class and gender in producing workplace health outcomes?
4 What do you understand by the statement that the 'state is constitutive of workplace health outcomes'?
5 In what sense can the development of workers' compensation policy and legislation in Australia be understood as part of a social democratic project to advance citizenship?
6 To what extent are employers and employees mutually served by the prevailing workers' compensation legislation and schemes?

Summaries of main points
at the ends of chapters help students to identify the most important issues covered in the chapter.

Sociological reflection exercises
at the end of each chapter are self-directed or class-based exercises that help students apply their learning and see the relevance of sociological analysis.

CHAPTER 6: WORKPLACE HEALTH ... 125

Further investigation

1 Adopt a sociological perspective to discuss the question of what causes workplace deaths and injuries in Australia.
2 What role has the state played in managing the health and financial consequences of workplace injuries and fatalities in Australia? Discuss with reference to at least one state or territory.

Further reading

Daykin, N. & Doyal, L. (eds) 1999, *Health and Work: Critical Perspectives*, Macmillan, London.
Mayhew, C. & Peterson, C. L. (eds) 1999, *Occupational Health and Safety in Australia*, Allen & Unwin, Sydney.
Peterson, C. L. 1999, *Stress at Work: A Sociological Perspective*, Baywood Press, Amityville, NY.
Peterson, C. L. (ed.) 2003, *Work Stress: Studies of the Context, Content and Outcomes of Stress. A Book of Readings*, Baywood Press, Amityville, NY.
Quinlan, M. 1988, 'Psychological and Sociological Approaches to the Study of Occupational Illness: A Critical Review', *Australia and New Zealand Journal of Sociology*, vol. 24, no. 2, pp. 189–206.
Whitehall II Study Team 2004, *Work, Stress and Health: The Whitehall II Study*, PCSU, London.

Web resources

Australian Safety and Compensation Council: <http://www.ascc.gov.au>
National Review into Model Occupational Health and Safety Laws: <http://www.national ohsreview.gov.au/>
Whitehall II Study: <http://www.ucl.ac.uk/whitehallII/>

Online case study • • • •
Visit the Second Opinion website to access relevant case studies.

Documentaries/films

Enough Rope with Andrew Denton (2006): 'Bernie and Karen Banton', Episode 10 July', ABC TV. Available online: <http://www.abc.net.au/tv/enoughrope/transcripts/s1679288.htm>
Blue Death (1988): 45 minutes. Four Corners, ABC TV. An award-winning documentary on the thousands of Australians who have died from preventable asbestos-related poisoning.

Toni Schofield

Discussion questions
can be approached in a variety of ways and allow students to revisit the key themes and ideas raised in each chapter.

Further investigation exercises
are essay-style questions that help students to prepare for examinations and other forms of assessment.

Further reading, Web resources, and Documentaries/films sections—NEW to this edition!—list chapter-specific books, websites, and documentaries and films to allow students to research and explore the topic further.

Acknowledgments

A book such as this is a team effort and once again I thank all of the contributors for producing chapters of high quality and consistency, and for making my job as editor a pleasurable one. This time I had the added luxury of a research assistant cum copy editor extraordinaire, Maria Freij, who has been fundamental to the production of the fourth edition and an absolute pleasure to work with. Thanks again to my dear friend and colleague Lauren Williams for ensuring my sensitivity to the work of health professionals.

In relation to the earlier editions, thanks to Helen Belcher for her willingness to provide invaluable feedback on drafts of various chapters; and my continuing gratitude to Lois Bryson and Deidre Wicks, who provided advice throughout the evolution of the first edition of the book for which I am forever grateful.

Thanks are also due to my publishers, firstly Jill Henry, Debra James, and more recently Katie Ridsdale and Rachel Saffer. Thanks also to Tim Campbell and the designer, Mary Mason.

Finally a special note of appreciation to Sue Jelovcan for her support, patience, and good humour during the production of this book, and also to our 3-year-old daughter 'Isabella' who has sharpened and enlivened my sociological gaze.

The authors and publisher are grateful to the following copyright holders for granting permission to reproduce various extracts and figures in this book: University of Queensland Press for permission to reproduce the figure from D. Gordon, *Health, Sickness and Society*, University of Queensland Press, Brisbane, 1976, p. 186, Figure 19; the Food and Agricultural Organization of the United Nations for reproduction of Figures 4.3 and 4.4; the World Health Organization for reproduction of Figure 4.5; the Australian Bureau of Statistics for Figure 5.1; the Australian Government Office for Women for reproduction of Table 7.1; the Commonwealth of Australia for reproduction of Table 15.1.

Every effort has been made to trace the original source of all material reproduced in this book. Where the attempt has been unsuccessful, the authors and publisher would be pleased to hear from the copyright holder concerned to rectify any omission.

Contributors

Fran Baum (PhD) is a Professor of Public Health at Flinders University, Foundation Director of the South Australian Community Health Research Unit and an Australian Research Council Federation Fellow. She is also Co-Chair of the Global Steering Council of the People's Health Movement (http://www.phmovement. org) and from 2005–08 was a Commissioner for the Commission on the Social Determinants of Health (http://www.who.int/social_determinants/en/) established by the World Health Organization. She is a Fellow of the Australian Academy of Social Science and the National Health Promotion Association and a past National President and Life Member of the Public Health Association of Australia. The third edition of her popular textbook *The New Public Health* was published in 2008.

Helen Belcher (PhD) is a Lecturer in the School of Humanities and Social Science at The University of Newcastle. She has a background in nursing and lectures nurses and allied health professionals. Her research interests include health sociology, health policy, and religion.

Alex Broom (PhD) is a Senior Lecturer in Sociology at The University of Sydney specialising in health and illness. His research interests include the sociology of cancer, gender and inequality, information technologies in healthcare, health systems in developing countries, and the sociology of complementary and alternative medicine. These specialisms have emerged from research projects in Australia, New Zealand, the United Kingdom, Pakistan, India, and Brazil.

Dorothy Broom (PhD) is a Professor at the National Centre for Epidemiology and Population Health (NCEPH), Australian National University (ANU), where she is involved in research on inequalities in health, the relationship between work and family health, and gendering health. She also supervises PhD candidates. She was formerly Convenor of Women's Studies at ANU, and is the author of a number of articles and books, including *Damned If We Do: Contradictions in Women's Health Care* (1991), *Double Bind: Women Affected by Alcohol and Other Drugs* (1994) and (with Jane Dixon) *The Seven Deadly Sins of Obesity: How the Modern World is Making Us Fat* (2007). In 1993 she was named Canberra Woman of the Year for distinguished service to the Australian Capital Territory's women's movement and to women's health. In 1994 she was made a Member of the Order of Australia for services to women and women's health.

Douglas Ezzy (PhD) is an Associate Professor of Sociology and Head of Discipline at the University of Tasmania. His research is driven by a fascination with how people make meaningful and dignified lives. His books include *Qualitative Research Methods* (1999) with Pranee Liamputtong, *Narrating Unemployment* (2001), *Qualitative Analysis* (2002), and *Teenage Witches* (2007) with Helen Berger (West Chester University).

Maria Freij (PhD) is a Social Researcher at the University of Newcastle, Australia, with interests in representations of health and identity. She has a PhD in Creative Writing and, in her other career, is a published poet. Her work appears in, among other journals, *Meanjin*, *Blue Dog*, *Overland Magazine*, *Softblow Poetry Journal*, and *Mascara*. Maria translates between French, Swedish, and English, especially poetry, and is interested in expatriate writing, grammar, and notions of identity and self in relation to place. She teaches Creative Writing and French at the University of Newcastle. Her poetry collection, *I Was Here*, won the Harri Jones memorial prize in 2007.

John Germov (PhD) is an Associate Professor of Sociology, Dean of Arts, and Head of the School of Humanities and Social Science at the University of Newcastle, Australia. John is a former President of TASA: The Australian Sociological Association (2002–04), established TASAweb and was its editor (1996–2005), is an Editorial Board Member for the *Journal of Sociology* and a former Executive Board member of the ISA: International Sociological Association (2002–06). John's books include: *A Sociology of Food and Nutrition: The Social Appetite* (with L. Williams; OUP 2008, 2004, 1999); *Public Sociology: An Introduction to Australian Society* (with M. Poole; Allen & Unwin, 2007); *Australian Youth: Social and Cultural Issues* (with P. Nilan & R. Julian; Pearson, 2007); *Histories of Australian Sociology* (with T. McGee; Melbourne University Publishing, 2005); *Get Great Marks for Your Essays* (Allen & Unwin, 2000, 1996), *Surviving First Year Uni* (with L. Williams; Allen & Unwin, 2001) and *Get Great Information Fast* (with L. Williams; Allen & Unwin, 1998).

Dennis Gray (MPH, PhD) is a Professor of Medical Anthropology and Deputy Director at the National Drug Research Institute (NDRI), Curtin University of Technology. He has worked in the areas of Indigenous and international health since the mid-1970s. In 1992, he established the Indigenous Australian Research Program at NDRI, which he continues to head. He has a theoretical interest in the structural determinants of Indigenous health and is committed to conducting research which has practical outcomes for Indigenous Australians. In 2006, his research team won a National Alcohol and Drug Award for Excellence in Research, and a Curtin University Vice-Chancellor's Award for Excellence.

Daphne Habibis (PhD) is Deputy Head of the School of Sociology and Social Work at the University of Tasmania. Her published works include *Social Inequality in Australia: Discourses, Realities and Futures* (2008) with Maggie Walter, and three editions of *Sociology: Themes and Perspectives* with van Krieken and others. Her interests in health research have focused on mental health in the areas of housing and service delivery. She is currently engaged in a national study on the housing implications of Indigenous patterns of mobility.

Clarissa Hughes (PhD) is a Research Fellow with the Department of Rural Health at the University of Tasmania. She has a background in sociology and a particular interest in utilising theoretical concepts and insights to strengthen practical efforts to improve health. Her main research interests include youth/child health, alcohol and other drugs, chronic illness, and mental health. She has published widely within health-related and social scientific journals, and has presented at national and international conferences. She is the first-named Chief Investigator for SNAP, which is the first Australian trial of the Social Norms Approach to Reducing Alcohol-related Harm Among Young People.

Roberta Julian (PhD) is an Associate Professor and Director of the Tasmanian Institute of Law Enforcement Studies at the University of Tasmania. She is a sociologist who has published widely in the areas of immigrant and refugee settlement, ethnicity and health, globalisation and diaspora, and the relationships between class, gender, and ethnic identity. She has published on Hmong identity and Hmong women in *Race, Gender and Class, Asian and Pacific Migration Journal,* and *Women's Studies International Forum.* She has recently completed an ARC-funded project on community policing and refugee settlement that focused on refugees from Africa. Her most recent books are *Australian Youth: Social and Cultural Issues* (with Pam Nilan and John Germov, Pearson 2007) and *Australian Sociology: A Changing Society (2e)* (with David Holmes and Kate Hughes, Pearson Longman 2007).

Helen Keleher (PhD) is a Professor and Head of the Department of Health Science in the School of Primary Health Care at Monash University. Her research has resulted in studies on mental health promotion, primary health care, and building capacity for health promotion in the workforce. She has co-authored evidence reviews on health promotion in cardiovascular disease, self-management in diabetes, and mental health promotion. Her teaching areas include health promotion, health systems and policy, and community capacity building. Currently, she holds an appointment to the Women and Gender Equity Knowledge Network of the World Health Organization's Commission on the Social Determinants of Health. She is the immediate past National Convenor of the Australian Women's Health Network and is a past Vice-President (Policy) of the Public Health Association of Australia.

Marilyn Poole (PhD) is an Associate Professor in Sociology at Deakin University. Although now retired and holding an honorary appointment, she continues to write and lecture and work in a voluntary capacity in programs and services for older people. She is co-editor of *A Certain Age: Women Growing Older* and *Public Sociology: An Introduction to Australian Society*, and editor of *Family*.

Katy Richmond (MA) is a former Senior Lecturer in Sociology and current Honorary Associate at La Trobe University. She has written on women in employment, women and deviance, homosexuality in prisons, and women and health. Her current research is on Aboriginal women's health. She was a founding member of TASA's Women's Section, was President of the Association in 1991–92, and in 2004 was a recipient of the Distinguished Service to Australian Sociology Award.

Sharyn L. Roach Anleu (PhD) is a Professor of Sociology at Flinders University, Adelaide, a Fellow of the Academy of Social Sciences in Australia, and a past president of The Australian Sociological Association. She was one of three editors of the *Journal of Sociology* (2001–04) and is the author of *Law and Social Change* (Sage, London) and four editions of *Deviance, Conformity and Control* (Pearson, Sydney) and numerous articles on deviance, legal regulation, and the criminal justice system. Sharyn is currently undertaking research with Professor Kathy Mack on judicial officers and their courts in Australia.

Sherry Saggers (PhD) is a Professor and Team Leader of a program on the social contexts of substance use at the National Drug Research Institute, Curtin University of Technology. An anthropologist, she was formerly Foundation Professor of Applied Social Science and Director of the Centre for Social Research at Edith Cowan University. She has conducted applied research among diverse populations throughout Australia, and published widely on Indigenous health and social issues, health and disability, and broadly in sociology.

Pauline Savy (PhD) has been a sociologist at the Albury-Wodonga campus of La Trobe University where her subjects included first year sociology, sociology of health and illness, and sociology of emotions. She now holds an honorary position at La Trobe University. Pauline's teaching, research, and community interests reflect her past professional nursing career working with aged and mentally ill people. Her publications concern the problem of voice for individuals marginalised by illness, stigma, and reduced capacity to give coherent accounts of their lives. Pauline is a co-author of the text *Sociology in Today's World*, 2008 (Thomson, Melbourne) and is an editor of the journal *Health Sociology Review*.

Anne-Maree Sawyer (PhD) is a Research Fellow in the School of Social Sciences at La Trobe University. She has taught sociology and social policy to undergraduate students, and also has extensive experience as a mental health social worker in both institutional and community-based settings. Her research interests include mental health policy and practice, social welfare, and narrative methodologies in social research.

Toni Schofield (PhD) works in the Faculty of Health Sciences at The University of Sydney. She conducts research in the field of health, equity, and social organisation and has worked extensively with community-based, state, and Commonwealth government agencies in developing policy and services in health. She is currently undertaking an ARC-funded investigation of the role of occupational health and safety legislation in New South Wales and Victoria in preventing major workplace injury and fatality.

Lauren Williams (PhD) is a Senior Lecturer and Program Convenor of Nutrition and Dietetics at the University of Newcastle, Australia. She holds tertiary qualifications in science, dietetics, social science, health promotion, and public health. Lauren has published journal articles and book chapters on her quantitative and qualitative research into weight gain, weight control practices, body acceptance in women, allied health, and rural health. Along with John Germov, she has co-edited *A Sociology of Food and Nutrition: The Social Appetite* (OUP 2008, 2004, 1999) and co-authored study skills books. With over 20 years of experience in the field of public health nutrition, Lauren is an Advanced Accredited Practising Dietitian, and an associate editor for the journal *Nutrition and Dietetics*.

Evan Willis (PhD) is a Professor of Sociology at La Trobe University in Melbourne. He has researched and taught in the medical sociology field for more than 30 years. His interests in the field cover medical technology, alternative medicine, occupational health and safety, and health care work. His first book, *Medical Dominance*, was voted by peers as one of the 10 most influential books in Australian sociology.

Abbreviations

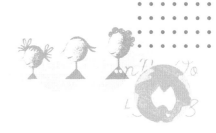

AA	Alcoholics Anonymous
ABS	Australian Bureau of Statistics
ACHA	Australian Community Health Association
AD[H]D	attention deficit [hyperactivity] disorder
AGPS	Australian Government Publishing Service
AHPA	Allied Health Professions Australia
AIDS	acquired immune deficiency syndrome
AIHW	Australian Institute of Health and Welfare
ALP	Australian Labor Party
AMA	Australian Medical Association
ARIA	Accessibility/Remoteness Index of Australia
ASCC	Australian Safety and Compensation Council
ASGC	Australian Standard Geographical Classification
ASRI	Australian Skills Recognition Information
ATSIC	Aboriginal and Torres Strait Islander Commission
BMA	British Medical Association
BMI	Body Mass Index
BRW	*Business Review Weekly*
Bt	*Bacillus thuringiensis*
CACPs	Community Aged Care Packages
CAM	complementary and alternative medicine
CCTs	Coordinated Care Trials
CHP	Community Health Program
CSDH	Commission on the Social Determinants of Health
DAA	Dietitians Association of Australia
DHFS	Department of Health and Family Services
DIMA	Department of Immigration and Multicultural Affairs
DIMIA	Department of Immigration and Multicultural and Indigenous Affairs
DOHA	Department of Health and Ageing
DNA	deoxyribonucleic acid
DRGs	Diagnosis Related Groups
DRS	Doctors Reform Society
DSM	*Diagnostic and Statistical Manual of Mental Disorders*
DSM-IV	Fourth edition of *Diagnostic and Statistical Manual of Mental Disorders*

DSM-IV-TR	Fourth (Text revised) edition of *Diagnostic and Statistical Manual of Mental Disorders*
DVA	Department of Veterans' Affairs
EBM	evidence-based medicine
ELSI	ethical, legal, and social implications (of the Human Genome Project)
EPC	Enhanced Primary Care
FAO	Food and Agriculture Organization
FDA	Food and Drug Administration
FSANZ	Food Standards Australia New Zealand
GDP	gross domestic product
GIO	Government Insurance Office
GM	genetic modification
GNI	gross national income
GP	general practitioner
HACC	Home and Community Care program
HGH	human growth hormone
HGP	Human Genome Project
HHSC	Hospitals and Health Services Commission
HIC	Health Issues Centre
HIV	human immunodeficiency virus
HPCA	Health Profession Council of Australia
HREOC	Human Rights and Equal Opportunity Commission
IHP	individualist health promotion
IMR	Infant mortality rates
MDGs	Millennium Development Goals
NAAFA	National Association to Advance Fat Acceptance
NACCHO	National Aboriginal Community Controlled Health Organisation
NAHOSN	National Allied Health Organisational Structures Network
NAHSWP	National Aboriginal Health Strategy Working Party
NAMI	National Alliance for the Mentally Ill
NATSIHC	National Strategic Framework for Aboriginal and Torres Strait Islander Health
NATSISS	National Aboriginal and Torres Strait Islander Social Survey
NCEPH	National Centre for Epidemiology and Population Health
NCHS	National Center for Health Statistics
NESB	non-English-speaking background
NHHRC	National Health and Hospital Reform Commission
NHMRC	National Health and Medical Research Council
NHPAs	National Health Priority Areas
NHS	National Health Strategy (Australia) or National Health Service (United Kingdom)

NOHSC	National Occupational Health and Safety Commission
NRRAHAS	National Rural and Remote Allied Health Advisory Service
NTDs	neural tube defects
OECD	Organization for Economic Cooperation and Development
ODI	official development assistance
OHS	occupational health and safety
OOS	occupational over-use syndrome
OSW	Office of the Status of Women
PBS	Pharmaceutical Benefits Scheme
PCPs	Primary Care Partnerships
PDD	premenstrual dysphoric disorder
PDRS	psychiatric disability rehabilitation support
PHC	primary health care
PHIAC	Private Health Insurance Administration Council
PKU	phenylketonuria
PMS	premenstrual syndrome
PTSD	post-traumatic stress disorder
RCTs	randomised control trials
RPBS	Repatriation Pharmaceutical Benefits Scheme
RRMA	Rural, Remote and Metropolitan Areas
RSI	repetition strain injury
RUSC	Rural Undergraduate Support and Coordination
RVCN	Royal Victorian College of Nurses
SARRAH	Services for Australian Rural and Remote Allied Health
SCHIP	State Children's Health Insurance Program
SCHP	structuralist-collectivist health promotion
SES	socio-economic status
SG	Superannuation Guarantee
TASA	The Australian Sociological Association
TCM	traditional Chinese medicine
TM	traditional medicine
TQM	Total Quality Management
VTNA	Victorian Trained Nurses' Association
WFS	World Food Summit
WHO	World Health Organization
WSO	World Sugar Organization

PART ONE

Health Sociology and the Social Model of Health

At the heart of health sociology is a belief that many health problems have social origins. The focus of health sociology is not on medical treatment or individual cures for ill health. While individuals suffer ill health and require health care, some of the causes and cures can often lie in the social context in which they live and work. Health sociology asks you to step outside the square and look beyond medical opinions by adopting a second opinion, which focuses on how health, illness, and the health care system are by-products of the way a society is organised.

This introductory part of the book provides an overview of health sociology: what it is, its major theoretical perspectives, and the types of health research it draws upon. Specifically, Part 1 consists of three chapters:

Chapter 1 Imagining Health Problems as Social Issues
Chapter 2 Theorising Health: Major Theoretical Perspectives in Health Sociology
Chapter 3 Researching Health: Methodological Traditions and Innovations

The health of the people is really the foundation upon which all their happiness and all their powers as a state depend.

BENJAMIN DISRAELI

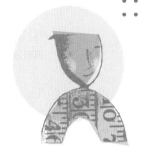

CHAPTER 1

Imagining Health Problems as Social Issues

Overview

- What is sociology and how can it be used to understand health and illness?
- What social patterns of health and illness exist?
- What is the social model of health and how does it differ from the medical model?

THE FOREST THROUGH THE TREES

We live in a health-obsessed age. We are bombarded with messages from health authorities, health professionals, and fitness gurus to 'do this' and 'not to do that'. Everywhere we turn we are urged to take individual responsibility for our health. Our personal experience of illness means that we tend to view it in an individualistic way—as a product of bad luck, poor lifestyle, or genetic fate. As individuals we all want quick and effective cures when we are unwell and thus we turn to medicine. Yet this is only part of the story. Even the highly individualised and very personal act of suicide occurs within a social context. In 2004–05, of the 2029 suicide-related deaths in Australia, more than 79 per cent of victims were male, with the highest rates occurring between the ages of 25 and 39 (AIHW 2008). In fact, the social patterning of suicide was first highlighted in the late nineteenth century by the sociologist Émile Durkheim (1858–1917). While Durkheim (1897/1951) acknowledged individual reasons for a person committing suicide, he found that suicide rates varied between countries and between different social groups within a country. By studying such social patterns, health sociology exposes the 'forest through the trees'—how individual health problems can be part of a social patterning of illness that have social origins and social solutions.

Introduction: the social origins of health and illness

This chapter introduces you to the sociological perspective and how it can be used to understand a wide range of health issues. Health sociology focuses on the social patterns of health and illness, such as the different health statuses between women and men, the poor and the wealthy, or the Indigenous and non-Indigenous populations, and seeks social, rather than biological or psychological, explanations. It provides a second opinion to the conventional medical view of illness derived from biological and psychological explanations, by exploring the social origins of health and illness—the living and working conditions that fundamentally shape why some groups of people get sicker and die sooner than others.

The social origins of health and illness can be clearly seen when we compare the life expectancy figures of various countries. As we all know, life expectancy in the least developed countries is significantly lower than that in industrially developed and comparatively wealthy countries such as Australia and the USA. For example, the average life expectancy at birth of people living in the least developed countries of the world is around 20 years less than that for developed countries such as Australia, which has an average life expectancy of 81.4 years (AIHW 2008; WHO 2008). As Table 1.1 shows, life expectancy varies among developed countries as well. Therefore, the living conditions of the country in which you live can have a significant influence on your chances of enjoying a long and healthy life.

Australian life expectancy is one of the highest in the world, second only to Japan. This is not due to any biological advantage in the Australian gene pool, but is rather a reflection of our distinctive living and working conditions. We can make such a case for two basic reasons. First, life expectancy can change in a short period of time, and in fact it did increase for most countries during the twentieth century. For example, Australian life expectancy has increased by more than 20 years since 1910 (AIHW 2008), which is too short a time frame for any genetic improvement to occur in a given population. Second, data compiled over decades of immigration shows that the health of migrants comes to reflect that of their host country over time, rather than their country of origin. The longer migrants live in their new country, the more their health mirrors that of the local population (Marmot 1999).

While the average Australian life expectancy figure is comparatively high, it is important to distinguish between different social groups within Australia. Life expectancy figures are crude indicators of population health and actually mask significant health inequalities among social groups within a country. For example, in Australia those in the lowest socio-economic group have the highest rates of illness and premature death, use preventive services less, and have higher rates of illness-related behaviours such as smoking (AIHW 2008). Furthermore, as Table 1.1 shows, life expectancy for Aboriginal Australians is around 20 years less than the national average. In fact, the current life expectancy of Aboriginal Australians is closer to that of Australians born in the early twentieth century (AIHW 2008). The indigenous population of New Zealand, the Māori, also have a lower life expectancy, around 8.5 years less than the national average.

Table 1.1 Life expectancy at birth, 2005

Country	Life expectancy	
	Men	Women
Australia	79.0	83.7
Aboriginal Australians*	59.0	65.0
Canada	78.0	82.7
France	76.8	83.9
Italy	77.9	83.8
Japan	78.7	85.5
New Zealand	77.5	81.9
Māori**	69.0	73.2
Sweden	78.7	83.0
United Kingdom	76.6	81.1
USA	75.3	80.4

* 1996–2001   ** 2000–02   Source: Adapted from AIHW 2008; Statistics New Zealand 2008

Introducing the sociological imagination: a template for doing sociological analysis

What is distinctive about the sociological perspective? In what ways does it uncover the social structure that we often take for granted? How is sociological analysis done? The American sociologist Charles Wright Mills (1916–62) answered such questions by using the expression **sociological imagination** to describe the distinctive feature of the sociological perspective. The sociological imagination is 'a quality of mind that seems most dramatically to promise an understanding of the intimate realities of ourselves in connection with larger social realities' (Mills 1959, p. 15). According to Mills, the essential aspect of thinking sociologically, or seeing the world through a sociological imagination, is making a link between 'private troubles' and 'public issues'.

As individuals, we may experience personal troubles without realising they are shared by other people as well. If certain problems are shared by groups of people, they may have a common cause and be best dealt with through collective action. As Mills (1959, p. 226) states, 'many personal troubles cannot be solved merely as troubles, but must be understood in terms of public issues ... public issues must be revealed by relating them to personal troubles.' The Australian sociologist Evan

sociological imagination
A term coined by Charles Wright Mills to describe the sociological approach to analysing issues. We see the world through a sociological imagination, or think sociologically, when we make a link between personal troubles and public issues.

Willis (2004) suggests that the sociological imagination consists of four interrelated parts:

1 *historical factors*: how the past influences the present
2 *cultural factors*: how culture impacts on our lives
3 *structural factors*: how particular forms of social organisation affect our lives
4 *critical factors*: how we can improve the current environment.

This four-part sociological imagination template is an effective way to understand how to think and analyse in a sociological way.

Figure 1.1 represents the sociological imagination template as a diagram that is easy to remember. Any time you want to analyse a topic sociologically, picture this diagram in your mind.

Figure 1.1 The sociological imagination template

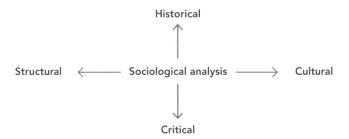

Sociological analysis involves applying these four aspects to the issues or problems under investigation. For example, a sociological analysis of why manual labourers have a shorter life expectancy would examine how and why the work done by manual labourers affects their health, by examining:

1 *historical factors*: to understand why manual workplaces are so dangerous
2 *cultural factors*: such as the cultural value of individual responsibility
3 *structural factors*: such as the way work is organised, the role of managerial authority, the rights of workers, and the role of the state
4 *critical factors*: such as alternatives to the status quo (increasing the effectiveness of occupational health and safety legislation, for instance).

By using the four parts of the sociological imagination template, you begin to 'do' sociological analysis. It is worth highlighting at this point that the template simplifies the process of sociological analysis. When analysing particular topics, it is more than likely that you will find that the parts overlap, making them less clear-cut than the template implies. It is also probable that for some topics, parts of the template will be more relevant and prominent than others—this is all to be expected.

The benefit of the template is that it serves as a reminder of the sorts of issues and questions a budding sociologist should be asking.

Is society to blame?
Introducing the structure–agency debate

As individuals we are brought up to believe that we control our own destiny, especially our health. It is simply up to each individual to 'do what they wanna do and be what they wanna be'. This belief ignores the considerable influence of society. Sociology makes us aware that we are social animals and are very much the product of our environment, from the way we dress to the way we interact with one another. We are all influenced by the **social structure**, such as our cultural customs and our **social institutions**. The idea of social structure serves to remind us of the social or human-created aspects of life, in contrast to purely random events or products of nature (López & Scott 2000).

Understanding the structure of society enables us to examine the social influences on our personal behaviour and our interactions with others. Yet to what extent are we products of society? How much **agency** do we have over our lives? Are we solely responsible for our actions or is society to blame? These questions represent a key debate in sociology, often referred to as the **structure–agency debate**. There is no simple resolution to this debate, but it is helpful to view structure and agency as interdependent—that is, humans shape and are simultaneously shaped by society. In this sense, structure and agency are not 'either/or' propositions in the form of a choice between constraint and freedom, but are part of the interdependent processes of social life. Therefore, the social structure should not automatically be viewed in a negative way, as only serving to constrain human freedom, since in many ways the social structure enables us to live, by providing health care, welfare, education, and work. As Mills maintained, an individual 'contributes, however minutely, to the shaping of this society and to the course of its history, even as he is made by society and by its historical push and shove' (1959, p. 6). Mills was clearly a product of the 'historical push and shove' of his social structure, as he uses the masculine 'he' to refer to both men and women—a usage now seen as dated and sexist.

Peter Berger long ago warned against depicting people as 'puppets jumping about on the ends of their invisible strings' (1966, p. 140). If we use the 'all the world's a stage and we are mere actors' analogy, we could liken life to a theatre in which we all play our assigned roles (father, mother, child, labourer, teacher, student, and so on). Whether it is how we are dressed as we walk down the street or how we present ourselves at a funeral, customs and traditions dictate expected modes of behaviour. In this sense we are all actors on a stage. Yet, we have the scope consciously to participate in what we do. We can make choices about whether simply to act, or whether to modify or change our roles and even the stage on which we live our lives.

social structure
The recurring patterns of social interaction through which people are related to each other, such as social institutions and social groups.

social institutions
Formal structures within society—such as health care, government, education, religion, and the media—that are organised to address identified social needs.

agency
The ability of people, individually and collectively, to influence their own lives and the society in which they live.

structure–agency debate
A key debate in sociology over the extent to which human behaviour is determined by social structure.

John Germov

Although we are born into a world not of our making and in countless ways our actions and thoughts are shaped by our social environment, we are not simply 'puppets on strings'. Humans are sentient beings—we are self-aware and thus have the capacity to think and act individually and collectively to change the society into which we are born. Structure and agency may be in tension, but they are interdependent—that is, one cannot exist without the other. Sociology is the study of the relationship between the individual and society; it examines how human behaviour both shapes and is shaped by society, or how 'we create society at the same time as we are created by it' (Giddens 1986, p. 11).

Social medicine and public health

Recognition of the social origins of health and illness actually occurred prior to the formal development of sociology as an academic discipline, and can be traced to the mid-nineteenth century, with the development of 'social medicine' (coined by Jules Guérin in 1848) or what more commonly became known as **public health** (sometimes referred to as social health, community medicine, or preventive medicine). At this time, infectious diseases such as cholera, typhus, smallpox, diphtheria, and tuberculosis were major killers for which there were no cures and little understanding of how they were transmitted. During the nineteenth century, a number of people such as René Villermé (1782–1863), Rudolph Virchow (1821–1902), John Snow (1813–58), Edwin Chadwick (1800–90), and Friedrich Engels (1820–95) established clear links between infectious diseases and poverty (Rosen 1972; Porter 1997).

Engels, Karl Marx's collaborator and patron, in *The Condition of the Working Class in England* (1845/1958), made a strong case for the links between disease and poor living and working conditions as an outcome of capitalist exploitation. He used the case of 'black lung', a preventable lung disease among miners, to make the point that 'the illness does not occur in those mines which are adequately ventilated. Many examples could be given of miners who moved from well-ventilated to badly ventilated mines and caught the disease. It is solely due to the colliery owners' greed for profit that this illness exists at all. If the coalowners would pay to have ventilation shafts installed the problem would not exist' (1845/1958, p. 281). Engels also noted the differences in the death rates between labourers and professionals, claiming that the squalid living conditions of the working **class** were primarily responsible for the disparity, stating that 'filth and stagnant pools in the working class quarters of the great cities have the most deleterious effects upon the health of the inhabitants' (1845/1958, p. 110).

In 1854, a cholera epidemic took place in Soho, London. John Snow, a medical doctor, documented cases on a city map and investigated all of the 93 deaths that had occurred within a well-defined geographical area. After interviewing residents

public health
Public policies and infrastructure to prevent the onset and transmission of disease among the population, with a particular focus on sanitation and hygiene such as clean air, water and food, and immunisation. Public health infrastructure refers specifically to the buildings, installations, and equipment necessary to ensure healthy living conditions for the population.

class (or social class)
A position in a system of structured inequality based on the unequal distribution of power, wealth, income, and status. People who share a class position typically share similar life chances.

he was able to establish that people infected with cholera had sourced their water from the same public water pump in Broad Street. Snow came to the conclusion that the water from the pump was the source of cholera, and at his insistence, the pump's handle was removed and the epidemic ceased (Snow 1855/1936; Rosen 1972; Porter 1997; McLeod 2000). This case is famous for being one of the earliest examples of the use of **epidemiology** to understand and prevent the spread of disease.

Virchow, often remembered in medical circles for his study of cellular biology, also made a clear case for the social basis of medicine, highlighting its preventive role when he claimed '[m]edicine is a social science, and politics nothing but medicine on a grand scale ... if medicine is really to accomplish its great task, it must intervene in political and social life ... The improvement of medicine would eventually prolong human life, but improvement of social conditions could achieve this result even more rapidly and successfully' (cited in Rosen 1972, p. 39 and Porter 1997, p. 415).

Virchow was a significant advocate for public health care and argued that the **state** should act to redistribute social resources, particularly to improve access to adequate nutrition. Therefore, social medicine and the public health movement grew from recognition that the social environment played a significant role in the spread of disease (Rosen 1972; Porter 1997). In other words, the infectious diseases that afflicted individuals had social origins that necessitated social reforms to prevent their onset (see Rosen 1972 and 1993 and Waitzkin 2000 for informative histories of social medicine, Porter 1997 for a very readable history of medicine in general, Bloom 2002 for a history of medical sociology, and White 2001).

In Britain, Chadwick was a key figure in the development of the first *Public Health Act* (1848) based on his 'sanitary idea'—that disease could be prevented through improved waste disposal and sewerage systems. In particular, he focused on removing cess pools of decomposing organic matter from densely populated areas, as well as on the introduction of high-pressure flushing sewers, and food hygiene laws to protect against food adulteration. Public health legislation in Australia was first introduced in Victoria in 1854, largely mirroring the British Act, with other colonies following suit (Reynolds 1995; Lawson & Bauman 2001). By the early twentieth century, public health had become part of the nation-building project in Australia, as efforts aimed at facilitating a fit, strong and patriotic 'race' of Australians mixed with ideas about **social Darwinism** and **eugenics** that were prevalent at the time (see Powles 1988; Crotty et al. 2000). In Australia and elsewhere, public health approaches were resisted by many doctors who viewed them as unscientific and as potentially undermining the need for medical services (Porter 1997; Waitzkin 2000). Such views had some popularity given the dominant laissez-faire political philosophy of the time, which supported only minor state intervention in economic and public affairs. Nonetheless, investment in public health was made, perhaps because infectious disease knew no class barriers (that is, it was worth spending money on the poor to prevent the spread of disease to the rich).

epidemiology/social epidemiology
The statistical study of patterns of disease in the population. Originally focused on epidemics, or infectious diseases, it now covers non-infectious conditions such as stroke and cancer. Social epidemiology is a sub-field aligned with sociology that focuses on the social determinants of illness.

state
A term used to describe a collection of institutions, including the parliament (government and opposition political parties), the public-sector bureaucracy, the judiciary, the military, and the police.

social Darwinism
The incorrect application of Charles Darwin's theory of animal evolution to explain social inequality by transferring his idea of 'survival of the fittest' among animals to 'explain' human inequality.

eugenics
The study of human heredity based on the unproven assumption that selective breeding could improve the intellectual, physical, and cultural traits of a population.

John Germov

Despite the influence of social medicine and the success of public health measures, health care would develop in an entirely different direction. The insights of social medicine would be cast aside for almost a century as the new science of **biomedicine** gained ascendancy.

The rise of the biomedical model

biomedicine/ biomedical model
The conventional approach to medicine in Western societies, based on the diagnosis and explanation of illness as a malfunction of the body's biological mechanisms. This approach underpins most health professions and health services, which focus on treating individuals, and generally ignores the social origins of illness and its prevention.

In 1878, Louis Pasteur (1822–96) developed the germ theory of disease, whereby illness was caused by germs infecting organs of the human body: a model of disease that became the foundation of modern medicine. Robert Koch (1843–1910) refined this idea through the doctrine of 'specific aetiology' (meaning specific cause of disease) through 'Koch's postulates': a set of criteria for proving that specific bacteria caused a specific disease (Dubos 1959; Capra 1982). The central idea was that specific micro-organisms caused disease by entering the human body through air, water, food, and insect bites (Porter 1997). This mono-causal model of disease, which came to be known as the medical or **biomedical model**, became the dominant medical paradigm by the early twentieth century. While early discoveries led to the identification of many infectious diseases, there were few effective cures. One of the earliest applications of the scientific understanding of infectious disease was the promotion of hygiene and sterilisation procedures, particularly in surgical practice, to prevent infection through the transmission of bacteria (Capra 1982). Until the early twentieth century, it had been common practice to operate on patients without a concern for hygiene or the proper cleaning and sterilisation of equipment, resulting in high rates of post-operative infection and death following surgery.

The biomedical model is based on the assumption that each disease or ailment has a specific cause that physically affects the human body in a uniform and predictable way, meaning that universal 'cures' for people are theoretically possible. It involves a mechanical view of the body as a machine made up of interrelated parts, such as the skeleton and circulatory system. The role of the doctor is akin to that of a body mechanic identifying and repairing the broken parts (Capra 1982). Throughout the twentieth century, medical research, training, and practice increasingly focused on attempts to identify and eliminate specific diseases in individuals, and thus moved away from the perspective of social medicine and its focus on the social origins of disease (Najman 1980).

Before the development of medical science, quasi-religious views of health and illness were dominant, whereby illness was connected with sin, penance, and evil spirits. Therefore, the 'body as machine' metaphor represented a significant turning point away from religious notions towards a secular view of the human body. Until this time, the dominant view had been to conceive the body and soul as a sacred entity beyond the power of human intervention. The influence of scientific discoveries, particularly through autopsies that linked diseased organs with symptoms observed before death, as well as Pasteur's germ theory, eventually endorsed a belief in the separation of body and soul. In philosophical circles, this view came to be known as mind/body dualism and is sometimes referred to as **Cartesian dualism** after the philosopher René Descartes (1590–1650). Descartes, famous for the saying 'I think therefore I am', suggested that although the mind and body interacted with one another, they were separate entities. Therefore, the brain was part of the physical body whereas the mind (the basis of individuality) existed in the spiritual realm and was apparent evidence of a God-given soul. Such a distinction provided the philosophical justification for secular interventions on the physical body in the form of medical therapies. Since the body was merely a vessel for the immortal soul or spirit, medicine could rightly practise on the body while religion could focus on the soul (Capra 1982; Porter 1997). The assumption of mind/body dualism underpinned the biomedical model, whereby disease was seen as located in the physical body, and thus, the mind, or mental state of a person, was considered unimportant.

Cartesian dualism
Also called mind/body dualism and named after the philosopher René Descartes, it refers to a belief that the mind and body are separate entities. This assumption underpins medical approaches that view disease in physical terms and thus ignore the psychological and subjective aspects of illness.

The limits of biomedicine

While the biomedical model represented a significant advance in understanding disease and resulted in beneficial treatments, it has come under significant criticism from both within medicine and from a range of social and behavioural disciplines such as sociology and psychology. The major criticism is that the biomedical model underestimates the complexity of health and illness, particularly by neglecting social and psychological factors (Powles 1973).

The idea of a specific cause for a specific disease, referred to as specific aetiology, only applies to a limited range of infectious diseases. As early as the 1950s, René Dubos (1959, p. 102) argued that 'most disease states are the indirect outcome of a constellation of circumstances rather than the direct result of single determinant factors'. Furthermore, Dubos noted that not all people exposed to an infectious disease contracted it. For example, we may all come into contact with someone suffering from a contagious condition like the flu, but only a few of us will get sick. Therefore, disease causation is more complex than the biomedical model implies and is likely to involve multiple factors such as physical condition, nutrition, and stress, which affect an individual's susceptibility to illness (Dubos 1959).

The biomedical model, underpinned by mind/body dualism and a focus on repairing the 'broken' parts of the machine-like body, can lead to the objectification of patients. Since disease is viewed only in physical terms, as something that can be objectively observed, treating 'it' takes primacy over all other considerations, and patients may become objectified as 'diseased bodies' or 'cases' rather than treated as unique individuals with particular needs. This form of criticism often underpins claims of doctors' poor interpersonal and communication skills. Such a situation is also related to what Fritjov Capra (1982) calls 'medical scientism'—that is, a reverence for scientific methods of measurement and observation as the most superior form of knowledge about understanding and treating disease. Therefore, patients' thoughts, feelings, and subjective experiences of illness are considered 'unscientific' and are mostly dismissed.

A further criticism of biomedicine is its **reductionism**. The development of medical science has led to an increasing focus on smaller and smaller features of human biology for the cause and cure of disease—from organs to cells to molecules and most recently to genes. By reducing its focus on disease to the biological, cellular, and genetic levels, medicine has ignored or downplayed the social and psychological aspects of illness, so that the experience of disease is treated as if it occurred in a social vacuum. Not only does this marginalise the importance of social support networks, it also ignores the role played by social factors such as poverty, poor working conditions, and discrimination in affecting an individual's physical and mental health.

A related outcome of reductionism has been an ever-growing number of medical specialists, such as cardiologists (heart specialists) and ophthalmologists (eye specialists), based on the assumption that each body part and function can be treated almost in isolation from the others. Such an approach has fuelled the search for 'magic bullet' cures, resulting in huge expenditure on medical drugs, technology, and surgery. It has also led to a curative and interventionist bias in medical care, often at the expense of prevention and non-medical alternatives.

Reductionism can also lead to **biological determinism**: a form of social Darwinism that assumes people's biology causes or determines their inferior social, economic, and health status. Biological determinism underpins most elitist, racist, and sexist beliefs. For example, some people argue that the poor are poor because they are born lazy and stupid. Such views have often been used to justify slavery and exploitation of Blacks, women, children, and workers; it is a very convenient 'explanation', particularly when those at the top of the social ladder espouse it. When people argue that social or health inequalities are biologically determined, the implication is that little can or should be done to change them.

A final criticism of the biomedical model is its tendency towards **victim-blaming** (Ryan 1971) by locating the cause and cure of disease as solely within the individual. As Capra states, 'Instead of asking why an illness occurs, and trying to remove the conditions that lead to it, medical researchers try to understand the biological mechanisms through which the disease operates, so that they can then interfere with them' (1982, p. 150). Therefore, the individual body becomes the focus of intervention, and health and illness become primarily viewed as individual responsibilities. A preoccupation with treating the individual has the potential to legitimate a victim-blaming approach to illness, either in the form of genetic fatalism (your poor health

reductionism
The belief that all illnesses can be explained and treated by reducing them to biological and pathological factors.

biological determinism
An unproven belief that individual and group behaviour and social status are an inevitable result of biology.

victim-blaming
The process whereby social inequality is explained in terms of individuals being solely responsible for what happens to them in relation to the choices they make and their assumed psychological, cultural, and/or biological inferiority.

is the result of poor genetics) or as an outcome of poor **lifestyle choices**. By ignoring the social context of health and illness and locating primary responsibility for illness within the individual, there is little acknowledgment of social responsibility—that is, the need to ensure healthy living and working environments.

The critique of the biomedical model above has necessarily been a generalisation and does not imply that all doctors work from within the confines of this model. In fact, many of the criticisms of the model have come from those within the medical profession itself. While it is now widely accepted that the causes of illness are multifactorial, it is still fair to claim that the biomedical model remains the dominant influence over medical training and practice to this day.

Rediscovering the social origins of health and illness

Thomas McKeown (1976, 1979, 1988), a doctor and epidemiologist, was one of the earliest authors to expose the exaggerated role of medical treatment in improving population health. McKeown argued that the medical profession and governments had overestimated the influence of medical discoveries on improvements in life expectancy during the twentieth century. McKeown (1976, 1979) found that mortality (death) from most infectious diseases had declined before the development of effective medical treatments, meaning that improvements in life expectancy were not substantially due to medical intervention. Similar findings have been reported in the USA (McKinlay & McKinlay 1977) and Australia (Gordon 1976; Lawson 1991). Figure 1.2 provides a graphic example of this, showing the declining rate of tuberculosis for Australia, which occurred before effective medical treatment. The same trend occurred in the United Kingdom and the USA in the period given. Graphs for most infectious diseases tell a similar story, aside from vaccination against smallpox and polio, indicating that the contribution of medicine to population-level improvements in life expectancy appear to have been smaller than is commonly assumed.

McKeown (1979) suggests that the major reason for the increase in life expectancy throughout the twentieth century was not due to medical treatments, but rather to rising living standards, particularly improved nutrition, which increased people's resistance to infectious disease. While McKeown's work highlighted the importance of social, non-medical interventions for improving population health, Simon Szreter (1988, p. 37) provides a more complex argument. He suggests that rather than the '"invisible" hand of rising living standards', it was the state's redistribution of economic resources that increased life expectancy through improved working conditions and a range of public health measures such as improved public housing, food regulation, education, and sanitation reforms.

lifestyle choices/ factors
The decisions people make that are likely to impact on their health such as diet, exercise, smoking, alcohol, and other drugs. The term implies that people are solely responsible for choosing and changing their lifestyle.

Figure 1.2 Decline in the number of tuberculosis and typhoid deaths in Australia

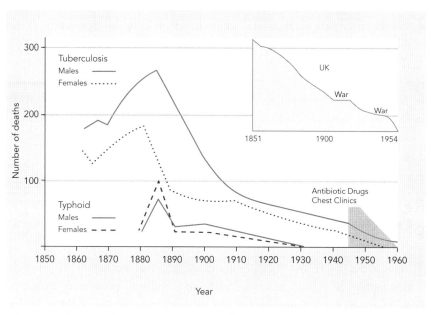

Source: Gordon 1976; after graph by H. Silverstone, Department of Social and Preventive Medicine, University of Queensland. Data from H. O. Lancaster and others.

While the exact contributions of public health measures, rising living standards, and medicine to improving population health is impossible to determine, the significance of McKeown's work and subsequent findings has been to highlight the importance of addressing the social origins of health and illness. As McKeown states, 'improvement in health is likely to come … from modification of the conditions which lead to disease, rather than from intervention in the mechanism of disease after it has occurred' (1979, p. 198).

It is important to note that McKeown himself was not anti-medicine, but wanted to reform medical practice so that it focused on prevention of what he saw were the new threats to health: 'personal behaviour', as evidenced through smoking, alcohol consumption, drug taking, poor diet, and lack of exercise. Therefore, he still viewed health care in individualistic terms, by focusing preventive efforts at the level of modifying the behaviour of individuals (see Box 1.1).

There is no denying the significant role medicine has played in the treatment of illness, particularly in trauma medicine, palliative care, and general surgery, as well as the prevention of illness through immunisation. Thus, the expertise of doctors lies in treating individuals once they are ill. Yet as we have seen, this is only part of the story and has tended to obscure the social origins of health and illness. The

BOX 1.1 Doing health sociology: from risk-taking to risk-imposing lifestyle factors

While the notion of 'lifestyle diseases' or 'diseases of affluence' is a clear indication of the social origins of illness, most disease prevention efforts have aimed to reform the individual rather than pursue wider social reform (often ignoring the fact that diseases of affluence tend to affect the least affluent much more). By solely targeting risk-taking individuals, there has been a tendency toward victim-blaming: ignoring the social determinants that give rise to risk-taking in the first place, such as stressful work environments, the marketing efforts of corporations, and peer group pressure. As Michael Marmot (1999, p. 1) incisively puts it, there is a need to understand the 'causes of the causes'. In other words, rather than just to focus on risk-taking individuals, there is also a need to address 'risk-imposing factors' and 'illness-generating social conditions' (Waitzkin 1983; Ratcliffe et al. 1984)—the social, cultural, economic, and political features of society that create unhealthy products, habits, and lifestyles.

World Health Organization (WHO) effectively acknowledged this limitation of biomedicine in 1946, when it included in its constitution the now-famous holistic definition of health as 'a state of complete physical, mental and social well-being and not merely the absence of disease or infirmity' (WHO 1946). This often-quoted definition implies that a range of biological, psychological, and social factors influence health. Furthermore, health is conceptualised as 'not merely the absence of disease', but rather in the positive sense of 'well-being'. While this definition has been criticised for its utopian and vague notion of 'complete well-being', it is of symbolic importance because it highlights the need for a broader approach to health than the biomedical model alone can deliver.

The widespread recognition of the biomedical model's limitations, from those within and outside the medical profession, has led to the development of a variety of multifactorial models, such as the biopsychosocial model (Engel 1977, 1980; Cooper et al. 1996), the web of causation model (MacMahon & Pugh 1970), and the ecological model (Hancock 1985). While these models represent a significant advance on the biomedical model in acknowledging the multiple determinants of health, to greater and lesser degrees they remain focused on health interventions aimed at the individual, particularly through lifestyle/behaviour modification and health education. What is required is an explicitly **social model of health** in order to propose effective health interventions at the population and community levels (Waitzkin 1983; Ashton & Seymour 1988; Baum 2008).

social model of health
Focuses on social determinants of health such as the social production, distribution, and construction of health and illness, and the social organisation of health care. It directs attention to the prevention of illness through community participation and social reforms that address living and working conditions.

John Germov

The social model of health

new public health
A social model
of health linking
'traditional' public
health concerns about
physical aspects of the
environment (clean air
and water, safe food,
occupational safety),
with concerns about
the behavioural, social,
and economic factors
that affect people's
health.

The social model of health, sometimes referred to as the **new public health** approach, focuses attention on the societal level of health determinants and health intervention. The two terms are used interchangeably by some authors, but have different disciplinary origins, with the new public health approach arising from the health sciences (particularly public health), and the social model drawn primarily from the field of health sociology. Some new public health approaches arising from the health sciences have been criticised by sociologists for an over-reliance on individualistic solutions in practice (see Lupton 1995; Petersen & Lupton 1996). Yet, there are significant examples of sociologically informed approaches that can make it problematical to draw distinctions between the two terms (see especially Beaglehole & Bonita 1997; Baggott 2000; Baum 2008). For our purposes we will use the term social model of health, as it better reflects the unique theories, research methods, and modes of analysis of health sociology discussed in this book.

The social model of health has been used as a general umbrella term to refer to approaches that focus on the social determinants of health and illness (see Broom 1991; Gillespie & Gerhardt 1995). As Dorothy Broom (1991, p. 52) states, 'the social model locates people in social contexts, conceptualises the physical environment as socially organised, and understands ill health as a process of interaction between people and their environments.' It is one of the aims of this book to map out in more detail what a social model of health entails. Table 1.2 contrasts the key features of the biomedical model with the social model to highlight the different foci, assumptions, benefits, and limitations of each. It is important to emphasise that the social model does not deny the existence of biological or psychological aspects of disease that manifest in individuals, or deny the need for medical treatment. Instead, it highlights that health and illness occur in a social context and that effective health interventions, particularly preventive efforts, need to move beyond the medical treatment of individuals. In exposing the social origins of illness, it necessarily implies that a greater balance between individual and social interventions is required, since the vast majority of health funding continues to be directed towards medical intervention. Therefore, the social model is not intended as a replacement for the biomedical model, but rather coexists alongside it.

The social model assumes that health is a social responsibility by examining the social determinants of individuals' health status and health-related behaviour. While the biomedical model concentrates on treating disease and risk-taking among individuals, the social model focuses on societal factors that are risk-imposing or illness-inducing (for example, toxic pollution, stressful work, discrimination, peer pressure), and in particular highlights the health inequalities suffered by different social groups based on class, gender, ethnicity, and occupation, to name a few. What should be clear from the comparison offered in Table 1.2 is that health issues have a number of dimensions.

Table 1.2 A comparison of biomedical and social models of health: key characteristics

	Biomedical model	Social model
Focus	Individual focus: acute treatment of ill individuals	Societal focus: living and working conditions that affect health
	Clinical services, health education, immunisation	Public health infrastructure and legislation, social services, community action, equity/access issues
Assumptions	Health and illness are objective biological states	Health and illness are social constructions
	Individual responsibility for health	Social responsibility for health
Key indicators of illness	Individual pathology	Social inequality
	Hereditary factors, sex, age	Social groups: class, gender, 'race', ethnicity, age, occupation, unemployment
	Risk-taking factors	Risk-imposing factors
Causes of illness	Gene defects and micro-organisms (viruses, bacteria)	Political/economic factors: distribution of wealth/income/power, poverty, level of social services
	Trauma (accidents)	Employment factors: employment and educational opportunities, stressful and dangerous work
	Behaviour/lifestyle	Cultural and structural factors
Intervention	Cure individuals via surgery and pharmaceuticals	Public policy
	Behaviour modification (non-smoking, exercise, diet)	State intervention to alleviate health and social inequalities
	Health education and immunisation	Community participation, advocacy, and political lobbying
Goals	Cure disease, limit disability, and reduce risk factors to prevent disease in individuals	Prevention of illness and reduction of health inequalities to aim for an equality of health outcomes
Benefits	Addresses disease and disability of individuals	Addresses the social determinants of health and illness
Criticisms	Disease focus leads to lack of preventive efforts	Utopian goal of equality leads to unfeasible prescriptions for social change
	Reductionist: ignores the complexity of health and illness	Over emphasis on the harmful side effects of biomedicine
	Fails to take into account social origins of health and illness	Proposed solutions can be complex and difficult to implement in the short-term
	Medical opinions can reinforce victim-blaming	Sociological opinions can underestimate individual responsibility and psychological factors

John Germov

The social model logically implies that any attempts to improve the overall health of the community need to address overall living and working conditions such as poverty, employment opportunities, working conditions, and cultural differences. The social model gives equal priority to the prevention of illness along with the treatment of illness and aims to alleviate health inequalities. Such issues necessitate community participation and state interventions, which include social services and public policies (such as workplace safety and pollution controls), that lie outside the strict confines of the health system or individuals' control. It must be acknowledged that this makes the interventions proposed by advocates of the social model more complex and difficult to achieve, given their broad thrust, long-term implications, and need for intersectoral collaboration.

The three main dimensions of the social model of health

The social model arose as a critique of the limitations and misapplications of the biomedical model. Sociological research and theorising, which underpins the social model of health, has comprised three main dimensions that are reflected in the structure of this book:

1   *The social production and distribution of health and illness*: highlights that many illnesses are socially produced. For example, illnesses arising from exposure to hazardous work practices are often beyond an individual's control and therefore need to be addressed at a societal level, such as through occupational health and safety legislation. Furthermore, there is an unequal social distribution of health, whereby some social groups suffer higher rates of morbidity and mortality. Therefore, a focus on the social production and distribution of health examines the role that living and working conditions can play in causing and alleviating illness.

social construction
Refers to the socially created characteristics of human life based on the idea that people actively construct reality, meaning it is neither 'natural' nor inevitable. Therefore, notions of normality/abnormality, right/wrong, and health/illness are subjective human creations that should not be taken for granted.

2   *The social construction of health and illness*: refers to how definitions of health and illness can vary between cultures and change over time, whereby what is considered a disease in one culture or time period may be considered normal and healthy elsewhere and at other times. For example, homosexuality was once considered a psychiatric disorder despite the lack of scientific evidence of pathology. It is no longer medically defined as a disorder; this is an example of how cultural beliefs, social practices, and social institutions shape, or construct, the ways in which health and illness are understood. Notions of health and illness are not necessarily objective facts, but can be **social constructions** that reflect the culture, politics, and morality of a particular society at a given point in time.

3   *The social organisation of health care*: concerns the way a particular society organises, funds, and utilises its health services. A central focus of study has been

the dominant role of the medical profession, which has significantly shaped health policy and health funding to benefit its own interests, largely to the detriment of preventive approaches and nursing, allied, and alternative health practitioners. Unequal relationships between the health professions can prevent the efficient use of health resources and the optimal delivery of health care to patients.

Conclusion

Question: What do you get when you cross a sociologist with a member of the Mafia?
Answer: An offer you can't understand.

Giddens 1996, p. 1

A common accusation made of sociology is that it is just common sense dressed up in unnecessary jargon. The subject matter of sociology is familiar, and as members of society it is easy to think we should all be experts on the subject. This familiarity can breed suspicion and sometimes contempt. All disciplines have specialist concepts to help classify their subject matter and sociology is no different. Sociological concepts, such as those you have been introduced to in this chapter, are used to impose a sense of intellectual order on the complexities of social life; they are a form of academic shorthand to summarise a complex idea in a word or phrase.

As this chapter has shown, to understand the complexity of health and illness, we need to move beyond biomedical approaches and incorporate a social model of health. Sociology enables us to understand the links between our individual experiences and the social context in which we live, work, and play. With a sociological imagination, seeing health problems as social issues can be a healthy way of opening up debate on a range of topics previously undiscussed.

Summary of main points

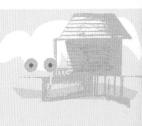

» Much of health sociology has arisen as a critique of the dominance of the medical profession and its biomedical model.

» Health sociology examines social patterns of health and illness, particularly various forms of health inequality, and seeks to explain them by examining the influence of society. When groups of people experience similar health problems, there are likely to be social origins that require social action to address them.

» The sociological imagination, or sociological analysis, involves four interrelated features—historical, cultural, structural, and critical—which can be applied to understand health problems as social issues.

» Health sociology challenges individualistic and biological explanations of health and illness through a social model of health that involves three key dimensions: the social production and distribution of health, the social construction of health, and the social organisation of health care.

Sociological reflection: a sociological autobiography

Apply the four parts of the sociological imagination template to explain the person you have become. In other words, write a short sociological autobiography by briefly noting the various things that have influenced you directly or indirectly in terms of your beliefs, interests, and behaviour.

» *Historical factors*: how has your family background or key past events and experiences shaped the person you are?
» *Cultural factors*: what role have cultural background, traditions, and belief systems played in forming your opinions and influencing your behaviour?
» *Structural factors*: how have various social institutions influenced you?
» *Critical factors*: have your values and opinions about what you consider important changed over time? Why/why not?

Repeat the sociological reflection, but this time apply the sociological imagination template to a health problem of interest to you. Briefly note any key points that come to mind under the four parts of the template. What insights can you derive by adopting a sociological imagination?

Discussion questions

1   How can illness have social origins? Give examples in your answer.
2   What are the advantages and limitations of the biomedical model?
3   What have been some of the consequences of the dominance of biomedical explanations for our understanding of health and illness?
4   Why did the insights of social medicine/public health approaches have such a limited influence over the development of modern medicine?
5   What are the three key dimensions of the social model of health? Provide examples of each in your answer. What are the advantages and limitations of the model?
6   In 1946, the World Health Organization defined health as 'a state of complete physical, mental and social well-being and not merely the absence of disease or infirmity'. Why might some groups regard this definition as 'radical' and utopian? Who might these groups consist of? What do you think of the definition?

Further investigation

1 The influence of the biomedical model is waning—the future belongs to public health. Discuss.
2 Illness is simply a matter of bad luck, bad judgment, or bad genetics. Critically analyse this statement by applying a sociological imagination to explore the social origins of illness.

Further reading

Australian Institute of Health and Welfare (AIHW) 2008, *Australia's Health 2008*, AIHW, Canberra. Available online: <http://www.aihw.gov.au/publications/index.cfm/title/10585>

Baum, F. 2008, *The New Public Health*, 3rd edn, Oxford University Press, Melbourne.

Blaxter, M. 2004, *Health*, Polity, Cambridge.

Bury, M. 2005, *Health and Illness*, Polity, Cambridge.

Cockerman, W. C. 2007, *Social Causes of Health and Disease*, Polity, Cambridge.

Gabe, J., Bury, M. & Elston, M. A. 2004, *Key Concepts in Medical Sociology*, Sage, London.

Marmot, M. & Wilkinson, R. (eds) 2006, *Social Determinants of Health*, 2nd edn, Oxford University Press. Oxford.

Nettleton, S. 2006, *The Sociology of Health and Illness*, 2nd edn, Polity, Cambridge.

Webster, A. 2007, *Health, Technology and Society: A Sociological Critique*, Palgrave Macmillan, London.

Web resources

Australian Bureau of Statistics: <http://www.abs.gov.au>

Australian Institute of Health and Welfare: <http://www.aihw.gov.au>

Medical Sociology (MedSoc) Study Group of the British Sociological Association: <http://www.britsoc.co.uk/medsoc/>

Medical Sociology Section of the American Sociological Association: <http://dept.kent.edu/sociology/asamedsoc/>

Public Health Association of Australia (PHAA): <http://www.phaa.net.au>

World Health Organization: <http://www.who.int.en>

Online case study • •
Visit the Second Opinion website to access relevant case studies.

Documentaries/films

The Trouble with Medicine (1993): 6 part documentary series (each around 55 minutes) dealing with various challenges and limitations relating to biomedicine, ABC TV, BBC TV & Thirteen-WNET.

References

Ashton, J. & Seymour, H. 1988, *The New Public Health: The Liverpool Experience*, Open University Press, Milton Keynes.

Australian Institute of Health and Welfare (AIHW) 2008, *Australia's Health 2008*, Cat. no. AUS 99, AIHW, Canberra.

Baggott, R. 2000, *Public Health: Policy and Politics*, Palgrave, Basingstoke.

Baum, F. 2008, *The New Public Health*, 3rd edn, Oxford University Press, Melbourne.

Beaglehole, R. & Bonita, R. 1997, *Public Health at the Crossroads*, Cambridge University Press, Cambridge.

Berger, P. L. 1966, *Invitation to Sociology: A Humanistic Perspective*, Penguin, Harmondsworth.

Bloom, S. 2002, *The Word as Scalpel: A History of Medical Sociology*, Oxford University Press, New York.

Broom, D. 1991, *Damned if We Do: Contradictions in Women's Health Care*, Allen & Unwin, Sydney.

Capra, F. 1982, *The Turning Point: Science, Society and the Rising Culture*, Simon & Schuster, New York.

Cooper, N., Stevenson, C. & Hale, G. (eds) 1996, *Integrating Perspectives on Health*, Open University Press, Buckingham.

Crotty, M., Germov, J. & Rodwell, G. (eds) 2000, '"A Race for a Place": Eugenics, Darwinism and Social Thought and Practice in Australia', Proceedings of the History & Sociology of Eugenics Conference, University of Newcastle, 27–28 April 2000, Faculty of Arts and Social Science, University of Newcastle, Newcastle.

Dubos, R. 1959, *Mirage of Health: Utopias, Progress, and Biological Change*, Harper & Row, New York.

Durkheim, E. 1897/1951, *Suicide: A Study in Sociology*, Free Press, Glencoe.

Engel, G. L. 1977, 'The Need for a New Medical Model: A Challenge for Biomedicine', *Science*, vol. 196, pp. 129–36.

Engel, G. L. 1980, 'The Clinical Application of the Biopsychosocial Model', *American Journal of Psychiatry*, vol. 137, no. 5, pp. 535–44.

Engels, F. 1845/1958, *The Condition of the Working Class in England*, trans. W. O. Henderson & W. H. Chaloner, Basil Blackwell, Oxford.

Giddens, A. 1986, *Sociology: A Brief but Critical Introduction*, 2nd edn, Macmillan, London.

Giddens, A. 1996, *In Defence of Sociology: Essays, Interpretations and Rejoinders*, Polity Press, Cambridge.

Gillespie, R. & Gerhardt, C. 1995, 'Social Dimensions of Sickness and Disability', in G. Moon & R. Gillespie (eds), *Society and Health: An Introduction to Social Science for Health Professionals*, Routledge, London, pp. 79–94.

Gordon, D. 1976, *Health, Sickness and Society: Theoretical Concepts in Social and Preventive Medicine*, University of Queensland Press, Brisbane.

Hancock, T. 1985, 'The Mandala of Health: A Model of the Human Ecosystem', *Family and Community Health*, November, pp. 1–10.

Lawson, J. S. 1991, *Public Health Australia: An Introduction*, McGraw-Hill, Sydney.

Lawson, J. S. & Bauman, A. E. 2001, *Public Health Australia: An Introduction*, McGraw-Hill, Sydney.

López, J. & Scott, J. 2000, *Social Structure*, Open University Press, Buckingham.

Lupton, D. 1995, *The Imperative of Health: Public Health and the Regulated Body*, Sage, London.

MacMahon, B. & Pugh, T. F. 1970, *Epidemiological Principles and Methods*, Little Brown, Boston.

Marmot, M. G. 1999, 'Introduction', in M. Marmot & R. G. Wilkinson (eds), *Social Determinants of Health*, Oxford University Press, Oxford.

McKeown, T. 1976, *The Role of Medicine: Dream, Mirage or Nemesis?*, Nuffield Hospital Trust, London.

McKeown, T. 1979, *The Role of Medicine: Dream, Mirage or Nemesis?*, Basil Blackwell, Oxford.

McKeown, T. 1988, *The Origins of Human Disease*, Basil Blackwell, Oxford.

McKinlay, J. B. & McKinlay, S. M. 1977, 'The Questionable Effect of Medical Measures on the Decline of Mortality in the United States in the Twentieth Century', *Milbank Memorial Fund Quarterly*, vol. 55, pp. 405–28.

McLeod, K. S. 2000, 'Our Sense of Snow: The Myth of John Snow in Medical Geography', *Social Science & Medicine*, vol. 50, pp. 923–35.

Mills, C. W. 1959, *The Sociological Imagination*, Oxford University Press, New York.

Najman, J. 1980, 'Theories of Disease Causation and the Concept of General Susceptibility', *Social Science & Medicine*, vol. 14A, pp. 231–7.

Petersen, A. & Lupton, D. 1996, *The New Public Health: Health and Self in the Age of Risk*, Allen & Unwin, Sydney, and Sage, London.

Porter, R. 1997, *The Greatest Benefit to Mankind: A Medical History of Humanity from Antiquity to the Present*, HarperCollins, London.

Powles, J. 1973, 'On the Limitation of Modern Medicine', *Science, Medicine and Man*, vol. 1, no. 1, pp. 1–30.

Powles, J. 1988, 'Professional Hygienists and the Health of a Nation', in R. MacLeod (ed.), *The Commonwealth of Science: ANZAAS and the Scientific Enterprise in Australasia 1888–1988*, Oxford University Press, Melbourne, pp. 292–307.

Ratcliffe, J., Wallack, L., Fagnani, F. & Rodwin, V. 1984, 'Perspectives on Prevention: Health Promotion vs Health Protection', in J. de Kervasdoue, J. R. Kimberley & G. Rodwin (eds), *The End of an Illusion: The Future of Health Policy in Western Industrialized Nations*, University of California Press, Berkeley, CA, pp. 56–84.

Reynolds, C. 1995, *Public Health Law in Australia*, Federation Press, Leichhardt.

Rosen, G. 1972, 'The Evolution of Social Medicine', in H. E. Freeman, S. Levine & L. G. Reeder (eds), *Handbook of Medical Sociology*, 2nd edn, Prentice Hall, Englewood Cliffs, NJ, pp. 30–60.

Rosen, G. 1993, *A History of Public Health*, Johns Hopkins University Press, New York.

Ryan, W. 1971, *Blaming the Victim*, Vintage, New York.

Snow, J. 1936/1855, *On the Mode of Communication of Cholera* [reprinted as *Snow on Cholera*], Hafner, New York.

Statistics New Zealand 2008, *Statistics New Zealand—Life Expectancy*. Available online: <http://www.stats.govt.nz/people/health/lifeexpectancy.htm>

Szreter S. 1988, 'The Importance of Social Intervention in Britain's Mortality Decline c. 1850–1914: A Re-interpretation of the Role of Public Health', *Society for the Social History of Medicine*, vol. 1, no. 1, pp. 1–37.

Waitzkin, H. 1983, *The Second Sickness: Contradictions of Capitalist Health Care*, Free Press, New York.

Waitzkin, H. 2000, *The Second Sickness: Contradictions of Capitalist Health Care*, 2nd edn, Rowman & Littlefield, Lanham.

White, K. (ed.) 2001, *The Early Sociology of Health and Illness*, 6 vols, Routledge, London.

World Health Organization (WHO) 1946, *Constitution of the World Health Organization*, WHO, Geneva.

World Health Organization (WHO) 2008, *Closing the Gap in a Generation: Health Equity through Action on the Social Determinants of Health*, Final Report of the Commission on Social Determinants of Health, WHO, Geneva.

Willis, E. 2004, *The Sociological Quest*, 4th edn, Allen & Unwin, Sydney

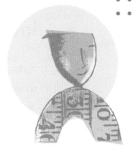

Theorising Health:
Major Theoretical Perspectives
in Health Sociology

J O H N
G E R M O V

Overview

- What is theory?
- Why is theory necessary?
- What are the main theoretical approaches in health sociology?

THEORY AND THE REAL WORLD

We often think of theory as somehow divorced from reality, but we actually make use of theories every day of our lives. For example, when some people suggest that violence on television or in the lyrics of popular music may lead to increased acts of violence in the wider community, they are espousing a theory of why things happen. People commonly espouse everyday theories for the differences between women and men, rich and poor, black and white, heterosexuals and homosexuals, to name but a few. Such theories can influence how people relate to one another, how tolerant they are of others, and whether they support social policies and laws aimed at addressing various forms of discrimination and inequality. So, rightly or wrongly, people have theories about how and why social life is the way it is. Such everyday theories or opinions are usually based on unacknowledged prejudices and lack reliable supporting evidence. What sets sociological theories (or social theories for short) apart from everyday opinions is that they attempt to explain social life by presenting a logical, detailed, and coherent account derived from systematically researched evidence.

Introduction

A theory is an explanation of how things work and why things happen. Theories allow us to make sense of our world—they provide answers to the 'how' and 'why' questions of life—by showing the way certain facts are connected to one another. This chapter provides an overview of the seven main theoretical perspectives in health sociology: functionalism, Marxism, Weberianism, feminism, symbolic interactionism, contemporary modernist approaches, and post-structuralism/postmodernism. It draws out the key features, assumptions, and concepts of these different theoretical approaches. Differences between theoretical perspectives are discussed, particularly with reference to the **structure–agency debate** and the different questions addressed by various perspectives. The chapter ends with a plea for theoretical pluralism and a caution against confusing perspectives with specific theories.

structure–agency debate
A key debate in sociology over the extent to which human behaviour is determined by social structure.

Theoretical perspectives in health sociology: an overview

> The Answer to the Great Question Of ... Life, the Universe and Everything ... Is ... Forty-two.
>
> Adams 1979, p. 135

As the above quote from *The Hitch-Hiker's Guide to the Galaxy* implies, the search for a 'theory of everything' is likely to be a futile task. Even if we could construct a theory that explains every imaginable social problem, public issue, or human action, its complexity is likely to be so great as to make it unusable. A theory attempts to simplify reality and generalise its common and related features relevant to the topic at hand. The sheer variety of social life and the diversity of human behaviour mean that there is no single sociological 'theory of everything'. As Fritjov Capra puts it, 'All scientific theories are approximations to the true nature of reality ... each theory is valid for a certain range of phenomena. Beyond this... new theories have to be found to replace the old one' (1982, p. 93).

As you read the chapters of this book and consult the wider literature, you will quickly become aware that there are many different and sometimes opposing social theories on a topic. Over the years, many social theories have been developed and advocated by sociologists, making it frustrating for those new to sociology to steer a course through the maze of theories that exist. One way to navigate through this theory maze is to start by grouping them into the following seven main theoretical perspectives or frameworks:

- structural functionalism
- Marxism

- Weberianism
- symbolic interactionism
- feminism
- contemporary modernism
- post-structuralism/postmodernism.

Theoretical perspectives are a form of shorthand to group similar theories of society together. Within each perspective there exist many individual theories developed by different authors, but they all tend to share the core features of the particular perspective. Any attempt to group theories in this way necessarily involves simplification as it becomes necessary to focus on the similarities within the one perspective at the expense of the differences between specific theories. For example, many Marxist theorists today would disagree with some of Karl Marx's ideas, but they nonetheless share the core assumptions and principles of a Marxist perspective.

A key distinction between theoretical perspectives is in relation to the structure–agency debate, with some perspectives favouring the structure side of the debate and others more the **agency** side. Figure 2.1 depicts sociological perspectives along a structure–agency continuum, with structuralist approaches at one end and agency approaches at the other. Structuralist approaches assume that **social structures**, such as the economic and political system, shape individual and group behaviour—that is, that they determine the type of person you are: how you think, feel, and act, as well as your chances of health, wealth, and happiness. Agency approaches maintain that society is fundamentally the product of individuals acting socially or collectively to make the society in which they live. These perspectives focus on small-scale aspects of social interaction, such as that which occurs in a classroom between teachers and students or between health professionals and patients, rather than focusing on the education or health system as a whole.

agency
The ability of people, individually and collectively, to influence their own lives, and the society in which they live.

social structure
The recurring patterns of social interaction through which people are related to each other, such as social institutions and social groups.

Figure 2.1 Theoretical perspectives along the structure–agency continuum

Structure				Agency
Marxism Functionalism Marxist/socialist feminism Radical feminism	Liberal feminism Critical theory	Contemporary moderism	Weberianism	Symbolic interactionism Post-structuralism/ Postmodernism Postmodern feminism

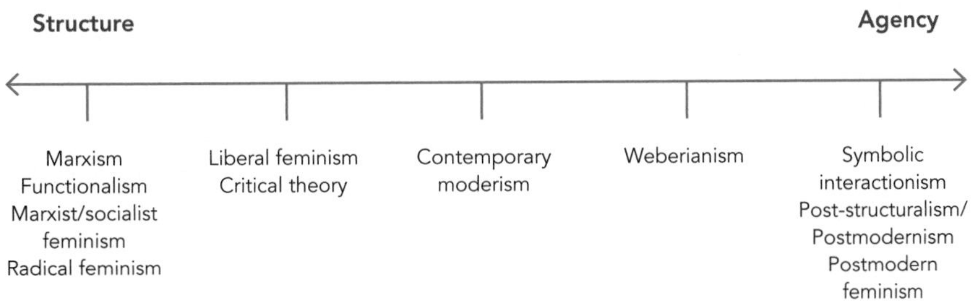

For our purposes here it is important to realise that most sociological theories fall between these two extremes—indeed many contemporary modernist social theories

attempt to integrate structure as well as agency. Few authors writing within any of the perspectives completely deny the roles that social structure or individuals play in any given social situation; nevertheless, a bias to one side of the continuum is usually displayed.

Key features of major theoretical perspectives

Table 2.1 summarises the key features of the major theoretical perspectives in health sociology and how 'at a glance' they apply to health issues. Greater detail on each perspective is provided in the remainder of the chapter.

Table 2.1 The seven major theoretical perspectives in health sociology

Theoretical perspective	Key theorists	Key concepts (see glossary)	Focus of analysis	Health example
Structural functionalism	Émile Durkheim Talcott Parsons Robert Merton	value consensus functional prerequisites sick role	Structuralist focus: shows how various parts of society function to maintain social order	The 'sick role' (social expectations of how doctors and patients should behave) exposes the management of illness as a social experience
Marxism	Karl Marx Friedrich Engels Vicente Navarro Howard Waitzkin	class conflict capitalism medical-industrial complex commodification of health care	Structuralist focus: shows how the unequal distribution of scarce resources in a capitalist society is based on class division and highlights who benefits and who is disadvantaged	Analyses the links between class and health status, and between class, medical power, and profit-maximisation
Weberianism	Max Weber George Ritzer Magali Larson Anne Witz	bureaucracy ideal type rationalisation McDonaldisation	Combines a primary focus on agency with structuralist tendencies: shows how the increasing regulation of social life takes place and may stifle human creativity; also explains the multiple forms of social inequality and social conflict	Examines how health professionals are increasingly subject to regulation and managerial control, producing greater efficiency and uniformity in health care delivery but potentially decreasing the effectiveness of patient care

Symbolic interactionism	George H. Mead Erving Goffman Herbert Blumer Howard S. Becker Anselm Strauss	the self labelling theory stigma total institutions negotiated order	Agency-focused: emphasises how individual and small-group interaction construct social meaning in everyday settings to construct and change social patterns of behaviour	Uncovers how and why certain forms of behaviour are treated as deviance, exposing the stigma, negative consequences, interactionism, and biased treatment of social groups whose behaviour is deemed 'abnormal' (e.g. homosexuality)
Feminism	Germaine Greer Ann Oakley Sylvia Walby Naomi Wolf Susan Bordo	patriarchy gender sexual division of labour	Consists of a range of strands that are either structuralist or agency focused; seeks to explain and address the unequal position of women in society	Exposes sexism, biological determinism, and gender inequality in health research, theory, and treatment
Contemporary modernism	Norbert Elias Ulrich Beck Pierre Bourdieu Anthony Giddens	figurations civilising processes habitus risk society reflexive modernity	A diverse group of social theories that attempt to integrate structure and agency	Explores how health risks are defined and acted upon by individuals, health professionals, and social institutions (e.g. government health promotion campaigns)

Functionalism (also known as structural functionalism or consensus theory)

Émile Durkheim (1858–1917), Talcott Parsons (1902–79), and Robert Merton (1910–2003) are the key theorists of structural functionalism, which is more commonly known simply as functionalism. Popular in the USA, this perspective studies the way social structures function to maintain social order and stability. Functionalism focuses on large-scale social processes and is based on the assumption that a society is a system of integrated parts, each of which have certain 'needs' (or **functional prerequisites**) that must be fulfilled for social order to be maintained. Hence, functionalists study various parts of society to understand how they interrelate and function to promote social stability and consensus.

The functionalist analysis of health care has been primarily influenced by the work of Parsons (1951), who viewed the health of individuals as a necessary condition of a stable and ordered society. He conceptualised illness as a form of **deviance**—that

functional prerequisites
A debated concept based on the assumption that all societies require certain functions to be performed for them to survive and maintain social order. Also known as functional imperatives.

deviance
Behaviour or activities that violate social expectations about what is normal.

sick role
A concept used by Talcott Parsons to describe the social expectations of how sick people are expected to act and of how they are meant to be treated.

biomedicine/ biomedical model
The conventional approach to medicine in Western societies, based on the diagnosis and explanation of illness as a malfunction of the body's biological mechanisms. This approach underpins most health professions and health services, which focus on treating individuals, and generally ignores the social origins of illness and its prevention.

• • **TheoryLink**
• • See Chapter 5
• • for a functionalist
• • perspective of health
• • inequality and Chapter
• • 19 for its approach on
• • professions.

capitalism
An economic and social system based on the private accumulation of wealth.

is, he viewed it as stopping people from performing various social roles, such as paid work and caring for children, which were essential to the functioning of society. In Parsons's terms, 'health is intimately involved in the functional prerequisites of the social system … too low a general level of health, too high an incidence of illness, is dysfunctional … because illness incapacitates the effective performance of social roles' (1951, p. 430).

For Parsons, illness disrupts the normal functioning of society, and thus it is important that the sick are encouraged to seek expert help, so that they return to health and can perform their social roles. The pathway to health was achieved through the **sick role**—that is, the social expectations that dictate how an individual sick person is meant to act and be treated.

According to Parsons, the sick role involves a series of rights and responsibilities. Once sick, it is the right of individuals to be exempted from their normal social roles such as those of the parent, employee, or student. This exemption from performing duties is legitimated by medical diagnosis and treatment. For example, students regularly have to provide medical certificates to support their case for not performing their student roles of turning up to class or submitting work on time. A further right of the sick person is not to be held personally responsible for the illness. Since illness is generally beyond individuals' control, they should be able to rely on others to care for them while they are ill. Sick people also have certain responsibilities. For example, they are expected to seek medical assistance and comply with the recommended treatment. Moreover, they are obliged to recover and resume their normal social duties.

The 'sick role' concept directs attention to the social nature of the illness experience and focuses attention on the doctor–patient relationship, but the importance of the concept also lies in the many critiques it has inspired as a result of its limited application to chronic, terminal, and permanently disabling conditions, as well as its uncritical acceptance of the role of the medical profession and its neglect of the limitations of the **biomedical model**.

Marxism (also known as conflict theory)

The term Marxism refers to a wide body of theory and political policies based on the writings of Karl Marx (1818–83) and Friedrich Engels (1820–95). Marx was a philosopher, economist, and sociologist. He was also politically active, and since his death his writings have not only inspired many sociologists, but have also laid the foundations for numerous political movements around the world. Marxism, also known as 'conflict theory', asserts that society is dominated by a conflict of interest between two social classes within **capitalist** societies—the bourgeoisie (the capitalist class) and the proletariat (the working class). The influence and contribution of Marxism in sociology is widespread, but the perspective's core concern remains that of class analysis, especially due to its emphasis on class conflict as the defining feature of social life and the catalyst of social change towards its desired goal of **socialism** and ultimately **communism**.

Much of Marx's theory has been reinterpreted and modified, and is now often referred to as neo-Marxism. The Marxist perspective of health and illness, reflected in the contemporary writings of Howard Waitzkin (1983, 2000), Lesley Doyal (1979), Vicente Navarro (1976, 1986), and Evan Willis (1989), focuses on the role of the medical profession and the impact of working and living conditions in capitalist society and how these contribute to illness. In particular, Marxist perspectives have highlighted that the exploitation of workers and the pursuit of profit can create dangerous work environments and poor living conditions, resulting in higher mortality and morbidity rates among the working class (see Chapters 5 and 6).

Marxist analyses of health care tend to focus on the professional power of doctors to serve class interests by placing profit-maximisation above access to optimal health care. Navarro and Waitzkin have been strong critics of the medical profession's individualistic focus and its continued reliance on the biomedical model. By locating the cause and treatment of illness in individuals and ignoring what Waitzkin (1983, 2000) calls 'illness-generating social conditions', the medical profession is viewed as performing an ideological function by masking the real causes of illness and thereby supporting the capitalist system. According to Navarro (1986, p. 35), in capitalist societies the influence of work on health 'is of paramount importance' since workers 'have no control over their work and, thus, over their lives, including their health'. In the Australian context, there has been significant research documenting workplace health hazards (see Chapter 6).

Australian sociologist Willis (1989) highlighted the profit-orientation and entrepreneurial ethos of the medical profession and its tendency to align itself with upper-class interests. For example, a significant section of the medical profession opposes forms of public health provision, as exemplified by the Australian Medical Association's (AMA) continued opposition to the Medicare system. Furthermore, fee-for-service, self-regulation, and the suppression of competition from other health practitioners (see Willis 1989) are indicative of medicine's alignment with 'the economic and ideological patterns of capitalism' (Connell 1988, p. 214). This has resulted in a commonality of lifestyles and interests between doctors and the upper class so that 'doctors as a group ... have particular political and economic interests they do not share with most of their patients: interests in maintaining a sharp division of labour in health care, in a substantial amount of public ignorance about health, and in seeing that self-help arrangements for health care remain marginal or ineffective' (Connell 1988, p. 214).

Weberianism

Max Weber (1864–1920) ranks along with Marx as one of the most influential theorists in sociology. Weber (1921/1968) produced a theory of society that acknowledges

socialism
A political ideology with numerous variations, but with a core belief in the creation of societies in which private property and wealth accumulation are replaced by state ownership and distribution of economic resources.

communism
A utopian vision of society based on communal ownership of resources, cooperation, and altruism to the extent that social inequality and the state no longer exist. Sometimes used interchangeably with socialism to refer to societies ruled by a communist party.

TheoryLink
Chapters 5 and 19 discuss Marxist approaches applied to health inequality and the medical profession.

the way in which people both shape and are shaped by the social structure. Weber's writings are extensive, but his major contributions concern his analysis of bureaucracy and his account of power and social inequality through the concepts of class, status, and party (political parties and pressure groups). Like Marx, Weber viewed class as important and believed that social conflict was a defining characteristic of increasingly complex societies. Rather than seeing two basic classes as in Marx's theory, Weber also considered the importance of the middle classes, which he saw as consisting of those occupational groups with qualifications and skills that provided them with market advantages (higher wages, prestige, and better working conditions) over those in manual occupations. Weber suggested that in addition to social class, status groups and parties were also a source of group formation and social inequality.

Status groups reflect cultural and sometimes legally conferred privileges, social respect, and honour. They are usually based on membership of specific professional, ethnic, and religious groups, and members tend to share common interests and lifestyles. Status group membership is often restricted through what Weber termed a process of **social closure**. While class and social status tend to be closely related, they need not be. Moreover, other groups, or parties in Weber's terms, could also serve the basis for collective interests and social inequality. Parties refer to groups attempting to wield power and include political parties, associations such as unions and professional bodies, as well as various interest/pressure groups.

In the health sector, Robert Alford's (1975) work on the competing interest groups is often cited. He argues that health policy and the delivery of health care are a compromise between three main vested interest groups: professional monopolists (doctors), corporate rationalists (public and private sector managers), and equal health advocates (various patient-rights groups). Alford, like many Weberians, acknowledges that some groups (such as doctors) are clearly dominant and exercise more power, but nonetheless maintains that other groups can and do exert influence.

Another strand of Weber's work concerns the process of **rationalisation**, which he considers was the overarching trend in society, epitomised by the growth of bureaucracy. Weber (1921/1968) predicted that the 'future belongs to bureaucratisation' (p. 1401) and described an **ideal type** bureaucratic organisation as having a highly specialised and hierarchical division of labour bounded by formal rules and regulations (see Weber 1921/1968, pp. 221–3). For Weber, bureaucracies are an effective response to social complexity and democracy by attempting to eliminate fraud, mismanagement, and inefficiency through conformity to standardised procedures. Despite what he acknowledges are the significant benefits of bureaucracy, he enunciates a fear that social life was to become so governed by objective and informal rules that people would become entrapped by an 'iron cage' of regulations that would limit their creativity and individuality. For example, health care delivery is increasingly subject to regulations and performance indicators so that health care

social closure
A term first used by Max Weber to describe the way that power is exercised to exclude outsiders from the privileges of social membership (in social classes, professions, or status groups).

● ● **TheoryLink**
● ● Chapter 18 discusses
● ● Alford's ideas further.

rationalisation
The standardisation of social life through rules and regulations.

ideal type
A concept originally devised by Max Weber to refer to the abstract or pure features of any social phenomenon.

becomes predictable and uniform, which may make health professionals more consistent in their treatment, but may also dehumanise interaction with patients and lessen the flexibility and quality of care provided (see Chapter 19).

Symbolic interactionism

Symbolic interactionism is associated with key theorists such as George Herbert Mead (1863–1931), Charles Cooley (1864–1929), Howard Becker (1928–), Erving Goffman (1922–82), Anselm Strauss (1916–96), and Herbert Blumer (1900–87). Blumer coined the term in 1937. The perspective arose as a reaction against structuralist approaches such as structural functionalism, which tends to view humans as simply responding to external influences. Instead, symbolic interactionists focus on agency and how people construct, interpret, and give meaning to their behaviour through interaction with others. The core philosophical assumption is that humans create reality through their actions and the meanings they give to them. Therefore, society is the cumulative effect of human action, interaction, and interpretation, and these are more significant than social structures, hence the focus of the perspective.

Symbolic interactionism provides a theoretical bridge between sociology and psychology by concentrating on small-scale social interaction and how this impacts on individuals' identity or image of themselves (often referred to as 'the self' or 'self-concept'). Cooley's (1906/1964) term 'the looking-glass self' encapsulates this approach, whereby the reactions of others influence the way we see ourselves and thus how we in turn behave. For example, if people regularly tell you that you are attractive and intelligent, this reaction can impact on what you believe and how you behave.

Symbolic interactionism emphasises that health and illness are perceived subjectively, and are **social constructions** that change over time and vary between cultures. Therefore, what is considered an illness is socially defined and passes through a social lens that reflects the culture, politics, and morality of a particular society at a particular point in time. Such a viewpoint has been used to great effect by interactionist theorists to expose many medical practices and opinions that are based on social (or moral), rather than biological, factors. Many interaction studies have also focused on patients' subjective experiences of illness, interactions between patients and health professionals, and interactions among health professionals (especially between doctors and nurses).

Becker (1963) argues that deviance is created through social interaction when certain behaviours or groups of people are labelled as deviant by social institutions such as the police, courts, and mental health authorities. **Labelling theory** examines the effect that being labelled deviant has for the individual concerned. Such an approach draws attention to how and why certain behaviours and groups of people are labelled deviant. For example, in the 1960s, African Americans involved in street protests or 'race riots' were labelled as exhibiting deviant, abnormal, and even

social construction
Refers to the socially created characteristics of human life based on the idea that people actively construct reality, meaning it is neither 'natural' nor inevitable. Therefore, notions of normality/abnormality, right/wrong, and health/illness are subjective human creations that should not be taken for granted.

labelling theory
Focuses on the effect that social institutions and health professions (such as the police, the courts, and psychiatry) have in labelling (defining and socially constructing) what is deviant.

TheoryLink   • •
Chapter 12 discusses   • •   • •
labelling theory further.   • •

John Germov

social control
Mechanisms that aim to induce conformity, or at least to manage or minimise deviant behaviour.

stigma
A physical or social trait, such as a disability or a criminal record, that results in negative social reactions such as discrimination and exclusion.

total institutions
A term used by Erving Goffman to refer to institutions such as prisons and asylums in which life is highly regulated and subjected to authoritarian control to induce conformity.

pathological behaviour. Labelling theory exposed the way that medicine (in this case psychiatry) could be used as an instrument of **social control** to constrain the actions of 'difficult' social groups (see Roach Anleu 1999).

Goffman (1961, 1963) examined **stigma** and focused attention on what he termed **total institutions** such as asylums. According to Goffman, people become stigmatised when they possess an attribute that negatively affects social interaction. He identified three forms of stigma: physical deformity, individual characteristics (mental disorder), and 'tribal' factors (based on 'race', ethnicity, and religion). In his terms, these resulted in tainted or 'spoiled identities', whereby social interaction was affected by negative traits associated with the particular stigma. For example, people may react to others with physical disabilities through outright discrimination or may treat them as if they were also mentally incompetent. A person diagnosed with schizophrenia may be treated as (and often called) a 'schizophrenic' as if that were the sole characteristic of who the individual is; the stereotype associated with the condition overrides the actual personality, actions, and achievements of the individual concerned.

Goffman's (1961) analysis of institutionalisation (the incarceration of people for some form of treatment or sanction) focused on the experience from the perspective of the 'inmates'. His observations of the interaction between inmates and institutional staff reflected the overt and covert forms of power relationships imbued in what he termed the 'total institution'. While such institutions served to impose highly regimented and authoritarian forms of conformity on inmates, often to the detriment of their personal and health needs, they also resulted in a hidden 'under-life' through which people kept a sense of their individual identity by resisting or undermining authority in secret ways (see also Scheff 1966). Goffman's insights on the negative affects of institutionalisation have had a wide social impact and did much to place the issue on the public agenda.

Feminism

Feminist perspectives in sociology first arose in the 1960s and were primarily aimed at addressing the neglect of gender issues and in some cases the blatant sexism of traditional sociological theories, exposing that most mainstream sociology was in fact 'male-stream' (Abbott et al. 2005). Women's experiences as workers, partners, carers, or victims of abuse were rarely studied or theorised. For example, most traditional theories of social class excluded the study of women and concentrated on fathers and sons, rather than mothers and daughters. Furthermore, some approaches perpetuated sexist assumptions about the role of women in society, such as Parsons's view of women as performing 'expressive roles' in society, fulfilling the 'function' of providing emotional care and support of men and families. Hence, feminist perspectives addressed the question 'What about the women?' and focused on social inequality between women and men.

patriarchy
A system of power through which males dominate households. It is used more broadly by feminists to refer to society's domination by patriarchal power, which functions to subordinate women and children.

Feminism is a broad social and intellectual movement that addresses many issues from a range of academic disciplines. There are many 'feminisms', most of which can be grouped into four 'schools of thought':

- liberal feminism
- radical feminism
- socialist and Marxist feminism
- post-structuralist feminism/post-feminism (postmodern feminism).

There are many comprehensive introductions to feminist perspectives (see Wearing 1996; Tong 1998; Beasley 1999; Abbott et al. 2005).

Despite the diversity of approaches, feminist perspectives all highlight the importance of **patriarchy**. Feminists argue that the social structure is patriarchal, with social institutions such as the legal, health, and education systems, as well as the wider culture, reflecting sexist values and supporting the privilege of men. They challenge biological assumptions about women's nature, highlighting that **gender** is a social construction and identifying gender-role socialisation and sex discrimination as keys to understanding inequality between the sexes.

Feminist perspectives of health care have underpinned the women's health movement and have drawn attention to:

- the **sexual division of labour** in health care, particularly the historical role of women healers, the subordination of female-dominated professions such as nursing, the performance of **emotional labour**, the role of women as informal carers outside the health system, and the effect of the increasing entry of women into the medical professions (Ehrenreich & English 1973, 1974, 1979; Hothschild 1979; Broom 1991; Gibson & Allen 1993; Pringle 1998; Wicks 1999)
- sexism and **biological determinism** in health care, particularly medical research and treatment, according to which much health research has been conducted on men and extrapolated to women, and women's specific health concerns have been under-researched or falsely assumed to be the result of their menstrual cycles (that is, women as 'helpless victims of their hormones') (Barrett & Roberts 1978)
- unwarranted and sometimes harmful interventions in the management of pregnancy, childbirth, contraception, reproductive technology, and gynaecological disorders (Frankfort 1972; Oakley 1980; Doyal 1995; Annandale & Clarke 1996)
- the issues of sexuality, rape, and domestic violence as key health issues requiring the need for appropriate health policies and specialised training of health workers (Doyal 1995; Abbott et al. 2005)
- body image and eating disorders (Wolf 1990; Bordo 1993; Bartky 1998; Williams & Germov 2008).

Today feminist perspectives and concerns are a central feature of sociology and health sociology in particular. Feminism has exposed the sexism and biological

gender/sex
This pair of terms refers to the socially constructed categories of feminine and masculine (the cultural identities and values that prescribe how men and women should behave), and the social power relations based on those categories, as distinct from the categories of biological sex (female or male).

sexual division of labour
Refers to the nature of work performed as a result of gender roles. In contemporary English-speaking societies, the stereotype is that of the male breadwinner and the female homemaker, even though this pattern is far from an accurate description of most people's lives.

emotional labour
Refers to the use of feelings by employees as part of their paid work. In health care, a key part of nursing work is caring for patients, often by providing emotional support.

biological determinism
An unproven belief that individual and group behaviour, and social status are an inevitable result of biology.

TheoryLink

Chapter 7 discusses gendered health and the contributions of various feminist writers.

determinism of medical approaches, and facilitated increasing attention on women's health rights in terms of health research, funding, and the provision of appropriate services (see Annandale 2004 for a review of feminist theories applied to health).

Contemporary modernist approaches: the theoretical synthesisers

modernity/ modernism

A view of social life that is founded upon rational thought and a belief that truth and morality exist as objective realities that can be discovered and understood through scientific means.

structuration

A concept developed by Anthony Giddens to indicate the interrelationship between **structure** and **agency**.

reflexive modernity

A term coined by Ulrich Beck and Anthony Giddens to refer to the present social era in developed societies, in which social practices are open to reflection, questioning, and change, and therefore in which social traditions no longer dictate people's lifestyles.

TheoryLink

Chapters 5 and 23 discuss these theories further.

Modernity refers to social life in the modern era or 'modern times', which is characterised by the rise of industrial society and the dominance of science and rationality over superstition and tradition. Marx, Weber, and Durkheim were some of the original (or classical) modernist social theorists who attempted to understand social change brought by industrialisation, capitalism, and rationalisation (Ritzer & Goodman 2004; Cuff, Sharrock & Francis 2005). Influenced by this tradition, though dealing with social life that has changed significantly since that of the classical theorists, contemporary theorists of modernity are a diverse group of writers who are difficult to classify because their work is a synthesis of various theories and concepts (notably drawn from Marxism, Weberianism, and functionalism). Key theorists include Norbert Elias (1897–1990), Anthony Giddens (1938–), Ulrich Beck (1944–), Jürgen Habermas (1929–), Pierre Bourdieu (1930–2002), and Manuel Castells (1942–), some of whom are often grouped under the banner of critical theory. The perspective of 'contemporary modernism' is thus a linguistic convenience to identify some of the shared concerns of these authors, a distinguishing feature of which is their attempt to integrate structure and agency; such as Giddens's **structuration** theory (Ritzer & Goodman 2004).

According to Giddens and Beck, we live in an era of **reflexive modernity** (Beck et al. 1994), whereby people's increased access to global travel, media, and information and communication technologies, along with increased rates of education (in developed countries at least) has displaced traditional values and modes of living with a multitude of lifestyle choices. While people are much freer to choose their lifestyles, values, and identities (Giddens 1991), they are also more conscious of the increased risks of social life in the face of environmental pollution, corporate corruption, and terrorism, which Beck (1992) argues is characteristic of living in a **risk society** (see also Beck 1999; Adam et al. 2000). In the context of health and illness, the contemporary modernist approaches discussed here can be applied to study health promotion, risk factors, and health-related behaviour.

Post-structuralism and postmodernism

The terms 'post-structuralism' and 'postmodernism' are often used interchangeably (Ritzer 1997), and, even though distinctions can be made between the two, for our purposes we will focus on their similarities and treat them as one (and for simplicity only use the term 'postmodernism'). Postmodernism arose in the 1980s and reflects a diverse range of social theories from many academic disciplines, making it difficult to categorise or treat systematically; however, to greater or lesser degrees, most social theorists who fall under the umbrella of postmodernism share the following key assumptions:

- The rejection of universal truths about the world, instead suggesting that reality is a social construction. Therefore, all theoretical perspectives (whether they be in the natural, health, or social sciences) reflect the vested interests of one group or another and thus all knowledge is merely a claim to truth, reflecting the subjectivity of those involved.

- The rejection of grand theories or **meta-narratives**: postmodern perspectives are critical of structuralist perspectives such as functionalism and Marxism, which suggest there is an overriding logic of social organisation. They dispute the existence or importance of unifying trends and structural determinants such as functional prerequisites, class conflict, patriarchy, or rationalisation.

- Since no perspective is neutral and there are no universal structural determinants of social life, postmodernists focus on how truth claims about the world are socially constructed. Thus, there is no single reality or ultimate truth, only versions or interpretations of what is 'real', 'true', 'normal', 'right', or 'wrong'. Postmodernists adopt a pluralist approach and claim that social life is characterised by fragmentation, differentiation, and subjectivity, reflecting people's differences in terms of their culture, lifestyle, and vested interests. Such a perspective supports tolerance of diversity, but can imply that 'almost anything goes'.

The main social theorists are Michel Foucault (1926–84), Jean-Francois Lyotard (1924–98), Jean Baudrillard (1929–2007), and Fredric Jameson (1934–). In sociology, the work of Foucault has had the most influence, especially his historical work on asylums, prisons, and hospitals, which uncovered how knowledge and power are used to regulate and control various social groups (see Box 2.1).

risk society
A term coined by Ulrich Beck (1992) to describe the centrality of risk calculations in people's lives in Western society, whereby the key social problems today are unanticipated hazards, such as the risks of pollution, food poisoning, and environmental degradation.

meta-analysis and meta-narratives
The 'big picture' analysis that frames and organises observations and research on a particular topic.

BOX 2.1 Doing health sociology: surveillance

Foucault's (1979) conceptualisation of the panopticon as a metaphor for his theory of surveillance and social control has been a key legacy of his work. The panopticon (all-seeing place) was developed by Jeremy Bentham in the eighteenth century as an architectural design for a prison, consisting of a central observation tower surrounded by circles of cells so that every cell could be observed simultaneously. According to Foucault:

All that is needed, then, is to place a supervisor in a central tower and to shut up in each cell a madman, a patient, a condemned man, a

... »

John Germov

worker, or a schoolboy ... [resulting in] a state of consciousness and permanent visibility that assures the automatic functioning of power ... in short, that the inmates should be caught up in a power situation of which they themselves are the bearers (1979, p. 200–1).

Therefore, control could be maintained by the assumption of being constantly under surveillance, so that individuals subjected to the disciplinary gaze were 'totally seen without ever seeing, whilst the agents of discipline see every-

thing, without ever being seen' (Foucault 1979, p. 202). The idea that social control of people's behaviour can be exerted in such an indirect and self-induced way has been a significant insight. For example, the wide promotion of the thin ideal of female beauty in Western societies results in panoptic effects whereby many women perceive themselves to be under constant body surveillance and undergo numerous disciplined activities with detrimental health consequences in an attempt to conform to the pressure to be thin (see Williams & Germov 2008).

Postmodernism has significantly influenced feminist perspectives. Postmodern feminism focuses on agency and subjectivity, exploring 'differences' among women in terms of class, religion, 'race', and ethnicity. Postmodern feminists stress that women use their agency to mediate, resist, and in some cases overcome patriarchy (see Butler 1990; Barrett & Phillips 1992; McNay 1992; Pringle 1995; Weedon 1997; Bartky 1998). In her book *Sex and Medicine*, Rosemary Pringle (1998) explores the impact that increasing numbers of female doctors are having on the organisation and delivery of health care. While not discounting the patriarchal basis of the medical profession, Pringle shows how female doctors are making a difference, and while 'struggles go on at a local level and outcomes vary' (1998, p. 222), their efforts have been primarily responsible for establishing the viability of women's health centres and addressing sexism in medical practice.

Conclusion

Despite the differences between the theoretical perspectives discussed here, the distinctions between specific social theories produced by individual authors are likely to be less clear-cut. As Judith Bessant and Rob Watts state (1999, p. 34), sociologists 'constantly "hover" between and in and out of different traditions', and specific social theories are not 'as neat or coherent' as grouping them into theoretical perspectives implies. While sociologists generally align themselves with particular perspectives, they tend to be in less disagreement than the differences between perspectives might imply. This is partly due to the fact that sociologists attempt to incorporate the insights of a range of perspectives into their specific social theory.

While the existence of so many perspectives can be challenging, new theories and perspectives are likely to continue to emerge. Social theories change over time as society itself changes and new knowledge, ideas, and capabilities emerge. This is as true of natural sciences as it is of the social sciences. In response to social change and the development of new insights, theories are regularly modified, reinterpreted, and even rejected.

It is worth noting that the theoretical perspectives presented in this chapter are more complex than can be discussed here. Furthermore, no attempt has been made to evaluate the theoretical perspectives, a feature beyond the scope of this introductory chapter. The aim has been to convey a basic understanding of some of the main assumptions, concepts, and approaches to explain the differences between perspectives and the insights they offer, and help lay the foundations of understanding for various sociological theories you will encounter in this text and the wider literature.

At this point it is important to sound a note of caution about the use and critique of sociological theories. This chapter began by using the framework of theoretical perspectives as a useful form of shorthand to convey the types of theories sociologists have developed. There is a danger then that when attempting to evaluate how well a specific social theory fits the evidence, the mistake is made of critiquing the general perspective to which the theory belongs, rather than assessing the insights of the specific theory itself. This is not an argument to ignore the various limitations of theoretical perspectives that many authors have exposed, but rather to warn against falling into the trap of dismissing a theory because it is allegedly guilty of all the sins of the perspective to which it is associated. A much healthier approach to adopt is a position of theoretical pluralism—that is, to accept that many theories have something to offer, even though you may have a preference for a certain theoretical perspective. Because different theoretical perspectives often address different levels of analysis and different issues, and attempt to find answers to varied questions, they should be viewed as potentially complementary rather than automatically oppositional (Turner 1995). It is up to you to judge how well a particular theory fits the researched evidence, based on your wider reading.

Summary of main points

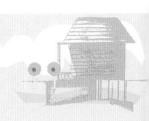

» Sociologists seek to interpret their findings by offering a 'how' and/or 'why' explanation—a theory—for what they seek to understand.

» There is often disagreement over which 'how' and 'why' explanations, or social theories, best explain certain aspects of social life. Just as there are people with different opinions, there are sociologists who offer different theories to explain social life.

» One way to understand the range of social theories that exists is to group the theories into seven main theoretical perspectives: functionalism, Marxism, Weberianism, symbolic interactionism, feminism, contemporary modernism, and post-structuralism/postmodernism.

» Differences between the theoretical perspectives are based on a range of philosophical assumptions and levels of focus, which direct attention to particular aspects of social life and how they should be investigated.

» The use of theoretical perspectives oversimplifies the reality of social theorising, so that some sociologists may adopt different theoretical positions according to the topic under study or may incorporate the insights of other perspectives into their own social theory.

» A specific social theory should not necessarily be discarded by being accused of the limitations of the theoretical perspective to which it belongs. While it is important to be aware of the underlying assumptions and limitations of theoretical perspectives, a specific social theory should always be evaluated on its merit.

Sociological reflection: what is your theory?

Sociological theories can help us understand how and why certain health problems exist. As this chapter has shown, most theories can be grouped into seven major theoretical perspectives:

1 functionalism
2 Marxism
3 Weberianism
4 symbolic interactionism
5 feminism
6 contemporary modernism
7 post-structuralism/postmodernism.

Which theoretical perspective do you prefer? Why? Identify some of the key insights into understanding health and illness that your preferred perspective provides.

Discussion questions

1 Why is theory necessary? Provide examples in your answer.
2 What are some of the limitations of adopting one theoretical perspective and ignoring others?

3 Which perspectives focus their attention on studying the interactions between health professionals and patients?

4 Marxist theorists suggest that health care is being increasingly commodified in Australia. In what ways? What factors do other perspectives highlight as important influences on health?

5 What insights into health issues and health care have feminist perspectives provided?

6 What insights do postmodern perspectives of health and illness provide?

Further investigation

1 Choose two of the perspectives discussed in this chapter and examine the similarities and differences in their approach to studying health and illness.

2 'The sick role is no longer applicable to the experience of illness and health care.' Discuss.

3 Compare modernist and postmodernist perspectives on a health issue of your choice.

Further reading

Annandale, E. 2004, *Feminist Theory and the Sociology of Health and Illness*, Routledge, London.

Bury, M. & Gabe, J. (eds) 2004, *The Sociology of Health and Illness: A Reader*, Routledge, London.

Cheek, J., Shoebridge, J., Willis, E. & Zadoroznyj, M. 1996, *Society and Health: Social Theory for Health Workers*, Longman, Melbourne.

Scambler, G. 2002, *Health and Social Change: A Critical Theory*, Open University Press, Buckingham.

Williams, S. J., Gabe, J. & Calnan, M. (eds) 2000, *Health, Medicine and Society: Key Theories, Future Agendas*, Routledge, London.

Web resources

SocioSite—Sociological Theories and Perspectives: <http://www.sociosite.net/topics/theory.php>

Online case study ● ● ●
Visit the Second Opinion website to access relevant case studies.

John Germov

Documentaries/films

Understanding Sociology (1998), 3 Volumes, Halo Vine Video, Middlesex, UK. Volume 1: Theory and Method (Classical sociology: positivism, interpretivism and realism), 42 minutes; Volume 2: Making Sense of Sociological Theory (Marxism, Functionalism and Interactionism), 58 minutes, and Volume 3: From Modernity to Postmodernity, 47 minutes. Available online:<http://www.halovine.com/socblurb.html>

References

Abbott, P., Wallace, C. & Tyler, M. 2005, *An Introduction to Sociology: Feminist Perspectives*, 3rd edn, Routledge, London.

Adam, B., Beck, U. & van Loon, J. (eds) 2000, *The Risk Society and Beyond: Critical Issues for Social Theory*, Sage, London.

Alford, R. R. 1975, *Health Care Politics: Ideological and Interest Group Barriers to Reform*, University of Chicago Press, Chicago.

Annandale, E. 2004, *Feminist Theory and the Sociology of Health and Illness*, Routledge, London.

Annandale, E. & Clarke, J. 1996, 'What is Gender? Feminist Theory and the Sociology of Human Reproduction', *Sociology of Health and Illness*, vol. 18, no. 1, pp. 17–44.

Barrett, M. & Phillips, A. 1992, *Destabilizing Theory: Contemporary Feminist Debates*, Polity Press, Cambridge.

Barrett, M. & Roberts, H. 1978, 'Doctors and their Patients', in C. Smart & B. Smart (eds), *Women, Sexuality and Social Control*, Routledge, London, pp. 41–52.

Bartky, S. L. 1998, 'Foucault, Femininity, and the Modernization of Patriarchal Power', in R. Weitz (ed.), *The Politics of Women's Bodies: Sexuality, Appearance and Behavior*, Oxford University Press, New York.

Beasley, C. 1999, *What is Feminism Anyway?*, Allen & Unwin, Sydney.

Beck, U. 1992, *Risk Society: Towards a New Modernity*, Sage, London.

Beck, U. 1999, *World Risk Society*, Polity Press, Malden, MA.

Beck, U., Giddens, A. & Lash, S. 1994, *Reflexive Modernization: Politics, Tradition and Aesthetics in the Modern Social Order*, Polity Press and Blackwell, Cambridge.

Becker, H. S. 1963, *Outsiders: Studies in the Sociology of Deviance*, Free Press, New York.

Bessant, J. & Watts, R. 1999, *Sociology Australia*, Allen & Unwin, Sydney.

Bordo, S. 1993, *Unbearable Weight: Feminism, Western Culture, and the Body*, University of California Press, Berkeley, CA.

Broom, D. 1991, *Damned if We Do: Contradictions in Women's Health Care*, Allen & Unwin, Sydney.

Butler, J. 1990, *Gender Trouble: Feminism and the Subversion of Identity*, Routledge, London.

Capra, F. 1982, *The Turning Point: Science, Society and the Rising Culture*, Simon & Schuster, New York.

Connell, R. W. 1988, 'Class Inequalities and "Just Health"', *Community Health Studies*, vol. 12, no. 2, pp. 212–17.

Cooley, C. H. 1964/1906, *Human Nature and the Social Order*, Scribner's, New York.

Cuff, E. C., Sharrock, W. W. & Francis, D. W. 2005, *Perspectives in Sociology*, 5th edn, Routledge, London.

Doyal, L. 1979, *The Political Economy of Health*, Pluto Press, London.

Doyal, L. 1995, *What Makes Women Sick: Gender and the Political Economy of Health*, Rutgers University Press, New Brunswick, NJ.

Ehrenreich, B. & English, D. 1973, *Witches, Midwives and Nurses*, Old Westbury Feminist Press, New York.

Ehrenreich, B. & English, D. 1974, *Complaints and Disorders: The Sexual Politics of Sickness*, Compendium, London.

Ehrenreich, B. & English, D. 1979, *For Her Own Good: 150 Years of Experts' Advice*, Pluto Press, London.

Foucault, M. 1979, *Discipline and Punish*, Penguin, Harmondsworth.

Frankfort, E. 1972, *Vaginal Politics*, Bantam Publishers, New York.

Gibson, D. & Allen, J. 1993, 'Phallocentrism and Parasitism: Social Provision for the Aged', *Policy Sciences*, vol. 26, pp. 79–98.

Giddens, A. 1991, *Modernity and Self-identity: Self and Society in the Late Modern Age*, Stanford University Press, Stanford, CA.

Goffman, E. 1961, *Asylums: Essays on the Social Situation of Mental Patients and Other Inmates*, Penguin, London.

Goffman, E. 1963, *Stigma: Notes on the Management of Spoiled Identity*, Prentice Hall, Englewood Cliffs, NJ.

Hothschild, A. R. 1979, 'Emotion Work, Feeling Rules and Social Structure', *American Journal of Sociology*, vol. 85, no. 3, pp. 551–75.

McNay, L. 1992, *Foucault and Feminism*, Polity Press, Cambridge.

Navarro, V. 1976, *Medicine under Capitalism*, Prodist, New York.

Navarro, V. 1986, *Crisis, Health and Medicine: A Social Critique*, Tavistock, London.

Oakley, A. 1980, *Women Confined*, Martin Robertson, Oxford.

Parsons, T. 1951, *The Social System*, Free Press, New York.

Pringle, R. 1995, 'Destabilising Patriarchy', in B. Caine & R. Pringle (eds), *Transitions: New Australian Feminisms*, Allen & Unwin, Sydney, pp. 198–211.

Pringle, R. 1998, *Sex and Medicine: Gender, Power and Authority in the Medical Profession*, Cambridge University Press, Cambridge.

Ritzer, G. 1997, *Postmodern Social Theory*, McGraw-Hill, New York.

Ritzer, G. & Goodman, D. J. 2004, *Sociological Theory*, 6th edn, McGraw-Hill, New York.

Roach Anleu, S. L. 1999, *Deviance, Conformity and Control*, 3rd edn, Longman, Melbourne.

Scheff, T. J. 1966, *Being Mentally Ill: A Sociological Theory*, Aldine, Chicago.

Tong, R. P. 1998, *Feminist Thought: A Comprehensive Introduction*, 2nd edn, Allen & Unwin, Sydney.

Turner, B. S. with Samson, C. 1995, *Medical Power and Social Knowledge*, 2nd edn, Sage, London.

Waitzkin, H. 1983, *The Second Sickness: Contradictions of Capitalist Health Care*, Free Press, New York.

Waitzkin, H. 2000, *The Second Sickness: Contradictions of Capitalist Health Care*, 2nd edn, Rowman & Littlefield, Lanham.

Wearing, B. 1996, *Gender: The Pain and Pleasure of Difference*, Addison Wesley Longman, Sydney.

Weber, M. 1968/1921, *Economy and Society*, Bedminster, New York.

Weedon, C. 1997, *Feminist Practice and Poststructuralist Theory*, 2nd edn, Blackwell, Cambridge, MA.

Wicks, D. 1999, *Nurses and Doctors at Work: Rethinking Professional Boundaries*, Allen & Unwin, Sydney.

Williams, L. & Germov, J. 2008, 'Constructing the Female Body: Dieting, the Thin Ideal and Body Acceptance', in J. Germov & L. Williams (eds), *A Sociology of Food and Nutrition: The Social Appetite*, 3rd edn, Oxford University Press, Melbourne, pp. 329–62.

Willis, E. 1989, *Medical Dominance*, revised edn, Allen & Unwin, Sydney.

Wolf, N. 1990, *The Beauty Myth*, Vintage, London.

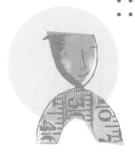

CHAPTER 3

Researching Health: Methodological Traditions and Innovations

DOUGLAS
EZZY

Overview

- What are the limitations of the major research methods used in biomedical studies such as evidence-based medicine, randomised control trials, and epidemiology?
- In what way do health sociologists address some of these limitations through qualitative approaches to the study of health and illness?
- What are some recent innovations in qualitative methods?

RESEARCHING DEPRESSION

The World Health Organization (2008) predicts that by 2020 depression will be the second most important cause of death for both sexes in all age groups. It is already the second most important cause of death amongst 15 to 44-year-old people of both sexes. This suggests two very important research questions: what causes depression, and, how should it be treated? The response to depression has been guided by the methods of medical research. However, there are two major problems with this response—and they both derive from inadequate methodological rigour. First, in the middle of the twentieth century, in response

to pressures to be 'scientific' and other political and cultural pressures, psychiatric research methods moved away from examining social factors and focused only on individuals. As a consequence 'psychiatry ... has retreated into a narrow, "medicalized" view of depression, ignoring, for the most part, the connection between depression and society' (Blazer 2005, p. 8). Poverty, gender, workplace stress, and a host of other social factors are clearly associated with depression. There has been little systematic research into these social aspects of depression. Second, pharmaceutical companies have spent vast amounts of money

··· 》

developing and assessing the efficacy of drugs for the treatment of depression. Very little money has been spent studying alternative responses to depression. Furthermore, a recent review of mostly unpublished clinical trials of drugs used to treat depression found that they were no more effective than a placebo in the treatment of mild to moderate depression, although they were effective in the treatment of severe depression (Kirsch et al. 2008). Given such complexities, a more sociological understanding of health research methods is required if depression is to be addressed adequately. This chapter discusses some of these key methodological issues.

Introduction

research methods
Procedures used by researchers to collect and investigate data.

randomised control trials (RCTs)
A biomedical research procedure used to evaluate the effectiveness of particular medications and therapeutic interventions. 'Random' refers to the equal chance of participants being in the experimental or control group (the group which receives a placebo or no treatment at all and is used for comparison), and 'trial' refers to the experimental nature of the method. RCTs are often mistakenly viewed as the best way to demonstrate causal links between factors under investigation, but tend to privilege biomedical over social responses to illness.

The **research methods** of health sociology are still profoundly shaped by biomedical research. Though the field of health sociology publishes its own journals and is increasingly contributing to health policy debates, the biomedical model strongly influences research into health issues. This is reflected by its dominance in the field of 'scientific' research, which covers nearly all aspects of health and illness. Although biomedical research methods such as **randomised control trials (RCTs)** are not part of health sociology's research methods, it is essential for health sociologists to understand the logic underpinning biomedical studies, and the consequences of the theoretical and political baggage they carry with them. The first section of this chapter discusses randomised control trials, **evidence-based medicine**, and the more public health oriented epidemiological research methods. The second section provides an overview of traditional **qualitative research**, introducing the distinctive logic of qualitative methods rather than discussing any particular tradition in detail. Third, recent innovations in qualitative methods are briefly outlined, pointing to the value of experimentation in methodologies.

The positivist tradition

Positivist research methodologies attempt to study the world through standardised procedures, which are allegedly uninfluenced by politics, subjectivity, or culture. Positivist methodologies, such as randomised control trials and epidemiological surveys, have proved to be very powerful methods for examining the efficacy of various health treatments and for identifying the risk factors associated with particular diseases. Positivist methodologies are not very useful for examining the actual way people experience illness, in terms of their personal meanings and interpretations. Positivist research is typically considered to be more important than other forms of research and, as a consequence, the cultural and interpretative dimensions of social life are often inadequately researched and understood. Further, supporters of positivist methodologies pretend that politics does not influence the research process and, as a consequence, are often blind to the power of the particular interest groups that these research methodologies serve.

Randomised control trials

Randomised control trials are a powerful way of demonstrating the efficacy of drugs and other biomedical interventions for diseases. An excellent example of an RCT is provided by Basil Hetzel (1995), who describes a trial of the injection of iodised oil for the prevention of cretinism in Papua New Guinea during the 1970s. The trial established that the children of mothers who had received a dose of iodine did not give birth to cretin infants, whereas women who had not received the iodine continued to produce children with cretinism. The trial was 'randomised' in the sense that whether a person received an iodine injection was decided randomly. This prevents the biasing influence of doctors, for example, choosing to give the medication to people whom they think may be more likely to benefit. It is a 'controlled' trial in the sense that a comparison group of people, who do not receive the medication but who are drawn from the same social group, is included in the trial. The benefit of the medication is then assessed by comparing the two groups, in which the only difference is whether they received the medication or not. RCTs are important because they allow cherished beliefs to be disproved. For example, the drug clofibrate was initially thought to be beneficial because it significantly reduced the level of cholesterol in the blood. It was used extensively to treat high cholesterol until an RCT demonstrated that it actually increased mortality (Sackett 1981).

Evelleen Richards (1988) provides an excellent account of the social and political nature of RCTs. She makes the strong claim that '[t]he randomised controlled clinical trial, no matter how tightly organized and evaluated, can neither guarantee objectivity nor definitively resolve disputes over contentious therapies or technologies' (Richards 1988, p. 686). She also provides a detailed analysis of the use of an RCT to test the efficacy of vitamin C as a cancer treatment. Two rival medical clinics were involved in examining the efficacy of vitamin C. One clinic argued for the value of vitamin C, not as a drug to kill cancer cells, but as a supplement to support the immune system's own suppression of the cancer tumours. The rival clinic was funded to conduct the trials, and evaluated the therapeutic value of vitamin C using criteria drawn from comparable trials of cytotoxic drugs. Not surprisingly, vitamin C was found to be ineffective, even though they did not actually 'attempt to evaluate the efficacy of vitamin C' (Richards 1988, p. 672). Richards

evidence-based medicine (EBM)
An approach to medicine that maintains all clinical practice should be based on evidence from randomised control trials (RCTs) to ensure treatment effectiveness and efficacy.

qualitative research
Research that focuses on the personal experiences and beliefs, subjective meanings and interpretations, of the participants being studied.

positivism
Research methods that attempt to study people in the same way that physical scientists study the natural world by focusing on quantifiable and directly observable events.

shows how the conduct of the published RCTs was clearly influenced by the theoretical and professional perspectives of the scientists involved.

As noted by Richards, the most telling criticism of the debate over vitamin C is that the clinic advocating the value of vitamin C was prevented from publishing further research, and was not given the opportunity to comment on the existing studies already published. This exposes the myth of disinterested and open scientific discussion. Richards (1988, p. 672) concludes, '[i]f the orthodox claim of the inefficacy of vitamin C in cancer treatment prevails … it will *not* be as the result of agreement or consensus brought about by the disinterested application of impersonal rules of experimental procedure' (original emphasis). She argues that the direct, or indirect, influence of big business with vested interests in maintaining control over expensive treatments and preventing the use of widely available, relatively cheap alternatives undermines the 'myth of objective evaluation' and ultimately the 'social authority of its practitioners' (Richards 1988, p. 686).

This criticism of one RCT does not, of course, demonstrate that all RCTs are unreliable. It does demonstrate that political and theoretical interests are inherent in the conduct of medical and health research. This is one of the central insights of the application of sociological theory to **biomedical** research methodology.

Evidence-based medicine (EBM)

Evidence-based medicine (EBM) is an extension of the privileging of RCTs, arguing that clinical practice should be based on evidence from RCTs, rather than other forms of evidence that are thought to be potentially more biased, and therefore less effective. However, RCTs and EBM are not as universally applicable and objective as claimed. Both are infused with political and theoretical biases that are unavoidable. While useful and rigorous within the parameters for which they are designed, they become problematic when it is forgotten, or ignored, that they cannot be used to assess all aspects of health and illness, particularly those relating to social, cultural, and interpretative dimensions of illness.

The underlying world view that privileges RCTs as the 'gold standard' against which all other methodologies must be assessed results in a failure to properly research, or understand, the dimensions of health and illness that cannot be studied utilising RCTs. It is difficult and quite unusual, for example, to conduct randomised control trials of the effects of clean water, or of poverty, or of international debt repayments, on the health of people. The rhetoric of RCTs and EBM focuses on the individual. There is little analysis of the social and cultural variables that profoundly shape the distribution of disease in contemporary society (White & Willis 1988). As such, EBM and RCTs do not represent the radical paradigm shift they are exalted to be by their advocates. Rather, they are an extension of the positivist, individualistic, politically driven model of science that has informed most of modern medical practice.

biomedicine/ biomedical model
The conventional approach to medicine in Western societies, based on the diagnosis and explanation of illness as a malfunction of the body's biological mechanisms. This approach underpins most health professions and health services, which focus on treating individuals, and generally ignores the social origins of illness and its prevention.

Similarly, RCTs are not a particularly useful way of understanding, for example, how people maintain hope during illness, or how people adjust to life after serious illness. The privileging of RCTs implicitly devalues the social and cultural aspects of the experience of illness. Can people be understood by only studying their bodies? The problematic nature of this somatic fundamentalism is clearest in the treatment of 'diseases' such as depression and mental illness, where huge sums of money are expended on new drugs, but by comparison relatively little research has been conducted on the social and cultural dimensions. It is not difficult to see the political interests of drug companies and doctors in producing this imbalance in research and, as a consequence, in treatment. Similarly, children in the USA are fifty times more likely to be diagnosed with attention deficit hyperactivity disorder (ADHD) than children in Britain and France, but the individualistic medical disease model means that the cultural and social factors that might generate these differences are rarely examined (Reid et al. 1993). Instead, research focuses on the efficacy of various drug treatments, or on locating the problem in the individual's biology, and is dominated by RCTs as a research methodology.

Epidemiology and public health research

In **public health** research, epidemiological surveys have been used to perform a similar function, becoming the 'scientific' standard. **Epidemiology** examines the distribution of diseases, and tries to identify the specific nature of the **risk factors** associated with the development of the disease. Epidemiological surveys are typically very large, and aim to generate statistically representative samples that can be used to generalise the findings to the general population. The aim is to identify risk factors that can then be targeted in both prevention and treatment of the disease (Daly et al. 1997).

Epidemiological surveys can be powerful tools for examining the distribution of a disease, and planning the nature of the response to it. For example, when the AIDS epidemic first came into public consciousness, prevention efforts were focused on the entire population, with the memorable and physically scarring image of the Grim Reaper in television advertising to encourage people to practise safe sex. Epidemiological research soon demonstrated that in Australia the main risk groups were sexually active homosexual men, and injecting drug users. This meant that prevention campaigns could be targeted on these groups, making more effective use of resources and greatly increasing the effectiveness of the prevention campaigns. Australia still has a very low level of HIV/AIDS infection, and this is largely a consequence of being well informed by epidemiological research, and having effective prevention policies in place, including safe-sex campaigns and needle exchanges.

Nevertheless, epidemiological research still privileges the aspects of social life that can be measured and statistically summarised. For example, in the excellent

public health/public health infrastructure
Public policies and infrastructure to prevent the onset and transmission of disease among the population, with a particular focus on sanitation and hygiene such as clean air, water and food, and immunisation. Public health infrastructure refers specifically to the buildings, installations, and equipment necessary to ensure healthy living conditions for the population.

epidemiology/social epidemiology
The statistical study of patterns of disease in the population. Originally focused on epidemics, or infectious diseases, it now covers non-infectious conditions such as stroke and cancer. Social epidemiology is a sub-field aligned with sociology that focuses on the social determinants of illness.

risk factors
Conditions that are thought to increase an individual's susceptibility to illness or disease such as abuse of alcohol, poor diet, or smoking.

research paper by the National Health Strategy (NHS), *Enough to Make You Sick*, an impressive variety of statistical evidence is utilised to demonstrate that '[o]n almost every measure, the health of Aborigines is poorer than the health of non-Aborigines' (NHS 1992, p. 86). The report convincingly demonstrates the effect of social structural factors on Aboriginal health, such as unemployment, poor education and housing, and lack of public infrastructure. It further suggests that these problems are a product of 'other factors such as dispossession, alienation, and racism' (NHS 1992, p. 97). Yet, there is little evidence provided for this explanation since these are cultural and interpretative factors that are difficult to quantify. Although the authors of the report are insightful enough to indicate the significance of these factors, they are unable to demonstrate them with epidemiological and survey data. The study of these factors requires a different methodology that explicitly examines people's meanings and interpretations.

The qualitative tradition

The logic, theoretical framing, and practice of qualitative methods are fundamentally different to those of the statistical approach of the positivist tradition. This is both a strength and a weakness of qualitative methods. It is a strength because qualitative methods enable an examination of the meanings and interpretations of illness that are inaccessible to traditional statistical methods. It is a weakness because positivist 'scientific' methods and rhetoric still dominate in the spheres of policy making, research funding, and the publishing of academic journals. Consequently, qualitative research, and many aspects of life that are only brought to light using qualitative methods, are routinely ignored and undervalued.

quantitative research
Research that focuses on the collection of statistical data.

purposive sampling
Refers to the selection of units of analysis to ensure that the processes involved are adequately studied, and where statistical representativeness is not required.

Qualitative research is different to **quantitative research** in two ways. First, qualitative researchers examine meanings. They explicitly examine how people interpret or make sense of their illness experience. Statistics reduces interpretations and evaluations to scales and numerical values. Qualitative researchers are interested in the stories, the ways that people make sense of their lives, and the way social interaction changes these meanings.

Second, qualitative methods typically use a very different sampling strategy. Good statistical studies attempt to draw representative samples, so that if 10 per cent of the participant sample reports something, the researchers can be confident that 10 per cent of the wider population will experience the same thing. The objective of qualitative sampling is not to make statistical generalisations, but to generalise about the nature of the experience. This is called **purposive sampling**. The aim is to be able to describe the processes, meanings, and interpretations that lie behind the different aspects of the experience. For example, in my study of mental health and unemployment, I describe the different types of stories that lead some people to report feeling depressed after losing a job and other people to report feeling much better about themselves after a losing a job (Ezzy 2000a). Survey research has already established that about one third of people who lose their job report feeling better, and two-thirds report feeling worse. My sample of unemployed people was not drawn randomly, to ensure statistical representativeness, but purposively, to ensure that I interviewed enough people from both groups so that the processes that lead to depression or hope were clearly understood. That is to say, the sample was chosen purposively to ensure that the different types of meanings of unemployment were properly understood, rather than being statistically representative of the general population of unemployed people (for a more detailed explanation see Rice & Ezzy 1999).

Similarly, Kathy Charmaz (1994) takes the basic statistical observation that men contract more serious and life-threatening chronic illnesses than women, and asks: what is it that is distinctive about the experience of illness for men? She is not interested in the statistical distribution of the illness of the men she studies. Rather, she examines the meanings, interpretations, and identity dilemmas that are characteristic of the men's illness experiences. The focus is on describing the social processes, not the statistical distributions. Charmaz asks her research questions in this way: 'What is it like to be an active, productive man one moment, and a patient who faces death the next? ... Which identity dilemmas does living with continued uncertainty pose for men? How do they handle them?' (Charmaz 1994, p. 271). Notice the structure of the questions. They are not about the distribution of illness experience, but about the process of making sense of illness; they explore meanings and interpretations. Only qualitative methods can answer these sorts of questions.

Charmaz (1994) shows how masculine identities tend to be active and problem-solving, emphasising personal power, autonomy, and bravery in the face of danger. When dealing with illness, these masculine identity strategies allow men to develop some distinctive coping strategies, but also prevent them from developing others. The emphasis on active problem-solving facilitates the recreation of new identities to replace those lost as a consequence of chronic illness. If it proves difficult to find a new active identity, the men find it difficult to develop and feel comfortable with identities that are less autonomous and less active. If satisfying alternative identities cannot be found, this can increase the likelihood of depression.

BOX 3.1 | Doing health sociology: a qualitative study of palliative care nurses

An excellent example of the tension between statistical methods and qualitative methods is provided by Patricia Boston's (1999) study of palliative care nurses. In Canada, a workload-

measurement statistical system had been implemented by nursing administrators. Under this system all aspects of the nurses' work were quantified in an attempt to plan nursing

...»

Douglas Ezzy

requirements and to increase efficiency of services. Based on a qualitative study using 50 long interviews, Boston shows that this attempt to objectively quantify and systematise nurses' work fails to deal with the nature of nursing care required in a multicultural environment. The problem that Boston identifies is not simply that the workload-measurement system has insufficient categories to cover the wide range of tasks that nurses consider part of their work; rather, Boston argues that it is impossible to quantify many aspects of nursing practice that involve intuitive and personalised ways of dealing with patients in a culturally complex environment. In particular, dealing with patients from diverse cultural backgrounds requires taking time to learn, understand, and accommodate culturally distinct responses to terminal illness, diagnosis, and rituals associated with death and dying. These processes are extremely difficult to quantify. As a consequence, 'that subjective "inner" knowledge, which necessarily involves prioritising cultural concerns, is left to "fall between the cracks"' (Boston 1999, p. 151). In short, statistical, categorical, and deductive methodologies for assessing and studying nursing practice miss many of the central tasks that nurses perform.

Evaluating the quality of research

The criteria for what constitutes 'good' research significantly change between quantitative and qualitative methods. In survey research, studies are designed to be valid (accurately to reflect what is being studied) and reliable (or repeatable, and subsequently verifiable). In contrast, qualitative researchers typically prefer to describe good research as 'rigorous'. Yet, should not qualitative research also aim to be valid and reliable? The problem with these terms is that they ignore the way in which social life is a product of interpretative processes. Qualitative researchers tend to prefer to use the term '**rigour**' to avoid the positivist overtones of the terms 'validity' and 'reliability'. The aim of rigorous research is to closely scrutinise the meanings and interpretations of the people being studied (Lincoln 1995). People's meanings change with time, and depending on who they are talking to. Qualitative methods try explicitly to engage with the fluidity of meanings and interpretations rather than to avoid them, as is attempted by quantitative research.

For example, the experience of living with HIV/AIDS in Australia was very different in the 1980s and early 1990s to what it was in the late 1990s. This was due to a number of factors, including the discovery of some at least partially effective treatments in 1996, a move away from a culture of fear, and declining death rates. This means that it is impossible to assess the reliability of research conducted in the early 1990s, such as Barry Adam and Alan Sears's (1996) excellent study of the

rigour
A term used by qualitative researchers to describe trustworthy research that carefully scrutinises and describes the meanings and interpretations given by participants.

experience of living with HIV. Although there are many similarities, living with HIV/AIDS is profoundly different today, as a consequence of the new treatments. It would be impossible to repeat their study (and thus to test its reliability) because meanings and interpretations have changed. Further, the aim of qualitative research is not accurately to measure meanings (validity); rather, it is to scrutinise these meanings closely, locating them in the complexity of the culture of which they are a part. Adam and Sears do this well, using extensive extracts from their interviews, focusing on the processes through which meanings are constructed, and demonstrating how the interpretative and subjective aspects of social life are formed. Meaning and the interpretative process are integral to qualitative methods, and rigorous research explicitly engages with this interpretative process.

Anne Kavanagh and Dorothy Broom (1997) provide an example of a qualitative study of women's understanding of an abnormal cervical smear-test result, drawing on long interviews with Australian women. Previous research has demonstrated a statistical link between an abnormal cervical smear result and psychological and sexual difficulties of various kinds. Kavanagh and Broom describe the experiences of the women during their interaction with the health care services that may contribute to these difficulties. In particular they show how the interaction during the medical encounter often created fear, and did not allow for the development of trust or for the women to gain an understanding of what was happening to them. While the women wanted to participate in decisions about their treatment, they found this difficult because doctors provided little information during the consultation and did not encourage them to ask questions. They conclude that 'the inherent power structure of medical practice combined with time pressures often make it difficult for doctors to give the detailed information and reassurance patients need when a diagnosis is distressing' (Kavanagh & Broom 1997, p. 1388). Their qualitative methodology allowed them to examine the experiences and interpretations the women gave to the medical encounter. This, in turn, can be used to make sense of the statistically observed relationships. Only a qualitative methodology can identify these interpretative processes and, as a consequence, suggest changes to the medical interaction that might alleviate them.

Analysis and reporting of qualitative research

Similarly, for qualitative research the structure of analysis and the nature of research reports are quite different to statistical studies. The analysis process does not aim to follow correct procedures to produce objective results, although good procedure is important. Rather, qualitative analysis methodologies such as thematic analysis (Kellehear 1993), **grounded theory** (Strauss & Corbin 1990), narrative analysis (Riessman 1993), and cultural studies (Alasuutari 1995) all aim to analyse data by

grounded theory
Usually associated with qualitative methods, it refers to any social theory that is derived from (or grounded in) empirical research of social phenomena.

interpreting them. The process of interpretation can be described, but it cannot be systematised. This difference is clearest in the computer packages developed to assist qualitative data analysis. These computer packages do not analyse the qualitative data for the researcher; rather, they assist the analysis through sophisticated search, coding, and filing mechanisms (Rice & Ezzy 1999). It is impossible to automate the process of qualitative data analysis, as can be done with statistics, because the process of interpretation and understanding is central to the analytic process. Similarly, qualitative research reports are difficult to produce as short summaries similar to those that appear in many medical journals. The reason for this is that the heart of qualitative research is in the detail. It aims to provide understanding of the meanings, the details that shape why people do what they do. To do this well requires long quotations and careful explanation of cultural and social context.

Celia Orona (1990) provides one of the clearest accounts of the process of analysing qualitative data using a grounded theory methodology. She emphasises the role of uncertainty and the exploratory nature of the analytic process. She describes how she read and reread her interviews so that she became immersed in the world of her participants. This process of imaginative participation is at the heart of good qualitative research. In this way it is possible genuinely to listen, hear, and be transformed by the voice of participants, and as a consequence, to discover new understandings. Orona emphasises the need to embrace uncertainty, to explore, and to use her intuition and creativity as part of the process of analysis. As she immersed herself in her data she began to see patterns and relationships, and began to build a theory of the experience of identity loss during Alzheimer's disease, which was the focus of her research.

This explicit engagement with personal subjectivity and the interpretative process may sound far from 'scientific' but the alternative is to pretend that you can avoid the interpretative process. Qualitative researchers are increasingly arguing that it is impossible to avoid the role of subjectivity in the research process. The aim is thus not to avoid subjectivity, but to engage in a dialogue with the participants in the research (Lincoln 1995). Rigorous qualitative research aims genuinely to hear the voices of the participants. To do so requires engaging in a dialogue in which we are honest about the influence of our own subjectivity on the research process.

Future directions: qualitative innovators

While qualitative research is increasingly becoming an accepted methodology, it is typically understood as a poor cousin to the 'stronger' statistical methods such as surveys and RCTs. However, some qualitative researchers are pushing their methodology even further away from the theory and practice of the positivist tradition. Influenced by the arguments of postmodernists, cultural studies, and **hermeneutics**, these practitioners argue for the explicit incorporation of politics and the subjectivity

hermeneutics
Study of the interpretation and understanding of texts.

of the researcher into the research process, the need to experiment with less formal modes of expression, such as poetry and performance, and a greater degree of engagement of participants in the research process (Lincoln 1995; Denzin 1997).

These qualitative innovations, of course, are deeply disturbing to those who espouse the more traditional methodologies. Some researchers still try to portray qualitative research as a 'scientific' method, and apply all the rhetoric and terms of the statistical methods to qualitative research (Green 1998). They believe that qualitative researchers should be objective, distancing themselves from their research, that the research should be validated and reliable, and that the report should not contain any account of the researcher's subjective experience, but be politically neutral, and written in the standard scientific format. The problem with this attempt to make qualitative methods 'scientific' is that it devalues the central process that qualitative methods aim to examine—the process of interpretation. While qualitative methods can be moulded to fit this scientific world view, researchers are increasingly arguing that such an approach is deceptive, and does not produce research that is as useful, insightful, respectful, or as politically appropriate as it could be (Denzin 1997; Ezzy 2001).

Sue Estroff (1995) draws on her study of chronic illness to demonstrate that qualitative interviews are not events in which objective information is gathered from subjects. People do not have 'objective' unchanging stories of events that they carry around in their heads that a qualitative research approach can simply 'gather' like measurements. Rather, people shape and change their stories, often unconsciously, to fit the particular interactive context. Interviews are moments of the co-creation of narratives (Estroff 1995); to pretend otherwise is to deceive ourselves as researchers. This does not, however, make interviews useless, just more complex to negotiate and requiring a more sophisticated theory (Holstein & Gubrium 1995).

Further, Estroff argues that interviews need to be seen as relationships that involve mutual obligations and responsibilities as the interviewer and interviewee attempt to make sense of the experience together. This leads to a number of complex ethical and political questions about the extent to which participants can or should be involved in the research process. Some qualitative researchers have attempted to include participants as co-researchers. Others take a more guarded approach.

Some qualitative innovators have experimented with other aspects of the research process, exploring new writing styles, and making the research the subject of the research. For example, Carolyn Ellis (1995; 1998) provides a detailed study of loss and illness through her **autoethnographic** account of her 10 year relationship with her dying partner. An autoethnography is, as the name implies, an **ethnographic** study that focuses on the experience of the researcher. 'Autoethnography blurs distinctions between social science and literature, the personal and the social, the individual and culture, self and other, and researcher and subject' (Ellis 1998, p. 49). Ellis's autoethnography *Final Negotiations* is a story-like account that at times feels like a

TheoryLink
See Chapter 2 for an overview of postmodernism.

autoethnography
An ethnography that focuses on the experience of the researcher.

ethnography
A research method that is based on direct observation of a particular social group's social life and culture—of what people actually do.

post-structuralism/ postmodernism
Often used interchangeably, these terms refer to a broad perspective that is opposed to the view that social structure determines human action, and instead emphasises a pluralistic world view that explores the local, the specific, and the contingent in social life.

popular autobiography, but which also demonstrates the influence of a careful social science approach to observation, analysis, and recording of experience. Ellis says that the aim of writing about her intimate experiences grew out of her frustration with traditional methodologies and reports that failed to engage with the detail of daily experiences of those living with chronic illness.

Autoethnography, the inclusion of participants as researchers, and various other innovations developed among qualitative researchers are hotly debated. Some argue that autoethnography is literature, not social research. Others point out that there is considerable value in experimenting with a variety of methodologies, analytic procedures, and writing styles in order better to understand social life, and to respond to the epistemological and methodological issues raised by the **postmodernists** (Richardson 1994). Box 3.2 provides a detailed example.

BOX 3.2 Doing health sociology: HIV/AIDS and autoethnography research

In my research on the experience of living with HIV/AIDS in Australia, I have focused on the relationship between religious belief, orientations towards the future, and people's sense of hope or depression (Ezzy 2000b). This study draws on all three types of research described above. It comprises a statistical survey, a qualitative study utilising traditional analytic strategies, and a report that takes a more novel approach by including a poem and some self-reflection.

The survey, involving 914 respondents and conducted in 1997, is a national representative survey of people living with HIV/AIDS in Australia. It includes a number of attitude scales, demographic variables, and questions about clinical indicators. The survey provided a number of important results; here, however, I focus only on the relationship between religious belief, future planning, and health status. Results from the survey show that religious belief is correlated with how people plan for the future. Surprisingly, people with religious

beliefs were more likely to plan for the short term. This seems a strange outcome, given that you might expect religious belief to be associated with hope and therefore with greater confidence about the future. Further analysis demonstrates that this holds irrespective of disease progression. That is to say, it could be argued that as people become more ill they are more likely to plan both for the short term and become religious. The survey data demonstrate that this is not the case (Ezzy 2000b). The data pose an interesting problem: why is it that people with HIV/AIDS tend to develop a religious orientation and plan for the short term?

In the qualitative part of the study I demonstrate that there are three types of responses to HIV/AIDS that revolve around different meanings of life, death, and the future (Ezzy 2000b). These types of response are linked to different stories about the future, and to different religious orientations. One story is of confidence in a long future that is typically secular, relying on the success of medical science for its optimism. A second story is of despair, anticipating a short life and an early death that is also secular. The third type of story is more complex. It is hopeful, but involves 'living with a philosophy of the present', in which the short term is celebrated. It is this narrative that is typically religious. Only qualitative research can identify the way that stories are constructed, and how these stories shape the way that people respond to illness. In a culture that often devalues the spiritual and religious dimensions of life, this study underlines the importance of spirituality, and particularly non-traditional spirituality, in helping people living with HIV/AIDS to come to terms with their illness.

Finally, in a subsequent paper I wrote a poem about confronting death (Ezzy 2002). One of the most confronting aspects of interviewing people living with HIV/AIDS was that I, as the interviewer, had to come to terms with my own sense of mortality. Poetry expresses some of the emotional, symbolic, and spiritual dimensions of experience that are often difficult to put into more traditional prose. While I do not advocate that sociologists should write only poetry, there is considerable value in exploring alternative ways of communicating the experiences of health and illness that we study, even if only as a small part of an overall research project.

Conclusion

Despite some authors' claims and assumptions to the contrary, no research methodology is objective or inherently superior to another. Each type of research method reflects particular philosophical, political, and theoretical interests that can influence the collection of data and their interpretation. This means that the privileging of biomedical research methods tends to benefit the political interests of those involved in biomedical professions and industries. This chapter advocates a more balanced approach and highlights the contributions of epidemiology, and traditional and innovative qualitative methodologies, to health research.

Summary of main points

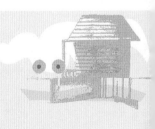

» Health research includes a number of different methodologies. Each methodology has its place and provides important and useful information about different aspects of contemporary experiences of health and illness.
» Some methodologies, such as RCTs, are considered more important than others and, as a consequence, our contemporary understandings of health tend to emphasise biomedical and individualistic responses to health.

Douglas Ezzy

» In contrast, epidemiological and qualitative methodologies informed by socio-logical theory recommend health policy responses that are more focused on social, cultural, and public health factors.

» No research methodology is objective. Each reflects particular political and theoretical interests.

» This chapter advocates a more balanced approach that values the contributions of epidemiology, and traditional and innovative qualitative methodologies, along-side the contributions of biomedical research.

Sociological reflection: researching HIV/AIDS

Why do people become infected with HIV/AIDS? This question can be answered in very different ways, depending on whether you adopt a medical, epidemiological, or a sociological framework. Can you suggest some answers from within these three different frameworks? Further, the framework adopted will shape the research methods funded to examine the epidemic. Can you describe some specific research projects that might be adopted by researchers from within the three different frameworks? What are some of the social and cultural factors that have shaped the development of the HIV/AIDS epidemic in Australia and other countries around the world and how might they be studied?

Discussion questions

1 What are the implications for public health of the privileging of randomised control trials?

2 What is evidence-based medicine (EBM)? What are some of the limitations of EBM?

3 Identify one health issue that can be addressed by epidemiological research and one that cannot.

4 What distinctive contribution do qualitative methods make to health research?

5 Why is qualitative research often ignored or undervalued in health research?

6 Why is it important to have alternative ways of studying, interpreting, and reporting research findings?

Further investigation

1 Find a recent journal article that reports a randomised control trial for the treatment of HIV/AIDS or tuberculosis. Drawing on sociological or public health

research that examines the same disease, provide a critical commentary on the first article, focusing on the role of social and economic factors that shape the distribution of the disease.

2   Why is it important to study meanings and culture in order to understand health in contemporary society? Draw on at least three published qualitative studies of a health issue to illustrate your argument.

Further reading

Alasuutari, P. 1995, *Researching Culture: Qualitative Method and Cultural Studies*, Sage, London.

Daly, J., Kellehear, A. & Glicksman, M. 1997, *The Public Health Researcher*, Oxford University Press, Melbourne.

Denzin, N. 1997, *Interpretive Ethnography*, Sage, London.

Ezzy, D. 2001, *Qualitative Analysis*, Allen & Unwin, Sydney.

Grbich, C. 1999, *Qualitative Research in Health: An Introduction*, Allen & Unwin, Sydney.

Rice, P. & Ezzy, D. 2005, *Qualitative Research Methods*, 2nd edition, Oxford University Press, Melbourne.

Walter, M. (ed.) 2006, *Social Research Methods: An Australian Perspective*, Oxford University Press, Melbourne.

Web resources

Resources for Methods in Evaluation and Social Research: <http://gsociology.icaap.org/methods>

SocioSite—Research Methodology and Statistics Section: <http://www.sociosite.net/topics/research.php>

Social Research Methods: <http://www.socialresearchmethods.net/>

Online case study • • •
Visit the Second Opinion website to access relevant case studies.

References

Adam, B. & Sears, A. 1996, *Experiencing HIV: Personal, Family and Work Relationships*, Columbia University Press, New York.

Alasuutari, P. 1995, *Researching Culture: Qualitative Method and Cultural Studies*, Sage, London.

Blazer, D. 2005, *The Age of Melancholy: 'Major Depression' and its Social Origins*, Routledge, New York.

Boston, P. 1999, 'Culturally Responsive Cancer Care in a Cost-constrained Work-Classification System: A Qualitative Study of Palliative Care Nurses.' *Journal of Cancer Education*, vol. 14, no. 3, pp. 148–53.

Charmaz, K. 1994, 'Identity Dilemmas of Chronically Ill Men', *The Sociological Quarterly*, vol. 35, pp. 269–88.

Daly, J., Kellehear, A. & Glicksman, M. 1997, *The Public Health Researcher*, Oxford University Press, Melbourne.

Denzin, N. 1997, *Interpretive Ethnography*, Sage, London.

Ellis, C. 1995, *Final Negotiations: A Story of Love, Loss, and Chronic Illness*, Temple University Press, Philadelphia.

Ellis, C. 1998, 'Exploring Loss through Autoethnographic Inquiry', in J. Harvey (ed.), *Perspectives on Loss: A Sourcebook*, Mazel, Brunner, pp. 49–62.

Estroff, S. 1995, 'Whose Story is it Anyway? Authority, Voice, and Responsibility in Narratives of Chronic Illness', in S. Toombs, D. Barnard & R. Carson (eds), *Chronic Illness: From Experience to Policy*, Indiana University Press, Bloomington.

Ezzy, D. 2000a, 'Fate and Agency in Job Loss Narratives', *Qualitative Sociology*, vol. 23, no. 1, pp. 121–34.

Ezzy, D. 2000b, 'Illness Narratives: Time, Hope and HIV', *Social Science & Medicine*, vol. 50, pp. 605–17.

Ezzy, D. 2001, *Qualitative Analysis*, Allen & Unwin, Sydney.

Ezzy, D. 2002, 'Finding Life through Facing Death', in B. Rumbold (ed.), *Spirituality and Palliative Care*, Oxford University Press, Melbourne.

Green, J. 1998, 'Commentary: Grounded Theory and the Constant Comparative Method', *British Medical Journal*, vol. 316, no. 7137, pp. 1064–5.

Hetzel, B. 1995, 'From Papua New Guinea to the United Nations', *Australian Journal of Public Health*, vol. 19, pp. 231–34.

Holstein, J. & Gubrium, J. 1995, *The Active Interview*, Sage, Beverly Hills, CA.

Kavanagh, A. & Broom, D. 1997, 'Women's Understanding of Abnormal Cervical Smear Test Results: A Qualitative Interview Study', *British Medical Journal*, vol. 314, pp. 1388–92.

Kellehear, A. 1993, *The Unobtrusive Researcher*, Allen & Unwin, Sydney.

Kirsch I., Deacon B., Huedo-Medina T., Scoboria A., Moore T. 2008, 'Initial Severity and Antidepressant Benefits: A Meta-analysis of Data Submitted to the Food and Drug Administration', *Public Library of Science Medicine*, vol. 5, no. 2, e45.

Lincoln, Y. 1995, 'Emerging Criteria for Quality in Qualitative and Interpretive Research', *Qualitative Inquiry*, vol. 1, pp. 275–89.

National Health Strategy 1992, *Enough to Make You Sick: How Income and Environment Affect Health*, AGPS, Canberra.

Orona, C. 1990, 'Temporality and Identity Loss due to Alzheimer's Disease', *Social Science & Medicine*, vol. 30, no. 11, pp. 1247–56.

Reid, R., Maag, J. & Vasa, S. 1993, 'Attention Deficit Hyperactivity Disorder as a Disability Category: A Critique', *Exceptional Children*, vol. 60, pp. 198–215.

Rice, P. L. & Ezzy, D. 1999, *Qualitative Research Methods: A Health Focus*, Oxford University Press, Melbourne.

Richards, E. 1988, 'The Politics of Therapeutic Evaluation: The Vitamin C and Cancer Controversy', *Social Studies of Science*, vol. 18, pp. 653–701.

Richardson, L. 1994, 'Writing: A Method of Inquiry', in N. Denzin & Y. Lincoln (eds), *Handbook of Qualitative Research*, Sage, Thousand Oaks, CA.

Riessman, C. 1993, *Narrative Analysis*, Sage, Newbury Park, CA.

Sackett, D. 1981, 'How to Read Clinical Journals, V: To Distinguish Useful from Useless or Even Harmful Therapy', *Journal of the Canadian Medical Association*, vol. 124, pp. 1156–62.

Strauss, A. & Corbin, J. 1990, *Basics of Qualitative Research*, Sage, London.

World Health Organization 2008, *Depression*. Available online: <http://www.who.int/mental_health/management/depression/definition/en/>,

White, K. & Willis, E. 1998, 'Evidence-Based Medicine and the Sociology of Medical Knowledge', paper presented at the Annual National Conference of the Australian Sociological Association, Brisbane.

The Social Production and Distribution of Health and Illness

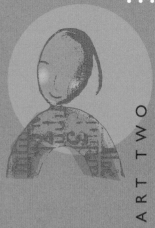

The chapters in Part 2 concern the first dimension of the social model of health introduced in Chapter 1: the social production and distribution of health. It is generally assumed that health and illness are simply undisputed facts, that medicine is best equipped to deal with health problems, and that illness is a matter of bad luck, fate, or individual responsibility. Health sociology debunks the myth that illnesses are solely the fault or responsibility of the individual. While health problems are experienced by individuals, they also have wider social determinants.

The chapters in this part address these issues by examining the evidence and explanations of health inequalities. The fact that there are significant social patterns in the distribution of health and illness, in which some groups of people suffer much higher rates of illness and premature death than others, implies not only that health inequalities have social origins, but also that the removal of such inequalities requires social action and social reform.

Part 2 is divided into seven chapters:

All animals are equal but some animals are more equal than others.

GEORGE ORWELL 1945, *Animal Farm*, p. 114

CHAPTER 4

Global Public Health

ALEX
BROOM
and
JOHN
GERMOV

Overview

- What are the major health problems experienced by people in the poorest countries?
- Why do global health inequalities persist despite the availability of effective interventions?
- What can be done to address global health inequality?

LIVE 8: THE BEGINNING OF AN END TO WORLD HUNGER AND POVERTY?

On 2 July 2005 a series of rock concerts were held across the world in the cities of London, Edinburgh, Philadelphia, Berlin, Paris, Rome, Moscow, Johannesburg, and Barrie (near Toronto). During the concert, actor and singer Will Smith led the combined audiences of the concerts to click their fingers simultaneously to represent the death of a child occurring every 3 seconds due to poverty. In Edinburgh, an estimated 225,000 people participated in a protest march and attended the concert. An estimated three billion people watched the telecast. The concerts were organised by Bob Geldof and marked the 20th anniversary of the dual Live Aid concerts held in London and Philadelphia that raised over US$200 million in 1985.

While Live Aid helped to raise global awareness of the African famine and provided short-term relief to millions, 20 years later the same problems continue to plague Africa—poverty, hunger, and preventable disease.

The 2005 LIVE 8 concerts did not aim to raise money in the form of charitable donations from the public; instead, they mobilised public pressure on the leaders of the G8 nations, who were to meet at Gleneagles in Scotland during 6–9 July. The G8 represents some of the world's wealthiest and most powerful countries and consists of the USA, Canada, the United Kingdom, France, Germany, Italy, Japan, and Russia. The concerts were part of a week of social activism that culminated in the LIVE 8 organisers

...»

presenting the G8 leaders with a 'LIVE 8 List' of names of people across the globe who signed their support (via the LIVE 8 website) for the 'Make Poverty History' campaign. Names from the list were randomly displayed on large screens during the concerts.

The LIVE 8 social protest held in 2005 was recognition that charity could only be a bandaid to addressing global poverty and that permanent structural changes in global affairs were required to solve the problem. The organisers called on the G8 nations to cancel all 'third world' debt, to double aid, and to implement policies to enable fair trade between developed and developing countries. On 7 July, the G8 leaders announced they would cancel the debt of 18 African nations and increase African aid to US$25 billion by 2010. While this was a significant achievement, the deal affected only half of the countries afflicted by debt and international trade rules were not greatly addressed. Furthermore, actual debt relief and increased funding has proved far slower to materialise than pledged in 2005.

Introduction

> There are only two families in the world, as my grandmother used to say: the haves and the have-nots.
>
> Sancho Panza in *Don Quixote de la Mancha*, Miguel de Cervantes (1605)

This chapter explores the social patterning of health and illness at a global level. The most severe health inequalities that exist today exist between countries not within them, and so much so, that your chances of illness, disability, and premature death vary greatly depending upon your country of residence. In developed countries, average life expectancy at birth is around 80 years compared to 45 years in sub-Saharan Africa (UNDP 2005). Infectious diseases that are treatable and preventable plague the poorest nations, but not the wealthiest ones. Such different **life chances** are avoidable and inequitable. As the World Health Organization's (WHO) Commission on the Social Determinants of Health (CSDH 2008, p. 1) pointedly states, the health inequalities between countries persist due to the:

> unequal distribution of power, income, goods, and services, globally and nationally, the consequent unfairness in the immediate, visible circumstances of people's lives—their access to health care, schools, and education, their conditions of work and leisure, their homes, communities, towns, or cities ... This unequal distribution of health-damaging experiences is not in any sense a 'natural' phenomenon but is the result of a toxic combination of poor social policies and programmes, unfair economic arrangements, and bad politics.

While the delivery of health care is important, solutions to global and national health inequalities lie with interventions that address the **social determinants of health**.

life chances
Derived from Max Weber, the term refers to people's opportunity to realise their lifestyle choices, which are often assumed to differ according to their social class.

social determinants of health
The economic, social, and cultural factors that directly and indirectly influence individual and population health.

In this chapter we review the extent of global health inequality, examine the major reasons for the perpetuation of such inequality, and explore some concrete examples of health interventions that are making a difference. Furthermore, we examine grassroots experiences of health in poor countries and the interplay of modern forms of medicine and traditional, indigenous health care practices.

Global health inequality

In thinking about inequalities between countries it is useful, albeit sometimes problematic, to group countries with similar living standards together. Traditionally, the world has been divided into three distinct socio-economic groups: first world countries (Australia, USA, UK, Japan, and others), second world (Russian Federation and former Eastern bloc countries), and the third world (poor countries in Asia, Africa, the Middle East and South America). The United Nations (UN) prefers the terms developed and developing countries; the World Bank uses the terminology of high and low-income countries; and the WHO uses a range of regional categories. Each is politically loaded in one way or another and as sociologists we need to be aware of the limitations of such categorical distinctions. For our purposes we will use the terms (economically) richer and poorer countries, following Robert Beaglehole and Ruth Bonita (2004), as this most clearly indicates the inequality (and often the relationship) between countries of the world. In utilising these categories we are referring to economics—not culture or history—indeed, some of the most 'rich' nations in these terms are the poorest economically.

The extent of global health inequality, particularly between rich and poor nations, has long been recognised. As Box 4.1 shows, declarations, goals, and plans of action have been produced by the UN over many years. Despite these plans and some progress, the extent of global health inequality remains unacceptably high. Most poor countries are yet to pass through the 'epidemiological transition' (Omran 1971), which refers to the changed pattern of disease in a country away from infectious disease to chronic, non-communicable, and lifestyle-related diseases (e.g. stroke, heart disease, cancer). Most infectious diseases are treatable and preventable, particularly through immunisation and improved living conditions.

BOX 4.1   Global health strategies: we have a plan...

The World Health Organization (WHO) was founded in 1948 following the endorsement of its constitution 2 years earlier, which included the famous holistic definition of health as 'a state of complete physical, mental and social well-being and not merely the absence of

...»

Alex Broom and John Germov

disease or infirmity' (WHO 1946). In 1978, the Alma-Ata Declaration called for an end to health inequality in and between countries and posited the goal of 'health for all the people of the world by the year 2000' (WHO 1978). This was followed by the Ottawa Charter for Health Promotion (WHO 1986), which reaffirmed the goal of 'health for all' by outlining a range of key strategies. In 1996, world leaders agreed to the World Food Summit Plan of Action, which outlined plans to meet a target of halving the number of undernourished people in the world by 2015. Further goals and targets to reduce poverty and inequality by 2015 were agreed upon in the United Nations Millennium Declaration (2000; see: http://www.un.org/millennium), which established the Millennium Development Goals. Most recently, the WHO's Commission on the Social Determinants of Health (CSDH 2008, p. 2) reaffirmed this commitment through three overarching recommendations to:

1   Improve daily living conditions
2   Tackle the inequitable distribution of power, money, and resources
3   Measure and understand the problem and assess the impact of action.

While such declarations, reports, goals, and strategies indicate a clear global awareness of the problem and what needs to be done, only small progress has been made, and much of this has stagnated or slowed in recent years.

Life expectancy

Figure 4.1 illustrates the changes in life expectancy between 1980–2003 for a number of countries and regions. While there has been a general improvement in life expectancy for many poor countries and regions, a significant gap between richer and poorer countries remains.

Amid some progress, it is worth noting that average life expectancy has worsened over recent decades in sub-Saharan Africa (mostly due to HIV/AIDS and conflict) and in the former socialist states of Eastern Europe (UNDP 2005). In the last 2 decades there have been many civil and between-country conflicts that have seen horrifying numbers of people killed. Conflicts in Kosovo, Rwanda, Afghanistan, Iraq, the Democratic Republic of the Congo, and the Darfur region of Sudan have resulted in genocide and millions of deaths, which have decimated communities and are clearly reflected in average life expectancy figures.

Life expectancy in the Russian Federation has declined markedly from 70 years in the mid-1980s to around 59 years for men; though the figure for women remains around 72 years. Much of this decline is explained by the social and economic restructuring that occurred in the wake of the collapse of the Soviet Union. This led to high rates of male unemployment and a reduction in expenditure on health and welfare services. Sub-Saharan Africa remains the most troubling region in terms of mortality and morbidity rates, with life expectancy approximating that of 1840 England. Since 1990, average life expectancy has declined to around 46 years (UNDP 2005). In addition to deaths from violent conflicts, the main cause of worsening life expectancy has been the spread of HIV/AIDS. In 2004, it was estimated that around 3 million Africans had died of AIDS, with 25 million of 38 million people infected with HIV residing in Africa.

Much of the increase in life expectancy noted in Figure 4.1 is due to improved infant and under-five child mortality rates (see Figure 4.2); there were 2 million fewer deaths in 2003 than in 1990. That said, child deaths for 2002 still occurred at a rate of one death every 3 seconds (UNDP 2005). In addition to malnutrition, many child deaths are from preventable diseases, such as measles, diphtheria, whooping cough, and tetanus—all of which can be addressed through immunisation (UNDP 2005).

Figure 4.1 Life expectancy improvements and disparities, 1980–2003

Figure 4.2 Under-five mortality rate (per 1000 live births), 1980–2003

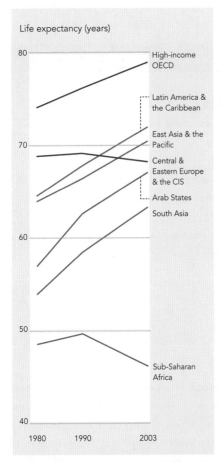

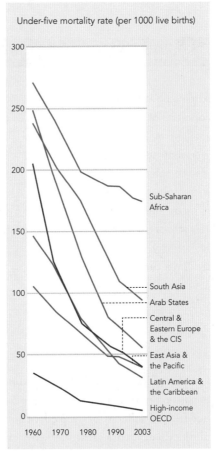

Source: UNDP 2005, p. 19

Source: UNDP 2005, p. 19

Alex Broom and John Germov

Global hunger

In 1996 at the World Food Summit (WFS), most governments agreed to the 2015 goal of halving the number of people in hunger from the 1990 level. This goal was reaffirmed by the Millennium Development Goals (MDGs) agreed to in 2000 (see Box 4.2), which aim to halve the proportion of undernourished people in the world. Very little progress has been made. The Food and Agriculture Organization of the United Nations (FAO 2006) estimates that during 2001–03, there were around 854 million people who were undernourished and faced life in a regular state of **food insecurity**—820 million in developing countries, 25 million in 'transition countries' (e.g. Balkan states and former Eastern Bloc nations), and 9 million in industrialised countries (see Figure 4.3). Progress has been negligible, with a small reduction in the proportion of undernourished people from 20 to 17 per cent occurring between 1990–92 and 2001–03. As Figure 4.4 shows, trends in the proportion of people who are undernourished vary by region, with improvements in some regions cancelled out by worsening conditions in other regions.

food security/ insecurity
Food security refers to the availability of affordable, nutritious, and culturally acceptable food. Food insecurity is a state of regular hunger and fear of starvation.

BOX 4.2   UN Millennium Development Goals by 2015

1   Eradicate extreme poverty and hunger: halve the proportion of people living on US$1/day and halve malnutrition.

2   Achieve universal primary education: ensure all children can complete primary school.

3   Promote gender equality and empower women: achieve gender equity in primary and secondary school completion.

4   Reduce child mortality: cut the under-five death rate by 75 per cent.

5   Improve maternal health: cut maternal mortality by 75 per cent.

6   Combat HIV/AIDS, malaria and other diseases: halt and reverse the proportion suffering these diseases.

7   Ensure environmental sustainability: cut by 50 per cent the proportion of people without access to safe drinking water and sanitation.

8   Develop a global partnership for development: reform aid and trade.

Source: United Nations 2008

It is widely accepted that the world produces enough food to feed the total population more than adequately (see Lappé et al. 1998; Lappé 2008). Despite this, hundreds of millions of people lack sufficient access to nutritious food, leading to nutritional deficiencies that affect physical and mental development, disease resistance, and life expectancy. Common examples are iodine and iron deficiencies, beriberi (lack of B vitamins), scurvy (lack of vitamin C), pellagra (lack of niacin), and rickets (lack

Figure 4.3 Undernourished people (millions) in the world, 2001–03

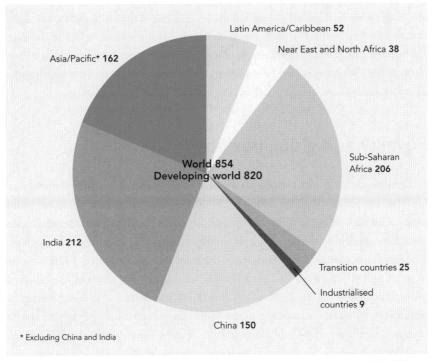

Source: FAO 2006, p.8

Figure 4.4 Changes in proportion of undernourished people, 1990–92 to 2001–03

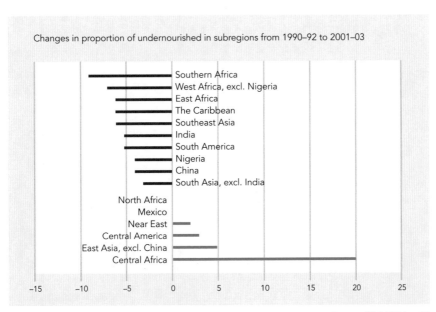

Source: FAO 2006, p.10

Alex Broom and John Germov

of vitamin D)—to name a few (Whit 2004). Amartya Sen (1990) identifies two forms of hunger: famine (caused by war and natural disasters) and the mostly hidden and less readily addressed 'endemic deprivation'. Sen was one of the earliest writers to argue that hunger persists due to insufficient wages or land to grow food, or lack of access to public programs that subsidise the cost of food and guarantee access to food as a basic human right. While there have been improvements in some regions of the world, as the above figures indicate, food insecurity persists to an unnecessary extent.

Poverty and globalisation

It is estimated that approximately 40 per cent of the world's population survives on US$2 or less per day (CSDH 2008, p. 21). As Figure 4.5 indicates, there are major regional differences in the number of people living on US$2/day, and there has been some improvement in the percentage of people living on this amount in most regions. The benefits of **globalisation** have clearly not been evenly distributed. India is a case in point as it is often cited as a globalisation success story in terms of its economic growth, primarily due to the development of its information and communication technology industries. According to the World Bank, India has the twelfth largest economy in the world (World Bank 2008). Yet, the benefits of economic growth have not been widely distributed to its population; under-five child death affects one child in eleven, and only 42 per cent of children are immunised (UNDP 2005).

globalisation
Political, social, economic, and cultural developments—such as the spread of multinational companies, information technology, and the role of international agencies—that result in people's lives being increasingly influenced by global, rather than national or local, factors.

Figure 4.5 Regional variation in the percentage of people in work living on US$2 per day or less

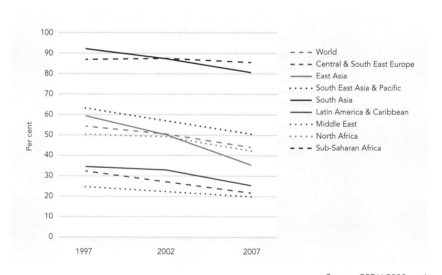

Source: CSDH 2008, p. 6

In 1980, the richest countries of the world, representing only 10 per cent of the global population, had a combined national income that was 60 times greater than the poorest countries; by 2005 the income gap had increased so that it was 122 times greater (CDSC 2008, p. 37). Figure 4.6 shows the extent of the unequal distribution of global income, depicted as a champagne glass, in which the richest 20 per cent of the global population (the wide top of the glass) own around 75 per cent of the world's income, while the bottom 40 per cent have around 5 per cent, and the poorest 20 per cent have only 1.5 per cent of global income. The bottom 40 per cent, approximately 2 billion people, represent those who are surviving on US$2 a day or less (UNDP 2005).

Figure 4.6 The champagne glass effect: the unequal distribution of world income

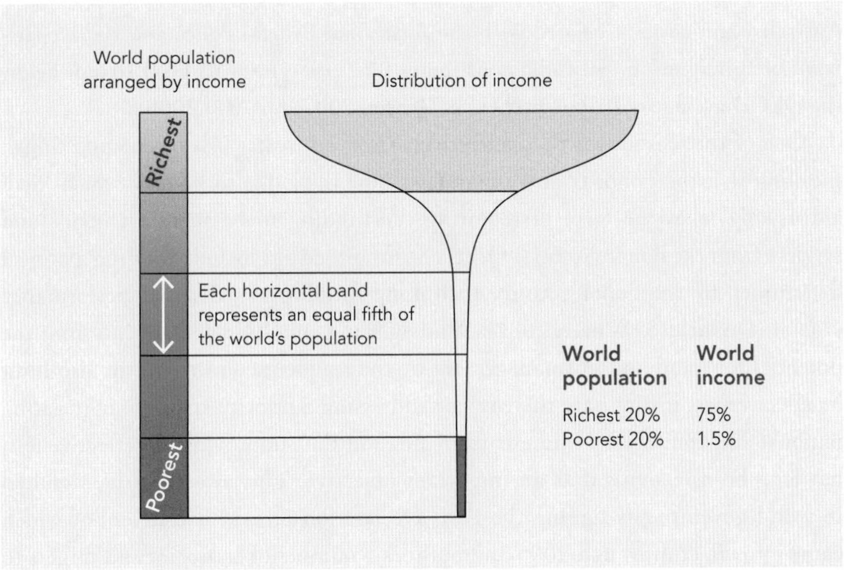

Source: Adapted from UNDP 2005

The politics of 'aid'

Let us remember that the main purpose of American aid is not to help other nations, but to help ourselves.

US President Richard Nixon (1968)

Aid, or official development assistance (ODA), is a contentious issue with many critics highlighting that the amount of aid provided is inadequate, but more importantly, that it is mostly ineffective and primarily used to benefit the national interest of the donor country. In 2004, global aid was estimated at around US$78 billion. While this is a significant figure, it should be treated with caution. Most countries are not meeting the preferred aid quantity commitment of 0.7 of gross national income (GNI), a target set in the 1990s and reaffirmed by the MDGs for 2015. The proportion of aid fell or stagnated throughout the 1990s so that for sub-Saharan Africa, aid fell from $24 per head in 1990 to $12 per head in 1999, but by 2003 had recovered to just under the 1990 level (UNDP 2005).

The USA is the largest aid donor in monetary terms, but its contribution represents only 0.16 per cent of its GNI, while other countries are proportionally contributing more. For example, Sweden, Norway, and Denmark have met the UN target of 0.7 per cent of GNI for many years (UNDP 2005). Australia provided AUD$3.7 billion of aid in 2008–09, though at least 1 billion of this was dedicated to cancelling Iraqi debt, university scholarships for foreign students studying in Australia, and costs associated with the Australian Federal Police and the Department of Immigration. Australia contributes 0.32 per cent of its GNI to aid, below the OECD average of 0.46 (Duxfield & Wheen 2007; AusAID 2008).

One of the reasons for the ineffectiveness of aid is that it is often conditional, meaning that the donor country mandates how the aid is to be used. Such 'tied' aid usually takes the form of requiring the funding to be spent on goods and services from the donor country. Others forms of tied aid include funding a project determined by the donor country or linking funding to particular performance criteria (Duxfield & Wheen 2007). While placing conditions on aid can limit the potential for fraud and mismanagement by the recipient country, it can also limit its effectiveness if funds are thereby not addressing a priority area. Disaggregating national and commercial interests from aid, and thus improving aid effectiveness, has long been recognised as an important objective. This awareness has resulted in world governments signing the Paris Declaration on Aid Effectiveness, which came into effect in March 2005 and outlines a number of strategies and targets to improve the quality and amount of aid provided. It is too early to determine if the Declaration is having a positive impact.

Examining rates of mortality and morbidity, malnutrition, and poverty is clearly critical for understanding and solving global health inequalities. Furthermore, access to biomedical expertise, medical technologies, and ongoing health care funding is vital if we are to improve the health and well-being of populations in poorer countries. Importantly, there are other factors that must be explored in order to shape our understanding of health and health care in such countries; these are culture, religion, and identity. Health is not just a matter of providing the 'best treatment'; it is also about cultural beliefs and cultural heritage. As such, for the remainder of this chapter we will focus on the roles of culture, identity, and history in shaping support for, and use of, different forms of medicine in poorer countries.

Medical pluralism and traditional practices

Unlike in the Australian context, in many poorer countries **biomedicine** is not the primary source of healthcare (WHO 2001). In fact, for many developing countries, traditional health practices are the status quo and biomedical treatments are new and even 'foreign' in cultural terms (Tovey et al. 2007). This is particularly the case in rural and remote areas of Asia and Africa where there may be no doctors or nurses within a few days' walk. As such, billions of people around the world rely, at least to some level, on traditional health practices including things like traditional Chinese medicine (TCM) and ayurveda (an Indian traditional medicine) (WHO 2001, 2005a). In India and China, many people would view practitioners of TCM or ayurveda in the same way as we view our local general practitioners; as the providers of general health care to the masses.

A key question that always emerges for sociologists is what we actually mean when we use certain words. 'Traditional' is a particularly good example as it is often used to describe biomedicine (i.e. the 'traditional' versus 'alternative' medicine) but yet it is also used to describe practices like TCM or ayurveda. In this chapter when we use the term traditional medicine (TM), we are referring to local knowledge, belief systems, and therapeutic practices that are generally used in poorer countries for health-related purposes (Tovey et al. 2007). Unlike, say, **complementary and alternative medicine (CAM)** in Western contexts (see Chapter 21), traditional medicines have often been the dominant means of treatment for health problems for centuries (e.g. traditional Chinese medicine in Chinese society), and in some cases, they continue to dominate health care beliefs and practices. Traditional medicine is thus characterised more by longevity, cultural specificity, religiosity, and often, but not always, by having indigenous roots (WHO 2001).

In recent times, the WHO has been promoting traditional health practices as one means of meeting the huge unmet health needs, as illustrated in the previous sections, of the populations in developing countries (WHO 2001, 2005a). TMs are viewed by many policy makers as culturally appropriate, relatively cheap (as compared to many biomedical treatments), and already available. As such, the WHO produced a Global Atlas of Traditional, Complementary and Alternative Medicine (TCAM) (WHO 2005a). This has in some ways set the agenda in terms of health policy to support the development of indigenous practices and biomedical facilities concurrently; however, although promising in theory, the idea of promoting therapeutic pluralism and integrating the traditional with modern, biomedical treatments is not as simple at a grassroots level (Tovey et al. 2007). As illustrated in the following sections, access to, and use of, health practices in pluralistic settings is often shaped by different forms of structural inequalities, often reinforcing the divides (gender, caste, religion etc.) already in place (Pal &

biomedicine/ biomedical model
The conventional approach to medicine in Western societies, based on the diagnosis and explanation of illness as a malfunction of the body's biological mechanisms. This approach underpins most health professions and health services, which focus on treating individuals, and generally ignores the social origins of illness and its prevention.

complementary and alternative medicine (CAM)
A broad term to describe both alternative medical practitioners and practices that may stand in opposition to orthodox medicine and also those who may collaborate with, and thus complement, orthodox practice (also referred to as integrative medicine).

Alex Broom and John Germov

Mittal 2004). As such, medicine, in its many forms, has come to reflect wider social forces and social problems which remain important for sociologists to study and critique.

Modernity, colonialism, and identity politics

The character of, and dynamics between, health practices in most developing contexts are embedded in particular historical events and socio-political processes. Countries in Asia, Africa, and South America, for example, were significantly influenced by **colonial** (and now post-colonial) rule (Arnold 2000), with health and illness closely linked to patterns of political struggle and resistance (Ecks 2004; Khan 2006; Reddy 2006; Sujatha 2007). Many forms of medicine were introduced by colonial rulers (both biomedical and alternative, e.g. homeopathy) and fundamentally shaped landscapes of therapeutic practice in individual nations (Arnold 2000). The forces of 'modernisation', Westernisation, and globalisation have each played important roles in shaping health and medicine in the developing world (Janes 1999). However, post-colonial struggle, nationalism, and the reinvention (or rediscovery) of tradition have played equally important roles (Ecks 2004). For example, for nations like India and China, traditional health care practices like Ayurveda, Unani and TCM remain key to their national heritage and identity politics. Medicine, in its many forms, has become an important expression of political and cultural relations both between economically richer and poorer countries and indeed between poorer countries (Khan 2006; Reddy 2006; Tovey et al. 2007). The global environment is complex: this is not simply a matter of 'Western' biomedical dominance but also involves the 'rediscovery' of traditional, indigenous medicine as an expression of post-colonial autonomy (Ecks 2004; Sujatha 2007). As such, while the 'project of **modernity**' (as some may call it) continues to influence the trajectory of health care in these countries (Janes 1999), so too do nostalgic and nationalistic notions of medicine as part of cultural identity and the rediscovery of the traditional as a key element of post-colonial identity.

For many nations **medical pluralism** is the norm, with a mix of potentially competing and even conflicting ideologies and practices around health and illness (Haram 1991; Sujatha 2007). While nationalism and post-colonial identity work sit well in theory, in practice, grassroots tensions often exist between practitioners of different forms of medicine and 'modern' versus 'traditional' health organisations. For example, in their study examining the dynamics between traditional healers (called Hakeems and Pirs) and doctors in Pakistan, Alex Broom and Philip Tovey (2007) found significant ideological conflict and often outright animosity between traditional practitioners and doctors in the context of treating cancer.

colonialism
A process by which one nation imposes itself economically, politically, and socially upon another.

modernity
A view of social life that is founded upon rational thought and a belief that truth and morality exist as objective realities that can be discovered and understood through scientific means.

medical pluralism
A general term that refers to the vast array of healing modalities across the globe, in particular to the increasing popularity of alternative therapies and their coexistence with biomedicine in Westernised societies.

BOX 4.3   Doing health sociology: traditionalism versus 'Westernisation'

Broom and Tovey's (2007) study provides an illustration of the potential conflict and animosity between traditional healers and doctors in Pakistan as shown in the accounts of cancer patients seeking treatment:

> Hakeems think that what they are doing is a justified and right treatment. Their method of treatment is a lengthy one. They often don't let patients visit doctors. (Female, 30 years, breast cancer)

Another respondent:

> Traditional healers say that if you want to be cut into pieces then go to doctors ... they say that doctors will harm you and cut into you and that it is not natural. (Male, 55 years, bladder cancer)

Another respondent:

> [Traditional healers] use very strong words for [doctors]; both traditional healers and doctors don't like each other. [Our healer] says in our community that both [hospital name] and [another hospital's name] kill people. (Female, 35 years, breast cancer)

As shown in the excerpts presented above, there exists significant conflict between healers and doctors in Pakistan, and similar dynamics can be found in other developing countries as 'modern' forms of medicine become an increasingly important part of health care delivery (Tovey et al. 2007). As such, while post-colonial autonomy and nationalistic sentiment may be embodied in the promotion of traditional practices (Arnold 2000; Ecks 2004; Khan 2006), at a grassroots level, there may be significant struggle and ideological conflict between traditional and biomedical practitioners. Furthermore, and as shown below, access to traditional versus modern forms of therapeutic practice can be more about social and economic status than actual preferences for particular therapeutic options.

Religion, caste, and gender: medical pluralism in context

In Western contexts, health care delivery is dominated by biomedical approaches and thus social inequality in relation to health is mostly considered to be about equity in access to general practitioners and hospitals. Furthermore, access is largely mediated by socio-economic status and ethnicity (the two are often intertwined). In the context of developing countries the situation is more complex. While socio-

Alex Broom and John Germov

economic status and ethnicity still play significant roles, geography (rural and remote areas), gender, religion, and caste are also influential. Furthermore, there is a distinction between what types of modalities different groups use. As such, it is not only about limited health services, but a divide between the types of modalities available (i.e. traditional medicines versus biomedical treatments) to different parts of the population. For example, in India, for most rural populations and the urban poor, traditional practitioners of Ayurveda and Unani are the only source of health advice and treatment (WHO 2005b). Use of a traditional practitioner may cost AUD$1 whereas treatment at a public or private hospital in India may cost AUD$2000. In a context where a large proportion of the population earn less than US$2 a day, there is no real choice. With serious illnesses such as cancer, treatment in a hospital may cost several times the annual wage of a reasonably well-off family. As such, families may have to consider whether paying for biomedical treatment is 'worth it' depending on the role or 'value' of the person who is ill (i.e. father, mother, or child). In such contexts, and with the importance of the 'breadwinner', inequality for women in terms of access to biomedical treatments for serious illnesses is a constant concern for policy makers. These kinds of concerns emerged in the study by Broom and Tovey shown in Box 4.4.

BOX 4.4 Doing health sociology: poverty and religiosity

In Broom and Tovey's (2007) research , cancer patients talked about who accesses which treatments in their community and why:

> Most of the people go to doctors; basically it is the matter of money. The wealthy people go to doctors and poor people go to Hakeems. (Male, 12 years, diagnosis unclear)

Another respondent:

> Poverty takes [people] to traditional healers. They ... know well that there are specialist doctors for the particular disease, but they are bound to go for traditional healing. People seek the treatments like Dam Darood, spiritual healing, as people are poor. They prefer self-medication and traditional healing because they don't have access to modern treatment ... If they seek the help of doctors [and the hospital] they have problems with accommodation, food etc. (Male, 37 years, fibrosarcoma)

Another respondent:

> We ... have firm belief in Dam Darood [traditional healing]. Islam gives you a complete code of life. So being an honest Muslim like others, I have a blind faith in Dam Darood. All diseases are caused by God's will, and I think prayer and Dam Darood do matter a lot for healing and [we use them for] any particular disease. (Husband of: Female, 47 years, breast cancer)

A key theme that emerged from this work was medicine as a form of distinction (Bourdieu 1979/1984); that health practices have become embedded in class and caste dynamics and therapeutic modalities (i.e. traditional versus biomedical) intertwined in key structures of social inequality (Tovey & Broom 2007). Poor people within these communities are opting for traditional practices due to the costs of biomedical treatment; a medico-cultural divide exists whereby consumption of certain practices is tied to social status. This is complicated further in contexts in which practices are intertwined with religious/spiritual beliefs and this is the case for many traditional medicines. For example, Hindus and Muslims use different forms of traditional medicine in India and Pakistan (i.e. Ayurveda and Unani respectively). Furthermore, healers may concurrently be religious mentors and thus the rejection of a treatment they may offer can result in community disapproval and even explicit anger from community healers (see Tovey et al. 2007). Using a practice can therefore be just as much about faith and illustrating your commitment to Islam, as for example, purely selecting the most 'effective' (in biomedical terms) treatment. As such, in many poorer countries there remains a certain acceptability of certain traditional practices as religiously based, rather than socio-economically driven. It is increasingly the case that the wealthier cohorts in developing countries use biomedicine and the poorer use traditional medicines. This suggests that WHO's policy of promoting TM may in fact be exacerbating a therapeutic divide between the rich and the poor.

Conclusion

In this chapter we have explored a range of issues facing poorer countries in terms of health and well-being. The most dire inequalities currently facing the world are for most of us 'out of sight and out of mind'. So, too, are major killers in the developing world like malaria, dengue fever, typhoid, and polio, as they have been eradicated in wealthier nations. The statistics, such as those presented in this chapter, make the health problems impacting on poorer countries seem huge, perhaps even insurmountable, but solutions are available for a relatively small cost. We already have the treatments available for many common conditions that cause premature death and thus what is needed is economic support and determination from richer nations. As we have emphasised, it is vital also to remember that it is much more complex than merely facilitating a biomedical, Western intervention. Such colonialist thinking results in fractures between implementing biomedical solutions and localised values and belief systems. While money and biomedical technologies/treatments are urgently needed, there is also a real need for a comprehensive understanding of the interplay of culture, identity, belief, and health. In a contest of globalisation and internationalisation, local belief systems and cultural values remain strong and are

Alex Broom and John Germov

vital to understanding experiences of disease and treatment choices. Without an understanding of cultural and social processes, we will never be able to support the amelioration of health problems in poorer countries successfully.

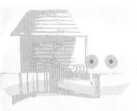

Summary of main points

» The social determinants of health are most significantly evidenced through the inequalities between richer and poorer nations.
» Despite the fact we have the ability to produce enough food to feed everyone on the planet, global hunger continues to plague millions each year due to poverty and a lack of global effort directed at redistributing sufficient resources.
» While aid can make a difference to poorer countries, much of it has limited effectiveness because it is used to serve the national interests of donor countries.
» Medical pluralism, particularly the use of complementary and alternative medicine (CAM) therapies in poorer countries, shows the importance of considering the role of culture, religion, and identity in effective and culturally appropriate health interventions.

Sociological reflection: does social protest make a difference?

What is your reaction to the LIVE 8 campaign? Do such social protests really make a difference in the long term? What are the benefits and limitations of such social activism?

Discussion questions

1 What are some of the major indicators of global health inequality?
2 What are some of the underlying causes of world hunger?
3 Why is aid political?
4 What are the benefits and limits of aid in addressing global health inequality?
5 What is medical pluralism? Give examples in your answer.
6 In what ways can complementary and alternative medicine (CAM) assist in addressing health inequality?

Further investigation

1   Consult the further reading and websites listed below and investigate some of the causes and proposed solutions to global poverty and hunger. Given the abundance of wealth that exists today, why is there a lack of substantial progress to address global health inequality?

2   Examine the evidence on progress (or lack thereof) towards the Millennium Development Goals.

3   Examine the impact of the Paris Declaration on improving the amount and effectiveness of aid.

Further reading

Baum, F. 2007, *The New Public Health*, 3rd edn, Oxford University Press, Melbourne.

Beaglehole, R. & Bonita, R. 2004, *Public Health at the Crossroads*, 2nd edn, Cambridge University Press, Cambridge.

Commission on the Social Determinants of Health (CSDH) 2008, *Closing the Gap in a Generation: Health Equity through Action on the Social Determinants of Health*, Final Report of the Commission on Social Determinants of Health, WHO, Geneva. Available online: <http://www.who.int/social_determinants/final_report/en/>

Lappé, F. M. 2008, 'World Hunger: Its Roots and Remedies', in J. Germov & L. Williams, (eds), *A Sociology of Food and Nutrition: The Social Appetite*, 3rd edn, Oxford University Press, Melbourne, pp. 27–57.

Wilkinson, R. 2005, *The Impact of Inequality: How to Make Sick Societies Healthier*, The New Press, New York.

Web resources

Focus on the Global South: <http://www.focusweb.org>

Food First/Institute for Food and Development Policy: <http://www.foodfirst.org>

Global Call to Action against Poverty: <http://www.whiteband.org/>

Global Health Reporting: <http://globalhealthreporting.org/>

Global Public Health: An International Journal for Research, Policy and Practice: <http://www.informaworld.com/smpp/title-content=t716100712>

International Forum on Globalization: <http://www.ifg.org>

Institute for Global Health: <http://www.globalhealth.vanderbilt.edu/>

Paris Declaration on Aid Effectiveness: <http://www.oecd.org/document/18/0,2340,en_2649_3236398_35401554_1_1_1_1,00.html>

State of Food Insecurity in the World (UN reports): <http://www.fao.org/sof/sofi/index_
en.htm>

UN Human Development Reports: <http://hdr.undp.org/en/reports/>

UN Millennium Development Goals: <http://www.undp.org/mdg/> and <http://www.
un.org/millenniumgoals/>

World Health Organization (WHO): <http://www.who.int/en/>

World Health Reports: <www.who.int/whr/en/>

● ● **Online case study**
Visit the Second Opinion website to access relevant case studies.

Documentaries/films

The Global Banquet: Politics of Food (2000): 56 minutes. A documentary examining the links between globalisation and world hunger. Available online: <http://www.olddog documentaries.com/vid_gb.html>

Life and Debt (2001): 86 minutes. Focusing on Jamaica, this documentary provides a critique of the impact of assistance from the World Bank and the International Monetary Fund (IMF). Available online: <http://www.lifeanddebt.org/>

Rx for Survival: A Global Health Challenge (2005): 336 minutes (6 parts). Narrated by actor Brad Pitt and filmed in over twenty countries, this documentary examines the causes and solutions to global health problems. Available online: <http://www.thefilm connection.org/films/424>

Silent Killer: The Unfinished Campaign against Hunger (2005): 60 minutes. Available online: <http://www.silentkillerfilm.org/>

References

Arnold, D. 2000, *Science, Technology and Medicine in Colonial India*, Cambridge University Press, Cambridge.

AusAID 2008, 'About Australia's Aid Program', *AusAID*. Available online: <http://www. ausaid.gov.au/makediff/default.cfm>

Beaglehole, R. & Bonita, R. 2004, *Public Health at the Crossroads*, 2nd edn, Cambridge University Press, Cambridge.

Bourdieu, P. 1979/1984, *Distinction: A Social Critique of the Judgement of Taste*, Routledge & Kegan Paul, London.

Broom, A. & Tovey, P. 2007, 'Inter-professional Conflict and Strategic Alliance between Traditional Healers and Oncologists in Pakistan', *Asian Journal of Social Science*, vol. 35, no. 4–5, pp. 608–25.

Commission on the Social Determinants of Health (SDH) 2008, *Closing the Gap in a Generation: Health Equity through Action on the Social Determinants of Health*, Final

Report of the Commission on Social Determinants of Health, WHO, Geneva. Available online: <http://www.who.int/social_determinants/final_report/en/>

Duxfield, F. & Wheen, K. 2007, *Fighting Poverty of Fantasy Figures: The Reality of Australian Aid*, AIDWATCH. Available online: <http://www.aidwatch.org.au/index. php?current=24&display=aw01084&display_item=1>

Ecks, S. 2004, 'Bodily Sovereignty as Political Sovereignty: "Self-care" in Kolkata, India', *Anthropology & Medicine*, vol. 11, pp. 75–89.

Food and Agriculture Organization of the United Nations (FAO) 2006, *The State of Food Insecurity in the World 2006*, United Nations, Rome.

Haram, L. 1991, 'Tswana Medicine in Interaction with Biomedicine', *Social Science and Medicine*, vol. 33, no. 2, pp. 167–75.

Janes, C. 1999, 'The Health Transition, Global Modernity and the Crisis of Traditional Medicine: The Tibetan Case', *Social Science & Medicine*, vol. 48, no. 12, pp. 1803–20.

Khan, S. 2006, 'Systems of Medicine and Nationalist Discourse in India: Towards "New Horizons" in Medical Anthropology and History', *Social Science & Medicine*, vol. 62, pp. 2786–97.

Lappé, F. M. 2008, 'World Hunger: Its Roots and Remedies', in J. Germov & L. Williams, (eds), *A Sociology of Food and Nutrition: The Social Appetite*, 3rd edn, Oxford University Press, Melbourne, pp. 27–57.

Lappé, F. M., Collins, J. & Rosset, P. 1998, *World Hunger: Twelve Myths*, 2nd edn, Grove Press, New York.

Omran, A.R. 1971, 'The Epidemiologic Transition: A Theory of the Epidemiology of Population Change', *The Milbank Memorial Fund Quarterly*, vol. 49, no. 4, pp. 509–38.

Pal, S. & Mittal, B. 2004 'Improving Cancer Care in India: Prospects and Challenges', *Asian Pacific Journal of Cancer Prevention*, vol. 5, pp. 226–8.

Reddy, S. 2006, 'Making Heritage Legible: Who Owns Traditional Medical Knowledge?', *International Journal of Cultural Property*, vol. 13, pp. 161–88.

Sen, A. 1990, 'Public Action to Remedy Hunger', *Arturo Tanco Memorial Lecture*, London, 2 August. Available online: <http://www.thp.org/reports/sen/sen890.htm>

Sujatha, V. 2007, 'Pluralism in Indian Medicine: Medical Lore as a Genre of Medical Knowledge', *Contributions to Indian Sociology*, vol. 41, pp. 169–202.

Tovey, P., Chatwin, J. & Broom, A. 2007, *Traditional, Complementary and Alternative Medicine and Cancer Care: An International Analysis of Grassroots Integration*, Routledge, London.

United Nations 2000, *United Nations Millennium Declaration*. Available online: <http:// www.un.org/millennium/>

United Nations 2008, *End Poverty 2015: Make it Happen*, 'UN Millennium Development Goals'. Available online: <http:// www.un.org/millenniumgoals/>

United Nations Development Programme 2005, *Human Development Report 2005. International Cooperation at the Crossroads: Aid, Trade and Security in an Unequal World*, UNDP, New York.

Whit, W. 2004, 'World Hunger' in J. Germov & L. Williams, (eds), *A Sociology of Food and Nutrition: The Social Appetite*, 2nd edn, Oxford University Press, Melbourne.

World Bank 2008, 'GDP 2007', *Quick Reference Tables*. Available online: <http://web.world bank.org/WBSITE/EXTERNAL/DATASTATISTICS/0,,contentMDK:20399244~menuPK:1504474~pagePK:64133150~piPK:64133175~theSitePK:239419,00.html>

World Health Organization 1946, *Constitution of the World Health Organization*, WHO, Geneva.

World Health Organization 1978, *Primary Health Care: Report of the International Conference on Primary Health Care*, Alma-Ata, USSR, 6–12 September, WHO, Geneva.

World Health Organization 1986, *Ottawa Charter for Health Promotion*, First International Conference on Health Promotion: The Move Towards a New Public Health, 17–21 November, Ottawa, Canada, and WHO, Geneva.

World Health Organization 2001, *Traditional Medicine Strategy 2002–2005, WHO*, Geneva.

World Health Organization 2005a, *WHO Global Atlas of Traditional, Complementary and Alternative Medicine*, WHO, Japan.

World Health Organization 2005b, *India, Core Health Indicators*, World Health Statistics, Geneva.

World Health Organization 2008, *World Health Report 2008. Primary Health Care: Now More than Ever*, WHO, Geneva.

CHAPTER 5

The Class Origins of Health Inequality

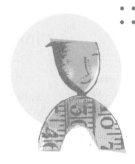

JOHN
GERMOV

Overview

- What is class?
- How can an understanding of class help to explain health inequality?
- What can be done to address class-based health inequality?

CLASS MATTERS

We all have some basic notion of class—we see it every day in the differences between low-priced and expensive cars, takeaway shops and fine-dining restaurants, public and private schools, and overcrowded and exclusive suburbs. In surveys over the years, Australians have regularly reported they believe that classes exist and have no trouble placing themselves into a class—only 5 per cent claim they have no class affiliation (Western & Baxter 2007). Debates over the importance of class focus on the extent to

which it determines your life chances—that is, your chances of social mobility, of gaining an education, and of getting a certain type of job. While most people acknowledge the existence of class, few recognise that health status is one of the clearest indicators of class inequality in Australia. Despite access to free public health services in Australia, working-class people have higher rates of death, illness, and disability as a result of their living and working conditions.

Introducing class

class (or social class)
A position in a system of structured inequality based on the unequal distribution of power, wealth, income, and status. People who share a class position typically share similar life chances.

Popular notions of **class** tend to focus on lifestyle differences, particularly fashion, as a social marker of status. While consumption patterns may indicate class member-ship in a general sense, they shed little light on how class differences are generated in the first place. This chapter discusses the concept of class, provides up-to-date evidence of class-based health inequality, and examines five main explanations of health inequality: artefact; natural/social selection; cultural/behavioural; materialist/ structural; and psychosocial/social capital explanations. The chapter ends with a discussion of a number of ways of tackling health inequality with the aim of achiev-ing equity in health outcomes.

Sociological analyses of class tend to focus on the underlying factors that produce and reproduce class differences. It is important to note that different theoretical per-spectives used by sociologists (as discussed in chapter 2) have resulted in continuing debate over appropriate definitions and theories of class, most of which focus on Erik Olin Wright's neo-Marxist and John Goldthorpe's neo-Weberian class models, but these debates are not addressed here (see Baxter et al. 1991; Goldthorpe 1996; Wright 1997, 2005; Crompton 1998; Crompton et al. 2000). To help clarify the concept of class, we will consider an admittedly simplified three-class model based on a hybrid of Marxist and Weberian perspectives in which class is defined according to three characteristics: ownership and control of scarce economic resources; ownership of marketable skills and qualifications; and wage labour.

The 'upper class' refers to those who own and/or manage economic resources (capital), such as raw materials, technology, and workplaces, and employ others to create profit for them. This group includes many senior executives who may not own a company, but nevertheless have access to the company's profit through share ownership, profit-sharing arrangements, and high incomes. Therefore, they con-trol how work is organised and carried out, including the power to hire and fire. The 'middle class' represents a diverse group of people who possess some form of qualification and skill that allows them to attract higher wages and better working conditions than unskilled workers, such as health professionals and teachers. This group can also include small-business owners and the self-employed. The 'working class' consists of unskilled manual and non-manual (blue and white collar) workers who gain employment solely by selling their labour power. Based on 2003 data from the Australian Survey of Social Attitudes (Western & Baxter 2007) we can construct the following three-class model of Australian society:

- upper class: 15 per cent
- middle class: 47 per cent
- working class: 38 per cent.

All class models have 'grey areas'. For example, whether a plumber is considered working class or middle class will depend on the particular class model used.

While it is relatively easy to divide the population into a class model statistically, it is important to remember that the concept of class is meant to reflect real-life groups of people who share similar living and working conditions. At this point, we need to clarify the difference between the terms 'class' and 'socio-economic status' (SES). These terms are often used interchangeably, but they do not mean the same thing. SES is determined by ranking people usually according to income, education, and occupation levels, and grouping them into corresponding high, medium, and low-SES groups. It is a relatively straightforward process to categorise people into SES groups, and this is why most of the **empirical** evidence of class inequality tends to be based on SES; this is often where the confusion arises between the two terms (see Connell 1977 and 1983 for more discussion of this issue). Measures of SES can only indicate levels of inequality in a society. It is a descriptive classification system and offers little insight in analysing how and why such inequality exists, effectively ignoring such questions by transforming 'the lived reality of class ... to an abstraction for the purpose of statistical treatment' (Connell 1977, p. 33). The 'lived reality' of class refers to people who are class conscious, have class-based values, lifestyles, and identities, and who mobilise politically as a class on certain issues (Connell & Irving 1992). To substitute SES for class ignores the key insight of class analysis—that the unequal distribution of wealth and power is embedded in the **social structure** and thus that class is not simply a label or status easily acquired or discarded.

empirical
Describes observations or research that is based on evidence drawn from experience. It is therefore distinguished from something based only on theoretical knowledge or on some other kind of abstract thinking process.

social structure
The recurring patterns of social interaction through which people are related to each other, such as social institutions and social groups.

Class inequality in Australia

One of the key indicators of class inequality is the distribution of wealth in a country. Figure 5.1 depicts the distribution of household wealth in Australia and shows that the average (mean) in 2005–06 was $563,000, but this figure is skewed by the relatively few high-wealth households. The better indicator of wealth distribution is the median figure (the mid-point at which half the population is either above or below). As shown in Figure 5.1, the median-wealth figure was much lower: $340,000 (ABS 2007).

Figure 5.2 shows the wealth distribution for Australia in 2005–06 by dividing the population into five quintiles (fifths of the population). Quintile 1 represents the top 20 per cent of the population (the wealthiest or most advantaged), and quintile 5 refers to the bottom 20 per cent of the population (the poorest or most disadvantaged). As Figure 5.2 indicates, the top 20 per cent own 61.1 per cent of the nation's wealth, the top 40 per cent own 81.1 per cent, and the top 60 per cent own 93.3 per cent. This means that the bottom 40 per cent account for only 6.7 per cent of all the known wealth in Australia. Such figures indicate that Australia is among the most unequal of countries and challenges the view that we live in a classless society.

John Germov

Figure 5.1 Distribution of household wealth in Australia, 2005–06

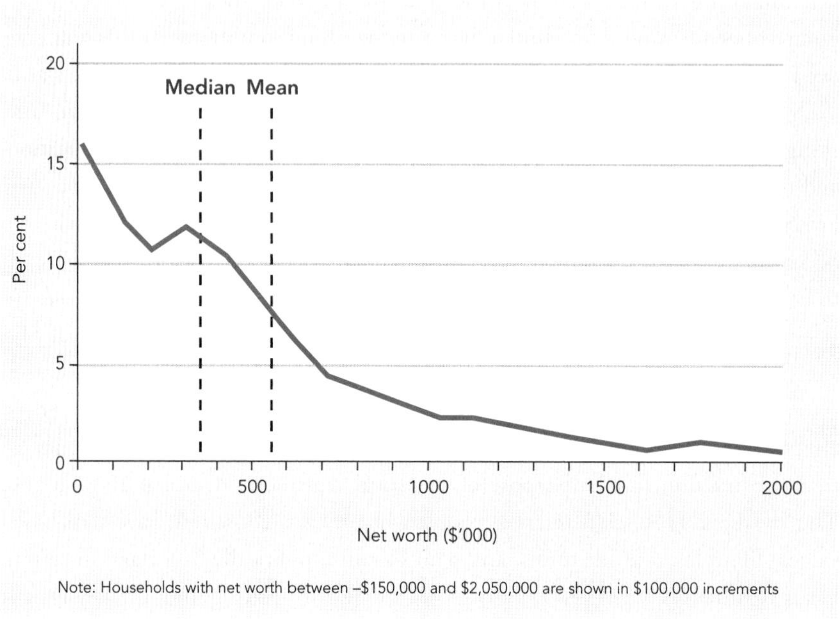

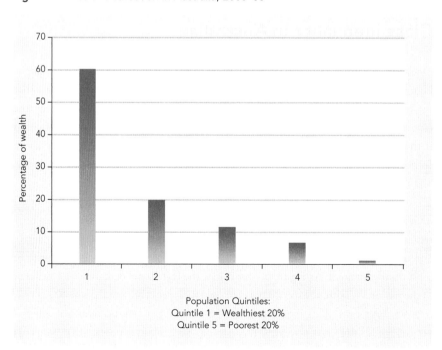

Note: Households with net worth between –$150,000 and $2,050,000 are shown in $100,000 increments

ABS data used with permission from the Australian Bureau of Statistics   *Source*: ABS 2007, p. 5

Figure 5.2 Wealth distribution in Australia, 2005–06

Population Quintiles:
Quintile 1 = Wealthiest 20%
Quintile 5 = Poorest 20%

Source: Adapted from ABS 2007, p. 11

Upper class or ruling class?

Each year, the *Business Review Weekly* (*BRW*) publishes a list of the richest 200 people and families in Australia. The cut-off point for entry to the top 200 has increased markedly over the years, rising from $10 million in 1984, to $45 million in 1995, to $200 million in 2008, indicating how well the rich have been doing in recent years. Between 1984 and 2008, the aggregate wealth of the richest 200 increased from $7.3 billion to $139.6 billion (more than a 19-fold increase); a third of which is accounted for by the top 10 'super rich' as shown in Table 5.1 (*BRW* 2008). It is worth noting that these figures are 'guesstimates', based on the officially declared assets and earnings of the wealthy, and as such are likely to significantly under-report the full extent of wealth. According to the *World Wealth Report* the combined wealth of individuals around the world was US$40.7 trillion in 2007 (Merrill Lynch & Capgemini 2008). The wealth of the super rich is difficult to fathom and the exponential rise in their wealth in the last two decades is historically without parallel.

Table 5.1 The top 10 super rich in Australia, individuals and families, 2008

Individual or family	Estimated wealth ($ billion)
Andrew Forrest	9.4
Frank Lowy	6.3
James Packer	6.1
Richard Pratt	5.5
Gina Rinehart	4.4
Harry Triguboff	3.3
John Gandel	3.2
Kerry Stokes	2.7
Smorgon family	2.4
Shi Zhengrong	2.3

Source: Adapted from BRW 2008

Debates about the upper class concern not only its wealth but also its influence—on whether it acts as a **ruling class**. While few theorists would argue that the upper class rules in a direct way, there is also little dispute that through their companies, the members of the upper class can affect investment, employment, and the stock market. In this way, their economic power provides them with significant political influence. The upper class may not pull the strings directly, but its members share similar interests. For example, they may pressure governments to adopt policies of low taxation and deregulation to aid the pursuit of profit maximisation, which tend to benefit those already well off. That said, there is no natural law of profit and wealth, and as recent history teaches us, social policies and taxation rates can work either to consolidate or redistribute wealth.

ruling class
This is a hotly debated term used to highlight the point that the upper class in society has political power as a result of its economic wealth. The term is often used interchangeably with 'upper class'.

John Germov

'race'
A term without scientific basis that uses skin colour and facial features to describe what are alleged to be biologically distinct groups of humans. Race is actually a social construction used to categorise groups of people and sometimes implies assumed (and unproven) intellectual superiority or inferiority.

ethnicity
Sociologically, the term refers to a shared cultural background, which is a characteristic of all groups in society. As a policy term, it is used to identify migrants who share a culture that is markedly different from that of Anglo-Australians. In practice, it often refers only to migrants from non-English-speaking backgrounds (NESB migrants).

gender/sex
This pair of terms refers to the socially construc-ted categories of feminine and masculine (the cultural identities and values that prescribe how men and women should behave), and the social power relations based on those categor-ies, as distinct from the categories of biological sex (female or male).

individualism/ individualisation
A belief or process supporting the primacy of individual choice, freedom, and self-responsibility.

Intersecting structures of inequality and the death of class

Class has been a central feature of sociological analysis, particularly the role that class plays in shaping individuals' beliefs, behaviour, and access to social rewards such as employment, education, and health (Western 2000). However, some authors argue that 'class is dead' in terms of its influence over individuals' lives and as the basis of the distribution of wealth and power. Others have criticised studies of class for ignoring or marginalising key social groups, such as the disabled, retirees, welfare recipients, the unemployed, and women not in paid work. Instead, it is argued that class has been replaced by social inequalities and power struggles based in **gender**, **'race'**, or **ethnicity**, and new social movements, such as gay rights, grey power, and environmental groups (for more on this debate see Eder 1993; Westergaard 1995; Pakulski & Waters 1996; Crompton 1998; Pakulski 2005; Wright 2005). Ulrich Beck (1992) suggests that a process of **individualisation** has overtaken class as the dominant marker of social distinction, whereby individual identity is now an outcome of lifestyle choice and consumption patterns (admittedly based on the ability to pay). According to Beck (1992, p. 131), tradition and family ties are no longer dominant in a 'post-class' society, so that individuals are free to construct their identity from a variety of lifestyle choices that are increasingly reflective of and 'dependent upon fashions, social policy, economic cycles and markets'. Therefore, class has lost its sub-cultural distinctiveness in the age of consumption as 'forms of perception become private and ahistorical' (Beck 1992, p. 235) and people actively construct their self-identity. The argument here is not that social inequality has decreased, but that class as a major determinant of social groups and individual identity has declined.

Jan Pakulski and Malcolm Waters (1996, p. 10) identify the following four key features of class analysis, arguing that each has diminished in importance in recent times:

1 *Economism*: class structure is an economic phenomenon based on the unequal ownership of productive capital and marketable skills that allows a minority to accumulate wealth.

2 *Groupness*: classes are real social groupings of people; these groupings result from conflict over social and economic rewards.

3 *Behavioural and cultural linkage*: members of a class share 'class consciousness', political preferences, similar interests, and lifestyles.

4 *Transformational capacity*: classes allow for collective action and can transform the social structure; class conflict is the central dynamic that shapes social life.

Given the huge increase in wealth among the rich in recent decades, it may appear curious that some authors are declaring the death of class. One way to accom-modate the insights of the 'death of class' argument is to reinvoke the distinction between objective and subjective notions of class, or, following Karl Marx (1818–83) among others, the difference between a class 'in itself' and a class 'for itself'

(Crompton 1998). A class 'in itself' refers to the objective dimension of class as the basis of social inequality. The unequal distribution of wealth, income, occupation, and education means that any population can be readily categorised into a social hierarchy of distinct classes.

It is one matter to identify an objectively defined class structure, but another issue altogether whether people are aware of their class membership and express characteristics of 'groupness', 'behavioural and cultural linkages', and 'transformational capacities', as noted by Pakulski and Waters above. A class 'for itself' refers to the subjective dimension of the lived reality of class in the form of social groups of people who share class consciousness and collective social identity and may engage in political action to promote social change. While the objective dimension of class remains as stark as ever, evidenced by the increasing gap between rich and poor, the subjective dimension of class as the basis of individual identity is less clear-cut and at the very least intersects with, and may have been overtaken by, group distinctions based on gender, 'race', ethnicity, and other social movements. This has led to the growing popularity of the term **social exclusion** to refer to socially disadvantaged groups (Levitas 2005; Pantazis et al. 2006; Abrams et al. 2007). The persistence of class-based patterns of illness and health-related behaviour suggests that both the objective and subjective dimensions of class are central to any analysis of health inequality.

Class and health inequality

If we accept that we should aim to live in a society that has an equality of health outcomes—that is, without health inequalities based on group membership such as class—then by current standards there is considerable room for improvement. Studies of morbidity (illness) and mortality (death) have consistently shown that the poor have the highest rates of illness and the shortest life expectancy. As Chapter 1 discussed, health inequality was a key focus of early **public health** efforts in the nineteenth century, particularly through the work of Friedrich Engels, Edwin Chadwick, and Rudolf Virchow (Engels 1845/1958; Rosen 1993; Porter 1997). Despite these early efforts, it was not until 1980 and the publication of *Inequalities in Health* (DHSS 1980) in the United Kingdom, commonly referred to as *The Black Report* after its chairman Sir Douglas Black, that interest in health inequality was renewed (see also Townsend & Davidson 1982; Whitehead 1987; Townsend et al. 1992). A further United Kingdom report, the *Independent Inquiry into Inequalities in Health* (Acheson 1998), reaffirmed the issue and resulted in dedicated government actions.

While a number of small Australian studies in the 1980s had found links between manual occupations and/or low socio-economic status and poor health, the most comprehensive evidence of health inequality was first presented in the government report, *Enough to Make You Sick: How Income and Environment Affect Health* (NHS 1992). In a detailed review of existing Australian research on health

social exclusion
A broad term used to encompass individuals and groups who experience persistent social disadvantage from a range of causes (poverty, unemployment, poor housing, *social* isolation etc.), preventing participation in social institutions and political processes.

public health
Public policies and infrastructure to prevent the onset and transmission of disease among the population, with a particular focus on sanitation and hygiene such as clean air, water and food, and immunisation. Public health infrastructure refers specifically to the buildings, installations, and equipment necessary to ensure healthy living conditions for the population.

inequality, *Socioeconomic Determinants of Health*, Gavin Turrell and colleagues (1999) state conclusively that 'socioeconomic differences in health are evident for both females and males at every stage of the life-course (birth, infancy, childhood and adolescence, and adulthood) and the relationship exists irrespective of how SES and health are measured' (Turrell et al. 1999, p. 33). Since then, the most up-to-date Australian health inequality data has come from the *National Health Survey 2001* (see Draper et al. 2004; Turrell et al. 2006).

Tables 5.2 and 5.3 present Australian data that clearly shows mortality and risk factor rates for both men and women aged between 25 and 64 are higher among those from the most disadvantaged areas, compared with those from the least disadvantaged areas (ABS 2002; AIHW 2004). For example, the stroke mortality rate was 93 per cent higher for males and 84 per cent higher for females in the most disadvantaged quintile, compared with the least disadvantaged quintile. Life expectancy at birth for the most disadvantaged quintile was 3.9 years lower for males and 2 years lower for females (AIHW 2004; Draper et al. 2004). As Table 5.3 shows, adults from

Table 5.2 Mortality rates for men and women aged 25–64 in the most disadvantaged quintile, compared with least disadvantaged quintile, Australia 1998–2000

	Men	Women
Heart disease	107% higher	170% higher
Lung cancer	102% higher	73% higher
Stroke	93% higher	84% higher
Accidents/injury	124% higher	103% higher

Source: Adapted from AIHW 2004

Table 5.3 Risk factor and chronic condition rates in the most disadvantaged quintile, compared with least disadvantaged quintile, Australia 2001

	Quintile 1 (least disadvantaged)	Quintile 5 (most disadvantaged)
Risk factors		
Current smoker	17.0	32.0
Sedentary/low exercise level	64.5	73.9
Overweight/obese	43.1	46.0
Low/no usual intake of fruit	44.1	50.7
Chronic conditions		
Diseases of the circulatory system	14.7	21.0
Diabetes	1.9	4.2
Arthritis	11.0	17.5

Source: Adapted from AIHW 2004; ABS 2002

the most disadvantaged areas have considerably higher rates of smoking, overweight/obesity, sedentary lifestyle, and chronic conditions such as diabetes and arthritis (AIHW 2003; O'Brien 2005; Turrell et al. 2006). The *National Health Survey 2001*, as with previous surveys (cf. NHS 1992), found that the most disadvantaged groups make the least use of preventive health services, most likely due to their inability to afford such services.

Explaining health inequality

The most common explanations of health inequality, as previously mentioned, can be grouped into five main categories:

1 artefact explanations
2 natural/social selection explanations
3 cultural/behavioural explanations
4 materialist/structural explanations
5 psychosocial/social capital explanations.

The first four were initially introduced in the *Black Report* (DHSS 1980) in Britain and were also discussed in the Australian report *Enough to Make You Sick* (NHS 1992). The fifth explanation is the most recent and has been influenced by the work of Michael Marmot and Richard Wilkinson (see Wilkinson 1996, 2005; Marmot 2004, 2006; Marmot & Wilkinson 2006).

Artefact explanations

The artefact explanation suggests that links between class and health are artificial and are the result of statistical anomalies or the inability to measure social phenomena accurately. This viewpoint is easily disputed by the vast amount of evidence based on various methods and classificatory schemes that have clearly found proof that health inequality exists. While the *Black Report* dismissed the artefact explanation as without basis, as Sally Macintyre (1997) suggests, what has been overlooked in the report is that the authors made the important point that the assumptions underpinning the way class and health are measured can influence the size of health inequality that is found.

Natural/social selection explanations

The *Black Report* also briefly discussed **social Darwinist** explanations that suggested that social and health inequality were due to biological inferiority. This viewpoint acknowledges the relationship between class and health, but explains it by assuming that inequality is 'natural' and thus inevitable, meaning nothing can or should be done about it. Such a viewpoint has been effectively dismissed by social science

social Darwinism
The incorrect application of Charles Darwin's theory of animal evolution to explain social inequality by transferring his idea of 'survival of the fittest' among animals to 'explain' human inequality.

John Germov

research, but Macintyre (1997) suggests there is a 'soft' version (her term) of this explanation that is still commonly ascribed to and has some explanatory power. The soft version suggests that social selection can play a part, whereby poor health early in life results in poor educational performance and occupational achievement. The central idea here is that people's health disadvantage (for example, disability) causes social disadvantage such as poverty. Most studies that have examined the social selection explanation have consistently found it can only account for a small percentage of people in groups who suffer health inequality. Furthermore, such an explanation neglects the structural causes of ill health to begin with, such as being born into a family already in poverty, which then leads to ill health and a cycle of disadvantage (such as that found among many Indigenous groups).

Cultural/behavioural explanations

Cultural/behavioural explanations focus on the individual to explain health inequality in the form of risk-taking or illness-related behaviour such as smoking, drug taking, excess alcohol consumption, and poor dietary intake as the primary causes of ill health. Such accounts have rightly been criticised for their **victim-blaming** and overly simplistic account of inequality. As Wilkinson (1996, pp. 21–2), among others, has forcefully argued, such views are unhelpful because:

> the underlying flaw in the system is not put right ... even when it comes to tackling the individual risk factors, it may sometimes be more effective to tackle them at a societal level ... to tackle the environment that establishes levels of exposure to risk.

A focus on changing the behaviour of individuals assumes they exist in a social vacuum, ignoring the social context, social relations, and social processes that affect their lives. As noted in Chapter 1, there are illness-inducing factors that lie outside of an individual's control, such as for example stressful work environments. The concept of the **risk society** (Beck 1992) epitomises the social basis of risk-imposing environments that impact on people's health and influence health-related behaviours. Therefore, a focus on the individual as the cause and cure of illness, particularly through behaviour modification (which has often been the prescription of much medical, **epidemiological**, and psychological research), will have limited success and also assumes that individuals have the time, resources, and motivation to change their lifestyle.

Macintyre (1997, p. 728) argues that the *Black Report* did discuss a 'more socially (rather than individually) based model of health-related behaviours'. For example, the report states that behaviour can also be viewed as 'embedded more within social structures; as illustrative of socially distinguishable styles of life, associated with, and reinforced by, class' (Townsend et al. 1999, p. 100). It is indeed true that the working class has higher rates of some health-damaging behaviour such as smoking

victim-blaming
The process whereby social inequality is explained in terms of individuals being solely responsible for what happens to them in relation to the choices they make and their assumed psychological, cultural, and/or biological inferiority.

risk society
A term coined by Ulrich Beck (1992) to describe the centrality of risk calculations in people's lives in Western society, whereby the key social problems today are unanticipated hazards, such as the risks of pollution, food poisoning, and environmental degradation.

epidemiology/social epidemiology
The statistical study of patterns of disease in the population. Originally focused on epidemics, or infectious diseases, it now covers non-infectious conditions such as stroke and cancer. Social epidemiology is a sub-field aligned with sociology that focuses on the social determinants of illness.

and working class people use preventive services less. The question of why there are class differences in health-related behaviour remains an issue that has received scant attention in sociological literature until recently. As Box 5.1 shows, research on lay perspectives of health inequality indicates the complex interrelationship between culture, social structure, and behaviour; finding that many disadvantaged people adopt a victim-blaming stance and deny a link between class and ill health (Blaxter 1993, 1997; Popay et al. 2003).

BOX 5.1 Doing health sociology: lay understandings of health inequality

In her review of research on lay conceptions of health and illness, Mildred Blaxter concluded that many disadvantaged people adopted individualistic explanations rather than linking poor living and working conditions to illness. According to Blaxter (1997, p. 754), '[t]o acknowledge "inequality" would be to admit an inferior moral status for oneself and one's peers: hence, perhaps, the emphasis on "not giving in to illness", which can be seen as a claim to moral equality even in the face of clear economic inequality'. Research by Jennie Popay and colleagues (2003, p. 22) reports similar findings, and suggests that 'strength of character and personal control are emphasised' in the face of social disadvantage, so that 'the way the individual responds to these will determine whether health is damaged.' Such views make sense in a culture based on individualism and the moral imperative of self-responsibility for health. Furthermore, as Popay and colleagues (2003, p. 22) state, 'the means to avoid ill health (framed in terms of individual resilience and strength of character) are, potentially at least, within an individual's control ... It is difficult to envisage what an effective individual response would be to any direct causal relationship between structural factors ... and ill health'. Therefore, disadvantaged people's tendency to deny the social origins of health inequality represents a rational response that avoids fatalism and offers the hope of self-determination.

Materialist/structural explanations

Materialist/structural explanations concern the role of social, economic, and political factors in determining the social distribution of health and illness. The basis of this view has been a focus on how poor living and working conditions—particularly poverty, discrimination, lack of educational and employment opportunities, inadequate nutrition and housing—directly influence illness. Materialist/structural explanations have been particularly addressed by Marxist and Weberian perspectives (see Waitzkin

TheoryLink

See Chapter 2 for a discussion of Marxism and Weberianism.

John Germov

1983, 2000; Connell 1988), which direct attention away from individualistic and victim-blaming accounts towards the basic class structure of society.

The value of class analysis and a structural approach to explaining health inequality is evident when examining the role played by employment and unemployment in understanding and addressing health inequality. For those who are employed, work can also be hazardous to health. For example, those employed in the mining industry have the highest occupational mortality and morbidity rates, followed by agriculture, manufacturing, construction, and transport and communication (Driscoll & Mayhew 1999; see Chapter 6). A growing literature has also documented the health consequences of unemployment, finding higher rates of chronic illness among the unemployed (see Mathers & Schofield 1998; Bartley et al. 1999).

There is continuing debate in this literature over whether unemployment leads to a deterioration of a person's health status or whether poor health status leads to unemployment, echoing the debate over social selection discussed above. Much of the literature on unemployment and health has been influenced by psychological perspectives, which tend to downplay economic insecurity in favour of psychosocial factors such as the impact of unemployment on social isolation, loss of identity, and anxiety, which allegedly increase illness-related behaviour. While these factors are without doubt important, a sociological analysis focuses on the underlying structural basis of unemployment and ill health, whereby low-income groups (Indigenous populations, recent migrants, and unskilled workers) are over-represented among the unemployed and have the poorest health status. According to Mathers and Schofield (1998, p. 181), there is clear evidence from a range of studies to show that the actual experience of unemployment 'has a direct effect on health over and above the effects of socioeconomic status, poverty, risk factors, or prior ill-health.'

Macintyre (1997, p. 740) notes that in the wider literature since the publication of the *Black Report*, the four explanations of health inequality discussed above have often been viewed as mutually exclusive, establishing false debates between 'artefact versus real differences', 'selection versus causation', and 'behaviour versus material circumstances'. Such 'either/or' debates have been unhelpful and she makes a clear case that even though the authors of the *Black Report* favoured the structural explanation, they still acknowledged the minor role of social selection and the role of cultural and behavioural factors. The focus on structural approaches and class analysis leads to policy prescriptions based on **social justice**, such as welfare measures to address poverty, improve workplace safety, and promote health-inducing work and public spaces (such as smoke-free environments). Class analysis has been less successful in explaining the continued difference in health-related behaviour among the poor. A more recent explanation has pointed to psychosocial factors and the lack of **social capital** as the basis for the persistence of health inequality in developed countries.

social justice
A belief system that gives high priority to the interests of the least advantaged.

social capital
A term used to refer to social relations, networks, norms, trust, and reciprocity between individuals that facilitate cooperation for mutual benefit.

Psychosocial/social capital explanations

An alternative explanation of health inequality has arisen from the work of social epidemiologists Marmot and Wilkinson (see Wilkinson 1996, 2005; Wilkinson & Marmot 1998, 2003; Marmot 2004, 2006; Marmot & Wilkinson 2006). While concerned with the social origins of illness, they have turned attention away from class analysis to a narrower focus on income inequality and psychosocial factors. The authors suggest that the widening income inequality accompanied by work intensification and unemployment has led to increased levels of stress, anxiety, insecurity, anger, and depression in the community, and that these psychosocial factors negatively impact on health not only among the poor, but also on those who experience relative inequality.

Marmot has been the principal researcher in what have become known as the Whitehall studies, which have examined the health of British civil servants since the 1960s and continue today (see Marmot et al. 1978; Marmot et al. 1991; Marmot et al. 1997; Marmot et al. 1999). The first study found a 'social gradient' in the mortality rate, whereby life expectancy increased for each employment level up to the top of the public service hierarchy. Participants in the initial study (all men) were grouped into four employment grades, with those in the bottom two grades found to have a life expectancy 4.4 years shorter than those in the top two grades (Marmot et al. 1978). Furthermore, the social gradient applied to a range of conditions such as stroke, cancer, and gastrointestinal disease (Marmot 2000).

There are two sociologically significant aspects to the findings arising from the Whitehall study. First, the social gradient of health continued along the whole occupational hierarchy, suggesting that health inequality did not only affect those in poverty, but also existed among relatively well-paid, white-collar workers. Second, **risk factors** only accounted for a small percentage of the social gradient. Risk factors such as being overweight, smoking, excessive alcohol consumption, and not exercising could not explain the health inequality between the occupational grades of the civil servants in the study (see Marmot et al. 1997; Marmot et al. 1999; Marmot 2000). In an attempt to discover what other determinants might be involved, the Whitehall II study (which included women) focused on the impact of stress on employee health, examining the extent of employee control and variety at work, and the role played by social support. The Whitehall II study also found a social gradient for morbidity among women as well as men, and its major conclusion was that those with less control over work had higher rates of heart disease, depression, and other health problems (see Marmot et al. 1991; Marmot et al. 1997; Marmot et al. 1999; Marmot 2000, 2004).

In *Unhealthy Societies*, Richard Wilkinson (1996) presents empirical evidence to support a thesis that societies with lower levels of income inequality have the

risk factors
Conditions that are thought to increase an individual's susceptibility to illness or disease such as abuse of alcohol, poor diet, or smoking.

gross domestic product (GDP)
The market value of all goods and services that have been sold during a year.

highest life expectancy. His argument is that once a country reaches a certain amount of wealth determined by **gross domestic product (GDP)** per capita (per head of population) and undergoes the 'epidemiologic transition' from infectious disease to chronic disease as the major cause of mortality, increases in national wealth have little impact on population health. For example, he notes that even though the GDP per head in the USA is almost twice that of Greece, life expectancy in Greece is higher (Wilkinson 1999; see also Wilkinson 1992; Wilkinson & Pickett 2006, 2007). Therefore, for developed countries, Wilkinson argues that it is not the total wealth of a society that is important, but rather the distribution of that wealth—the more egalitarian it is, the better the life expectancy and hence the less likelihood of health inequality: there is a 'strong relationship between income distribution and national mortality rates. In the developed world, it is not the richest countries which have the best health, but most egalitarian' (Wilkinson 1996, p. 3).

Wilkinson's work has spawned a significant literature debating the merits of his study and its conclusions. While some studies have supported his findings (see Kaplan et al. 1996; Kennedy et al. 1996), others have cast doubt on the accuracy and strength of his claims. For example, in a significant study by Ken Judge and colleagues (1998), statistical associations between income inequality and population health were found to be small, posing 'a serious challenge to those who believe that the relationship is a very powerful one' (Judge et al. 1998, p. 578).

The work of Marmot and Wilkinson extends the health inequality debate beyond a focus on the most socio-economically disadvantaged groups. Instead, they highlight that a social gradient or continuum of health inequality exists, whereby health gradually worsens as you move down the social hierarchy, so that each social group has worse health than the one above it. For these authors, relative inequality is linked to poorer health, even for employed white-collar workers, who by definition are not poor or exposed to hazardous work environments. Therefore, it is not only the working class or the poor who experience health inequality, but groups along the whole social hierarchy. Though these findings are yet to be confirmed in Australia, they suggest that materialist/structural explanations offer an incomplete account of health inequality. Subsequently, a range of authors spearheaded by Marmot and Wilkinson has focused on psychosocial factors as the main explanation of health inequality.

Social capital and the psychosocial thesis: an evaluation

The 'psychosocial thesis' is a neo-functionalist perspective that proposes societies with greater income inequality have less social cohesion or social capital. The idea of social cohesion or social capital is a reworking of Émile Durkheim's (1893/1984,

1897/1951) concept of social solidarity. More recently the concept of social capital has been advanced in the work of Pierre Bourdieu (1986), Jonathon Coleman (1988), and Robert Putnam (1993) and has been popularised in Australia by Eva Cox (1995) and Fran Baum (Baum et al. 2000; Bush & Baum 2001; Baum 2002). Social capital refers to social relations and networks that exist among social groups and communities and that provide access to resources and opportunities for mutual benefit. Social capital depends on a high level of community participation, altruism, trust, and an expectation of reciprocity. It has been suggested that the lack of social capital or social cohesion explains why certain social groups adopt health-damaging behaviour. The assumption is that access to social capital will lead to improved health outcomes by lowering stress, providing outlets for social interaction and opportunities for enhancing control over one's life through democratic participation in community life (Winter 2000a, 2000b).

Putnam (1993) and Cox (1995) envisage social capital as a collective property of specific communities or society as a whole, rather than an attribute or trait possessed by individuals. For Cox (1995, p. 46), social capital involves an 'interplay of state and community', and has been a useful concept for counteracting the negative effects of economic rationalism, which she claims has undermined communities by fostering insecurity and anxiety. High levels of social capital are reflected in altruistic activities such as volunteer work that contributes to the welfare of others. Putnam (2000, p. 331) goes so far as to claim that 'if you belong to no groups but decide to join one, you cut your risk of dying over the next year by half.'

Michael Woolcock (1998, p. 195), while supportive of the social capital concept, suggests that it is often used in an uncritical and imprecise way, resulting in a handy catch-all concept that 'risks trying to explain too much with too little'. The vague nature of the concept and its intangible qualities (trust, reciprocity) have allowed it to be used by both progressive and conservative political groups, notably the World Bank, a key proponent of the concept (Kawachi & Berkman 2000). Conservative commentators (see Coleman 1988) conceptualise social capital as a property of individuals whereby social disadvantage is viewed as being overcome by individuals engaging in volunteer work, joining associations, and making the most of their own support networks. In this formulation, social capital becomes a code word for mutual obligation and individual responsibility. Therefore, social capital can be used to support **economic rationalist** policies of cutting expenditure on the **social wage** and public health by placing an increased emphasis on community and family responsibility and voluntary work. It is interesting to note that working class examples of social capital, such as collective action through union involvement, tend to be ignored and are rarely taken into account as evidence of social cohesion and democratic participation in community life by psychosocial proponents (Muntaner & Lynch 1999). Proponents of social capital also downplay the possibility that it can have negative implications, whereby communities and membership of certain

TheoryLink
See Chapter 2 for a discussion of functionalism.

economic rationalism/economic liberalism
Terms used to describe a political philosophy based on small-government and market-oriented policies, such as deregulation, privatisation, reduced government spending, and lower taxation.

social wage
Government spending on health, social security, education, and housing (often referred to as welfare spending).

clubs and associations can be used for the social exclusion of others such as ethnic minorities. It is even possible to view the close-knit and mutually supportive nature of criminal gangs as exhibiting strong social capital—a particularly unhealthy scenario (Muntaner et al. 2001).

Social capital resembles community development approaches advocated in the 1970s and fits well with current health promotion efforts that advocate empowering individuals to participate in community activities (Baum et al. 2000); however, these have often met with limited success because they ignored the important role that economic resources and public policies play in facilitating community development and fostering notions of social capital (Winter 2000b; Muntaner et al. 2001; Szreter & Woolcock 2004). High rates of poverty and unemployment in a community are unlikely to facilitate social cohesion. As Putnam states (1993, p. 42), '[s]ocial capital is not a substitute for effective public policy but rather a prerequisite for it and, in part, a consequence of it.' Public policies that facilitate employment opportunities, social services, and access to social institutions such as education set the conditions for social capital and health-enhancing environments.

Bringing class analysis back in: the structure–agency debate and health behaviour

structure–agency debate
A key debate in sociology over the extent to which human behaviour is determined by social structure.

The benefit of the psychosocial/social capital approach is its engagement with the **structure–agency debate** (see Chapter 1). Theories of health inequality have tended to be vague on the issue of class patterns of health-related behaviour, particularly the 'poor behaviour of the poor'. There has been little detailed examination of the processes through which the social structure shapes individuals' health-related behaviour (Macintyre 1997; Cockerham 2005). The psychosocial/social capital explanation provides some insights into the dynamic relationship between structure and agency, establishing pathways between the experience of inequality and health-damaging behaviour.

Even though Marmot and Wilkinson both acknowledge the need to address structural issues such as poverty, unemployment, and income redistribution, their preferred policy prescriptions have focused on facilitating social cohesion (trust, reciprocity, cooperation, community participation), rather than political and economic change, downplaying the class relations that create income inequality in the first place (Muntaner & Lynch 1999; Coburn 2000; Lynch 2000). As David Coburn (2000) argues, there is an implicit assumption that wider reform, such as income redistribution to decrease inequality, is beyond reach. Instead, attention is focused on psychosocial factors at the level of the individual and the community in which people live, rather than the wider structural factors such as the social and economic policies pursued by governments. By marginalising the role of public policy in both undermining and creating social capital, there is the potential to fall into the trap of a 'community-level version of "blaming the victim"' (Muntaner & Lynch 1999, p. 59). For example, issues of work intensification and occupational health and safety are marginalised in the discussion of psychosocial factors such as stress, anxiety, and depression. Furthermore, it is likely that social capital is more extensive in middle-class and upper-class communities, where individuals have the time and resources to contribute to and participate in community life. Therefore, social capital may be important for psychosocial health, but the lack of a class analysis in the social capital literature undermines its value as an explanatory concept.

Conclusion: towards health equity or health equality?

The link between the working class and high rates of morbidity and mortality is now undisputed, but it remains fair to say that aside from poverty and work-related conditions, the reasons for class-based health inequality, particularly health-damaging behaviours, remain unclear. The social patterning of behaviour clearly indicates that it is not simply an outcome of individual choice—there are social processes at work. Individual behaviour occurs in a social context of living and working conditions that create exposure to health-enhancing or damaging environments.

In much of the health-inequality literature the five explanations discussed here have often been contrasted as either/or propositions—considerable effort has gone into supporting or refuting a particular theory over all others. While no single theory has offered an adequate explanation, a way forward is offered by a multifactorial approach that addresses structural, cultural, and psychosocial factors (Vågerö & Illsley 1995; Macintyre 1997). Only such theoretical pluralism can effectively deal with the range of social and psychological determinants of health inequality.

At this point it is important to make a distinction between health inequality and health inequity (Whitehead 1990, 1992; Harris et al. 1999; Baggott 2000). While the terms 'inequality' and 'inequity' are often used interchangeably, '[n]ot all in-equalities are necessarily inequitable' (Baggott 2000, p. 221). For example, some people can run faster than others or are more industrious at their work. Such inequalities would rarely be seen as unfair or inequitable. In the same vein, health inequality is inevitable given genetic variation, lifestyle choices, and socio-economic differences among the population. Therefore, health inequality refers to the different health statuses associated with various social groups, particularly in terms of class, gender, age, ethnicity, and indigeneity. Health inequity refers to whether such inequality is unfair and avoidable. In other words, it concerns whether health outcomes are the result of everyone having equal opportunity to be optimally healthy or whether they are due to inadequate income, education, food, and health care. Given that there is no universally accepted understanding of what is equitable or fair, there

John Germov

remains considerable debate as to appropriate goals and interventions to address health inequality.

Margaret Whitehead (1995, 2007) suggests there are four 'policy levels' at which interventions to address health inequality can occur:

1 strengthening individuals through health education to encourage health-enhancing behaviour
2 strengthening communities by facilitating social cohesion to enable collective action to address health hazards and establish health-conducive environments
3 improving living and working conditions through better access to safer work-places, nutritious food, affordable recreation facilities, and preventive services
4 encouraging macroeconomic and cultural change through income maintenance for those in poverty; education and training to prevent long-term poverty; and income redistribution through welfare and taxation policies to reduce overall rates of inequality.

Whitehead (1995) acknowledges that all policy levels are necessary to ensure a comprehensive approach to addressing health inequalities; however, she cautions against an over-reliance on health education and suggests that it is often the lack of time and resources available to the poor that prevents them from adopting healthier lifestyles—something that can be addressed by the other three levels of policy intervention. Health interventions should be guided by a social justice imperative so that the ultimate goal is the maximisation of the health status of the most disadvantaged (Rawls 1970; Connell 1988). Until this aspect of the social structure is addressed, it is unlikely that little will change in respect of class and health inequality.

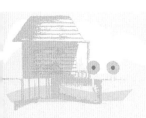

Summary of main points

» Although class is a major form of social inequality, there are other important intersecting structures of inequality based on gender, 'race', ethnicity, and other social groups, such as youth and the aged. While there is disagreement in the wider literature between objective (class 'in itself') and subjective (class 'for itself') notions of class, with some suggesting class in subjective terms 'is dead', class is still strongly associated with health status.

» Numerous studies using different research methods and forms of measurement have consistently found that the working class (or low-SES groups) have higher rates of mortality and morbidity.

» Recent studies have also exposed a social gradient of health, whereby a continuum of health inequality exists from top to bottom of the occupational and income hierarchy.

» There are five main explanations of health inequality: artefact; natural/social selection; cultural/behavioural; materialist/structural; and psychosocial/social capital explanations.

» Health inequality can be reduced through social justice strategies that address class inequality through structural change in the economy, the workplace, and the community.

Sociological reflection: addressing class-based health inequality

Whitehead (1995) suggests there are four 'policy levels' through which health inequality can be addressed:

» strengthening individuals
» strengthening communities
» improving access to essential facilities and services
» encouraging macroeconomic and cultural change.

What do you think needs to be done to minimise class differences in health status? Think of examples for each of the four policy levels and reflect on how effective these might be. Why might some levels of intervention be focused on more than others?

Discussion questions

1   What class do you belong to? Do you believe class has influenced your beliefs, lifestyle, and life chances?

2   In what ways might the upper class in Australia also be considered a ruling class? Think of some real-life examples in your response.

3   In what ways can class analysis shed light on why health inequality exists? What are the limits of class analysis?

4   What are the benefits and limitations of psychosocial/social capital explanations of health inequality?

5   Why do members of the working class exhibit higher rates of health-damaging behaviour?

6   Given that there are social patterns of health-related behaviour, to what extent are individuals responsible for their health?

John Germov

Further investigation

1 Equal access to health care does not lead to equal health outcomes. Discuss.
2 Compare and contrast the neo-functionalist approach of psychosocial/social capital explanations of health inequality with the neo-Marxist approach. Which provides the best fit in explaining health inequality in Australia?
3 Health education as a policy response to addressing health inequality individualises the social origins of illness. Discuss.
4 'Not all inequalities are necessarily inequitable' (Baggott 2000, p. 221). Discuss with reference to class-based health inequality.

Further reading

Bartley, M. 2004, *Health Inequality: An Introduction to Theories, Concepts and Methods*, Polity, Cambridge.

Cockerham, W. C. 2007, *Social Causes of Health and Disease*, Polity, Cambridge.

Draper, G., Turrell, G. & Oldenburg, B. 2004, *Health Inequalities in Australia: Mortality*, Health Inequalities Monitoring Series no. 1, AIHW Cat. no. PHE 55, Queensland University of Technology and AIHW, Canberra.

'Health Inequalities and the Psychosocial Environment', 2004, *Social Science & Medicine*, Special issue, vol. 58, no. 8.

Marmot, M. 2004, *Status Syndrome: How your Social Standing Directly Affects your Health and Life Expectancy*, Bloomsbury, Oxford.

Marmot, M. 2006, 'Health in an Unequal World', *Lancet*, vol. 368, pp. 2081–94. Available online: <http://www.globalhealth.vanderbilt.edu/Documents/Lancet06.pdf>

Marmot, M. & Wilkinson, R. (eds) 2006, *Social Determinants of Health*, 2nd edn, Oxford University Press, Oxford.

Pusey, M. 2003, *The Experience of Middle Australia: The Dark Side of Economic Reform*, Cambridge University Press, Melbourne.

Stilwell, F. & Jordan K. 2007, *Who Gets What? Analysing Economic Inequality in Australia*, Cambridge University Press, Melbourne.

Turrell, G., Stanley, L., de Looper, M. & Oldenburg, B. 2006, *Health Inequalities in Australia: Morbidity, Health Behaviours, Risk Factors and Health Service Use*, Health Inequalities Monitoring Series no. 2, AIHW Cat. no. PHE 72, Queensland University of Technology and AIHW, Canberra.

Waitzkin, H. 2000, *The Second Sickness: Contradictions of Capitalist Health Care*, 2nd edn, Rowman & Littlefield, Lanham.

Wilkinson, R. 2005, *The Impact of Inequality: How to Make Sick Societies Healthier*, The New Press, New York.

Wright, E. O. (ed.) 2005, *Approaches to Class Analysis*, Cambridge University Press, Cambridge.

Web resources

Inequality.org (USA): <http://www.demos.org/inequality/>
International Society for Equity in Health: <http://www.iseqh.org>
NATSEM: National Centre for Social and Economic Modelling: <http://www.canberra. edu.au/centres/natsem/>
UK Department of Health—Health Inequalities: <http://www.dh.gov.uk/en/Public health/Healthinequalities/index.htm>
Whitehall II study: <http://www.ucl.ac.uk/whitehallII/>

Online case study • • •
Visit the Second Opinion
website to access
relevant case studies.

Documentaries/films

People like Us: Social Class in America (2001): 124 minutes. A documentary depicting people's experiences of class in everyday life.

References

Abrams, D., Christian, J. & Gordon, D. (eds) 2007, *Multidisciplinary Handbook of Social Exclusion Research*, John Wiley & Sons, Chichester.

Australian Bureau of Statistics 2002, *National Health Survey 2001: Summary of Results*, Cat. no. 4364.0, ABS, Canberra.

Australian Bureau of Statistics 2007, *Household Wealth and Wealth Distribution, 2005–06*, Cat. no. 6554.0, ABS, Canberra.

Acheson, D. 1998, *Independent Inquiry into Inequalities in Health*, Stationery Office, London.

Australian Institute of Health and Welfare 2003, *Indicators of Health Risk Factors: The AIHW View*, AIHW Cat. no. PHE 47, AIHW, Canberra.

Australian Institute of Health and Welfare 2004, *Australia's Health 2004*, AIHW, Canberra.

Baggott, R. 2000, *Public Health: Policy and Politics*, Palgrave, Basingstoke.

Bartley, M., Ferrie, J. & Scott, S. M. 1999, 'Living in a High-unemployment Economy: Understanding the Health Consequences', in M. Marmot & R. G. Wilkinson (eds), *Social Determinants of Health*, Oxford University Press, Oxford, pp. 81–104.

Baum, F. 2002, *The New Public Health*, 2nd edn, Oxford University Press, Melbourne.

Baum, F., Palmer, C., Modra, C., Murray, C. & Bush, R. 2000, 'Families, Social Capital and Health', in I. Winter (ed.), *Social Capital and Public Policy in Australia*, Australian Institute of Family Studies, Melbourne, pp. 250–75.

Baxter, J., Emmison, M. & Western, M. 1991, *Class Analysis and Contemporary Australia*, Macmillan, Melbourne.

Beck, U. 1992, *Risk Society: Towards a New Modernity*, Sage, London.

Blaxter, M. 1993, 'Why do Victims Blame Themselves?', in A. Radley (ed.), *Worlds of Illness: Biographical and Cultural Perspectives of Health and Disease*, Routledge, London.

Blaxter, M. 1997, 'Whose Fault is it? People's own Conceptions of the Reasons for Health Inequalities', *Social Science & Medicine*, vol. 44, no. 6, pp. 747–56.

Bourdieu, P. 1986, 'The Forms of Capital', in J. Richardson (ed.), *Handbook of Theory and Research for the Sociology of Education*, Greenwood Press, New York, pp. 241–58.

Bush, R. & Baum, F. 2001, 'Health Inequities, Community and Social Capital', in R. Eckersley, J. Dixon & J. Douglas (eds), *The Social Origins of Health and Well-being*, Cambridge University Press, Melbourne, ch. 13, pp. 189–204.

Business Review Weekly (*BRW*) 2008, 'Rich 200', May 29–July 2.

Coburn, D. 2000, 'Income Inequality, Social Cohesion and the Health Status of Populations: The Role of Neo-liberalism', *Social Science & Medicine*, vol. 51, no. 1, pp. 135–46.

Cockerham, W. C. 2005, 'Health Lifestyle Theory and the Convergence of Agency and Structure', *Journal of Health and Social Behavior*, vol. 46, no. 1, pp. 51–67.

Coleman, J. 1988, 'Social Capital in the Creation of Human Capital', *American Journal of Sociology*, vol. 94, pp. 95–120.

Connell, R. W. 1977, *Ruling Class, Ruling Culture*, Cambridge University Press, Cambridge.

Connell, R. W. 1983, *Which Way is Up? Essays on Sex, Class and Culture*, Allen & Unwin, Sydney.

Connell, R. W. 1988, 'Class Inequalities and "Just Health"', *Community Health Studies*, vol. 12, no. 2, pp. 212–17.

Connell, R. W. & Irving, T. H. 1992, *Class Structure in Australian History: Poverty and Progress*, 2nd edn, Longman Cheshire, Melbourne.

Cox, E. 1995, *A Truly Civic Society: Boyer Lectures 1995*, ABC Books, Sydney.

Crompton, R. 1998, *Class and Stratification: An Introduction to Current Debates*, 2nd edn, Polity Press, Cambridge.

Crompton, R., Devine, F., Savage, M. & Scott, J. (eds) 2000, *Renewing Class Analysis*, Blackwell, Oxford.

Department of Health and Social Security 1980, *Inequalities in Health*, Report of a Working Group Chaired by Sir Douglas Black, DHSS, London.

Draper, G., Turrell, G. & Oldenburg, B. 2004, *Health Inequalities in Australia: Mortality*, Health Inequalities Monitoring Series no. 1, AIHW Cat. no. PHE 55, Queensland University of Technology and AIHW, Canberra.

Driscoll, T. & Mayhew, C. 1999, 'Extent and Cost of Occupational Injury and Illness', in C. Mayhew & C. L. Peterson (eds), *Occupational Health and Safety in Australia*, Allen & Unwin, Sydney, pp. 28–51.

Durkheim, É. 1893/1984, *The Division of Labor in Society*, trans. W. Halls, Free Press, New York.

Durkheim, É. 1897/1951, *Suicide*, Free Press, New York.

Eder, K. 1993, *The New Politics of Class: Social Movements and Cultural Dynamics in Advanced Societies*, Sage, London.

Engels, F. 1958/1845, *The Condition of the Working Class in England*, trans. W. O. Henderson & W. H. Chaloner, Basil Blackwell, Oxford.

Goldthorpe, J. 1996, 'Class and Politics in Advanced Industrial Societies', in D. J. Lee & B. S. Turner (eds), *Conflicts About Class*, Longman, London.

Harris, E., Sainsbury, P. & Nutbeam, D. (eds) 1999, *Perspectives on Health Inequity*, Australian Centre for Health Promotion, University of Sydney, Sydney.

Judge, K., Mulligan, J. & Benzenval, M. 1998, 'Income Inequality and Population Health', *Social Science & Medicine*, vol. 46, nos 4–5, pp. 567–79.

Kaplan, G. A., Pamuk, E., Lynch, J. W., Cohen, R. D. & Balflour, J. L. 1996, 'Income Inequality and Mortality in the United States', *British Medical Journal*, vol. 312, pp. 999–1003.

Kawachi, I. & Berkman, L. 2000, 'Social Cohesion, Social Capital, and Health', in L. F. Berkman & I. Kawachi (eds), *Social Epidemiology*, Oxford University Press, New York, pp. 174–90.

Kennedy, B. P., Kawachi, I. & Prothrow-Stith, D. 1996, 'Income Distribution and Mortality: Cross-sectional Ecological Study of the Robin Hood Index in the United States', *British Medical Journal*, vol. 312, pp. 1004–7.

Levitas, R. 2005, *The Inclusive Society? Social Exclusion and New Labour*, Palgrave Macmillan, Basingstoke.

Lynch, J. 2000, 'Income Inequality and Health: Expanding the Debate', *Social Science & Medicine*, vol. 51, no. 3, pp. 1001–5.

Macintyre, S. 1997, 'The Black Report and Beyond: What are the Issues?', *Social Science & Medicine*, vol. 44, no. 6, pp. 723–45.

Marmot, M. G. 2000, 'Social Determinants of Health: From Observation to Policy', *Medical Journal of Australia*, vol. 172, 17 April, pp. 379–82.

Marmot, M. G. 2004, *Status Syndrome: How your Social Standing Directly Affects your Health and Life Expectancy*, Bloomsbury, Oxford.

Marmot, M. G. 2006, 'Health in an Unequal World', *Lancet*, vol. 368, pp. 2081–94. Available online: <http://www.globalhealth.vanderbilt.edu/Documents/Lancet06.pdf>

Marmot, M. G., Bosma, H., Hemingway, H., Brunner, E. & Stansfeld, S. 1997, 'Contribution of Job Control and Other Risk Factors to Social Variations in Coronary Heart Disease Incidence', *Lancet*, July 26, vol. 350, no. 9073, pp. 235–9.

Marmot, M. G., Davey Smith, G., Stansfield, S., Patel, C., North, F., Head, J., White, I., Brunner, E. & Feeney, A. 1991, 'Health Inequalities among British Civil Servants: The Whitehall II Study', *Lancet*, vol. 337, no. 8754, pp. 1387–93.

Marmot, M. G., Rose, G., Shipley, M. & Hamilton, P. J. S. 1978, 'Employment Grade and Coronary Heart Disease in British Civil Servants', *Journal of Epidemiology and Community Health*, vol. 32, pp. 244–9.

Marmot, M. G., Siegrist, J., Theorell, T. & Feeney, A. 1999, 'Health and the Psychosocial Environment at Work', in M. Marmot & R. G. Wilkinson (eds), *Social Determinants of Health*, Oxford University Press, Oxford.

Marmot, M. G. & Wilkinson, R. (eds) 2006, *Social Determinants of Health*, 2nd edn, Oxford University Press, Oxford.

Mathers, C. D. & Schofield, D. 1998, 'The Health Consequences of Unemployment: The Evidence', *Medical Journal of Australia*, vol. 168, pp. 178–82.

Merrill Lynch & Capgemini 2008, *World Wealth Report 2008*, Merrill Lynch, Pierce, Fenner & Smith Incorporated and Capgemini.

Muntaner, C. & Lynch, J. 1999, 'Income Inequality, Social Cohesion, and Class Relations: A Critique of Wilkinson's Neo-Durkheimian Research Program', *International Journal of Health Services*, vol. 29, no. 1, pp. 59–81.

Muntaner, C., Lynch, J. & Davey Smith, G. 2001, 'Social Capital, Disorganized Communities and the Third Way: Understanding the Retreat from Structural Inequalities in Epidemiology and Public Health', *International Journal of Health Services*, vol. 31, no. 2, pp. 213–37.

National Health Strategy 1992, *Enough to Make You Sick: How Income and Environment Affect Health*, AGPS, Canberra.

O'Brien, K. 2005, *Living Dangerously: Australians with Multiple Risk Factors for Cardiovascular Disease*, Bulletin no. 24, AIHW Cat. no. AUS 57, AIHW, Canberra.

Pakulski, J. 2005, *Globalising Inequalities: New Patterns of Social Privilege and Disadvantage*, Allen & Unwin, Sydney.

Pakulski, J. & Waters, M. 1996, *The Death of Class*, Sage, London.

Pantazis, C., Gordon, D. & Levitas, R. (eds.) 2006, *Poverty and Social Exclusion in Britain: The Millennium Survey*, Policy Press, Bristol.

Popay, J., Bennett, S., Thomas, C., Williams, G., Gatrell, A. & Bostock, L. 2003, 'Beyond "Beer, Fags, Egg and Chips"? Exploring Lay Understandings of Social Inequalities in Health', *Sociology of Health & Illness*, vol. 25, no. 1, pp. 1–23.

Porter, R. 1997, *The Greatest Benefit to Mankind: A Medical History of Humanity from Antiquity to the Present*, HarperCollins, London.

Putnam, R. 1993, *Making Democracy Work: Civic Traditions in Modern Italy*, Princeton University Press, Princeton.

Putnam, R. 2000, *Bowling Alone: The Collapse and Revival of American Community*, Simon & Schuster, New York.

Rawls, J. 1970, *A Theory of Justice*, The Clarendon Press, Oxford.

Rosen, G. 1993, *A History of Public Health*, Johns Hopkins University Press, New York.

Szreter, S. & Woolcock, M. 2004, 'Health by Association? Social Capital, Social Theory, and the Political Economy of Public Health', *International Journal of Epidemiology*, vol. 33, no. 4, pp. 650–67.

Townsend, P. & Davidson, N. (eds) 1982, *Inequalities in Health: The Black Report*, Penguin, Harmondsworth.

Townsend, P., Davidson, N. & Whitehead, M. (eds) 1992, *Inequalities in Health: The Black Report and the Health Divide*, Penguin, London.

Turrell, G., Oldenburg, B., McGuffog, I. & Dent, R. 1999, *Socioeconomic Determinants of Health: Towards a National Research Program and a Policy and Intervention Agenda*, Centre for Public Health Research, School of Public Health, Queensland University of Technology, Brisbane.

Turrell, G., Stanley, L., de Looper, M. & Oldenburg, B. 2006, *Health Inequalities in Australia: Morbidity, Health Behaviours, Risk Factors and Health Service Use*, Health Inequalities Monitoring Series no. 2, AIHW Cat. no. PHE 72, Queensland University of Technology and AIHW, Canberra.

Vågerö, D. & Illsley, R. 1995, 'Explaining Health Inequalities: Beyond Black and Barker', *European Sociological Review*, vol. 11, pp. 219–41.

Waitzkin, H. 1983, *The Second Sickness: Contradictions of Capitalist Health Care*, Free Press, New York.

Waitzkin, H. 2000, *The Second Sickness: Contradictions of Capitalist Health Care*, 2nd edn, Rowman & Littlefield, Lanham.

Westergaard, J. 1995, *Who Gets What? The Hardening of Class Inequality in the Late Twentieth Century*, Polity Press, Cambridge.

Western, M. 2000, 'Class in Australia in the 1980s and 1990s', in J. M. Najman & J. S. Western (eds), *A Sociology of Australian Society*, 3rd edn, Macmillan, Melbourne, pp. 68–88.

Western, M. & Baxter, J. 2007, 'Class and Inequality in Australia', in J. Germov & M. Poole (eds) *Public Sociology: An Introduction to Australian Society*, Allen & Unwin, Sydney, pp. 215–36.

Whitehead, M. 1987, *The Health Divide: Inequalities in Health in the 1980s*, Health Education Council, London.

Whitehead, M. 1992, 'The Concepts and Principles of Equity and Health', *International Journal of Health Services*, vol. 22, no. 3, pp. 429–45.

Whitehead, M. 1990, *The Concepts and Principles of Equity and Health*, World Health Organization Regional Office for Europe, Copenhagen.

Whitehead, M. 1995, 'Tackling Inequalities: A Review of Policy Initiatives', in M. Benzeval, K. Judge & M. Whitehead (eds), *Tackling Inequalities in Health: An Agenda or Action, King's Fund*, London.

Whitehead, M. 2007, 'A Typology of Actions to Tackle Social Inequalities in Health', *Journal of Epidemiology and Community Health*, vol. 61, pp. 473–8.

Wilkinson, R. G. 1992, 'Income Distribution and Life Expectancy', *British Medical Journal*, vol. 304, pp. 165–8.

Wilkinson, R. G. 1996, *Unhealthy Societies: The Afflictions of Inequality*, Routledge, London.

Wilkinson, R. G. 1999, 'Putting the Picture Together: Prosperity, Redistribution, Health, and Welfare', in M. Marmot & R. G. Wilkinson (eds), *Social Determinants of Health*, Oxford University Press, Oxford, pp. 256–74.

Wilkinson, R. G. 2005, *The Impact of Inequality: How to Make Sick Societies Healthier*, The New Press, New York.

Wilkinson, R. & Marmot, M. (eds) 1998, *The Solid Facts: Social Determinants of Health*, World Health Organization, Copenhagen.

Wilkinson, R. & Marmot, M. (eds) 2003, *The Solid Facts: Social Determinants of Health*, 2nd edn, World Health Organization, Copenhagen.

Wilkinson, R. G. & Pickett, K. E. 2006, 'Income Inequality and Population Health: A Review and Explanation of the Evidence', *Social Science & Medicine*, vol. 62, no. 7, pp. 1768–84.

Wilkinson, R. G. & Pickett, K. E. 2007, 'The Problems of Relative Deprivation: Why Some Societies do Better than Others', *Social Science & Medicine*, vol. 65, no. 9, pp. 1965–78.

Winter, I. (ed.) 2000a, *Social Capital and Public Policy in Australia*, Australian Institute of Family Studies, Melbourne.

Winter, I. 2000b, 'Major Themes and Debates in the Social Capital Literature: The Australian Connection', in I. Winter (ed.), *Social Capital and Public Policy in Australia*, Australian Institute of Family Studies, Melbourne, pp. 7–42.

Woolcock, M. 1998, 'Social Capital and Economic Development: Toward a Theoretical Synthesis and Policy Framework', *Theory & Society*, vol. 27, pp. 151–208.

Wright, E. O. 1997, *Class Counts: Comparative Studies in Class Analysis*, Cambridge University Press, Cambridge.

Wright, E. O. (ed.) 2005, *Approaches to Class Analysis*, Cambridge University Press, Cambridge.

CHAPTER 6

Workplace Health

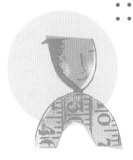

T O N I
S C H O F I E L D

Overview

- What is workplace health?
- Why is workplace health a significant social problem?
- What are the main social responses to workplace health problems?

WORKPLACE INJURY

Liz, a registered nurse, was working alone on an afternoon shift at Bailey Cottage, part of a complex of supported accommodation and nursing facilities for adults with intellectual disability. Each nurse working in the complex had a personal duress alarm and each cottage had an alarm attached to the wall. These alarms were linked to location lights, which would light up if an alarm had been pressed, enabling staff to identify the cottage in which assistance was required. During Liz's shift, one of the residents of the cottage, Barry, had an angry and abusive outburst. Liz activated her personal alarm to summon other staff. They arrived promptly at the cottage and gave Barry some medication to settle him down.

Liz subsequently went to the nurses' office to complete a report of the incident—a requirement of her work when such events occurred. Barry unexpectedly entered the office as she did so and began punching and kicking her. Liz immediately activated her duress alarm but in the nurses' office it was not connected to any signalling light. Consequently, when two nurses heard it and responded, they were at first unable to find its source. By the time they did arrive at the scene, Liz had already been seriously assaulted.

Immediately following the incident Barry was removed from Bailey Cottage and placed in a more secure unit. Liz sustained severe physical injuries, including extensive bruising and broken ribs, and was diagnosed as suffering a post-traumatic stress injury. She was off work for over two months. One of the nurses who responded to Liz's alarm was also diagnosed with post-traumatic stress syndrome and had a period off work, returning to work on graded hours.

Introduction

This chapter discusses what workplace health is and why it is a significant social problem. There is great public interest relating to workplace health since it influences individual and family costs and the economy in general. Workplace injuries and fatalities happen to a large extent and are of many different types. Further, there is inequity in the distribution of workplace injury and death by occupation, industry, and sex.

Incidents like the one that occurred at Bailey Cottage are not unique. Assaults on nurses by patients and/or their families are surprisingly common. In such situations, a person who commits such an assault may be charged with a criminal offence, but the nurse's employer may also be charged for a breach of occupational health and safety law, depending on the state or territory in which such an offence occurs. Liz's experience, in fact, is based on real-life circumstances in which a large employer within the health and disability services industry was fined over $200,000 by an industrial court judge and ordered to pay the prosecution's costs (see NSW Industrial Relations Commission Decisions 2005). As Liz's case highlights, any injury, illness, or fatality incurred by an employee while at work is a workplace health matter and subject to costly legal sanctions against employers if the health impact is significant. Yet, workplace injuries, illnesses, and deaths are not only of intense legal interest; they also attract regular media coverage frequently provoking wide-ranging community concern and even moral outrage. These responses reflect some of the depth of the public interest in workplace health. They also underlie what is recognised as a major social and public policy problem not only in Australia but in other, comparable, countries belonging to the Organization for Economic Co-operation and Development (OECD), which includes most members of the European Union, Japan, the United Kingdom, the USA, Australia and Canada. This interest is evident in the complex policy and legislative arrangements designed to regulate and minimise workplace injury and fatality in most of these countries (see Malmberg 2003).

A large part of the public interest in serious workplace injuries and deaths derives from the personal and financial costs that individuals and their families incur if they are badly injured or killed at work. The case of the now deceased Bernie Banton is a good example. Bernie developed asbestosis from working in the manufacturing of asbestos products for the company, James Hardie. The following extract of a televised conversation between Bernie, his wife, Karen, and the ABC interviewer, Andrew Denton (ABC TV 2006), provides a glimpse of the personal and family costs of such a disease.

ANDREW DENTON: You worked at Hardies for six years… Was there any talk then about the dangers of asbestos?

BERNIE BANTON: Yes, there was talk about the danger of asbestos, but they never, ever told us that it would kill you.

ANDREW DENTON: The group you worked with were known as the 'Snowmen'. Why was that?

BERNIE BANTON: Because we were covered from head to toe with the white dust of asbestos... all you could see was our eyes.

...

ANDREW DENTON: ...Of the 137 people you worked with at James Hardie BI, how many are still alive?

BERNIE BANTON: Nine.

Such an experience does not only mean reduced financial security for disabled workers but it often involves a radical diminishment in the quality of life of those who are seriously injured and of family members as well, as it did for Bernie Banton and his family (see ABC TV 2006). Financial, interpersonal, and emotional hardship becomes a way of life (Schofield 2005). The extent and severity of the personal and family costs imposed by serious workplace injury and death are depressingly well documented (see Haines 1997; Mayhew & Peterson 1999; Dorman 2000; Royal Australasian College of Physicians 2001; NOHSC 2004). In the USA, one large study found that most of the calculable costs of workplace injury and death were incurred by workers (80 per cent) with the remainder being shared roughly between employers (11 per cent) and consumers (9 per cent) through higher prices (Leigh et al. 1996 cited in Mylett & Markey 2007, p. 20). In Australia, injured workers' share of total financial costs of workplace injury and death is estimated to be less than half that of their US counterparts—reportedly less than 40 per cent of the total (NOHSC 2004). Yet the ruinous impact of severe workplace injuries and deaths in Australia remains a major social problem, as the costs to the national economy demonstrate.

These costs are estimated to be huge. Most such estimates are based on the 'financial drain on the nation's productive capacity' (Purse 2005, p. 8). In 2004, the cost of work-related injury and death in Australia was calculated to be at least $34 billion per year—around 5 per cent of gross domestic product (NOHSC 2004, p. 23). Direct costs include workers' compensation premiums paid by employers to insurance companies, direct payments to injured workers, legal costs, and fines paid to government agencies and the courts. Indirect costs include those associated with equipment damage, disruption of work and decreased productivity, and recruitment and training of replacement workers (Mylett & Markey 2007).

The vast economic expense of workplace injuries and deaths, of course, reflects their widespread and regular occurrence. They are extensive. According to the Australian Safety and Compensation Council (ASCC), located in the Common-wealth Department of Education, Employment and Workplace Relations, there were 162 notified work-related fatalities in Australia over the 12-month period, 2006–07 (ASCC 2007, p. 4). The overwhelming majority of these occurred in workplaces but

30 of them happened on public roads and elsewhere, usually involving 'rollovers of mobile mechanical equipment such as tractors, forklifts and construction vehicles' (ASCC 2007, p. 4). The ASCC figure for workplace deaths is extremely conservative because it involves significant exclusions which the Council itself recognises. These include work-related deaths for which workers' compensation claims were not lodged, deaths from diseases contracted while at work, such as asbestosis, deaths arising in the course of commuting to or from work, and in several states, work-related deaths caused by vehicle accidents on public roads such as rollovers of mobile mechanical equipment. (In some states these deaths are the responsibility of the police and not occupational health and safety authorities, so they do not appear in work-related deaths.) Accordingly, it has been estimated that the real number of deaths from work-related causes is closer to 2000 than 200 per year (NOHSC 2004, p. 3).

Work-related deaths are neither randomly nor evenly distributed throughout the workforce, rather, they are significantly more concentrated in particular industries and occupations. In Australia, the most deadly workplaces, in terms of fatalities per 100,000 workers, are found in four main industries (in descending order): i) mining, ii) agriculture, forestry, and fishing, iii) transport and storage, and iv) construction. The construction industry, however, accounts for the largest number of deaths (more than 25 per cent) among workers by industry (ASCC 2007, p. 5).

Workplace injuries, of course, are far more common than work-related fatalities. The ABS (2006) calculates that in the year to June 2006, 690,000 people who were employed over that period incurred a work-related injury. This amounts to around 6.5 per cent of the workforce (ABS 2006, p. 4). Almost two-thirds (63 per cent) of those who sustained work-related injuries were men. Thus the rate of workplace injury among men was 74 per 1000, while among women it numbered 51 per 1000 —an outcome of the gender-differentiated pattern of employment that prevails in Australia and that is addressed in more detail below.

The most common types of injuries recorded were sprains or strains (30 per cent), followed by cuts or open wounds, and chronic joint or muscle conditions (each 19 per cent) (though again the pattern for sex-based groups was differentiated). In relation to the immediate causes of work-related injury, most were sustained 'through lifting, pushing or pulling an object (32 per cent or 218,400), hitting, being hit or cut by an object (27 per cent or 183,100), falls on the same level (9 per cent or 59,500) and repetitive movements (8 per cent or 56,500)' (ABS 2006, p. 7).

As the ABS figures on the types and causes of work-related injury suggest, most workplace injuries occur in industries and occupations that involve a high degree of manual work and hazardous conditions. So the *industries* with the highest work-related injury rates were agriculture, forestry, and fishing (109 per 1000 employed people), manufacturing (87 per 1000 employed people), and construction and mining (each 86 per 1000 employed people) (ABS 2006, p. 6). The industries with the lowest rates were finance and insurance (19), property and business services (36), and communication services (37). Correspondingly, the *occupations* with the highest rates of people who experienced a work-related injury were production and transport workers (108 per 1000 employed people), tradespersons and related workers (107 per 1000 employed people), and labourers and related workers (106 per 1000 employed people) (ABS 2006, p. 5).

The over-representation of men in the industries and occupations with the highest rates of work-related injury accounts for most of the sex difference in the overall workplace injury rates. The majority of women's work-related injuries also derive from their participation in manual work but in industries in which they are massively over-represented by comparison with men. These are accommodation, cafés and restaurants, retail services, and health and community services (ABS 2006). Men who are employed in these industries have a markedly lower rate of work-related injuries primarily because they do not perform the kinds of work that are physically injurious.

The industries and occupations that incur the greatest rates of work-related injury for both men and women also involve a greater rate of shift work. This is significant because shiftwork is strongly associated with higher work-related injury rates. According to the ABS (2006), 27 per cent of those who incurred a work-related injury in the period 2005–06 were shift workers even though they comprise only 16 per cent of all employed people. Clearly, shiftwork is a major workplace hazard.

So workplace injury and fatality are not likely to happen randomly among members of the workforce. Workplace health damage is patterned, with inequity being a major feature of the pattern. Those employed at the lower levels of the occupational hierarchy—in jobs that involve lots of physical work—are generally low paid, with hours of employment that are less socially conducive (that is, outside the normal 9–5 shift), and more work-intensive (more than 40 hours per week). Such jobs are more 'precarious' (Quinlan et al. 2001; Quinlan 2007), and permit little autonomy or control over the tasks required—workers are much more likely to be injured, made ill, or killed at work. The distribution of workplace health, then, is characterised by major socio-economic inequality (Whitehead 2007; Baum 2008). And while some employed women carry a substantial proportion of this burden, most of it is borne by particular groups of employed men.

How are we to make sense of, or explain, this inequitable distribution of workplace injury and fatality from a sociological perspective? A pattern such as this one is widely understood among sociologists as reflecting the dynamics of **class** (see Chapter 5) in relation to the organisation and distribution of paid work in countries such as Australia. These dynamics basically take the shape of a hierarchy between those who do the work of paid employment and those who create it through their investment—either public or private. A further group of participants is often brought in to assist in organising and managing work. People involved in work creation, organisation, and management, are able to exercise control over employees and derive

class (or social class)
A position in a system of structured inequality based on the unequal distribution of power, wealth, income, and status. People who share a class position typically share similar life chances.

significant economic and social benefits in doing so. Generous financial rewards and organisational power are customary features of the package. Workplace injuries and deaths are not. These are largely the preserve of the lower level employees who carry a greater risk of death and serious injury. These workers are not employed to provide advice about the work they do, the conditions under which they work, or how it should be done. Such concerns are the 'prerogative' of employers and managers, and are usually fiercely defended by the latter as their exclusive territory (McIntyre 2005). Excluding workers from participating in the design and management of their work, and exercising 'managerial prerogative', is a major mechanism of workforce control by employers and managers (Ronnmar 2006). Yet, recent research suggests that where the social organisation and management of work encourage employees' participation, including in arrangements to prevent workplace injuries, then workplace health outcomes are more likely to be better (Frick 2004; Walters 2004).

Interestingly, the class processes at work in the inequitable distribution of workplace injury and death also get played out at the same time as what sociologists call **gender** dynamics (see Chapter 7). These factors, combined with those of class, lead to a greater proportion of men rather than women being killed and seriously injured at work. Like their class-based counterparts, gender dynamics are also embedded in the processes associated with the distribution and organisation of paid work. They are mainly played out through making the 'reproductive distinction' (Connell 2002)—or sex difference—a criterion for who gets to do what jobs and when, how, and with what remuneration. Mining and agricultural work, for example, is now performed almost exclusively by men, but until the early nineteenth century in Britain, the reproductive distinction was of little consequence in such employment (Pahl 1984). In Britain, the 'coal mining industry was several hundred years old by the nineteenth century' (Bartrip & Burman 1983, p. 13), and men, women, and children were all recruited to work in it. The exclusion of women from entry into mining and other industrial work in Britain occurred in the first half of the nineteenth century when organised labour (comprised almost entirely of men), supported by government, prevented women and children from competing with men (Barrett & McIntosh 1982; Walby 1986). This development coincided with the spread of eighteenth century religious and cultural factors that saw the home as the proper place for women and children (Davidoff & Hall 1983).

Such developments involved the assertion of the reproductive distinction as a basic principle of workplace organisation and job allocation. Its subsequent and widespread application has resulted in what sociologists have called the gender-based segregation of employment (Walby 1986; Crompton & Harris 1998; Preston & Whitehouse 2004). This has become an international and enduring phenomenon and one that is especially pronounced in Australia (Preston and Whitehouse 2004). Underpinned by the enactment of the reproductive distinction in employment, it is this process that accounts for the higher rate of major workplace injury and fatality

gender/sex
This pair of terms refers to the socially constructed categories of feminine and masculine (the cultural identities and values that prescribe how men and women should behave), and the social power relations based on those categories, as distinct from the categories of biological sex (female or male).

among men (Schofield 2007a). Combined with class dynamics, it ensures that men in working class jobs are those worst affected. This is not to say that women are immune from health damage arising from gender-segregated employment. As the statistics outlined above show, women employed to do repetitive and/or heavy physical tasks are much more likely to be injured at work than both men and women employed in middle-class jobs—those that are professional, technical, or managerial. For example, occupational over-use syndrome (OOS)—or repetition strain injury (RSI) as it used to be called—is a workplace 'disease' that is significantly higher among women employed as, for example, cleaners, mail sorters, assembly workers, call centre operators, data processing operators, cash register operators, meat processors, sewing machinists, typists, and workers engaged in repetitive clerical work (Bohle & Quinlan 2000). Migrant women from non-English-speaking backgrounds who are employed in 'blue collar' occupations with the highest prevalence (trades, labouring, and related) have been especially at risk (Clapham et al. 1992).

While workplace injury and deaths in Australia are extensive and costly, they have nevertheless decreased markedly over the last century, particularly since the 1970s (Mayhew & Peterson 1999). One of the main reasons for this decline is that the Australian economy has restructured and many of the hazardous jobs, especially in manufacturing, have gone offshore or relocated to 'developing' countries. Recent international comparisons of rates of workplace fatality and 'accidents'—or incidents in the workplace causing three days' or more absence from work—suggest that the Australian pattern is now comparable to that of world leaders in occupational health and safety—the Scandinavian countries of Denmark, Norway, and Sweden (Hamalainen et al. 2006 cited in Mylett & Markey 2007). As Table 6.1 shows, the fatality and accident rates per 100,000 workers in Australia and Norway are almost identical, while in Denmark they are marginally higher and in Sweden, a bit lower.

Table 6.1 Injuries resulting in fatalities and lost time

Country	Fatalities	Fatality rate per 100 000 workers	Accident rate per 100 000 workers
Australia	275	3.2	2 434
New Zealand	61	3.5	2 699
Norway	72	3.2	2 446
Denmark	90	3.4	2 561
China	73 615	10.5	8 028
Spain	1 177	8.9	6 803
Sweden	77	1.9	1 469
United Kingdom	225	0.8	632
United States	6 821	5.2	3 959

Source: Mylett and Markey 2007, p. 21; adapted from Hamalainen et al. 2006

Toni Schofield

state
A term used to
describe a collection
of institutions,
including the
parliament
(government and
opposition political
parties), the public-
sector bureaucracy,
the judiciary, the
military, and the
police.

While economic restructuring has played a central role in reducing Australian workplace injuries and deaths, so, too, have interventions by governments and other agencies that comprise what sociologists call the **state**. Such interventions generally involve the development and implementation of public policy and legislation to prevent workplace deaths and serious injuries by regulating potentially injurious and lethal workplace practices, substances, equipment, conditions, and processes. This kind of public action was initiated in the English-speaking world between 1833 and 1864 with the British Factory Acts (Doyal 1979). Similar legislation was enacted in Australia as the colonial economy gradually industrialised in the late nineteenth century. Today, apart from governments, the main agencies through which the state participates in regulating workplace health are public administrative organisations, such as WorkCover in NSW and WorkSafe in Victoria, and the system of courts, judges, and lawyers that is sanctioned to prosecute those who breach the laws. The state is thus integrally involved in determining the kind of paid work that can be legally conducted and in what ways. From a sociological perspective, the state's role in this arena is not simply one of neutral arbitrator. Rather, the state and its actions are constitutive of the kinds of work that are acceptable, the conditions under which work is conducted, and the patterns of health associated with it.

At the same time, the state's participation in work and health has significant implications for the workforce as industrial citizens (McCallum 2005). In regulating workplaces to prevent health damage to employees, the state in effect recognises that such workers are more than participants in a labour market. State recognition of this kind, as German social theorist Axel Honneth (1995, 2007) proposes, means that workers are understood to be individuals with rights to 'safe' workplaces and to legal and financial redress if they are seriously injured. Such rights usually only prevail in democratic societies where individual participation is understood and valued as a foundation for a fair and equitable way of life (ABS 2004). Obstructing or limiting individuals' participation in employment through injuring or disabling them in the workplace amounts to a breach of industrial rights in a democratic society.

Social responses to workplace health problems

So what are the main social responses to the problem? There is state Occupational Health & Safety (OHS) legislation (state/territory governments make policy and legislation that is administered through bureaucratic agencies and the courts to prevent and deter workplace injury), and there are state/territory workers' compensation and rehabilitation schemes. As outlined above, the state directly influences the extent and severity of workplace injuries and deaths. It does so directly and explicitly by enacting and implementing (or administering) OHS legislation and regulations. In Australia, this process is conducted at state and territory levels. So, for example, the workplace health of employees in New South Wales is governed by the *NSW Occupational Health and Safety Act 2000*. In Victoria, employees are covered by the *Victorian Occupational Health and Safety Act 2004* and in Queensland by the *Queensland Workplace Health and Safety Act 1995*. The variations in OHS legislation throughout Australia have been criticised as creating barriers to improved national workplace health outcomes and economic productivity. In response, the current Commonwealth Rudd Labor Government plans to establish national model occupational health and safety laws to promote greater 'harmonisation' in the state's approach to workplace health regulation (Australian Government 2008).

Despite state and territory variations in OHS law and regulation, all jurisdictions aim to minimise and prevent workplace injury and death. Some sociologists interpret the involvement of the law in workplace health as a form of **social control** by the state (Roach-Anleu 2000). Central to this approach is the idea of deterrence, that is, that prosecutions and hefty fines, imposed on those found guilty of breaching OHS legislation and regulations, will stop or minimise further breaches (Australian Institute of Criminology 2004). This approach is informed by the idea of OHS breaches as criminal activity and those who infringe the law as criminals. Others involved in the study of OHS legislation acknowledge its broad impact as social control but they view it as part of a 'regulatory pyramid of enforcement' (see Ayres & Braithwaite 1992; Johnstone 2004). According to this approach, the base of the pyramid is comprised of techniques to persuade employers to comply with OHS laws and standards (information, education, and advice), while the ascent towards the 'pointy end' is accompanied by increasingly severe punishments designed to deter OHS offences.

It is evident, though, that no one really knows exactly what overall impact the state's legal and regulatory interventions have on preventing or deterring workplace injury and fatality (Schofield 2007b). As international researchers have pointed out, employment injury statistics are extremely unreliable indicators of the impact of legislation and regulation because it is impossible to isolate a specific outcome given the diverse number of other influences reflected in such measures (Hutter 2002; Simpson 2002). It is nevertheless clear, as mentioned previously, that the state is a key player in workplace health. According to some sociologists influenced by French social theorist Michel Foucault, the state's centrality in workplace health is achieved through the system of governance (Hunt & Wickham 1994) the state imposes on workplaces through its OHS legislative and regulatory interventions. From this perspective, governance is effective in securing the state's tenure in workplace health because it involves the exercise of power and dominance. It does so through the deployment of specialised types of knowledge (legal and technical) that most employers, especially in the small business sector, and employees do not have.

Workplace health regulation is not the only means by which the state is involved in dealing with workplace injury. It also plays a key role in managing the problem of

social control
Mechanisms that aim to induce conformity, or at least to manage or minimise deviant behaviour.

injury and incapacitation incurred by workers. It does so through legislation and programs referred to as workers' compensation and rehabilitation. Like their counterparts in OHS regulation, workers' compensation and rehabilitation schemes vary by state and territory in Australia. The first Australian workers' compensation legislation, entitled the *Workmen's Compensation Act 1900*, was passed in South Australia (Purse 2005). Other states soon followed. In New South Wales, for example, workers' compensation was established through a series of Acts from 1910–26 (Cass 1983). The 1926 Act removed the obligation on injured employees to prove that their employment caused their injury. Prior to this, injured employees had to prove employer negligence. The 1926 Act and its counterparts in other states granted injured workers an automatic right to compensation. As such, in legal terms, it was a 'no-fault' scheme. This early legislation reflected public acknowledgment that employers were obliged to accept responsibility for some of the costs of workplace injury (Purse 2005).

The main objective of the early workers' compensation schemes was to ensure income replacement and coverage of medical and other costs for injured workers and their dependants. As noted above, the health and financial costs of workplace injury to individuals and their families can be devastating. Prior to the introduction of workers' compensation legislation in early twentieth century Australia, the victims of serious workplace injury and death, and their family dependants, were often consigned to poverty and charity for survival (Bohle & Quinlan 2000). It was not until organised labour was able to influence and participate in policy and law making, and the allocation of public resources, that seriously injured workers and their dependants were entitled to 'no-fault' income replacement and financial redress for the pain and losses incurred as a result of the injury. This occurred in Australia primarily as a result of trade union demands for parliamentary representation and legislative reform for working, importantly, men. 'The emergence of the Australian Labor Party during the 1890s was a direct expression of these demands' (Purse 2005, p. 10). Significantly, employed women, many of whom were engaged in a range of dangerous jobs in the early twentieth century (Frances & Scates 1993), were not eligible for workplace injury compensation under the new legislation. They were not working men—a further example of the reproductive distinction at work in determining access to social resources.

The first workers' compensation schemes, providing income and payment of medical and ancillary costs to workers laid off from work because of injury, were funded through insurance premiums that employers were compulsorily required to pay under legislation. In New South Wales at that time, workers' compensation premiums were paid to, and managed by, the New South Wales Government Insurance Office (GIO). Employers throughout Australia are still required to make such contributions but they are now managed by a range of insurance companies, predominantly in the private sector (see below). Until the 1980s, workers' compensation was administered by the state through public sector agencies such as the

New South Wales Workers' Compensation Commission established under the 1926 Act to hear all disputes and to regulate and license insurers (Cass 1983).

BOX 6.1 **Doing health sociology: exposing the myth of the 'accident-prone worker'**

Individualistic explanations have figured prominently in explaining workplace health problems, such as the myth of 'kangaroo paw' during the 1980s (referring to Australian workers' alleged predilection to falsely claim workers' compensation for RSI). Michael Quinlan (1993) suggests that such **victim-blaming** views have a long history, and were particularly legitimated from the 1950s onwards through the work of industrial psychologists, who attempted to 'explain' workplace illness as the result of **accident proneness**. Despite years of research, no specific personality traits identifying the 'accident-prone' worker independent of workplace conditions were substantiated. While human error plays a role in workplace injuries, it is usually the result of long hours, high noise levels, poor training, or pressure to produce a certain rate of output that leads to errors being made. Industrial psychologists can face a conflict of interest if employers pay their wage, and their training means that the solutions they offer tend to be individualistic—attempting to modify worker behaviour rather than recommending safer equipment or changes in staffing and shift work.

Key players in the process were the legal and medical professions. Their participation in workers' compensation is sometimes described as the medico-legal management of workplace injury. Some have commented that doctors served as 'gatekeepers' (Quinlan & Bohle 1991, p. 273) to the provisions offered under workers' compensation, and that they continue to do so. As such, doctors are involved in what sociologists describe as the legitimation of workplace injury (Willis 1986; Grbich et al. 1998). The specific practices of this process include identifying and confirming the presence of workplace injury or disease, assessing its severity, and determining its impact on injured workers' physical capacities. Legal professionals are involved in the legitimation process in different ways. Until the 1980s, these consisted largely of adversarial negotiations between legal representatives of an employer (or insurance company) and an employee. These usually occurred in courtroom assessments about whether a worker's injury was caused in the course of employment, the severity of the injury, the extent of permanent disablement and loss, and the amount of compensation to which the injured worker was entitled. Such proceedings were carried out under common law provisions which were separate from workers' compensation legislation. They were a significant mechanism in negotiating the industrial rights of employees. But, as explained further below, dramatic changes in workers'

victim-blaming
The process whereby social inequality is explained in terms of individuals being solely responsible for what happens to them in relation to the choices they make and their assumed psychological, cultural, and/or biological inferiority.

accident proneness
A term invented by industrial psychologists to 'explain' workplace injury and illness. It is based on the false and unproven assumption that workers are careless and malingering, and are therefore solely responsible for accidents.

Toni Schofield

compensation legislation throughout Australia since the 1980s have seen the role of common law and lawyers greatly diminished.

From the very inception of 'no-fault' workers' compensation in Australia, employers complained vehemently and regularly through their state parliamentary representatives about the 'burden of cost' imposed by compulsory workers' compensation (Considine 1991; O'Loughlin 2005). By the 1980s, many employers were threatening to take their investment offshore because the costs of employment, particularly workers' compensation, were rendering business decreasingly profitable. First in Western Australia, followed by Victoria, South Australia, and New South Wales, state governments introduced new workers' compensation legislation specifically to address employers' grievances. The *Workers' Compensation and Rehabilitation Act 1981* (WA), the *Accident Compensation Act 1985* (Vic), the *Workers' Compensation and Rehabilitation Act 1986* (SA), and the *Workers' Compensation Act 1987* (NSW) were passed and heralded a markedly different approach to the public management of workplace injury and compensation (Bohle & Quinlan 2000). At the heart of the new approach were two key features: the return of injured workers to the workplace, and the curtailment of lump-sum payments and injured workers' access to common law. If injured workers were obliged to return to employment after incurring an injury, they would not be reliant on workers' compensation payments, thereby reducing workers' compensation payouts and premiums for employers. More constrained access to lump-sum and common-law payments would also reduce employers' costs.

As a way of offsetting the diminishment in injured employees' rights associated with more limited access to lump-sum payments and common law, the workers' compensation legislative reforms of the 1980s introduced compulsory workplace-based or occupational rehabilitation for seriously injured workers. This was intended not only to reduce the number of injured workers dependent on compensation payments—decreasing the burden of cost to employers—but also to provide opportunities for injured workers to continue to participate in employment. Greater workforce participation, it was proposed by policy makers, would address and resolve the financial and social marginalisation—manifest in experiences of a more restricted social life, mental and emotional difficulties, family breakdown, and so on—that injured workers frequently experienced as a result of their exclusion from paid work and reliance on compensation benefits. Rehabilitation professionals—such as rehabilitation counsellors, physiotherapists, and occupational therapists—would work with the injured worker's treating doctor and the employer to assist the injured worker to return to work, preferably to the same workplace in which the injury occurred. While on compensation and undergoing rehabilitation, injured workers would be paid a fixed weekly amount generally based on the pre-injury award rate for a period of around 26 weeks. Injured workers' claims and payments would be administered by a private insurance company that was an authorised workers' compensation fund manager.

The workers' compensation reforms of the 1980s ushered in a vastly different public approach to managing work injury. Despite consistent government reviews and revisions of the reforms throughout the 1990s and early 2000s, the basic features of the approach remain the same. Some sociologists have described it as 'state-regulated therapeutic management' (O'Loughlin 2005, p. 30) because in the place of access to legal redress for injury, workers are obliged to participate in programs and services administered by health professionals. They are now accorded the status of 'therapeutic clients' (O'Loughlin 2005, p. 30) rather than industrial citizens. In addition, as further sociological research suggests (Parrish & Schofield 2005), seriously injured workers are required to negotiate their entitlements, such as access to rehabilitation and other health services, through a complex administrative process controlled by large insurance corporations. For many who are seriously injured at work this has meant that compensation has become a complex and fraught form of state-regulated welfare governed by corporate imperatives and procedures (Parrish & Schofield 2005). This outcome derives primarily from the fact that the clients of the insurance companies are employers who pay workers' compensation premiums. Accordingly, insurance companies prioritise the objectives of their clients—to minimise premium costs—rather than providing adequate and appropriate services to compensation claimants.

Conclusion

Workplace injuries, illnesses, and deaths continue to be a major social and public policy concern in Australia despite significant improvements in workplace health over the last century. One of the most pronounced features of the pattern of work-place injury and fatality in Australia, and in comparison to other countries, is persistent inequality. This derives basically from the role of class and gender dynamics in the distribution of paid work and its organisation and management. The state—primarily through occupational health law and regulation—interacts in these processes, directly contributing to workplace health outcomes. At the same time, the state has played a vital role in managing the consequences of workplace injury and death through the establishment of workers' compensation schemes. From a social perspective, public attempts to reduce and prevent workplace injury and death, and to provide support for injured workers and their families, may be understood as part of a social democratic project to advance **industrial citizenship**; however, recent workers' compensation policy developments pose serious barriers to achieving such a goal.

industrial citizenship
The right of workers to unionise and take collective action such as strikes, protests, and negotiation over improved pay and working conditions.

Toni Schofield

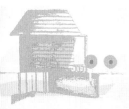

Summary of main points

» Workplace injury, disease, and death continue to be a significant health problem in Australia and elsewhere, resulting in significant personal, social, and economic costs.

» There are around 2000 work-related deaths each year, taking into account accidents and disease.

» A conservative estimate of the economic cost of work-related injury and death suggests it represents at least $34 billion per year in Australia.

» There is a social distribution of work-related health deaths, injuries, and disease, which are highest in particular industries and occupations.

» Systematic public health responses to workplace health problems have been relatively recent, such as OHS legislation, and compensation and rehabilitation schemes.

» Sustained improvement in workplace health continues to flounder on the fundamental conflict of interest between workers' health and profit-maximisation.

Sociological reflection: improving OHS

Workplace health continues to be viewed as an economic burden and many employers and governments have been unwilling substantially to encroach upon managerial prerogative to address ongoing OHS problems.

» What else could employers and governments do to reduce workplace health problems?

Discussion questions

1 Why is workplace health a significant social issue?

2 What does it mean to say that workplace health is inequitable?

3 What do you understand about the role of class and gender in producing workplace health outcomes?

4 What do you understand by the statement that the 'state is constitutive of workplace health outcomes'?

5 In what sense can the development of workers' compensation policy and legislation in Australia be understood as part of a social democratic project to advance citizenship?

6 To what extent are employers and employees mutually served by the prevailing workers' compensation legislation and schemes?

Further investigation

1 Adopt a sociological perspective to discuss the question of what causes workplace deaths and injuries in Australia.

2 What role has the state played in managing the health and financial consequences of workplace injuries and fatalities in Australia? Discuss with reference to at least one state or territory.

Further reading

Daykin, N. & Doyal, L. (eds) 1999, *Health and Work: Critical Perspectives*, Macmillan, London.

Mayhew, C. & Peterson, C. L. (eds) 1999, *Occupational Health and Safety in Australia*, Allen & Unwin, Sydney.

Peterson, C. L. 1999, *Stress at Work: A Sociological Perspective*, Baywood Press, Amityville, NY.

Peterson, C. L. (ed.) 2003, *Work Stress: Studies of the Context, Content and Outcomes of Stress. A Book of Readings*, Baywood Press, Amityville, NY.

Quinlan, M. 1988, 'Psychological and Sociological Approaches to the Study of Occupational Illness: A Critical Review', *Australia and New Zealand Journal of Sociology*, vol. 24, no. 2, pp. 189–206.

Whitehall II Study Team 2004, *Work, Stress and Health: The Whitehall II Study*, PCSU, London.

Web resources

Australian Safety and Compensation Council: <http://www.ascc.gov.au>

National Review into Model Occupational Health and Safety Laws: <http://www.national ohsreview.gov.au/>

Whitehall II Study: <http://www.ucl.ac.uk/whitehallII/>

Online case study
Visit the Second Opinion website to access relevant case studies.

Documentaries/films

Enough Rope with Andrew Denton (2006): 'Bernie and Karen Banton', Episode 10 July', ABC TV. Available online: <http://www.abc.net.au/tv/enoughrope/transcripts/s1679288.htm>

Blue Death (1988): 45 minutes. Four Corners, ABC TV. An award-winning documentary on the thousands of Australians who have died from preventable asbestos-related poisoning.

Toni Schofield

References

ABC TV 2006, 'Bernie and Karen Banton, Episode 10 July', *Enough Rope with Andrew Denton*. Available online: <http://www.abc.net.au/tv/enoughrope/transcripts/s1679 288.htm>

Australian Bureau of Statistics 2004, *Measures of Australia's Progress: Democracy, Governance and Citizenship*, Cat. no. 1370.0, ABS, Canberra.

Australian Bureau of Statistics 2006, *Work-Related Injuries, Australia, 2005–2006*, Cat. no. 6324, ABS, Canberra.

Australian Government 2008, *National Review into Model Occupational Health and Safety Laws: Issues Paper*. Available online: <http://www.nationalohsreview.gov.au/>

Australian Institute of Criminology 2004, 'Understanding Deterrence', *AICrime Reduction Matters*, no. 27. Available online: <http://www.aic.gov.au>

Australian Safety and Compensation Council 2007, *Statistical Report Notified Fatalities, July 2006 to June 2007*, Commonwealth of Australia, Canberra.

Ayres, I. & Braithwaite, J. 1992, *Responsive Regulation: Transcending the Deregulation Debate*, Oxford University Press, NY.

Barrett, M. & McIntosh, M. 1982, 'The "Family Wage"', in E. Whitelegg et al. (eds) *The Changing Experience of Women*, Martin Robertson, Oxford.

Bartrip, P. W. J. & Burman, S. B. 1983, *The Wounded Soldiers of Industry: Industrial Compensation Policy 1833–1897*, Clarendon Press, Oxford.

Baum, F. 2008, *The New Public Health*, 3rd edn, Oxford, Melbourne.

Bohle, P. & Quinlan, M. 2000, *Managing Occupational Health and Safety: A Multidisciplinary Approach*, 2nd edn, Macmillan, Melbourne.

Cass, G. 1983, *Workers' Benefit or Employers' Burden?: A History of Workers' Compensation in NSW 1880–1926*, Industrial Relations Research Centre, UNSW, Kensington.

Clapham, K., Schofield, T. & Alcorso, C. 1992, *Managing the Work Injury of Women from Non-English Speaking Backgrounds*, Report to the National Women's Consultative Council, AGPS, Canberra.

Connell, R.W. 2002, *Gender*, Polity Press, Cambridge.

Considine, M. 1991, *The Politics of Reform: Workers' Compensation from Woodhouse to Workcare*, Centre for Applied Social Research, Deakin University, Geelong.

Crompton, R. & Harris, F. 1998, 'Explaining Women's Employment Patterns: "Orientations to Work" Revisited', *British Journal of Sociology*, vol. 49, no. 1, pp. 118–36.

Davidoff, L. & Hall, C. 1983, 'The Architecture of Public and Private Life: English Middle-class Society in a Provincial Town 1780–1850', in D. Fraser and A. Sutcliffe (eds), *The Pursuit of Urban History*, Edward Arnold, London.

Dorman, P. 2000, *The Economics of Safety, Health and Well-being at Work: An Overview*, ILO:41, Geneva.

Doyal, L. 1979, *The Political Economy of Health*, Pluto Press, London.

Frances, R. & Scates, B. 1993, *Women at Work in Australia from the Gold Rushes to World War II*, Cambridge University Press, Melbourne.

Frick, K. 2004, 'Organisational Development for Occupational Health and Safety Management' in L. Bluff, N. Gunningham & R. Johnstone (eds), *OHS Regulation for a Changing World of Work*, Federation Press, Sydney.

Grbich, C., McGartland, M. & Polgar, S. 1998, 'Regulating Workers' Compensation: The Medico-legal Evaluation of Injured Workers in Victoria', *Australian Journal of Social Issues*, vol. 33, no. 3, pp. 241–63.

Haines, F. 1997, *Corporate Regulation: Beyond 'Punish or Persuade'*, Clarendon Press, Oxford.

Hamalainen, P., Takala, J. & Saarela, K.L. 2006, 'Global Estimates of Occupational Accidents', *Safety Science*, vol. 44, pp. 137–56.

Honneth, A. 1995, *The Struggle for Recognition: The Moral Grammar of Social Conflicts*, Polity Press, Cambridge.

Honneth, A. 2007, *Disrespect: The Normative Foundations of Critical Theory*, Polity Press, Cambridge.

Hunt, A. & Wickham, G. 1994, *Foucault and Law: Toward a Sociology of Law as Governance*, Pluto Press, London.

Hutter, B.M. 2002, *Regulation and Risk: Occupational Health & Safety on the Railways*, Oxford University Press, Oxford.

Johnstone, R. 2004, 'Rethinking OHS Enforcement' in L. Bluff, N. Gunningham & R. Johnstone (eds), *OHS Regulation for a Changing World of Work*, Federation Press, Sydney.

Malmberg, J. (ed.) 2003, *Effective Enforcement of EC Labour Law*, Kluwer Law International, The Hague.

Mayhew, C. & Peterson, C. 1999, 'Introduction: Occupational Health and Safety in Australia', in C. Mayhew & C. Peterson (eds), *Occupational Health and Safety in Australia*, Allen & Unwin, Sydney.

McCallum, R. 2005, 'Industrial Citizenship', in J. Isaac and R. D. Lansbury (eds) *Labour Market Deregulation: Rewriting the Rules*, Federation Press, Sydney.

McIntyre, D. 2005, '"My Way or the Highway": Managerial Prerogative, the Labour Process and Workplace Health', *Health Sociology Review*, vol. 14, no. 1, pp. 59–68.

Mylett, T. & Markey, R. 2007, 'Worker Participation in OHS in New South Wales (Australia) and New Zealand: Methods and Implications', *Employment Relations Record*, vol. 7, no. 2, pp. 15–30.

National Occupational Health and Safety Commission 2004, *The Cost of Work-Related Injury for Australian Employers, Workers and the Community*, NOHSC, Canberra.

NSW Industrial Relations Commission Decisions (2005) *Inspector de Leon-Stacey v The State of NSW (DADHC)*, NSWIRComm 131, April 2005. Available online: <http://www.austlii.edu.au/au/cases/nsw/NSWIRComm/2005/131.html>

O'Loughlin, K. 2005, 'From Industrial Citizen to Therapeutic Client: The 1987 Workers' Compensation "Reforms"', *Health Sociology Review*, vol. 14, no. 1, pp. 21–32.

Pahl, R.E. 1984, *Divisions of Labour*, Basil Blackwell, Oxford.

Parrish, M. & Schofield, T. 2005, 'Injured Workers' Experiences of the Workers' Compensation Claims Process: Institutional Disrespect and the Neoliberal State', *Health Sociology Review*, vol. 14, no. 1, pp. 33–46.

Preston, A. & Whitehouse, G. 2004, 'Gender Differences in Occupation of Employment within Australia', *Australian Journal of Labour Economics*, vol. 7, no. 3, pp. 309–28.

Purse, K. 2005, 'The Evolution of Workers' Compensation Policy in Australia', *Health Sociology Review*, vol. 14, no. 1, pp. 8–20.

Quinlan, M. (ed.) 1993, *Work and Health*, Macmillan, Melbourne.

Quinlan, M. 2007, 'Organisational Restructuring/Downsizing, OHS Regulation and Worker Health and Well-being', *International Journal of Law and Psychiatry*, vol. 30, no. 4–5, pp. 385–99.

Quinlan, M. & Bohle, P. 1991, *Managing Occupational Health and Safety: A Multidisciplinary Approach*, Macmillan, Melbourne.

Quinlan, M., Mayhew, C. & Bohle, P. 2001, 'The Global Expansion of Precarious Employment, Work Disorganisation, and Consequences for Occupational Health: A Review of Recent Research', *International Journal of Health Services*, vol. 31, no. 2, pp. 335–414.

Roach-Anleu, S. L. 2000, *Law and Social Change*, Sage, London.

Ronnmar, M. 2006, 'The Managerial Prerogative and the Employee's Obligation to Work: Comparative Perspectives on Functional Flexibility', *Industrial Law Journal*, vol. 35, no. 1, pp. 56–74.

Royal Australasian College of Physicians 2001, *Compensable Injuries and Health Outcomes*, RACP, Sydney.

Schofield, T. 2005, 'Introduction: The Impact of Neoliberal Policy on Workplace Health', *Health Sociology Review*, vol. 14, no. 1, pp. 5–7.

Schofield, T. 2007a, 'Men's Health and Illness' in M. Flood, J. Kegan-Gardiner, B. Pease, and K. Pringle (eds), *Routledge International Encyclopedia of Men and Masculinities*, Routledge, London.

Schofield, T. 2007b, 'Deterring Workplace Deaths and Injuries: Legal Sanctions and Outcomes or Institutional Process?' in B. Curtis, S. Matthewman & T. McIntosh (eds) *Public Sociologies: Lessons and Trans-Tasman Comparisons: TASA/SAANZ 2007 Joint Conference Proceedings*, Department of Sociology, The University of Auckland.

Simpson, S. 2002, *Corporate Crime, Law & Social Control*, Cambridge University Press, Cambridge.

Walby, S. 1986, *Patriarchy at Work: Patriarchal and Capitalist Relations in Employment*, Polity Press, Cambridge.

Walters, D. 2004, 'Workplace Arrangements for Worker Participation in OHS' in L. Bluff, N. Gunningham & R. Johnstone (eds), *OHS Regulation for a Changing World of Work*, Federation Press, Sydney.

Whitehead, M. 2007, 'A Typology of Actions to Tackle Social Inequalities in Health', *Journal of Epidemiology and Community Health*, vol. 61, no. 6, pp. 473–8.

Willis, E. 1986, 'Commentary: RSI as a Social Process', *Community Health Studies*, vol. 10, no. 2, pp. 210–19.

CHAPTER 7

Gender and Health

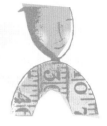

DOROTHY
BROOM

Overview

- What does gender contribute to the understanding of health and illness?
- What have been the origins and main activities of the women's health movement and the men's health movement?
- What factors underlie the different medical treatment given to women and men who have the same health conditions?

MORTALITY RATES IN THE SOVIET UNION

Contrary to mortality patterns internationally, mortality in the former Soviet Union has been rising in recent years. Researchers have been puzzled by this anomalous trend, but because the rise has occurred chiefly among adult men, part of the explanation must be sought in the gendered lives of the population. The question is: how do Russian women and men differ in the nature of their daily lives, paid and unpaid work, recreation and relaxation, sociability and social networks, family and other personal relationships? Somehow, these factors apparently expose men and women to very different risks of the serious illnesses and injuries that lead to premature death. Of course, gender is not operating by itself; there have also been dramatic transformations in the political environment, the economy, and in the opportunity structure that shapes access to the resources necessary to protect and promote health. Deterioration in infrastructure (agricultural and industrial plant and machinery, for example) also appears relevant. However, the stark sex difference suggests that these significant structural dimensions are expressed and experienced very differently in the lives of Russian women and men—so differently that they can make the literal difference between life and death.

Introduction

Because **gender** is such a significant dimension of social difference in contemporary Western societies, we tend to take it for granted. It is hard to imagine that gender could be less socially important or organised very differently from the familiar patterns that we see every day. So it can be surprising to learn that, while gender is socially recognised in all known societies, there is wide historical and cultural variation in the way it is expressed and experienced. In every society, at least some work is allocated on the basis of gender; this allocation is called the **sexual division of labour**. In some societies, females and males undertake sharply differentiated activities, and may be physically segregated for substantial periods, either because of social **norms** or as a consequence of the sexual division of labour. In other societies, children of both sexes are treated in much the same ways, but gender difference becomes important in adolescence or early adulthood. In many cultures, only a few activities are specific to one sex, and the sexual division of labour is minimal. Men dominate overtly in certain cultures; elsewhere, the lives and powers of the two sexes are largely balanced and complementary. In developed economies, the norms and symbols that govern gender tend to vary according to class, subculture, and ethnicity. And everywhere, gender patterns are dynamic: they change over time.

Indeed, the terms themselves are continually contested. In the early 1970s, a distinction was drawn between sex (biological) and gender (psychosocial) (Oakley 1972). Subsequent theoretical discussions have unsettled that clear dichotomy (Gatens 1983; Walsh 2004), and although the contrast is still often invoked, in this chapter the words are used without any reliance on a sharp distinction. A particular central—but often neglected—component of gender is its capacity to consider relevant power structures (Sen et al. 2007).

In the context of such variation and fluidity, making useful generalisations about gender and health is a challenging task. As with both class and ethnicity, the relationship between health and gender is a complex interaction among material circumstances, physical entities, cultural processes, and social organisation. The discussion here concentrates on the interplay between health and gender in Australia and in similar contemporary developed societies.

gender/sex
This pair of terms refers to the socially constructed categories of feminine and masculine (the cultural identities and values that prescribe how men and women should behave), and the social power relations based on those categories, as distinct from the categories of biological sex (female or male).

sexual division of labour
Refers to the nature of work performed as a result of gender roles. In contemporary English-speaking societies, the stereotype is that of the male breadwinner and the female homemaker, even though this pattern is far from an accurate description of most people's lives.

norms
Expectations about how people ought to act or behave, sometimes based in cultural values.

BOX 7.1 Doing health sociology: gendering medical training

For decades, many women feared and avoided pelvic examinations and pap smears because of their doctors' lack of skill or sensitivity. The women's health movement and the health consumers' movement lobbied together for the greater involvement of consumers in medical

· · · ≫

Dorothy Broom

training. As a result, in recent years, some medical schools have employed women as tutors to train doctors to perform these procedures respectfully, and so as to make them as comfortable as possible. A few medical schools include tutors who are examined by medical students, and give feedback to the trainees on how to improve. Despite considerable initial resistance, evaluations indicate that these tutorials are effective learning processes, sensitising trainee doctors regarding the impact of their behaviour on their patients as well as equipping them with improved technical skills.

These arrangements arise from a socio-political analysis of medical encounters and an explicit challenge to traditional models of medical expertise and professional power. They invest authority and power in people who have previously been the objects (and occasionally the victims) of normal medical practice.

Gendered health

gendered health
A term used to acknowledge the different experiences and exposures to health and illness that result from gender.

On the face of it, one might think there is little to explain about the link between gender and health. Humans have sexually specific organs and processes, and malfunction in those organs and processes *is* the relationship between gender and health. Females can get breast and cervical cancer; males can get testicular and prostate cancer. According to this view, the rest of health is just human, not gendered. A discussion of sexually specific complaints hardly exhausts the topic. Many of the conditions that occur in both sexes appear more often in one sex than the other, or they occur at very different ages. For example, stomach cancer is much more common among males than females whereas cardiovascular disease is common in both sexes but tends to occur at later ages among women than among men. These kinds of comparisons suggest that the health of women and men is a product of many elements, and not only reproductive organs. The sexes differ in the types of lives that they typically live, and these differences can influence health. That is, gender is a significant and complex element in the social production of health and illness.

Disease and death: sex comparisons

Except for a very few nations (mostly in South Asia), there are slightly more females in the population than males because women typically live longer than men (Kane 1991), and this is true for contemporary Australia. The Australian population is evenly balanced (50.2 per cent female), but because female life expectancy exceeds male life expectancy by nearly five years , there are proportionally more women in the older population (twice as many women as men aged 85 years and over) (Australian Government Office for Women 2007, pp. 3–4). The gender gap in longevity is gradually closing as male life expectancy has been improving more rapidly than female. Life expectancy for the Indigenous population is markedly shorter than for the total Australian population, but sex differences in longevity prevail among Indigenous as well as non-Indigenous people (see Chapter 8). The main causes of death are largely similar for both sexes, and sexually specific diseases contribute only a small proportion of the overall death rate as is evident in Table 7.1. Dementia looms larger as a cause of death among women than men (because of the higher proportion of women among the elderly), while lung cancer still causes proportionally more deaths among men than women (although this gap has been narrowing).

Table 7.1 Leading causes of death, all ages, 2004

Cause of death	Female		Males	
Ischaemic heart disease	11 424	17.8%	13 152	19.2%
Cerebrovascular disease	7 215	11.3%	4 826	7.1%
Other heart disease	4 272	6.7%	3 290	4.8%
Dementia and related disorders (women)/ diabetes (men)	3 253	5.1%	1 869	2.7%
Breast cancer/prostate cancer	2 641	4.1%	2 761	4.0%
Lung cancer	2 531	3.9%	4 733	6.9%
Chronic obstructive pulmonary disease	2 213	3.5%	2 986	4.4%
Colorectal cancer	1 911	3.0%	2 215	3.2%
Pneumonia and influenza (women)/suicide (men)	1 883	2.9%	1 661	2.4%

Source: Australian Government Office for Women 2007, p.38

Depending on how health is measured, health surveys usually find that the majority of the adult population has some health problem or other at any given time, though many of these health problems are comparatively minor, such as headaches or colds, but substantial proportions of people have a long-term health condition (lasting six months or more). While some of these are minor problems such as visual deficiencies that are readily managed, some are disabling sensory or mobility impairments, or life-threatening diseases such as cancer. In Australia's 2004–05 National Health Survey (NHS), females reported more health problems generally, as well as more diagnosed long-term conditions (ABS 2006).

Excluding hospitalisation related to pregnancy, women and men are equally likely to be admitted to hospitals, but women are more likely to go to the doctor, even when pregnancy-related consultations are omitted, and they are also more likely to consult other health service providers such as chemists, physiotherapists,

Dorothy Broom

and chiropractors. For example, in the 2004–05 NHS, 26 per cent of women and 20 per cent of men had visited a GP in the previous 2 weeks (ABS 2006).

Analyses of such statistics have identified a paradox: women have higher rates of illness, but men die younger. This apparent paradox is at least partly a consequence of oversimplifications—attempts to make sweeping generalisations about the sexes —such as 'women get sick; men die'. On closer inspection, the statistics are not so contradictory. Men tend to experience comparatively higher rates of several life-threatening conditions and **risk factors** such as alcohol abuse and dangerous driving. Women, on the other hand, have relatively high prevalence of painful, unpleasant, but not lethal, conditions such as migraines and arthritis. For example, according to most measures, psychological distress appears to be more common among women than among men (AIHW 1996), but men die from suicide more frequently than women. Furthermore, over the life course, there are variations in certain conditions. Younger men are more likely than younger women to have elevated blood pressure, but by the age of 65, more women are hypertensive. Such variations mean that we must regard simple contrasts between the sexes with caution, since they can conceal as much as they disclose (Macintyre et al. 1996).

An emphasis on sex differences tends to focus our attention on those health conditions for which simple contrasts can be drawn. But in many respects, the sexes are more alike than different, and variations within gender categories (by age or ethnicity, for example) may be more significant. As we have seen in Table 7.1, cancers and cardiovascular disease are the major causes of mortality for all adults. Although there are sex contrasts in the distribution of specific malignancies, cancer is a major threat to the survival and health of adults of both sexes. Everyone falls prey to colds and the flu, and long-term health problems such as sensory impairment can affect anyone. The fact that both sexes can get a condition—even that they get it equally frequently—does not necessarily mean that gender is irrelevant to that condition. Instead, we must look to more subtle patterns to detect the interplay between health and gender, as gender can shape both exposures to health problems and the experience of illness.

risk factors
Behaviours such as poor diet, smoking, or abuse of alcohol that are thought to increase an individual's susceptibility to illness or disease.

Gendered exposures

While the main causes of many illnesses remain uncertain, others have clearly identified risk factors. Smoking is a well-known hazard for a range of serious diseases, and smoking behaviour is sexually differentiated. Among Australians over the age of 18, more men than women smoke daily—19 per cent compared to 16 per cent— and in the past this sex difference was very much more marked (AIHW 2007). Consequently, it is not surprising that more men than women die from lung cancer. Smoking also contributes to the higher male rates of premature morbidity and mortality from cardiovascular and respiratory diseases. Indeed, some writers have suggested that a substantial portion (perhaps half) of the sex difference in longevity may be attributable to smoking (Waldron 1995). While smoking prevalence has gradually declined, the decline began earlier and has been more dramatic among males, and some surveys now find that smoking is more common among adolescent girls aged 14–19 (16 per cent) than in boys of a similar age (14 per cent) (AIHW 2007, p. 6). These comparisons illustrate a dynamic interaction between gender and exposure to a major illness risk factor. Most of the illness effects of current exposure will appear many years in the future, when the relationship between smoking (the 'exposure') and gender may have changed yet again. If young women continue to take up smoking, the sex difference in lung cancer will probably diminish further or even disappear. Already, deaths from lung cancer among women are nearly as common as deaths from breast cancer, although not yet as common as lung cancer deaths among males, which are nearly twice as numerous as deaths from prostate cancer (ABS 2004).

Certain occupations are significant sources of injury and disease, and the sexual division of labour has tended to concentrate men in the occupations in which such hazards are greatest. Construction, mining, waterside work, and farming are examples of comparatively hazardous occupations mainly done by men. Few female-dominated occupations are as dangerous, although the health hazards of women's work (such as office jobs, nursing, and unpaid household and caregiving work) are often harder to detect and may be underestimated (Broom 1986; Doyal 1995; Strazdins & Broom 2004). The nature of the hazards may also differ. For example, the low levels of autonomy, pay, and other rewards in many female-dominated jobs may contribute to women's poor mental health. Such work conditions are known to be related to comparatively poor mental and physical health (Bosma et al. 1997).

Exercise is a health-beneficial behaviour that helps prevent a wide range of significant illnesses, and most young children engage in regular vigorous activity. However, a persistent sex difference emerges in adolescence. Consequently, more adult men (33 per cent) are exposed to the beneficial health effects of moderate or high levels of exercise than are women (26 per cent) (ABS 2006). While physical activity generally improves health, some forms of exercise, particularly contact sports, also expose participants to injury.

The tendency for women to reduce their involvement in exercise may contribute to the fact that more adult women than men are obese, although more men than women are categorised as overweight (AIHW 2004). Being underweight is more prevalent among females. These comparisons point to the fact that both exercise and eating patterns are, to some extent, gendered. The prevalence of disordered eating among young women is a well-known example (MacSween 1993).

Males, especially young men and adolescents, are more likely to engage in a range of dangerous activities such as risky driving, contact sports, and physical aggression.

Dorothy Broom

Consequently, males suffer higher rates of accidental and non-accidental injury. There is considerable debate about gender differences in exposure to violence and its health consequences (Hurst 1996). Males are the main perpetrators of physically violent acts, but they are not the main victims of all kinds of violence (Fletcher 1995). The most visible kinds of violence—such as mugging, street assault, and fights in public places—usually involve males as both aggressor and victim. But sexual assault and domestic violence are overwhelmingly crimes against women, and they constitute a serious threat to the health of many women. In the USA, 'domestic violence is the leading cause of injury among women of reproductive age' (World Bank 1993, p. 50), and women appear to be at particularly high risk when they are pregnant (Stark & Flincraft 1991; Gazmararian et al. 1996). Despite uncertainty regarding exact numbers, the overall picture is similar in Australia and in many other developed societies (Taft et al. 2004). A woman is in more danger of being attacked (ABS 1996b) or killed (Easteal 1993) by a man she knows—particularly by her husband or former partner—than by a stranger. For example, the Women's Safety Survey reported that 338,700 women were victims of physical violence, and 180,400 of these assaults were committed by the women's partners or former partners, nearly three times as many as those where the attacker was a stranger (67,300) (ABS 1996b, p. 19). Australian research has found that 'intimate partner violence is responsible for more ill health and premature death in Victorian women under the age of 45 than any other of the well-known risk factors, including high blood pressure, obesity and smoking' (VicHealth 2004, p. 8). Ninety per cent of all domestic violence deaths were women (Sherrard et al. 1994, p. 42). In summary, women's and men's vulnerability to violence is sharply differentiated and socially situated.

Gendered experiences

The example of violence points directly to a consideration of how gender shapes the experience of health conditions. A particular injury, such as a concussion or laceration, may be physically the same, regardless of how one was injured, but the personal meaning and social consequences will be very different depending on whether the injury was sustained in a car accident, a mugging by a stranger, a pub fight with a drinking companion, or an attack by one's intimate partner. The first three of those sources of injury are likely to be singular or relatively rare events, to be publicly recognised, and to receive immediate assistance. By contrast, 'wife bashing' is apt to be repeated and escalating, shrouded in shame and secrecy, and often concealed from health care workers. Indeed, the source of injury is frequently undetected, even when injuries are so severe that the victim presents at an emergency service (Roberts 1994). While any injury can leave emotional scars, the psychological impact of being attacked by a parent or loved and trusted partner is particularly devastating and personally debilitating. Because females are typically shorter and lighter than males, and are less likely to have learned skills of self-defence, women are often poorly equipped to protect themselves if their partner becomes violent. In the rare instance in which a man is attacked by a female partner, other elements of shame and denial may enter the picture because of the implicit insult to masculine power and strength. Thus, the experience of violent assault is highly variable and contains important gender dimensions. Even public violence among males is gendered insofar as displays of toughness and aggression are often considered markers of masculinity, so that men and boys who try to avoid violent behaviour may be victimised themselves (Plummer 1999).

Another area shaped by gender is the diagnosis and treatment of heart disease. Research in the USA, Britain, and Australia suggests that cardiovascular symptoms may be investigated less thoroughly and treated less intensively in women than they are in men (Ayanian & Epstein 1991; Steingart et al. 1991). Sometimes the difference may reflect excessive intervention in the treatment of men (Bicknell et al. 1992), or variations in living arrangements and mortality before admission (Sonke et al. 1996), while other studies suggest that certain women may miss out on potentially beneficial therapies (Tobin et al. 1987; Lawlor et al. 2001). Although some researchers believe that women's high mortality after a heart attack is accounted for by pre-existing risk factors, this does not fully explain the sex discrepancies (Feibach et al. 1990), and there is evidence of systematic underdiagnosis and undertreatment of women. The failure to pursue symptoms vigorously would be an understandable result of the erroneous belief that women do not get heart disease, or that they get it only in advanced old age. This might make doctors less likely to suspect heart disease in a woman, and hence less likely to investigate it thoroughly or manage it appropriately when it occurs (McKinlay 1996). It may also promote the belief among women and their families that heart disease is not a women's health problem, and therefore that the risk factors or symptoms are not important. Surprisingly, although these issues have been studied for two decades, very recent research shows that doctors still tend to diagnose and manage patients with symptoms of heart attack differently, leading to the identification of a pattern the researchers called 'gendered ageism' (Arber et al. 2006).

Similar gender differences have been documented in admissions to intensive care units and in the treatment of a range of critical illnesses (Fowler et al. 2007). A popular impression prevails—perhaps shared by doctors—that men are prone to ignore symptoms, and that their elevated mortality is a consequence of their reluctance to seek medical care, but systematic research does not consistently confirm that idea (Macintyre 1999). Instead, American and British studies found that women who have symptoms of a heart attack are more likely than men to delay seeking care (Meischke et al. 1993; Emslie et al. 2001; Martin et al. 2004). Researchers now suspect that heart disease (and perhaps other illnesses) may be characterised by different symptoms in females and males, so that clinical definitions of 'classic cases' derived from males could contribute to under-diagnosis of women. While such

Dorothy Broom

factors may account for delays and failures in diagnosing, they would not explain inadequate treatment of women once a diagnosis has been achieved.

Even such apparently trivial illnesses as colds and flus may be experienced in ways that are organised and given meaning by gender (Macintyre 1993). For example, because of women's responsibilities for unpaid domestic work (Bittman 1991) and their concentration in casual employment (with no paid sick leave), they may find it particularly difficult to stay in bed when they are ill. Married men are more likely to be in full-time employment and hence to be unavailable to supply domestic care to ailing family members, but when those same men get sick, they may have paid sick-leave as well as a supportive wife. These patterns, and the lifelong habits and material circumstances to which they contribute, are particularly important with regard to the care of people with severe or chronic illness. Among older people, women are twice as likely as men to live alone and hence to have no co-resident who can care for them when they are sick or frail. Women are more likely to need care from outside the household at some time during their lives, and so have a different interest in state-funded services (Gibson & Allen 1993; OSW 1999).

Many of the patterns described above are inflected by other social variables such as **class**, **'race'**, and **ethnicity**. For example, in some cultures, the expectation that health care will be supplied by members of the family (usually women) obstructs access to health and community services delivered by agencies or professionals. In Australia, when family members cannot supply needed support, ill and elderly migrants can be disadvantaged by their reluctance to use the services they need.

Class has been found to correlate with most measures of health: better health is consistently associated with higher status. The relationship between health and socio-economic status prevails for both sexes, but the relative importance of various elements of social and material circumstances is, to an extent, distinctive for women and men (Arber 1991; Macintyre 1997; Broom 2008). It has been difficult to establish appropriate measures of status for the whole population because of women's interrupted labour-force involvement and part-time employment to accommodate child rearing. All these examples show how the experience of illness may be gendered in subtle and complex ways, even for conditions that are not sexually specific. They also illustrate how the relationship between health and gender can be complicated by other dimensions of social difference (see the other chapters in this section of the book for further detail).

Responding to gendered health and illness

For many years, it was commonly assumed that the gendered patterning of disease and death was a simple 'fact of nature' that humans could do little or nothing about. Culture and medicine constantly modify facts of nature. Many health problems lead

---

class (or social class)
A position in a system of structured inequality based on the unequal distribution of power, wealth, income, and status. People who share a class position typically share similar life chances.

'race'
A term without scientific basis that uses skin colour and facial features to describe what are alleged to be biologically distinct groups of humans. Race is actually a social construction used to categorise groups of people and sometimes implies assumed (and unproven) intellectual superiority or inferiority.

ethnicity
Sociologically, the term refers to a shared cultural background, which is a characteristic of all groups in society. As a policy term, it is used to identify migrants who share a culture that is markedly different from that of Anglo-Australians. In practice, it often refers only to migrants from non-English-speaking backgrounds (NESB migrants).

to severe illness, injury, or death if they are not treated, but in most societies they are not allowed to run their course if they can be controlled. The best approaches to gendered health are less obvious than how to treat post-operative infection or catastrophic bleeding. It is one thing to describe the way gender interacts with health and illness; it is quite another to determine when those interactions are creating problems, and to discern how individuals, communities, and societies might respond constructively.

A problem identified over three decades ago has been referred to as **sexism in medicine**. Originally this term pointed to the sexual division of labour in medical care where most doctors were men and nearly all nurses were women. Nursing is still mainly a female profession, but the medical workforce is now much more gender balanced, particularly among primary care doctors, although most medical specialties are still male-dominated (Chur-Hansen & Elliott 2007). Another early concern focused on the 'sexist' behaviour of some doctors. Far from signalling a constructive sensitivity to the potential relevance of gender, sexism in medicine included behaviour that was at best objectionable and at worst dangerous. Anecdotal evidence was substantiated by systematic research showing that doctors sometimes did not interact appropriately with their women patients (Broom-Darroch 1978). They failed to hear or accept women's accounts of their symptoms and did not inform women about unwanted effects of drugs and other therapies. Furthermore, doctors have been prone to label women's problems as psychiatric or psychosomatic rather than 'real' (Barrett & Roberts 1978). The movement of substantial numbers of women into medicine does not automatically improve care for women, due to medical socialisation. Still, there is evidence that the changing sex ratio is also changing aspects of medical culture in ways that may diminish some of the most offensive and harmful aspects of sexism in medicine (Pringle 1998).

Historically, women in Australia have had difficulty getting access to birth-control services (Matthews 1984), especially if doctors felt that those women (young, unmarried, divorced, or disabled) should not be sexually active. The advent of family planning services and women's health centres has substantially alleviated the problem in most metropolitan areas, but it remains a significant health issue in many nations and in some rural areas of Australia.

Research

Service providers striving to give women the best possible care have been handicapped by limited medical research on women and their health problems. Until recently, men and other male animals have been the main, or only, subjects of most studies of disease, diagnostic procedures, management, therapy, and prevention (Melbourne District Health Council 1990). Often, even when women are included, no analysis by gender is reported (Greenberger & Marts 2000). One consequence

sexism in medicine Refers to doctors' discriminatory and harmful treatment of women by ignoring women's health concerns in medical research and intervention, not informing women of the availability of other treatments or the side effects of drugs/ therapies, and labelling of women's problems as 'psychosomatic' rather than 'real'.

has been the comparative neglect of many women's health concerns, except those that are directly relevant to fertility (Eckerman 1999), which is arguably the women's health domain of most interest to men. Consequently, often relatively little is known about how non-reproductive disorders may manifest themselves differently in women and men, how risk factors may vary, or how the sexes may differ in their response to therapeutic interventions such as drugs (Woosley et al. 2000).

While these deficiencies persist (Vidaver et al. 2000), they are gradually being addressed by the growth in gender-specific research, and by major longitudinal initiatives such as the 'Million Women' study in the UK and the 15-year Women's Health Initiative in the USA (Finnegan 1996) which included **randomised control trials** of the effects of diet and hormone replacement therapy in preventing breast and colorectal cancer, heart disease, and osteoporosis (for current information see <http://www.nhlbi.nih.gov/whi/>). In the 1990s, the Australian Government sought to remedy the neglect of women's health research by funding a major longitudinal study, beginning data collection in 1996 (Brown et al. 1996). The study recruited more than 40,000 respondents in three age cohorts to investigate such issues as reproductive health problems, access to services, stress, and time use.

The exclusion of women from research has significant implications for population health. For example, a number of drugs originally approved for general use have later been found to affect men and women quite differently, in some instances necessitating their withdrawal from the market, most frequently when they are belatedly found to be ineffective for or harmful to women (Woosley et al. 2000). Furthermore, a variety of non-lethal but difficult women's health conditions, such as endometriosis, remain poorly understood. Also, concerns that have been identified by women, such as overweight, poverty (Redman et al. 1988), and violence (Jones 1996), were for many years not considered as 'health' issues by researchers and largely escaped scrutiny.

Getting masculinity on the agenda

Perhaps a surprising aspect of the traditional perspective is that it has neglected masculinity—as well as femininity—in health and health research. This may seem paradoxical in light of the male domination of medicine, the focus on males in research, and the privileging of the male body as normal. But it is less surprising when we note that these processes have occurred without being explicitly theorised, and hence until recently, there was no conscious or thoughtful attention to masculinity *per se*. While men have featured in medical research and often in **health promotion** campaigns (Keleher 2004), there was little effort to consider how masculinity may figure in health and disease; the example of smoking has already been introduced. Although it was mainly a male activity for several decades, few people except advertisers have paid attention to its function as a means of confirming

---

randomised control trials (RCTs)
A biomedical research procedure used to evaluate the effectiveness of particular medications and therapeutic interventions. 'Random' refers to the equal chance of participants being in the experimental or control group (the group which receives a placebo or no treatment at all and is used for comparison), and 'trial' refers to the experimental nature of the method. RCTs are often mistakenly viewed as the best way to demonstrate causal links between factors under investigation, but tend to privilege biomedical over social responses to illness.

health promotion
Any combination of education and related organisational, economic, and political interventions designed to promote behavioural and environmental changes conducive to good health, including legislation, community development, and advocacy.

and displaying certain forms of masculinity. More interest in the gender—not to mention class—implications of smoking, and hence of quitting, might have reduced men's smoking sooner.

Efforts to promote dietary change and exercise must also take gender seriously if they are to be effective. Alcohol consumption and drunkenness have been socially accepted behaviours for men, and are almost required in some circles of adolescent and young adult men. They are also becoming common among some young women. The similar prevalence of tobacco use or drunkenness should not be assumed to have the same meanings, social sources, or consequences for women and men (Broom 2008). For example, women were originally recruited to smoke when smoking prevalence was very high among men; and while prevalence has declined in both sexes, the decline has been much more rapid among males than females. Young people who take up smoking now do so in a very different social and symbolic environment. The social and sexual signification of smoking continues subtly to shape tobacco use in gender-specific ways (Nichter et al. 2006; Gilbert 2007). For example, it appears that young males have more alternative ways (such as sport) to establish attractive adolescent identities, whereas young females may risk appearing 'uptight' to their peers if they do not smoke (Plumridge et al. 2002).

In recent years, increased awareness of the pertinence of masculinity to health has stimulated a dramatic rise in research (Robertson 2003) and commentary on a wide range of issues, including policies (Smith 2007) and services (Bentley 2006). There are now books devoted to the topic (Robertson 2007) as well as several specialist journals, and new teaching and research programs have been established. These initiatives promise to enhance the basis on which fully elaborated approaches to gendered health can be developed.

Because gender is so much a part of the taken-for-granted world (Connell et al. 1999), it is easy to rely on anecdotes and stereotypes to interpret gendered patterns in health without realising that it is happening. For example, it is popular to refer to male risk-taking behaviour; but such generalised allusions are of much less value than information on *which* males take risks, which risks in what circumstances, how their masculinity might be implicated in their behaviour, or how masculinity might be mobilised to diminish risk. A positive example is available in a study that investigated the culture surrounding particular sports, whose participants were more liable to engage in violent behaviour, as a way of understanding the specific dynamics involved in a stereotyped form of male health risk (Greager 2007).

Another striking exception to the tendency to ignore or oversimplify masculinity has been the case of homosexual men dealing with HIV/AIDS. Their efforts have been distinguished by a focus on the lives of specific groups of men, and they have sought to transform prevention into a positive and pleasurable part of gay masculinity. Indeed, recent increases in HIV incidence suggest it may be time to revisit and perhaps revise the strategies in light of social change and related behaviour change.

Dorothy Broom

Research into how HIV was originally controlled in Australia may supply valuable directions for the appropriate incorporation of gender in future research.

These examples point to the need for six major shifts in order to improve research (including applied research) on health:

1   the inclusion of women in clinical trials and epidemiological research
2   routine analyses of health and medical data by gender
3   the investigation of health issues to which women and men themselves give priority
4   an understanding that 'women's health' and 'men's health' include conditions beyond reproduction
5   the study of women's and men's health in their own right, and not simply in comparison with each other or when disease prevalence differs by sex
6   the study of how particular forms or aspects of gender (specific masculinities and femininities) are distinctively related to health.

The women's health movement

By some accounts, contemporary sensitivity to the relationship between gender and health was initially created by the renascent women's movement, beginning in the late 1960s (Broom & Doyal 2004). Since that time, what might loosely be termed the **women's health movement** has worked to change the face of health services for women, and there is now substantial evidence of such change. Participants in this movement were the first to identify sexism in medicine (discussed above), and many of the movement's early activities were efforts to overcome sexism. Women have advocated innovations such as:

women's health movement
A term broadly used to describe attempts to address sexism in medicine by highlighting the importance of gender in health research and services. Achievements include women's community health centres and Australia's 1989 National Women's Health Policy.

• improvements and expansion in health services
• safer, cheaper, and more accessible contraceptives
• better access to terminations of pregnancy
• changes in medical education and increases in the number of women in medical practice
• encouragement of multidisciplinary teams in the delivery of health care
• fostering support groups to enable women to help one another.

All of these are occurring, at least to an extent.

In contemporary Australia, perhaps the single most visible manifestation of the movement is the existence of several dozen predominantly community-based, feminist-influenced women's health centres. At the time of writing, these centres are located in every state and territory, mostly in large urban areas, but some are in regional centres, country towns, and smaller cities. They have come into being largely as a result of community-based action that has sought to establish services that are controlled by women and more appropriate to women's needs, as defined by women themselves (Broom 1991). Because they are now such a familiar part of the Australian health care landscape, readers may be surprised to learn that their origins were highly contentious. Despite the fact that most of the activities of women's health centres do not duplicate those supplied by mainstream medicine (Broom 1997), doctors in private practice feared that centres would compete for their clientele, or they objected to the employment of what they thought were 'unqualified' women's health workers. Several women's health centres were opened with minimal funding and relied heavily on volunteer labour and donations of money and materials. A few centres were notorious for their political radicalism, but almost all have sought to influence the mainstream, recognising that most women will obtain most health services from conventional sources. Reliance on government funding, a commitment to serving the most vulnerable clients, and the desire to encourage doctors and hospitals to become more 'woman friendly' are all issues that have confronted women's health centres with dilemmas and challenges: how are they to preserve their feminist independence and still be respectable enough to exert influence on the mainstream? They were partially legitimised as a strategy of the National Women's Health Policy (Gray 1998) and have become better established since the first centres opened in 1974. Nevertheless, and despite their long waiting lists, opposition persists and some commentators now claim that they have become obsolete.

Governments respond

Governments—both state and Commonwealth—have responded to women's community-based action by developing women's health strategies, policies, and programs. Much of this activity took place during the 1980s and 1990s, with particular focus on the National Women's Health Policy (Commonwealth Department of Community Services and Health 1989) and the program for its implementation. Despite their apparent legitimacy, such developments have not been without their critics. During the early 1990s, considerable energy was expended defending a complaint against women's health initiatives and services brought by a male doctor (then employed by the Commonwealth Department of Health). The complaint used the *Sex Discrimination Act 1984* (Cwlth) to assert that women's health services discriminate against men. It was heard by the President of the Human Rights and Equal Opportunity Commission (HREOC) in 1991 and 1992, and the decision upheld the lawfulness of special women's health activities (Broom 1994). Nevertheless, by the mid-1990s, diminished resources for health, reallocation of previously targeted women's health funding, and an increasingly conservative political climate, began to accomplish what the discrimination complaint could not: the partial winding-back of women's health services. It is unclear what impact—if any—might result from further political changes.

Dorothy Broom

The Fourth World Congress on Women in Beijing brought women's health issues to an international forum (Van Wijk et al. 1996). Globally, a very broad range of common principles in health care (universal access, gender sensitivity, and appropriateness) were identified. The most urgent health needs, however, are nationally and locally specific. The emphasis in developing countries is on clean water, adequate fuel for cooking and heat, secure food supplies, and basic maternal and infant health. In developed countries, the focus tends to be more on dignity in medical treatment, participation in decision-making, better care for chronic conditions such as cancer, and reducing inequalities in access to services. Clearly there can be overlap on many issues—such as access to safe means of fertility control and real choice about when to use them—but most priorities tend to be specific rather than universal.

Men's health: progress or threat?

men's health
Running parallel to women's health initiatives, the men's health movement recognises that certain elements of masculine identity and behaviour can be hazardous to health.

The emerging focus on **men's health** in Australia and other English-speaking countries follows the women's health movement by about twenty years (Sabo & Gordon 1995; Primary Health Care Group 1996; Baker 2001). It has benefited from a number of the theoretical and political developments that resulted from the women's health movement, but identifies distinctive issues and strategies (Fletcher 1995). For example, goals such as reducing drink-driving and other highly risky behaviours are central elements on a men's health agenda, particularly for young men. Suicide is an urgent priority. Early detection of unhealthy weight, high blood pressure, and other 'lifestyle' risk factors forms the focus of relatively recent health promotion targeting middle-aged men, including screening checks at workplaces.

Specific subgroups of men have particular needs, as is evident from the activities of gay men in relation to HIV/AIDS. Resonating with women's health initiatives, men's health advocates have identified the importance of investigating the role of masculinity in men's health, recognising that certain elements of masculine identity and behaviour can be hazardous to health. For Indigenous men, the threats of morbidity and premature mortality from substance abuse, violence, and complications of diabetes loom very large (Rowley et al. 2008). These insights suggest that improving men's health will entail slow and careful shifts in understandings of what it means to be a man in contemporary society.

In Australia, seven Commonwealth-sponsored national men's health conferences have been held since 1995. The conference in 2003 combined the 5th National Men and Boys' Health Conference with the 3rd National Indigenous Male Health Convention. A national centre of excellence in male reproductive health (Andrology Australia) was established with Commonwealth funding in 1999, and at the 7th National Men's Health Conference in 2007, the Freemasons launched 'Foundation 49' to promote men's health and a new men's health research centre in Adelaide. Initial steps towards a national men's health policy (Primary Health Care Group 1996) were taken in the mid-1990s at the direction of the then Commonwealth Health Minister, Carmen Lawrence. Although a change of government halted the process (Lumb 1997, 2003), several states have subsequently taken modest initiatives. A variety of school and community-based health training and education, and health promotion programs have also been developed to target men's health issues, including parenting. Both the Australian Medical Association (AMA) and the Royal Australian College of General Practitioners (RACGP) now have official statements on men's health.

Some women's health advocates are nervous about men's health initiatives. The anxiety is provoked in part by the stark realities of tiny budgets for community health activities, and a perception that resources for men's health will be taken from hard-won, vulnerable, and poorly funded women's health programs. Such fears are inflamed by episodes such as the discrimination case brought before the HREOC, summarised previously, and by the rhetoric of a few individuals who assert that the accomplishments of women's health services have been made at the expense of men's health. Some commentators argue that women's health initiatives rely on feminist claims that women are 'victims' and that women are 'sicker' than men. These critics of women's health go on to assert that it is not women but men whose health is disadvantaged by sex, that attention to women's health is misplaced and the focus should be shifted to men. As we have seen above, such generalisations about which sex is 'sicker' are unlikely to be informative empirically, and they are still less likely to work to improve the health of men or women.

Most men's health advocates see neither women nor women's health services as enemies. They are aware that both lay people and health professionals—both women and men—are now beginning to explore how various forms of masculinity may enhance or detract from men's health. Mothers and wives who become aware of neglected health problems in their sons and husbands have been among those who have stimulated the increased activity and awareness of diseases such as testicular cancer. Equally important, attention to the relationship between gender and health stands to benefit both women and men.

Future directions: towards a gendered understanding of health

In the future we may have to think of gender as a much more complicated concept than the simple dichotomous variable to which most of us are accustomed. Some writers now suggest that it is time to move towards gender-specific approaches that 'provide greater interpretive richness and give full voice to the complexity of the socially constructed meaning of gender' (Kunkel & Atchley 1996, p. 295). We must remember that such dimensions as 'race', ethnicity, and age are all implicated in gender in ways that cannot be reduced to binary thinking. A person is not Black at one moment and male the next: he is always a Black male (among many other things). The implications of such connections present challenges to accurate and constructive research about health and gender, and to the development and delivery of appropriate health promotion and medical care services. Complex models may be awkward and more intellectually demanding than a simple bivariate model, but greater complexity promises more fruitful and ultimately more practical ways of thinking about contemporary social life and the health patterns with which it is inextricably entangled. A productive analysis of gender involves taking both masculinity and femininity seriously, and appreciating that gender is an aspect of every person's individual experience and social life. Femininity and masculinity are complex sources of risks and benefits, simultaneously—but differently—constraining and empowering.

Broad social, political, and economic change, the accomplishments of the women's health movement, and the emergence of activity regarding men's health, have all altered the context in which health is created and managed. They have also effected subtle shifts in the meanings of gendered subject positions. For example, from the embattled beginnings of the women's health movement in the early 1970s, women's health has become more 'mainstream' and established, despite its continuing vulnerability, and the identities of all the actors (participants, supporters, and opponents) are modified by these developments (Singleton 1996). Approaches to funding health services and measuring their productivity are also in considerable flux throughout the developed world. All these and other changes have altered fundamental aspects of the way health and gender are understood, and therefore the way research, services, and advocacy will proceed in the future. While it is not clear how or by whom the next phase will be defined, it seems likely that revised assumptions and alliances will be necessary, and that attention to gender—not simply to women—will be a feature of developing understandings of health. If that is so, it will not be before time.

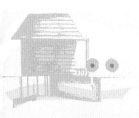

Summary of main points

» The typical way of life of each sex differs, and these differences can influence health. The statement that 'women get sick; men die' is an oversimplification. Men experience comparatively higher rates of life-threatening conditions, while women have a relatively high prevalence of some painful, but not lethal, conditions. Binary gender contrasts must be treated with caution since they can conceal as much as they disclose.

» A number of studies have shown that sexism in medicine has resulted in objectionable and harmful treatment of women by doctors, such as doctors ignoring women's accounts of their symptoms, not informing women about unwanted effects of drugs and other therapies, labelling women's problems as 'psychosomatic' rather than 'real', and failing to diagnose and treat serious illnesses in women.

» Until recently, men have been the main subjects of most medical research. Such bias is based on an assumption that the 'normal' body is not subject to such processes as hormonal cycling, pregnancy, lactation, or menopause, and that females can therefore be excluded from research.

» The women's health movement has advocated safer, cheaper, and more accessible contraceptives; better access to terminations of pregnancy; changes in medical education and increases in the number of women in medical practice; encouragement of multidisciplinary teams in the delivery of health care; women's health centres; and the National Women's Health Policy.

» Most men's health advocates see neither women nor women's health services as enemies. Attention to gender and health stands to benefit both women and men.

» Social change—including changes prompted by the advocacy of women's and men's health activists—are altering the environment in which health policy is developed, health services are delivered, and health and illness are experienced.

Sociological reflection: gender and smoking

Smoking rates among teenaged women in Australia are very similar to those among similarly aged men. How therefore can gender still be relevant to understanding adolescent smoking? How is experimenting with cigarettes different for young women and men? What about refusing offers to smoke? What about becoming a regular (rather than experimental or occasional smoker)? How does smoking operate to support certain gendered social relations and undermine others? What about gendered personal identities? What does smoking or sharing cigarettes symbolise to and say about young men? Young women?

Discussion questions

1   In what ways is gender an important factor in determining the exposure to, and experience of, health and illness?

2   Why is the statement 'women get sick; men die' an oversimplification of the link between gender and health?

Dorothy Broom

3   What are some examples of 'sexism in medicine' and how can it be addressed?

4   Can you summarise some of the explanations of why sexual assault and domestic violence are overwhelmingly perpetrated by men against women?

5   Why is the women's health movement necessary?

6   Why is the men's health movement necessary?

Further investigation

1   How successful has the women's health movement and the entry of increasing numbers of women into the medical profession been in addressing 'sexism in medicine'?

2   Examine the ways in which femininity and masculinity result in gendered exposures and gendered experiences of health and illness.

Further reading

Annandale, E. & Hunt, K. (eds) 2000, *Gender Inequalities and Health*, Open University Press, Buckingham.

Broom, D. H. 1991, *Damned if We Do: Contradictions in Women's Health Care*, Allen & Unwin, Sydney.

Doyal, L. 1995, *What Makes Women Sick: Gender and the Political Economy of Health*, Macmillan, London.

Ehrenreich, B. & English, D. 1979, *For Her Own Good: 150 Years of Experts' Advice*, Pluto Press, London.

Fee, E. & Krieger, N. (eds) 1994, *Women's Health, Politics, and Power: Essays on Sex/Gender, Medicine, and Public Health*, Baywood, New York.

Robertson, S. 2007, *Understanding Men and Health: Masculinities, Identity and Well-being*, Open University Press/McGraw Hill, Berkshire.

Rosenfeld, D. & Faircloth, C. A. 2006, *Medicalized Masculinities*, Temple University Press, Philadelphia.

Sabo, D. & Gordon, D. F. (eds) 1995, *Men's Health and Illness: Gender, Power and the Body*, Sage, Thousand Oaks, CA.

Web resources

Australian Longitudinal Study of Women's Health: <http://www.alswh.org.au/>

Australian Women's Health Network: <http://www.awhn.org.au/>

International Journal of Men's Health
<http://www.mensstudies.com/content/120391/>
Journal of Men's Health
<http://www.elsevier.com/wps/find/journaldescription.cws_home/714640/description#
description >
Men's Bibliography by Michael Flood: <http://mensbiblio.xyonline.net/>
National Centre for Epidemiology and Population Health: <http://nceph.anu.edu.au/>
Women's Health Initiative (USA): <http://www.nhlbi.nih.gov/whi/>

Online case study
Visit the Second Opinion
website to access
relevant case studies.

Documentaries/films

Dance Me to My Song (1998): 101 minutes. An Australian film directed by Rolf de Heer; about a woman dealing with cerebral palsy and her belligerent carer.

The Shape of Water (2006): 70 minutes. A documentary narrated by Susan Sarandon about five women striving for social justice in their developing countries. Available online: <http://www.theshapeofwatermovie.com/>

References

Arber, S. 1991, 'Class, Paid Employment and Family Roles: Making Sense of Structural Disadvantage, Gender and Health Status', *Social Science & Medicine*, vol. 32, no. 4, pp. 425–36.

Arber, S., McKinlay, J., Adams, A., Marceau, L., Link, C. & O'Donnell, A. 2006, 'Patient Characteristics and Inequalities in Doctors' Diagnostic and Management Strategies Relating to CHD: A Video-simulation Experiment', *Social Science & Medicine*, vol. 62, no. 1, pp. 103–15.

Australian Bureau of Statistics 1996b, *Women's Safety Australia*, Cat. no. 4128.0, ABS, Canberra.

Australian Bureau of Statistics 2004, *AusStats: Year Book Australia*, ABS. Available online: <www.abs.gov.au>

Australian Bureau of Statistics 2006, *2004–05 National Health Survey: Summary of Results*, Cat. no. 4364.0, ABS, Canberra.

Australian Institute of Health and Welfare 1996, *Australia's Health 1996*, AGPS, Canberra.

Australian Institute of Health and Welfare 2004, *Australia's Health 2004*, AIHW, Canberra.

Australian Institute of Health and Welfare 2007, *Statistics on Drug Use in Australia 2006: Drug Statistics Series no. 18*, Cat. no. PHE80, AIHW, Canberra.

Australian Government Office for Women 2007, *Women in Australia 2007,* Commonwealth of Australia, Canberra.

Ayanian, J. Z. & Epstein, A. M. 1991, 'Differences in the Use of Procedures between Men and Women', National Men's Health Conference, AGPS, Canberra, pp. 100–11.

Baker, P. 2001, 'The International Men's Health Movement', *British Medical Journal,* vol. 323, no. 7320, pp. 1014–15.

Barrett, M. & Roberts, H. 1978, 'Doctors and their Patients', in C. Smart & B. Smart (eds), *Women, Sexuality and Social Control,* Routledge, London, pp. 41–52.

Bentley, M. 2006, 'A Primary Care Approach to Men's Health in Community Health Settings: It's Just Better Practice', *Australian Journal of Primary Health,* vol. 12, no. 1, pp. 21–6.

Bicknell, N. A., Pieper, K. S., Lee, K. L., Mark, D. B., Glower, D. D., Pryor, D. B. & Calif, R. M. 1992, 'Referral Patterns for Coronary Artery Disease Treatment: Gender Bias or Good Clinical Judgment?', *Annals of Internal Medicine,* vol. 116, no. 10, pp. 791–7.

Bittman, M. 1991, *Juggling Time: How Australian Families Use Time,* Office of the Status of Women, Canberra.

Bosma, H., Marmot, M. G., Hemingway, H., Nicholson, A. C., Brunner, E. & Stansfeld, S. A. 1997, 'Low Job Control and Risk of Coronary Heart Disease in Whitehall II (Prospective Cohort) Study', *British Medical Journal,* vol. 314 (22 February), pp. 558–65.

Broom, D. 1986, 'The Occupational Health of Houseworkers', *Australian Feminist Studies,* vol. 2, pp. 15–34.

Broom, D. 1991, *Damned if We Do: Contradictions in Women's Health Care,* Allen & Unwin, Sydney.

Broom, D. 1994, 'Taken Down and Used against Us', in C. Waddell and A. R. Petersen (eds), *Just Health: Inequality in Illness, Care and Prevention,* Churchill Livingstone, Melbourne, pp. 397–405.

Broom, D. 1997, *There Should Be More: Women's Use of Community Health Facilities,* National Centre for Epidemiology and Population Health, Canberra.

Broom, D. H. 2008, 'Gender in/and/of Health Inequalities', *Australian Journal of Social Issues,* in press.

Broom, D. H. & Doyal, L. 2004, 'Sex and Gender in Health Care and Health Policy', in J. Healy and M. McKee (eds), *Health Care: Responding to Diversity,* Oxford University Press, Oxford.

Broom-Darroch, D. 1978, 'Power and Participation: The Dynamics of Medical Encounters', PhD thesis, Australian National University, Canberra.

Brown, W., Bryson, L., Byles, J., Dobson, A., Manderson, L., Schofield, M. & Williams, G. 1996, 'Women's Health Australia: Establishment of the Australian Longitudinal Study on Women's Health', *Journal of Women's Health,* vol. 5, no. 5, pp. 467–72.

Chur-Hansen, A. & Elliott, T. E. 2007, 'Medical Education and the Medical Workforce in Australia', *Journal of Continuing Education in the Health Professions*, vol. 272, no. 1, pp. 34–5.

Commonwealth Department of Community Services and Health 1989, *National Women's Health Policy: Advancing Women's Health in Australia*, AGPS, Canberra.

Connell, R. W., Schofield, T., Walker, L., Wood, J., Butland, D., Fisher, J. & Bowyer, J. 1999, *Men's Health: A Research Agenda and Background Report*, Commonwealth Department of Health and Aged Care, Canberra.

Doyal, L. 1995, *What Makes Women Sick: Gender and the Political Economy of Health*, Rutgers University Press, New Brunswick, NJ.

Easteal, P. W. 1993, *Killing the Beloved: Homicide Between Adult Sexual Intimates*, Australian Institute of Criminology, Canberra.

Eckerman, E. 1999, 'Towards a New Gendered and "Differentiated" Social Epidemiology', in L. Hancock (ed.), *Analysing Health Policy*, Allen & Unwin, Sydney.

Emslie, C., Hunt, K. & Watt, G. 2001, 'Invisible Women? The Importance of Gender in Lay Beliefs about Heart Problems', *Sociology of Health & Illness*, vol. 23, no. 2, pp. 203–33.

Feibach, N. H., Viscoli, C. M. & Horwitz, R. I. 1990, 'Differences between Women and Men in Survival after Myocardial Infarction', *Journal of the American Medical Association*, vol. 263, no. 8, pp. 1092–6.

Finnegan, L. P. 1996, 'The NIH Women's Health Initiative: Its Evolution and Expected Contributions to Women's Health', *American Journal of Preventive Medicine*, vol. 12, no. 5, pp. 292–3.

Fletcher, R. 1995, *An Introduction to the New Men's Health*, University of Newcastle, Newcastle, NSW.

Fowler, R. A., Sabur, N., Li, P., Juurlink, D. N., Pinto, R., Hladunewich, M. A., Adhikari, N. K. J., Sibbald, W. J. & Martin, C.M. 2007, 'Sex- and Age-based Differences in the Delivery and Outcomes of Critical Care', *Canadian Medical Association Journal*, vol. 177, no. 11, pp. 1513–19.

Gatens, M. 1983, 'A Critique of the Sex/Gender Distinction', in J. Allen & P. Patton (eds), *Beyond Marxism? Interventions After Marx*, Intervention Publication, Leichhardt, pp. 139–157.

Gazmararian, J. A., Lazorick, S., Spitz, A. M., Ballard, T. J., Saltzman, L. E. & Marks, J. S. 1996, 'Prevalence of Violence Against Pregnant Women', *Journal of the American Medical Association*, vol. 275, pp. 1915–20.

Gibson, D. & Allen, J. 1993, 'Phallocentrism and Parasitism: Social Provision for the Aged', *Policy Sciences*, vol. 26, pp. 79–98.

Gilbert, E. 2007, 'Constructing "Fashionable" Youth Identities: Australian Young Women Cigarette Smokers', *Journal of Youth Studies*, vol. 10, no. 1, pp. 1–15.

Gray, G. 1998, 'How Australia Came to have a National Women's Health Policy', *International Journal of Health Services*, vol. 28, no. 1, pp. 107–25.

Greager, D. A. 2007, 'Unnecessary Roughness? School Sports, Peer Networks, and Male Adolescent Violence', *American Sociological Review*, vol. 72 (October), pp. 705–24.

Greenberger, P. & Marts, S. A. 2000, 'Women in NIH-funded Research Studies: There's Good News, and There's Bad News', *Journal of Women's Health & Gender-Based Medicine*, vol. 9, no. 5, pp. 463–4.

Hurst, D. 1996, 'Men's Violence and Men's Health: Some Recent Worldwide Trends', in Commonwealth Department of Human Services and Health (ed.), *Proceedings of the National Men's Health Conference*, AGPS, Canberra, pp. 125–32.

Jones, W. K. 1996, 'Centres for Disease Control and Prevention', *American Journal of Preventive Medicine*, vol. 12, no. 5, p. 410.

Kane, P. 1991, *Women's Health: From Womb to Tomb*, Macmillan, London.

Keleher, H. 2004, 'Why Build a Health Promotion Evidence Base about Gender?', *Health Promotion International*, vol. 19, no. 3, pp. 277–9.

Kunkel, S. R. & Atchley, R. C. 1996, 'Why Gender Matters: Being Female is not the Same as Not Being Male', *American Journal of Preventive Medicine*, vol. 12, no. 5, pp. 294–6.

Lawlor, D. A., Ebrahim, S. & Davey Smith, G. 2001, 'Sex Matters: Secular and Geographical Trends in Sex Differences in Coronary Heart Disease Mortality', *British Medical Journal*, vol. 323, no. 7312, pp. 541–5.

Lumb, P. 1997, 'An Early Death? Australian Men's Health Policies', in A. Huggins (ed.), *Second National Men's Health Conference: Conference Proceeding*, Curtin University of Technology, Perth, pp. 194–200.

Lumb, P. 2003, 'Why is Men's Health and Well-being Policy not Implemented in Australia?', *International Journal of Men's Health*, vol. 2, no. 1, pp. 73–88.

Macintyre, C. 1999, 'From Entitlement to Obligation in the Australian Welfare State', *Australian Journal of Social Issues*, vol. 34, no. 2, pp. 103–29.

Macintyre, S. 1993, 'Gender Differences in the Perceptions of Common Cold Symptoms', *Social Science & Medicine*, vol. 36, no. 1, pp. 15–20.

Macintyre, S. 1997, 'The Black Report and Beyond: What are the Issues?', *Social Science & Medicine*, vol. 44, no. 6, pp. 723–45.

Macintyre, S., Hunt, K. & Sweeting, H. 1996, 'Gender Differences in Health: Are Things Really as Simple as they Seem?', *Social Science & Medicine*, vol. 42, no. 4, pp. 617–24.

MacSween, M. 1993, *Anorexic Bodies: A Feminist and Sociological Perspective on Anorexia Nervosa*, Routledge, London.

Martin, R., Lemos, K., Rothrock, N., Bellman, S. B., Russell, D., Tripp-Reimer, T., Lounsbury, P. & Gordon, E. 2004, 'Gender Disparities in Commonsense Models of Illness among Myocardial Infarction Victims', *Health Psychology*, vol. 23, pp. 345–53.

Matthews, J. J. 1984, *Good and Mad Women: The Historical Construction of Femininity in Twentieth Century Australia*, Allen & Unwin, Sydney.

McKinlay, J. B. 1996, 'Some Contributions from the Social System to Gender Inequalities in Heart Disease', *Journal of Health and Social Behaviour*, vol. 37, pp. 1–26.

Meischke, H., Eisenberg, M. S. & Larsen, M. P. 1993, 'Prehospital Delay Interval for Patients Who Use Emergency Medical Services', *Annals of Emergency Medicine*, vol. 22, no. 10, pp. 1597–601.

Melbourne District Health Council 1990, *A Sliver—Not Even a Slice*, District Health Councils of Victoria, Melbourne.

Nichter, M., Nichter, M., Lloyd-Richardson, E. E., Flaherty, B., Carkoglu, A. & Taylor, N. 2006, 'Gendered Dimensions of Smoking among College Students', *Journal of Adolescent Research*, vol. 21, no. 3, pp. 215–43.

Oakley, A. 1972, *Sex, Gender and Society*, Sun Books, Melbourne.

Office of the Status of Women. 1999, *Women in Australia*, OSW, Canberra.

Plummer, D. 1999, *One of the Boys: Masculinity, Homophobia, and Modern Manhood*, Haworth Press, Binghamton, NY.

Plumridge, E. W., Fitzgerald, L. J. & Abel, G. M. 2002, 'Performing Coolness: Smoking Refusal and Adolescent Identities', *Health Education Research*, vol. 17, no. 2, pp. 167–79.

Primary Health Care Group 1996, *Draft National Men's Health Policy*, Commonwealth Department of Human Services and Health, Canberra.

Pringle, R. 1998, *Sex and Medicine: Gender, Power and Authority in the Medical Profession*, Cambridge University Press, Cambridge.

Redman, S., Hennrikus, D. J., Bowman, J. A. & Sanson-Fisher, R. W. 1988, 'Assessing Women's Health Needs', *Medical Journal of Australia*, no. 148, pp. 123–7.

Roberts, G. L. 1994, *Domestic Violence Victims in a Hospital Emergency Department*, Department of Psychiatry, University of Queensland, St Lucia.

Robertson, S. 2003, 'Men Managing Health', *Men's Health Journal*, vol. 2, no. 4, pp. 111–13.

Robertson, S. 2007, *Understanding Men and Health: Masculinities, Identity and Well-Being*, Open University Press/McGraw Hill, Berkshire.

Rowley, K. G., O'Dea, K., Anderson, I., McDermott, R., Saraswati, K., Tilmouth, R., Roberts, I., Fitz, J., Wang, Z., Jenkins, A., Best, J. D., Wang, Z. & Brown, A. 2008, 'Lower than Expected Morbidity and Mortality for an Australian Aboriginal Population: 10-year Follow-up in a Decentralised Community', *Medical Journal of Australia*, vol. 188, no. 5, pp. 283–7.

Sabo, D. & Gordon, D. F. (eds) 1995, *Men's Health and Illness: Gender, Power and the Body*, Sage, Thousand Oaks, CA.

Sen, G., Ostlin, P. & George, A. 2007, *Unequal, Unfair, Ineffective and Inefficient: Gender Inequity in Health—Why it Exists and How We Can Change It (Final Report to the WHO Commission on Social Determinants of Health: Women and Gender Equity Knowledge Network)*, Karolinska Institutet, Stockholm.

Sherrard, J., Ozanne-Smith, J., Brumen, I. A., Routley, V. & Williams, F. 1994, *Domestic Violence: Patterns and Indicators*, Monash University, Melbourne.

Singleton, V. 1996, 'Feminism, Sociology of Scientific Knowledge and Postmodernism: Politics, Theory and Me', *Social Studies of Science*, vol. 26, pp. 445–68.

Smith, J. A. 2007, 'Addressing Men's Health Policy Concerns in Australia: What Can Be Done?', *Australia & New Zealand Health Policy*, vol. 4, no. 20, pp. 1–4. Available online: <http://www.anzhealthpolicy.com/content/4/1/20>

Sonke, G. S., Beaglehold, R., Stewart, A. W., Jackson, R. & Stewart, F. M. 1996, 'Sex Differences in Case Fatality Before and After Admission to Hospital After Acute Cardiac Events: Analysis of Community Based Coronary Heart Disease Register', *British Medical Journal*, vol. 313, pp. 853–5.

Stark, E. & Flincraft, A. 1991, 'Spouse Abuse', in M. Rosenberg & A. Finley (eds), *Violence in America: A Public Health Approach*, Oxford University Press, New York, pp. 161–81.

Steingart, R. M., Packer, M., Hamm, P., Colianese, M. E., Gersh, B., Geltman, E. M. et al. 1991, 'Sex Differences in the Management of Coronary Artery Disease', *New England Journal of Medicine*, vol. 325, no. 4, pp. 226–30.

Strazdins, L. M. & Broom, D. H. 2004, 'Acts of Love (and Work): Gender Imbalance in Emotional Work and Women's Psychological Distress', *Journal of Family Issues*, vol. 25, no. 3, pp. 356–78.

Taft, A. J., Watson, L. F. & Lee, C. 2004, 'Violence against Young Australian Women and Association with Reproductive Events: A Cross-sectional Analysis of a National Population Sample', *Australian and New Zealand Journal of Public Health*, vol. 28, no. 4, pp. 324–9.

Tobin, J. N., Wassertheil-Smoller, S., Wexler, J. P., Steingart, R. M., Budner, N., Lense, L. & Wachspress, J. 1987, 'Sex Bias in Considering Coronary Bypass Surgery', *Annals of Internal Medicine*, vol. 107, pp. 19–25.

Van Wijk, C. M. T. G., Van Vliet, K. P. & Kolk, A. M. 1996, 'Gender Perspectives and Quality of Care: Towards Appropriate and Adequate Health Care for Women', *Social Science & Medicine*, vol. 43, no. 5, pp. 707–20.

VicHealth 2004, *The Health Costs of Violence: Measuring the Burden of Disease Caused by Intimate Partner Violence (Summary of findings)*, Victorian Health Promotion Foundation, Melbourne.

Vidaver, R. M., Lafleur, B., Tong, C., Bradshaw, R. & Marts, S. A. 2000, 'Women Subjects in NIH-funded Clinical Research Literature: Lack of Progress in both Representation and Analysis by Sex', *Journal of Women's Health & Gender-Based Medicine*, vol. 9, no. 5, pp. 495–504.

Waldron, I. 1995, 'Contributions of Changing Gender Differences in Behavior and Social Roles to Changing Gender Differences in Mortality', in D. Sabo & D. F. Gordon (eds), *Men's Health and Illness: Gender, Power and the Body*, Sage, Thousand Oaks, CA, pp. 22–45.

Walsh, M. 2004, 'Twenty Years Since "A Critique of the Sex/Gender Distinction": A Conversation with Moira Gatens', *Australian Feminist Studies*, vol. 19, no. 44, pp. 213–24.

Woosley, R. L., Anthony, M. & Peck, C. C. 2000, 'Biological Sex Analysis in Clinical Research', *Journal of Women's Health & Gender-Based Medicine*, vol. 9, no. 9, pp. 933–4.

World Bank 1993, *World Development Report 1993: Investing in Health*, Oxford University Press, New York.

ACKNOWLEDGMENT

I am grateful to James A. Smith for information regarding AMA and RACGP statements on men's health and for several references on men's health research and policy initiatives.

Dorothy Broom

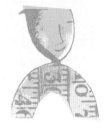

CHAPTER 8

Indigenous Health: The Perpetuation of Inequality

**DENNIS
GRAY
and
SHERRY
SAGGERS**

Overview

- What is the extent of Indigenous health inequality?
- What has been done to address this inequality?
- Why do health inequalities persist?

AN INDIGENOUS LIFE

Mary is 70 years old and one of the few Indigenous people of her generation still living. She is a battler who has lived a hard life. Under the old assimilation policy, she was taken from her Aboriginal mother and put in a 'home'—the memories of which still induce occasional bouts of depression. Her husband Jack, who was 4 years older than Mary, died at the age of 46 of smoking-related lung cancer. For a long period before his death—after being evicted from a pastoral station at around the time that 'equal wages' and 'drinking rights' were introduced—he drank heavily. Mary had five children, two of whom are dead—one boy died from diarrhoea at the age of 18 months, and another boy died in a car accident when he

was 22 years old. She loves them all, but of the three living children, she is most proud of Ron, who is a successful artist living interstate.

Mary moved to the city just over 20 years ago, where she lives in a three-bedroom housing commission house. The house is also occupied by her daughters Joan and Margaret, Joan's 'man' Ken, and five of Joan's and Margaret's six children. Initially, this arrangement was to have been temporary, but since Ken lost his job it has become a financial necessity. Mary shares one bedroom with Margaret, Ken and Joan have the second bedroom, and Jenny and Karen (Margaret's 20- and 18-year-old daughters) share the third bedroom with Donna (Ken and Joan's 15-year-old). To provide sleeping accommodation for Ken junior and John—their 13- and 9-year-old boys—Ken and Joan set up an old caravan in the yard.

The house was not designed for this many people. Although Mary and her daughters do their best, it is almost impossible to keep the place clean, and, with all the wear and tear, fittings such as fly screens are broken and the septic tank often overflows. In these circumstances, infections such as colds and flu are frequent occurrences and in the past one or other of the kids has picked up lice and spread them to other family members. Also, there is no room for the kids, who are still at school, to do their homework.

Ken used to count himself as 'one of the lucky ones'. Unlike many of the Aboriginal men in the neighbourhood, he had a job—as a storeman at a freight terminal. He used to say, 'It don't pay much, but it stops me from goin' nuts an' keeps me off the piss'. One day, he injured his back helping his brother put an engine in an old car and could no longer work. 'It gives me the shits,' he says. 'I've worked 'ard all me life and now people treat me like a bludger.' Since the accident, Ken has started drinking heavily—a source of conflict between him and Joan's family.

As well as worrying about Ken's drinking, Mary is also concerned about the use of other drugs by some of her 'grannies' (grandchildren). 'Ganja' (cannabis) and, to a lesser extent, 'ice' (methamphetamine) are available in the local community and she knows that Jenny and Karen have occasionally used them.

With the income they receive from social security entitlements, no one in the family goes hungry. However, because it is difficult to cook for so many at once, or for everyone to be in the kitchen, they eat a lot of fast food, which the kids love. Mary knows that too much of this food is not good for them, particularly without vegetables. She tries to supplement the fast food with fruit, but on their income this is expensive.

For a long time now, Mary has been considerably overweight; she finds it difficult to get around, and she has diabetes, one consequence of which is failing eyesight. Nevertheless, until about 5 years ago Mary was active on the committee of the local Aboriginal child-care centre that she helped to establish. 'It's important to do things for the young people,' she says, 'we 'ad nothin'. No decent education. No good jobs. Always poor. Always battlin'. Same for me kids—'cept maybe for Ronnie. But we gotta keep tryin'. Do things ourselves. Make it better for the grannies.'

Introduction

Mary is not simply a statistic. Her story represents the life experiences of many Indigenous people in this country, and it helps to explain why too many Indigenous people are sick and die early. In this chapter we attempt to reveal the 'public issues' behind these intensely 'personal troubles' (Mills 1959, p. 14).

Dennis Gray and Sherry Saggers

Evidence of Indigenous health inequality

Despite calls going back almost three decades, there is still no comprehensive national system for the collection of data on the health of Indigenous Australians. Nevertheless, the data that are available provide dramatic evidence of the health inequalities faced by Indigenous people. A key indicator of this is life expectancy, which measures '... the average number of years a person of a given age and sex can expect to live, if current age–sex–specific death rates continue to apply throughout his or her lifetime' (ABS & AIHW 2008, p. 154). Based on data for the period 1996–2001, life expectancy at birth for all Australian males and females was estimated to be approximately 77 and 82 years respectively; for Indigenous Australian males and females the expectancies were approximately 17 years less (ABS & AIHW 2008, p. 154).

The main causes of mortality among Indigenous and non-Indigenous Australians are similar: cardiovascular diseases; external causes such as accidents, poisoning, and violence; respiratory disorders; various forms of cancer; and diseases of the digestive system, but in the period 2002–05, Indigenous people died from these causes between 1.5 and 4.3 times the rates among non-Indigenous people. In addition, the mortality rate for endocrine, nutritional, and metabolic diseases (excluding diabetes) was 7.5 times greater among Indigenous men and 10.1 times greater among Indigenous women, and for diabetes was 10.8 and 14.5 times greater for Indigenous men and women (ABS & AIHW 2008, p. 161).

Hospitalisation data are key indicators of morbidity (sickness). In 2005–06, for all conditions the rate of hospitalisations among Indigenous people was over twice as great as that among non-Indigenous Australians. The most common reasons for hospitalisation were injury and accidents, respiratory disease, diseases of the digestive system, mental and behavioural disorders, and kidney dialysis, and, additionally for women, complications of pregnancy and childbirth. In the particular case of kidney dialysis, the rate of hospitalisation was 13.5 times as great as that in the non-Indigenous population (ABS & AIHW 2008, p. 108).

Hospitalisations are only an indicator of ill health. They do not include the heavy burden of illness that is either treated in other settings or that goes untreated. As well as particular illnesses *per se*, a number of underlying **risk factors** are of concern. These include **alcohol misuse**, smoking, and obesity. In addition to medical awareness, understanding the higher prevalence of these problems requires a 'sociological imagination' (Mills 1959).

Alcohol misuse is a major health risk factor among all Australians but its impact is heightened among Indigenous people. Despite some variation in the methods used and the resulting estimates (Chikritzhs & Brady 2006), various studies have concluded—although Indigenous Australians are more likely to be either lifetime abstainers or to have given up drinking—that those who do drink are likely to do so at levels which pose risks for their health. The most recent National Drug Strategy

risk factors
Conditions, such as alcohol misuse, smoking, and poor diet, that are thought to increase an individual's susceptibility to illness or disease.

alcohol misuse
Excessive consumption of alcohol leading to health and/or social problems.

Household Survey found that 21.3 per cent of Indigenous people do not currently drink, 38.7 per cent drink at levels likely to cause risk or high risk to their health in the short term, and 22.7 per cent drink at levels likely to cause risk or high risk to their health in the long term. Comparable percentages for the non-Indigenous population are 16.1 per cent, 20.5 per cent, and 9.7 per cent (AIHW 2005). These high rates of consumption are reflected in mortality and hospitalisation rates, and in social problems such as violence, sexual assaults, neglect of children, crime, and threats to culture and tradition.

In the Australian population as a whole, tobacco smoking has been identified as the largest single preventable cause of death and disease and it accounted for 15 per cent of all deaths in 1998 (ABS 2006). In the Indigenous population—where the prevalence of smoking is double that among non-Indigenous people—its impact is even greater. It underlies the higher rates of stroke, heart disease, lung cancer, and respiratory diseases such as emphysema.

Indigenous people are more likely to be exposed to violence than non-Indigenous people—much of which is under-reported. In 2005–06, Indigenous males were 6 times, and Indigenous females were 33 times, more likely to be hospitalised for assault-related injuries (ABS & AIHW 2008, p. 126). Self-harm—including suicide and attempted suicide—also occurs more frequently among Indigenous people (ABS & AIHW 2008, p. 169).

Linked to issues of self-harm are broader questions in relation to mental health. Of particular relevance here are the experiences of the **'stolen children'**. The report of the National Inquiry into the Separation of Aboriginal and Torres Strait Islander Children and their Families estimated that in the years 1910–70, between one in three and one in ten children were forcibly removed from their families (HREOC 1997). Many of those people and their descendants have suffered and continue to suffer a wide range of mental health and social problems related to those experiences. A national study found that rates of depression, self-harm, and suicide are considerably higher among Indigenous people; substance misuse, domestic violence, child abuse, and disadvantage were additional risk factors; and that 'trauma and grief were seen as overwhelming problems' (Swan & Raphael 1995, p. 1).

All of the above demonstrate vividly the extent to which health inequalities are experienced by Indigenous people. Most people have an opinion about why these inequalities persist, despite increasing allocations of funds to health care. As sociologists, we need to examine how ill health is socially produced and maintained.

Social production of Indigenous ill health

Sociological, as opposed to **biomedical**, explanations of ill health attempt to throw light on why people from different social groups are differentially—rather than randomly—afflicted by disease and illness. Numerous studies have demonstrated

'stolen children'
Children who were forcibly removed from their families during the nineteenth and twentieth centuries by the agents of government in order to assimilate them into mainstream Australia.

biomedicine
The conventional approach to medicine in Western societies, based on the diagnosis and explanation of illness as a malfunction of the body's biological mechanisms. This approach underpins most health professions and health services, which focus on treating individuals, and generally ignores the social origins of illness and its prevention.

relationships between health status and social indicators such as class, ethnicity, and gender. One of the most dramatic illustrations of this is provided by the 'Whitehall study' from the United Kingdom. The study found that male civil servants in the lowest employment grade had a mortality rate that was four times higher than that among those in the highest grade, and there was a clear social gradient affecting total mortality and all major causes of death (Wilkinson & Marmot 2003). Similar inequalities based on socio-economic disadvantage have been demonstrated in Australia (Turrell & Mathers 2000).

Among Indigenous Australians, in 2006 the average household income (adjusted for differences in family size) was $362 compared to $642 among non-Indigenous people. Similarly, in the same year, only 4 per cent of Indigenous people aged 25–65 years had a diploma or advanced diploma and only 5 per cent had a university degree (compared to 9 per cent and 21 per cent among non-Indigenous Australians) (ABS & AIHW 2008, pp. 11 & 19). Given the socio-economic disadvantage reflected in these figures, poor Indigenous health status should come as no surprise (Carson et al. 2007).

Racism, too, has been implicated as a key determinant of ill health (Paradies 2006). For example, Indigenous Australians who reported racist experiences in a rural Western Australian town were more likely to have poorer mental health, physical health, and self-reported general health (Larson et al. 2007).

Despite such findings, **health discourses** are dominated by theories attributing much ill health to the risky behaviour of individuals (Brown & Bell 2006; Baum 2007). The trouble with this type of analysis is that it ignores the demonstrated links between health and socio-economic status and blames those least able to take control of their lives and institute healthy practices (Wilkinson & Marmot 2003).

The importance of social factors in the production of Indigenous Australian ill health is further highlighted by looking at comparative data from Canada and New Zealand. The patterns are distressingly similar. What underlie them are common colonial histories involving the **dispossession** and subsequent marginalisation of indigenous peoples.

Colonialism and dispossession

The invasion and subsequent settlement of Australia by the British was justified by the legal fiction of **terra nullius**, under which particular territories were declared 'unoccupied'. The term reveals the **ethnocentric** belief that the Indigenous occupants of the continent had no claim to the land, because they did not exploit it as Europeans would. With a population estimated at 750,000, and consisting of groups with hundreds of distinct languages and cultures, Indigenous peoples maintained a hunter-gatherer existence in highly diverse environments. Unlike sedentary agriculturalists, Indigenous Australians depended upon large tracts of land for their foraging, and

health discourses
A domain of language use that is characterised by common ways of talking and thinking about health.

dispossession
The removal of people from land they regard as their own.

terra nullius
A Latin term used by the British legally to define Australia as an unoccupied land belonging to no one and therefore open to colonisation.

ethnocentric
Viewing others from one's own cultural perspective, with an implied sense of cultural superiority based on an inability to understand or accept the practices and beliefs of other cultures.

their relationship to that land was cemented in a complex network of sacred stories and rituals.

Evidence from early historical accounts and studies among contemporary hunter-gatherers, indicates that the health status of the Indigenous Australians at the time of the British invasion was better than that of most people then living in Britain. This does not mean, however, that they were free from disease. Parasitic and infectious diseases were present, although experienced far less frequently than in settled populations, and people would have experienced various physical injuries. To cope with these problems an elaborate **traditional medical system** was developed.

The traditional medical system was not equipped, of course, to deal with the health consequences of the colonial invasion. Within a few years of European settlement, the basics of good health—such as adequate shelter and nutrition—were no longer available to many Indigenous people. Understanding the historical context in which dispossession, depopulation, and the disintegration of traditional societies occurred is fundamental to an understanding of the current health status of Indigenous people in this country.

The colony of New South Wales was founded with the twin aims of providing a dumping ground for convicts and thwarting French colonial intentions. It was expected that the colony would become economically self-supporting as soon as practically possible. The availability of convict labour meant that Indigenous labour was largely superfluous to colonial requirements. The colonists were instructed by the British Government to live at peace with Indigenous peoples.

Initial dispossession occurred around early settlement sites and nearby rural areas, and it was in those locations that the disastrous impacts of introduced diseases such as smallpox were soon described. As this process continued, within 150 years of the first European settlement, the Indigenous population was decimated under the impact of introduced diseases and direct frontier violence. It is important to note that this process of dispossession and its consequences did not occur without resistance (Reynolds 1995). This has continued to the present and has included pastoral strikes (by shearers and others), freedom rides, and the establishment of a Tent Embassy in front of Parliament House to protest against the lack of Indigenous sovereignty (Ginsberg & Myers 2006).

Australian economic development is largely based upon the exploitation of natural resources appropriated from Indigenous peoples. The private sector has primarily been concerned to remove Indigenous people from their land in order to facilitate that development and maximise returns on its capital investment. Except in the agricultural industry and, to a lesser extent, the pearling and sealing industries—where their labour was required—Indigenous people have been marginal to this economic development. On one hand, government policy has been to appropriate, or sanction the appropriation of, land and to curb any resistance to it; on the other hand, it has been to attempt to ameliorate the effects of this appropriation.

traditional medical system
Indigenous beliefs and practices about health and illness.

Dennis Gray and Sherry Saggers

Institutionalisation and beyond

The governing of Indigenous peoples proved problematic from the start. Historical reviews of government policy towards Indigenous Australians reveal some recurring themes: the need for 'protection' from both the violence of Europeans and the 'uncivilised' influences of traditional life, the persistent economic dependence of the original inhabitants on their colonial masters, and the overriding need for Indigenous people more closely to resemble other Australians (Lawrence & Gibson 2007). 'Protecting' and 'civilising' were attempted initially through the creation of government reserves and Christian missions, established during the nineteenth century. This first half of the twentieth is well known for the 'stolen generations' of children taken from their families to these centres. However, the **institutionalisation** of much larger numbers of Indigenous people through more mundane processes such as the rationing of food and clothing is less well known (Rowse 1998).

These unhealthy relationships remained in place until the 1950s, when the gradual implementation of the **assimilation** policy saw the revocation of many of these settlements and missions. Under assimilation policies, Indigenous people were expected to become indistinguishable from non-Indigenous Australians, with the same rights and responsibilities as other citizens. At the heart of this policy was the assumption that harmonious relationships between Black and White Australians could only be achieved by 'breeding out Aboriginality' (Brock 1993, pp. 14–19). Commencing in the mid-1960s, the inherently racist assimilation policy was replaced by policies, first, of 'integration', then '**self-determination**' and 'self-management', which allowed for the expression of cultural difference and for the right of Indigenous people to have some degree of control over their destinies.

In recent times Indigenous governance has remained highly contentious, with a return to the assimilationist paternalism of the past in an attempt to address persistent inequality. In 2004, 'Shared Responsibility Agreements' were promoted as the 'new way of doing business' with Indigenous Australia. Under these agreements, the Howard Coalition Government committed to provide particular services or investment in return for behavioural change. In Mulan, a remote community in the East Kimberley in Western Australia, for instance, this involved the provision of two petrol bowsers in return for rubbish collection and regular washing of children's faces (Lawrence & Gibson 2007). In 2007—purportedly in response to a report on child abuse (Wild & Anderson 2007), but largely ignoring the report's recommendations—the Howard Coalition Government conducted a military-style intervention in the Northern Territory involving child health checks, restrictions on alcohol, and compulsory quarantining of welfare payments. At the same time it passed the *Northern Territory National Emergency Response Act 2007* which overrode provisions of the *Racial Discrimination Act 1975* which would have made some elements of the intervention illegal. While many Indigenous people have argued

institutionalisation
A process by which the lives of individuals are regulated in every way, and which creates dependent relationships between the institutionalised person and authority figures.

assimilation
A policy term referring to the expectation that Indigenous people and migrants will 'shed' their culture and become indistinguishable from the Anglo-Australian majority.

self-determination
A government policy designed to ensure that Indigenous communities decide the pace and nature of their future development.

that issues such as child protection warrant urgent attention, most do not support what they see as a stripping away of their hard-won citizenship rights in the name of service provision (Altman & Hinkson 2007). In addition to these actions, under the Howard Government, Australia was one of four nations (along with the USA, Canada, and New Zealand) which voted against the 'Declaration on Rights of Indigenous Peoples', adopted by the United Nations in September 2007 (UN News Service 2007).

It remains to be seen how the election of the Rudd Labor Government in late 2007 might change Indigenous policy; however, the 'national apology' as the first order of business for the new government was an important symbolic start.

History and political economy of alcohol in Indigenous Australia

Alcohol is widely acknowledged by Indigenous Australians as contributing to their very poor health. It is also clear that substance misuse, like illness, is socially produced and Indigenous people's relationship with alcohol has been shaped by their position in Australian society.

The early British colonists consumed large amounts of alcohol and introduced it in commercial quantities to Indigenous Australians (Lewis 1992). While initially cautious towards it, some Indigenous people soon developed a taste for alcohol, and colonists used it 'unconsciously or consciously as a device for seducing Indigenous people to engage economically, politically and socially with the colony' (Langton 1993, p. 201). For many Indigenous Australians, as for other people, intoxication was a pleasurable experience, but as they were dispossessed of their lands, their societies undermined, and they were increasingly marginalised, some turned to excessive alcohol consumption both as a way of dealing with the consequent psychological trauma and as one of the few pleasures available.

The relationship between high levels of alcohol misuse and socio-economic deprivation observed in the broader society is reproduced within the Indigenous population. For example, a national study of Indigenous people found that the unemployed and those on low incomes were more likely to be high-risk drinkers (ABS & AIHW 1999, p. 55); and a local study of Indigenous young people found that those who were unemployed were 13 times more likely to be frequent users of alcohol and other drugs than those who were still at school, in training, or employed (Gray et al. 1996).

For some Indigenous people, drinking is about not accepting inequalities. For much of the nineteenth and twentieth centuries, consumption of alcohol by or the sale of alcohol to Indigenous people was illegal; though some employers obtained exemptions to these laws and other Europeans profited from the illicit sale of alcohol

norms
Expectations about how people ought to act or behave.

colonialism
A process by which one nation imposes itself economically, politically, and socially upon another.

Indigenous community-controlled health services
Independent local organisations, controlled and managed by Indigenous people, which provide a range of services to meet the needs of their particular communities.

Pharmaceutical Benefits Scheme (PBS)
The publicly funded federal government scheme that subsidises the cost of prescribed medicines in Australia.

to Indigenous people. Exemptions to these laws were granted to Indigenous people who became citizens. This association and coincidence of the repeal of prohibitionary legislation, with the granting of citizenship to all Indigenous people in the various state and territory jurisdictions in the 1960s, meant that for at least some Indigenous people to be intoxicated without legal sanction became a strong expression of equality (Brady 2007). For some, public intoxication was also a form of protest against the imposition of non-Indigenous laws and social **norms** (Sackett 1988).

The pattern of drinking among Indigenous Australians is similar to that observed in countries such as New Zealand and Canada among peoples who are both ethnically and culturally diverse. What accounts for the pattern are their similar histories of **colonialism**, dispossession, and marginalisation. The demand for alcohol growing out of this history is further fuelled by global and local factors that ensure that alcohol is relatively cheap and easily available (Saggers & Gray 1998).

Indigenous communities acknowledge the harm that excessive alcohol use causes, and many have developed programs to tackle the issues of both demand and supply. In 1999–2000, across Australia, 177 Indigenous community-controlled organisations were conducting 226 intervention projects directly targeting alcohol and other drug misuse. These organisations included **Indigenous community-controlled health services**, but in addition other such services also provided a more general range of alcohol and other drug intervention (Gray et al. 2002). Indigenous people are also insisting that government agencies, such as liquor licensing authorities, pay more attention to their demands that alcohol be restricted. These actions demonstrate that Indigenous people are not hapless victims of broader political and economic forces, but their relative powerlessness must nevertheless be acknowledged (Saggers & Gray 1998).

Addressing Indigenous ill health: rhetoric and reality

Interventions aimed at reducing Indigenous health inequalities have been undertaken by Indigenous people themselves and by governments. To understand these interventions and their impact, it is necessary to know something about the structure of the Australian health care system and the way in which it is financed.

Except in some rural and remote areas, most primary medical care in Australia is provided by private practitioners. This care is funded privately through medical insurance and direct payment to providers, and publicly though rebates from the national health insurance scheme, Medicare (see Chapter 18), and the subsidisation of medications through the **Pharmaceutical Benefits Scheme (PBS)**. However, work by John Deeble and his colleagues (1998) showed that—largely because of the inaccessibility or inappropriateness of services—the level of Medicare and PBS funding accessed by Indigenous people was out of line with the greater burden of morbidity they faced.

Hospital care is provided by private organisations and by state or territory health departments, although, outside urban areas, there are few private hospitals. In some rural and remote areas, public hospitals also provide primary medical care. Hospital care is also privately and publicly funded. Public funding of state hospitals is largely provided by the Australian Government under Medicare agreements and from the financial resources of the states themselves.

In contrast, public health services (including some aspects of **primary health care (PHC)**) are almost exclusively provided by the government and non-government sectors. Again, this is funded from state or territory financial resources and by Commonwealth Government grants.

Public health infrastructure has greater impact on health status than the provision of health services. Housing, which is particularly important, is provided by both the private and public sectors. Water and electricity supply, and waste disposal services, are provided by state and local governments, with financial grants from the Commonwealth, and with a 'user pays' component. Indigenous people, as a result of poverty and location, generally have less access to such infrastructure than do non-Indigenous people, and this contributes significantly to their poor health status.

Since the mid-1990s, both Liberal–National and Labor Commonwealth Governments have sought to shift some of the burden of financing the health care system, particularly for primary medical and hospital care, from the public sector to private individuals. However, the cost of private health insurance remains beyond the means of many Australians. Governments have also sought to increase the 'user pays' component of utility services. This cost-shifting further restricts the access of Indigenous people to health services and infrastructure.

The World Health Organization's Alma-Ata Declaration (WHO 1978) stated that to be effective, primary health care should be affordable, accessible, appropriate, and acceptable. To varying degrees, and despite attempts to address them, most private and mainstream medical and health services fail to meet these criteria with regard to Indigenous people.

Indigenous people have taken significant initiatives to address the shortcomings of mainstream health services. In 1971, the first Aboriginal medical service was established in the inner Sydney suburb of Redfern. Since the establishment of the Redfern service, the number of Indigenous community-controlled health services has expanded considerably. The National Aboriginal Community Controlled Health Organisation (NACCHO), which represents these services, has 137 member organisations and 30 affiliates. As well as providing primary medical care, they conduct a range of health promotion and public health activities. NACCHO has played a leading role in representing the interests of its members to governments, and developing health policy and standards of care. In addition to health services, there

primary health care (PHC)
Both the point of first contact with the health care system and a philosophy for delivery of that care.

public health/public health infrastructure
Public policies and infrastructure to prevent the onset and transmission of disease among the population, with a particular focus on sanitation and hygiene such as clean air, water, and food, and immunisation. Public health infrastructure refers specifically to the buildings, installations, and equipment necessary to ensure healthy living conditions for the population.

Dennis Gray and Sherry Saggers

are over 150 Indigenous-controlled organisations providing services to prevent or treat the misuse of alcohol and other drugs. These include night patrols, sobering-up shelters, counselling programs, and residential treatment centres (Gray et al. 2002). Importantly, in Australia and elsewhere, it has been shown that—when adequately supported and resourced—community control enhances both the acceptability and effectiveness of health care.

Funding for Indigenous community-controlled organisations comes from a variety of sources including grants from state and territory and Commonwealth Government agencies, from Medicare rebates, and from charitable organisations. Importantly, resourcing of these organisations also includes significant amounts of time provided voluntarily by community members.

Major government initiatives aimed at alleviating Indigenous ill health are a relatively new phenomenon. It was not until the late 1960s and early 1970s that state and territory governments began to introduce special Aboriginal health programs. The focus of these was upon health education and promotion campaigns and making mainstream health services more accessible and acceptable to Indigenous people. At the same time, the Commonwealth Government began to provide funds to the states and territories to support those initiatives. Through the then newly formed Department of Aboriginal Affairs (later to become the Aboriginal and Torres Strait Islander Commission, or ATSIC), the Commonwealth also began to fund the newly emerging community-controlled health services, and housing and community infrastructure projects. Importantly, these funds were intended to supplement, not replace, the services that the states and territories were obligated to provide.

In 1973, the Commonwealth Departments of Health and of Aboriginal Affairs developed a rudimentary Ten Year Plan for Aboriginal Health. In the absence of agreements with the states, the Plan was never implemented (Australian Indigenous HealthInfoNet 2004; Grant et al. 2008).

The initiatives of the late 1960s and 1970s did have some positive impact; however, a 1979 report on Aboriginal Health by the House of Representatives Standing Committee on Aboriginal Affairs highlighted the continuing poor health status of Indigenous people. This was attributed to unsatisfactory environmental and housing conditions, socio-economic factors, and the provision of inappropriate health services. It also questioned the commitment of some state governments to improving Indigenous health. The Committee's recommendations focused upon improvements to the physical environment and the provision of essential services as well as the upgrading of health services, including a greater role for community-controlled services. While the Committee identified the importance of underlying socio-economic factors, it made no recommendations to address them.

Over the following decade, gains in Indigenous health status remained modest. To address this, the Commonwealth Government established a Working Party which consulted widely and developed a National Aboriginal Health Strategy

Working Party (NAHSWP 1989). In 1990, with some modification, the Working Party's recommendations were endorsed by a Council of Commonwealth and State Ministers for Health and Aboriginal Affairs; and the Commonwealth announced that, over the following five years through ATSIC, it would provide an additional $232 million to implement the strategy. The bulk was to be allocated for essential services infrastructure but some was to be allocated to Indigenous community-controlled health services (Australian Indigenous HealthInfoNet 2004).

An evaluation of the NAHS found that the National Council of Aboriginal Health—established to oversee implementation of the NAHS—lacked political support. Furthermore, all governments had grossly underfunded the NAHS and thus the NAHS had never been adequately implemented. As a result there had been 'minimal gains in the appalling state of Aboriginal health' (ATSIC 1994, pp. 2–3). The evaluation team also reported that 'at least a quarter of Commonwealth Aboriginal specific expenditures appear to substitute for expenditures which otherwise would occur within mainstream services' (ATSIC 1994, p. 84).

In 1995, the responsibility for administering funds for Indigenous health and substance-abuse programs was transferred from ATSIC to a new Office of Aboriginal and Torres Strait Islander Health Services (now the Office for Aboriginal and Torres Strait Islander Health) within what is now the Australian Government Department of Health and Ageing. Since that time, at the national level, there have been a number of initiatives to address Indigenous health (Australian Indigenous HealthInfoNet 2004). In 1995–96 a series called 'Framework Agreements' was put in place in each state and territory. Under these, joint planning forums and a National Aboriginal and Torres Strait Islander Health Council were established. Changes were also made to the acts of parliament relating to the Pharmaceutical Benefits Scheme and Medicare to facilitate improved access to pharmaceuticals and funding of health care interventions. A 10 year *National Strategic Framework for Aboriginal and Torres Strait Islander Health* was introduced in 2003 (NATSIHC 2003), followed in 2004 by a *National Strategic Framework for Aboriginal and Torres Strait Islander Peoples' Mental Health and Social and Emotional Well-Being 2004–2009* (Social Health Reference Group 2004).

These initiatives led to increased funding and some positive outcomes. However, they are not without their critics. It has been argued that—despite the rhetoric surrounding them—Indigenous input into decision-making is constrained and funding has not been commensurate with need (Grant et al. 2008). For example, in 2004–05, $1.17 was spent on Indigenous health for every $1.00 spent on non-Indigenous health, and there had been little change in that ratio in 10 years (Deeble et al. 2008). As long ago as 1991, the Commonwealth Grants Commission stated that 'the poorer health status of Indigenous people, and their greater reliance on the public health care system, would justify at least a doubling of the average per capita expenditure on non-Indigenous people' (Commonwealth Grants Commission 2001). As these figures show, this has clearly not happened.

BOX 8.1 Doing health sociology: the personal and the public

Our theoretical interests in the structural determinants of health have found practical expression in work that we and our colleagues at the National Drug Research Institute have undertaken in collaboration with Indigenous community-controlled organisations.

There is clear evidence nationally and internationally that the level of alcohol consumption is closely related to its availability. In our applied work, we have examined strategies that are used to promote the sale of alcohol to Indigenous people; examined the effectiveness of strategies, such as liquor licensing restrictions, which seek to reduce availability; and documented the attitudes of both Indigenous and non-Indigenous Australians to such restrictions. We have also appeared as expert witnesses in liquor licensing court hearings.

This research has had impact at a range of levels. For example, it has been used by Indigenous organisations effectively to address alcohol misuse in their communities; informed policy documents such as the Northern Territory Government's Alcohol Framework; been used as background to the development of the *National Drug Strategy Aboriginal and Torres Strait Islander People's Complementary Action Plan*; and through membership by one of the authors (Gray) on the National Indigenous Drug and Alcohol Committee—the peak advisory body on Indigenous substance misuse issues—the work continues to inform national policy.

Conclusion

The inequalities in Indigenous health are a consequence of fundamental structural inequalities related to the dispossession of Indigenous people and their continued economic and political marginalisation. The 'common sense' ideology of neo-liberalism obscures those structural inequalities by proclaiming that individuals are responsible for their own 'successes' and 'failures'. In also proclaiming that all should be treated equally, it militates against solutions, for *nothing more assures the perpetuation of inequality than the equal treatment of unequal individuals*.

The inadequacy of funding for Indigenous health programs reflects what has occurred in other areas of Indigenous affairs. Indigenous people striving for self-determination and social equality have been undermined. In 2004, ATSIC was abolished. The elected Commission was replaced by a non-representative National Indigenous Council and its service activities were 'mainstreamed'. Under the Howard Coalition Government there was a call for a 'new paternalism' and the Northern Territory 'intervention' was introduced without consultation with Indigenous people, provisions of the *Racial Discrimination Act* were overridden, and an attack was made on Indigenous land rights.

At the time of writing, a new Labor Government has been elected, an 'apology' offered to Indigenous people, and there are moves afoot to establish a new elected Indigenous advisory body. These are positive steps. However, it remains to be seen whether the new government will make the investment necessary to alleviate Indigenous disadvantage. A recent report has shown that—while there have been undoubted improvements—without a more vigorous program to address them, Indigenous inequalities will be perpetuated into the foreseeable future (Altman et al. 2008).

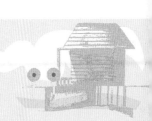

Summary of main points

» While the causes of illness and death among Indigenous and non-Indigenous Australians are similar, the rates of hospitalisation and death among Indigenous people are much greater.

» Tobacco, alcohol, and other drug misuse make a significant contribution to Indigenous ill health.

» Patterns of health and illness in any population reflect social inequalities such as ethnicity, social class, and gender.

» The contemporary ill health of Indigenous people must be located in the historical context of colonialism and continuing inequalities.

» On one hand, government policy has been to appropriate, or sanction, the appropriation of Indigenous land and resources. On the other, it has been to attempt to ameliorate the effects of this appropriation.

» Reducing Indigenous health inequalities requires both addressing the underlying structural determinants and providing health services that are accessible, appropriate, affordable, and acceptable to Indigenous people.

» For more than three decades there has been a gap between the rhetoric and reality of Indigenous health policy, with insufficient attention and resources directed to the fundamental inequalities experienced by Indigenous people.

Sociological reflection: blaming the victims

Consider the way in which beliefs that 'individuals are responsible for their own health' and that 'all individuals should be treated the same', converge with racism to lay the blame for poor Indigenous health on Indigenous people themselves.

Dennis Gray and Sherry Saggers

Discussion questions

1 How is health inequality measured, and what evidence is there of inequalities between Indigenous and non-Indigenous Australians?
2 Discuss the historical context of the social production of contemporary Indigenous health, including some assessment of the traditional Indigenous health system.
3 Describe the past and present impact of the reserve and mission system on the health of Indigenous people.
4 What have been some of the key policies designed to improve Indigenous health over the past thirty years?
5 What are some of the major differences between mainstream health services and those that are community controlled?
6 Why has change in Indigenous health and social indicators been so slow?

Further investigation

1 Discuss the demand for and supply of alcohol to Indigenous people in a historical context, and the efforts by Indigenous communities to address substance misuse.
2 What do contemporary political debates about the 'stolen generation' and reconciliation have to do with the status of Indigenous health in the past and present?

Further reading

Carson B., Dunbar T., Chenhall R. & Baille R. (eds) 2007, *The Social Determinants of Indigenous Health*, Allen & Unwin, Sydney.
Couzos, S. & Murray R. (eds) 2008, *Aboriginal Primary Health Care*, 3rd edn, Oxford University Press, Melbourne.
Saggers, S. & Gray, D. 1998, *Dealing with Alcohol: Indigenous Usage in Australia, Canada and New Zealand*, Cambridge University Press, Melbourne.

Web resources

Aboriginal and Torres Strait Islander Social Justice (HREOC): <http://www.hreoc.gov.au/social_justice/index.html>
Centre for Aboriginal Economic Policy Research: <http://www.anu.edu.au/caepr/>
Cooperative Research Centre for Aboriginal Health: <http://www.crcah.org.au/>
National Drug Research Institute, Curtin University of Technology: <http://www.ndri.curtin.edu.au/>

● ● ● **Online case study**
Visit the Second Opinion website to access relevant case studies.

Documentaries/films

Crossing the Line (2005): 56 minutes. A documentary about the experiences of two young, white medical students who go to work in a remote Aboriginal community and find their personal and professional beliefs challenged.

Minymaku Way (2001): 52 minutes. A film about an Indigenous Women's Council and how these women are addressing problems in their remote communities, such as petrol sniffing, and how they are working together with non-Indigenous women.

Rabbit Proof Fence (2002): 94 minutes, directed by Phillip Noyce. A film set in 1931 that traces the experiences of three young Aboriginal girls who escape from being trained as domestic servants after being taken from their homes.

The Tracker (2002): 94 minutes, directed by Rolf de Heer. Set in 1922, the film tells the story of two white men pursuing a fugitive with the help of an Indigenous 'tracker'.

Vote Yes For Aborigines (2007): 52 minutes. This documentary examines the 1967 Referendum and its contemporary relevance for Aboriginal citizenship rights.

Why Me? (2007): 56 minutes. A documentary exploring the 'stolen generation' by focusing on how the lives of five children were affected by the government policy to forcibly remove Indigenous children from the families and culture.

Yolngu Boy (2000): 85 minutes. A film about three Aboriginal teenagers struggling with questions about identity as they deal with the tensions between being part of today's youth culture and part of Indigenous culture.

References

Aboriginal and Torres Strait Islander Commission 1994, *The National Aboriginal Health Strategy: An Evaluation*, ATSIC, Canberra.

Altman, J. & Hinkson, M. (eds) 2007, *Coercive Reconciliation: Stabilise, Normalise, Exit Aboriginal Australia*, Arena Publications, Melbourne.

Altman, J., Biddle, N. & Hunter, B. 2008, 'The Challenge of "Closing the Gaps"', in *Indigenous Socioeconomic Outcomes*, Centre for Aboriginal Economic Policy Research, Australian National University, Canberra.

Australian Bureau of Statistics 2006, *Tobacco Smoking in Australia: A Snapshot, 2004–05*, Cat. no. 4831.0.55.001, ABS, Canberra.

Australian Bureau of Statistics & Australian Institute of Health and Welfare 1999, *The Health and Welfare of Australia's Aboriginal and Torres Strait Islander Peoples: 1999*, ABS & AIHW, Canberra.

Australian Bureau of Statistics & Australian Institute of Health and Welfare 2008, *The Health and Welfare of Australia's Aboriginal and Torres Strait Islander Peoples: 2008*, Cat. no. 4704.0, ABS & AIHW, Canberra.

Australian Indigenous HealthInfoNet. 2004, *Major Developments in National Indigenous Health Policy Since 1967*. Available online: <http://www.healthinfonet.ecu.edu.au/html/html_programs/programs_policy/reviews/programs_policies_timelines.htm>

Australian Institute of Health and Welfare 2005, '2004 National Drug Strategy Household Survey: Detailed Findings', *Drug Statistics Series No.16*, AIHW, Canberra.

Baum, F. 2007, 'Cracking the Nut of Health Equity: Top Down and Bottom Up Pressure for Action on the Social Determinants of Health', *Promotion & Education*, vol. 14, no. 2, pp. 90–5.

Brady, M. 2007, 'Equality and Difference: Persisting Historical Themes in Health and Alcohol Policies Affecting Indigenous Australians', *Journal of Epidemiology and Community Health*, vol. 61, pp. 759–63.

Brock, P. 1993, *Outback Ghettos: Aborigines, Institutionalisation and Survival*, Cambridge University Press, Melbourne.

Brown, T. & Bell, M. 2006, 'Off the Couch and on the Move: Global Public Health and the Medicalisation of Nature', *Social Science & Medicine*, vol. 64, pp. 1343–54.

Carson B., Dunbar T., Chenhall R. & Baille R. (eds), 2007, *The Social Determinants of Indigenous Health*, Allen & Unwin, Sydney.

Chikritzhs, T. & Brady, M. 2006, 'Fact or Fiction? A Critique of the National Aboriginal and Torres Strait Islander Social Survey 2002', *Drug and Alcohol Review*, vol. 25, pp. 277–87.

Commonwealth Grants Commission 2001, *Report on Indigenous Funding*, Commonwealth Grants Commission, Canberra.

Deeble, J., Agar, J. S. & Goss, J. 2008, *Expenditures on Health for Aboriginal and Torres Strait Islander Peoples 2004–05*, Cat. no. HWE 40, AIHW, Canberra.

Deeble, J., Mathers, C., Smith, L. et al. 1998, *Expenditures on Health Services for Aboriginal and Torres Strait Islander People, Australian Institute for Health and Welfare*, Department of Health & Family Services and National Centre for Epidemiology and Population Health, Canberra.

Ginsberg, F. & Myers, F. 2006, 'A History of Aboriginal Futures', *Critique of Anthropology*, vol. 26, no. 1, pp. 27–45.

Grant, M., Wronski, I., Murray, R. B. & Couzos, S. 2008, 'Aboriginal Health and History', in S. Couzos and R. Murray (eds), *Aboriginal Primary Health Care*, 3rd edn, Oxford University Press, Melbourne, pp. 1–28.

Gray, D., Morfitt, B., Williams, S., Ryan, K. & Coyne, L. 1996, *Drug Use and Related Issues Among Young Aboriginal People in Albany*, National Centre for Research into the Prevention of Drug Abuse, Curtin University of Technology, Perth.

Gray, D., Sputore, B., Stearne, A., Bourbon, D. & Strempel, P. 2002, *Indigenous Drug and Alcohol Projects: 1999–2000*, Australian National Council on Drugs, Canberra.

Human Rights and Equal Opportunity Commission, 1997, *Bringing Them Home: Report of the National Inquiry into the Separation of Aboriginal and Torres Strait Islander Children and Their Families*, Human Rights and Equal Opportunity Commission, Canberra.

Langton, M. 1993, 'Rum, Seduction and Death: "Aboriginality" and Alcohol', *Oceania*, vol. 63, no. 3, pp. 195–206.

Larson, A., Gillies, M., Howard, P. J. & Coffin 2007, 'It's Enough to Make You Sick: The Impact of Racism on the Health of Aboriginal Australians', *Australian and New Zealand Journal of Public Health*, vol. 31, no. 4, pp. 322–9.

Lawrence, R. & Gibson, C. 2007, 'Obliging Indigenous Citizens?', *Cultural Studies*, vol. 21, pp. 650–71.

Lewis, M. 1992, *A Rum State: Alcohol and Public Policy in Australia 1788–1988*. Australian Government Publishing Service, Canberra.

Mills, C. W. 1959, *The Sociological Imagination*, Oxford University Press, New York.

National Aboriginal Health Strategy Working Party 1989, *A National Aboriginal Health Strategy*, Australian Government Printer, Canberra.

National Aboriginal and Torres Strait Islander Health Council 2003, *National Strategic Framework for Aboriginal and Torres Strait Islander Health*, NATSIHC, Canberra.

Paradies, Y. 2006, 'A Systematic Review of Empirical Research on Self-reported Racism and Health', *International Journal of Epidemiology*, vol. 35, no. 4, pp. 888–901.

Reynolds, H. 1995, *Aboriginal Resistance to the European Invasion of Australia*, 2nd edn, Penguin, Ringwood.

Rowse, T. 1998, *White Flour, White Power: From Rations to Citizenship in Central Australia*, Cambridge University Press, Melbourne.

Sackett, L. 1988, 'Resisting Arrests: Drinking, Development and Discipline in a Desert Context', *Social Analysis*, vol. 24, pp. 66–77.

Saggers, S. & Gray, D. 1998, *Dealing with Alcohol. Indigenous Usage in Australia, New Zealand and Canada*, Cambridge University Press, Melbourne.

Social Health Reference Group, for the National Aboriginal and Torres Strait Islander Health Council and National Mental Health Working Group 2004, *National Strategic Framework for Aboriginal and Torres Strait Islander Peoples' Mental Health and Social and Emotional Well-Being 2004–2009*, Department of Health and Ageing, Canberra.

Swan, P. & Raphael, B. 1995, *Ways Forward: National Consultancy Report on Aboriginal and Torres Strait Islander Mental Health, Part 1 & 2*, Australian Government Publishing Service, Canberra.

Turrell, G. & Mathers, C. D. 2000, 'Socioeconomic Status and Health in Australia', *Medical Journal of Australia*, vol. 172, pp. 434–8.

UN News Service. 2007, *United Nations Adopts Declaration on Rights of Indigenous Peoples.* Available online:<http://www.un.org/apps/news/story.asp?NewsID=23794&Cr=indig enous&Cr1>

Wild, R. & Anderson, P. 2007, 'Ampe Akelyernemane Meke Mekarle, "Little Children are Sacred"', *Report of the Northern Territory Board of Inquiry into the Protection of Aboriginal Children from Sexual Abuse*, Northern Territory Government, Darwin.

Wilkinson, R. & Marmot, M. 2003, *Social Determinants of Health: The Solid Facts*, 2nd edn, WHO, Copenhagen.

World Health Organization 1978, *Declaration of Alma-Ata*, International Conference on Primary Health Care, Alma-Ata, USSR, 6–12 September 1978, WHO, Geneva.

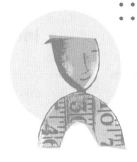

CHAPTER 9

Ethnicity, Health, and Multiculturalism

ROBERTA
JULIAN

Overview

- What does the research evidence tell us about the health of Australia's ethnically diverse population?
- How important is ethnicity (or culture) in determining health outcomes for Australia's ethnically diverse population?
- How can the Australian health care system provide culturally and linguistically appropriate health care services to all Australians?

REFUGEE HEALTH

In February 2006, the *Sydney Morning Herald* reported on two cases that demonstrated the problems experienced by refugees in accessing appropriate health care services in Australia. One was the tragic case of a 2-year-old refugee child from Burundi who had died of a treatable disease in an apartment in Sydney. The child and his family had recently arrived in Australia with medical records that outlined the child's medical condition, but the child had become ill within a few days of arrival and his parents had not known how to contact emergency services. The other case

was that of an adult refugee from Sudan who was an amputee without legs. He lived in a first-floor apartment where he had to crawl up the stairs and rely on passers-by to carry his wheelchair for him. The *Sydney Morning Herald* reported that 'he had made many requests for medical help which resulted in him being referred to a GP, who gave him some tablets. What he really wanted was prosthetic legs and he could not ... find out how to contact the right health services' (Sheikh-Mohammed et al. 2006; *Sydney Morning Herald* 2006a, 2006b).

Introduction

immigrants
A term for those in the population who were born in another country, which is sometimes extended to the descendants of immigrants through the terms 'second-generation' and 'third-generation' immigrants. However, this usage confuses the term and obscures the key fact that those born overseas have a set of immigrant experiences that their descendants do not have.

ethnic minorities
Ethnic groups that are not the dominant ethnic group in a society. Unlike the term 'ethnic group', it highlights the power differences between different ethnic groups in society.

social construction
Refers to the socially created characteristics of human life based on the idea that people actively construct reality, meaning it is neither 'natural' nor inevitable. Therefore, notions of normality/abnormality, right/wrong, and health/illness are subjective human creations that should not be taken for granted.

Australia is one of the most ethnically diverse countries in the world today (ABS 2005). In 2004, almost one-quarter of the total population was born overseas with more than half of these **immigrants** born in a non-English-speaking country (AIHW 2006, p. 235). In addition, one out of every five persons is a second-generation Australian (Khoo et al. 2002, p. 9). As two-fifths of the Australian population are immigrants or the children of immigrants, it is not surprising that there has been a growing interest in issues relating to the health and illness of Australia's **ethnic minorities** (Stevens 2001; Allotey et al. 2002; Allotey 2003; Manderson & Allotey 2003; Multicultural Mental Health Australia 2004; Karantzas-Savva & Kirwan 2004; Centre for Culture, Ethnicity and Health 2005; Romios et al. 2007). This interest has arisen as service providers have had to address the needs of Australians whose understandings of health and illness are 'different' from those of the Anglo-Australian majority. Within this context, migrants are often viewed as 'people with problems' because they do not fit neatly into the culture and structure of the Anglo-Australian health care system. This pragmatic interest has led policy developers and service providers to examine the work of sociologists and anthropologists, who have long had an interest in the social and cultural factors influencing health (see, for example, Kleinman 1980, 1988; Kleinman & Good 1985).

This chapter adopts a sociological perspective to explore issues relating to the health of Australia's ethnically diverse population. It discusses the **social construction** of health, illness, and **ethnicity**, and examines the relationship between ethnicity, **class**, and health. Importantly, this discussion is located within the socio-historical context of Australia's immigration program which has profoundly affected patterns of structural inequality and cultural difference in Australian society. The chapter concludes with a critical discussion of Australia's health care system in the context of **multiculturalism**.

The social and cultural construction of health and illness

'Health' and 'illness' are terms that we typically take for granted. We know what it means to be healthy, and we know when someone is ill. We tend to assume that these are objective facts: states of the body and the mind that can be measured against what is 'normal', but sociologists and anthropologists have shown us that health and illness are social constructions; they are not objectively defined. Thus, definitions of 'health' and 'illness', and understandings of appropriate health care vary over time and across cultures. For example, in Australia during the 1950s and 1960s, many childhood diseases, such as measles, were defined as 'normal'. Thus children were encouraged to interact with others who had the virus so that they would be exposed and 'get the measles', but now, since the development of new medical knowledge—in this case a vaccine—measles is defined as a serious illness and children are encouraged to avoid exposure to the virus (Manderson & Reid 1994).

Furthermore, in any society, some people have more power than others to define health and illness. Some members of society are the custodians of 'legitimate' medical knowledge, while others, who do not have specialist knowledge, are encouraged to define health and illness in the same ways as the 'experts'. In Australian society, the dominant cultural model of health and illness is that of **biomedicine**, and the 'experts' are health professionals such as doctors. The structure of the health care system (for example, hospitals and general practice) reflects the dominance of this model; it locates these medical 'experts' in positions of power. In other societies, though, there may be a different model of health and illness. Among the Hmong in Laos, for example, health and illness are believed to have organic and/or inorganic causes. The medical 'experts' are the shamans. They have the power to interact with the spirits, and their involvement is crucial in the ritual management of illness (Rice 1994; Adler 1996; Julian & Easthope 1996; Fadiman 1997).

Health and illness are thus social constructions. Different cultures have different understandings of health and illness, and people within societies are differentially located with respect to access to 'expert' knowledge in this area. Cultural understandings and the structure of health care both play important parts in determining health and illness.

Ethnic groups in Australia

It is relatively easy to comprehend that there are significant cultural differences between different societies, but it is also important to recognise the existence of **cultural diversity** within a single society. Diversity can arise from a range of factors such as class, **gender**, sexuality, **'race'**, and ethnicity.

Studies of ethnic groups in Australia have demonstrated that differences exist with respect to cultural understandings of health and illness. For example, the Hmong, whose beliefs and practices are outlined above, are an ethnic group in Australia. The Vietnamese believe that physical and emotional illness is caused by an imbalance in the forces of *am* and *duong* (similar to the Chinese *yin* and *yang*). One cause of mental illness is believed to be possession by ancestral spirits who have been offended and have become angry (Lien 1992). Among Latin Americans, the word *susto* refers to illnesses associated with unexpected experiences of fright that produce symptoms such as loss of appetite, nervousness, and depression. According to folklore, it is caused by 'the separation of the spiritual element from the physiological element of the person' (Allotey 1998, p. 70; see also Holloway 1994). Similarly,

ethnicity
Sociologically, the term refers to a shared cultural background, which is a characteristic of all groups in society. As a policy term, it is used to identify migrants who share a culture that is markedly different from that of Anglo-Australians. In practice, it often refers only to migrants from non-English-speaking backgrounds (NESB migrants).

class (or social class)
A position in a system of structured inequality based on the unequal distribution of power, wealth, income, and status. People who share a class position typically share similar life chances.

multiculturalism
A policy term referring to the expectation that all members of society have the right to equal access to services, regardless of 'race', ethnicity, culture, or religion. It is based on the recognition that all people have the right to maintain their cultural beliefs and identity while adhering to the laws of the nation state.

Roberta Julian

biomedicine/ biomedical model
The conventional approach to medicine in Western societies, based on the diagnosis and explanation of illness as a malfunction of the body's biological mechanisms. This approach underpins most health professions and health services, which focus on treating individuals, and generally ignores the social origins of illness and its prevention.

cultural diversity
A term used to refer to the existence of a range of different cultures in a single society. In popular usage, it typically refers to ethnic diversity, but sociologically the term can equally refer to differences based on gender, social class, age, disability, and so on.

gender/sex
This pair of terms refers to the socially constructed categories of feminine and masculine (the cultural identities and values that prescribe how men and women should behave), and the social power relations based on those categories, as distinct from the categories of biological sex (female or male).

traditional healing practices among West Africans are based on the belief that illness can be caused by 'things we see and things we don't see', such as hereditary curses, breach of sexual taboos, witchcraft, and spirit possession (Nyagua & Harris 2008).

Different ethnic groups may also have different expectations of what constitutes appropriate treatment. These will, in part, reflect different cultural understandings of the causes of health and illness. For example, in the post-partum (following birth) period, a Vietnamese mother must not leave the house for 30–40 days, must not speak loudly, must not clean her teeth with a toothbrush, must not read or strain her eyes, and must not wash her hair or have a bath for at least a week, in some cases a month (Tran 1994). West Africans who are used to going to a traditional healer will expect questions to be asked about their ancestry and they will expect a solution to be proposed (for example, being given a protective amulet to wear). They are likely to be confused and dissatisfied if the response they receive is limited to assistance from a social worker or counsellor (Nyagua & Harris 2008). Even among ethnic groups in which a biomedical model is taken for granted, there may be cultural differences in expectations of appropriate medical or health care, and in appropriate ways of articulating and managing pain. Salvadorans, for example, are used to general practitioners treating a wide range of illnesses with injections and are therefore often dissatisfied with the oral treatment that predominates in the Australian health system (Macintyre 1994). Greek and Italian mothers vocalise pain during childbirth more than do mothers from Vietnamese cultural backgrounds—a fact that, in the past, often led nursing staff to assume (incorrectly) that the former were exaggerating their pain, while the latter 'don't feel pain like we do' (Manderson & Reid 1994).

Clearly, an adequate understanding of the ethnic patterning of health and illness must take into account the cultural factors influencing the ways in which different ethnic groups understand, experience, and manage illness. In the quest to demonstrate the significance of 'culture' among ethnic groups, a number of problems have arisen that have confounded rather than contributed to our understanding of the cultural influences on health and illness. First, culture has been equated with minority ethnicity. In other words, it has been assumed that 'culture' has an impact on health for ethnic minorities, but Anglo-Australian views of health and illness are viewed as 'scientifically based' and therefore not influenced by culture. Such a view is **ethnocentric**. Second, 'culture', 'ethnicity' and 'race' have been reified in explanations of immigrant health (Manderson & Reid 1994; Braun et al. 2007). In other words, 'ethnic' culture is invoked as the major (if not the only) factor affecting differential patterns of health and illness among different ethnic groups. Such 'culturalist' explanations fail to examine the significance of alternative factors, such as class, gender, and age, which may be more important variables than 'culture' or 'ethnicity' in the incidence, diagnosis, and treatment of some illnesses (Collins 2004).

In order to overcome these problems, cultural analyses of health and illness need to be balanced with structural analyses. Ethnic groups differ not only in terms of culture but also, and perhaps more importantly, in terms of their social location—that is, in terms of their location in the structure of social inequality. It is possible to identify a hierarchy of ethnic groups on the basis of indicators such as income, occupation, education, and access to goods and services such as health. Clearly, ethnicity and class are interrelated.

One of the major debates in research on the ethnic patterning of health and illness has focused on the relative significance of ethnicity in relation to class. Such debates are often represented as 'culturalist' versus 'structuralist' (or '**materialist**'); researchers (for example, Manderson & Reid 1994; Smaje 1996) have pointed to the futility of such debates. Both class and ethnicity are significant structural dimensions of Australian society. As such, it is important to examine the ways in which class and ethnicity are interrelated and thus interact to produce differential health outcomes, rather than addressing each as separable from the other and attempting to determine which is more important. It is significant that sociological analysis opens up the opportunity to examine the interaction of other structural variables, particularly gender, age, and sexuality, all of which have a significant impact on health.

The socio-historical context

The structure of ethnic relations in contemporary Australia, and thus the ethnic patterning of health and illness, is the outcome of a series of socio-historical processes. One of the most significant events in Australian history in terms of its impact on Australian society has been the postwar immigration program (Jamrozik et al. 1995; Jupp 1999, 2002). The outcome of this program is a 'multicultural' society, characterised by cultural diversity as well as structural inequality between different ethnic groups (Vasta & Castles 1996; Jupp 2001, 2002; White et al. 2003; Ho & Alcorso 2004).

Australia's immigration program

In the aftermath of the Second World War, the Australian Government embarked on a mass immigration program with the catch-cry 'populate or perish'. The first Minister for Immigration, Arthur Calwell, was committed to the goal of racial purity and promised to accept 10 British immigrants for every 'foreigner' (Collins 1991). As this goal proved difficult to achieve, migrants were accepted from other sources but were selected on the basis of an ethnic preference hierarchy. Since 1945, Australia has accepted over five million people from over a hundred countries (Collins 1991; Castles 1992). With the dismantling of the White Australia Policy in the 1970s, the proportion of people who were of European descent declined; since 1976, 35 to 40

'race'
A term without scientific basis that uses skin colour and facial features to describe what are alleged to be biologically distinct groups of humans. Race is actually a social construction used to categorise groups of people and sometimes implies assumed (and unproven) intellectual superiority or inferiority.

ethnocentric
Viewing others from one's own cultural perspective, with an implied sense of cultural superiority based on an inability to understand or accept the practices and beliefs of other cultures.

materialist analysis
An analysis that is embedded in the real, actual, material reality of everyday life.

per cent have come from Asian countries (Jupp 1999, p. 120). This 'ethnic shift' away from European origins is associated with an increase in immigrants from Asia, the Middle East, and Africa, and is likely to continue in the future (Jupp 2002). The types of immigrants entering Australia have also varied over the years, with an increasing emphasis on skilled and business immigration since the 1980s (Collins 1996; Jupp 2002; DIMA 2006), and a fluctuation in the humanitarian program which accounted for 19 per cent of the immigrant intake in 1985 and 6 per cent in 1991 (ABS 2004–05, pp. 5 and 9).

The conditions under which immigrants arrived and settled in Australia, as well as the characteristics of the immigrants themselves, have led to the pattern of cultural diversity and social inequality that exists in Australia today. A number of aspects are important to note.

First, not all immigrants establish visible **ethnic communities** in Australia, and none is totally segregated from mainstream Australian society. Furthermore, the assumption that an ethnic community exists on the basis of a shared aspect of 'ethnic culture' such as language or citizenship (for example, a Salvadoran community or an African community) is erroneous. It assumes homogeneity where it may not exist by overlooking differences based on class, gender, and political orientation within the social category (Langer 1998; Centre for Culture, Ethnicity and Health 2005). This is an important fact to keep in mind when examining support structures for those suffering ill health.

Second, while immigrants are spread throughout the class structure in Australia, the labour force is segmented along lines of ethnicity and gender (Ho & Alcorso 2004) with Australian-born and postwar Anglophone male migrants over-represented in the 'primary' labour market and postwar non-Anglophone migrant women concentrated at the 'bottom of the heap' in shrinking jobs in the manufacturing sector, such as in the clothing, footwear, and textile industries (Collins 1991, 1996). Notably, though, this pattern of labour market segmentation has altered over the last 20 years as a consequence of economic restructuring and changes in the immigration program. Many immigrants arriving from Asian countries since the 1990s have been highly skilled and qualified managers and professionals who have been employed in 'primary' sector jobs (Jupp 2002; ABS 2004). The immigrant workforce is thus becoming increasingly bimodal with clustering at the upper and lower levels of the labour market (Castles & Miller 1998; Ho & Alcorso 2004).

Third, refugees have very high rates of unemployment and welfare dependency compared with those born in Australia and with other immigrants (Viviani et al. 1993; Healey 1996; Colic-Peisker & Tilbury 2006, 2007). Many of these refugees are highly qualified but lack the documentation and/or English language skills to translate this into skilled employment (Jupp 2002).

Finally, demographic factors affect the experiences of immigrants. The early postwar immigrants now constitute an ageing population and there is a growing

ethnic communities
Those ethnic groups that have established a large number of ethnic organisations, thus providing a shared context for interaction between members. Only some ethnic groups develop the institutional structure that enables them to become ethnic communities.

number of second- and third-generation Australians. While there is evidence to suggest that non-English-speaking background (NESB), second-generation Australians have achieved upward social mobility, such observations must be treated with caution. It is important to recognise the wide variation in rates of mobility between different ethnic groups and the higher-than-average unemployment rates among migrant youth (Castles & Miller 1998; Collins et al. 2000; Windle 2004).

Clearly, when exploring the relationship between ethnicity and health, it is important to examine ethnicity not only as a cultural phenomenon associated with lifestyle and identity, but also as it impacts on social location and thus on **life chances**. In other words, ethnicity is both a cultural and a structural dimension of society. It is the nexus between the two that determines the health of the Australian population.

The health of Australia's ethnically diverse population

What does the research evidence tell us about the health of Australia's ethnically diverse population? As the following review of research shows, the effects of ethnicity cannot be separated from the effects of immigrant status, class, gender, and age; rather, ethnicity interacts with each of these factors, meaning their effect can be different for different ethnic groups (see Kai 2003).

Mortality and morbidity

Most research on the ethnic patterning of health begins by noting that the on-arrival health status of immigrants is generally better than that of the Australian-born population. In general, levels of mortality for immigrants tend to be lower than those for the Australian-born population (Singh & de Looper 2002; AIHW 2006) and immigrant populations often have lower rates of disability, lower lifestyle-related **risk factors** and lower hospitalisation rates (AIHW 2006).

There are a number of explanations given for this. One is known as the 'healthy migrant effect' (Singh & de Looper 2002, p. 9) that results from two main factors: a self-selection process and a government selection process. While a self-selection process cannot be proven, it is likely that the population of migrants seeking work in another country would be healthier than the general population, which also includes those not in the labour market (Smaje 1996; AIHW 2006). With respect to the latter, in the case of Australia, the superior health outcomes of migrants are the direct effect of a selection process that involves stringent health tests as part of the process of applying for permanent residence (Wooden et al. 1994). Importantly, the initial lower mortality rates among immigrants decline with length of residence in

life chances
Derived from Max Weber, the term refers to people's opportunity to realise their lifestyle choices, which are often assumed to differ according to their social class.

risk factors
Conditions, such as alcohol misuse, smoking, and poor diet, that are thought to increase an individual's susceptibility to illness or disease.

Australia so that over time 'the health status of immigrants ... tends to converge towards that of the native-born population' (AIHW 2006, p. 238).

One hypothesised explanation—both of differential mortality rates between immigrants and the Australian-born population, and of the increase in mortality rates with length of residence among immigrants—focuses on the effect of different lifestyles, particularly in relation to diet. Research has shown that Southern European immigrants consume less animal fat and protein than the Australian-born population and that diets begin to look more like the Australian norm with length of residence. Interestingly, research has also shown that, for some birthplace categories, mortality rates do not converge on the rate for the Australian-born population: differential rates are sometimes maintained, even after 15 years of residence in Australia (AIHW 2004).

The complex relationship between genetic, environmental, and lifestyle risk factors is evident in an examination of the prevalence of diabetes among different ethnic groups. Thirty-five per cent of Australians who reported having diabetes in 2001 were born overseas. Research has shown that males born in the Middle East and North Africa have a prevalence rate 3.6 times that of Australian-born males (Holdenson et al. 2003) and Greek and Italian migrants are 3 times more likely than the Australian born to have Type 2 diabetes (Hodge et al. 2004; ABS 2004–05, p. 25). Importantly, the AIHW (2006, p. 238) notes that 'for migrants the changes in diet and physical activity have been implicated in their increased risk'.

Mental health

epidemiology
The statistical study of patterns of disease in the population. Originally focused on epidemics, or infectious diseases, it now covers non-infectious conditions such as stroke and cancer. Social epidemiology is a sub-field aligned with sociology that focuses on the social determinants of illness.

Epidemiological studies in the postwar period demonstrated a high level of psychiatric disorder, such as depression and schizophrenia, among immigrants (Wooden et al. 1994). Current estimates suggest that 250,000 first-generation adult Australians from culturally and linguistically diverse backgrounds experience some form of mental disorder in any 12-month period (Multicultural Mental Health Australia 2004). At the same time, statistics for 2001–02 show lower rates of hospitalisation for the overseas born than the Australian born for a number of mental disorders such as schizophrenia, depressive episodes, and sleep disorders (AIHW 2008) and under-representation in service usage (Multicultural Mental Health Australia 2004). These apparently contradictory findings are explained, in part, by the significance of cultural factors in mental disorders. Researchers stress that cultural factors influence the personal meanings and experiences of illness, help-seeking behaviour, and treatment receptiveness (Guerin et al. 2004; Karasz 2005; Minas et al. 2007). In addition, other researchers have noted the problematic nature of Western psychiatry's criteria for, and diagnosis and treatment of, mental illness in the context of higher rates of Asian immigration (Jayasuriya et al. 1992).

Settlement experiences have been found to contribute to mental illness (Davis 2000; Beiser & Hou 2001; Costa & Williams 2002). These include employment and accommodation difficulties, downward social mobility, separation from family and social networks, and communication problems as a result of language difficulties (National Health Survey 1993; Manderson & Allotey 2003), as well as **racism** and discrimination (Jayasuriya et al. 1992). Importantly, research has consistently found that socio-economically disadvantaged ethnic groups have higher rates of mental disorders than socio-economically advantaged ethnic groups (Minas 1990).

Theoretical explanations

How important is ethnicity (or culture) in determining health outcomes for Australia's ethnically diverse population? Are class or gender more powerful determinants of health than ethnicity? Do the experiences of migration and settlement, rather than ethnicity *per se*, distinguish the health profiles of immigrants from those of the Australian-born population? The answers to these questions have direct implications for appropriate health care policies based on principles of equality and **social justice**.

A number of arguments have been presented to explain the research findings discussed above. Culturalist explanations, which emphasise the significance of ethnicity as the major cause of health outcomes, predominate within the Australian discourse. These types of explanations take two basic forms: first, there are 'explanations' based on simplistic accounts of cultural difference. These so-called 'explanations' do not examine the complex ways in which culture influences health; rather, they tend to assume that people with particular ethnic backgrounds are more likely to exhibit certain illnesses simply as a function of their 'ethnicity'. This view is evident, for example, in references to the 'Mediterranean back' or in the belief that Southern European women experience more pain during childbirth than women from Asian countries. Such views, in addition to taking an overly simplistic view of ethnicity and/or culture, homogenise people of a similar ethnic background and reify culture, thereby contributing to the perpetuation of racist and **cultural stereotypes** (Braun et al. 2007). They are of little value in addressing the health care needs of Australia's ethnically diverse population.

Second, there are more sophisticated culturalist explanations of health outcomes, and these focus on the processes of interaction between patient and health care provider. In other words, they recognise the importance of cultural differences in the meaning of health and illness among people of different ethnic backgrounds, as well as the effects of these in diagnosis and treatment. Such explanations often incorporate a critique of the biomedical model that is taken for granted in the Anglo-Australian health system. More specifically, such explanations emphasise the problems that arise through cultural misunderstandings and poor communication.

racism
Beliefs and actions used to discriminate against a group of people because of their physical and cultural characteristics.

social justice
A belief system that gives high priority to the interests of the least advantaged.

cultural stereotypes
Shared images of the members of an ethnic group that are often negative and are based on a simplistic, overgeneralised, and homogeneous view of an 'ethnic' culture.

Roberta Julian

structuralist explanations
Explanations that locate causality outside of the individual. For instance, these may include one's social class position, age, or gender.

● ● ● **TheoryLink**
● ● ● See Chapter 2 for a
● ● ● discussion of Marxist,
● ● ● Weberian, and feminist
● ● ● perspectives.

In contrast to culturalist explanations, materialist or **structuralist explanations** stress the significance of social location as the major causal factor in health outcomes. Such explanations emphasise the role of one or more of the following aspects of social location: social class, gender, age, and immigrant status. Once again, there are two main types of structuralist accounts. The first tends to dismiss the significance of ethnicity as a causal factor altogether. Such explanations usually view health outcomes as a function of social class position, typically associated with a Marxist perspective. If the influence of other factors is acknowledged at all, these are viewed as secondary. For example, according to this type of account, the high incidence of work-related injuries among immigrants would be explained in terms of the over-representation of immigrants in dangerous working-class occupations.

The second type of structuralist account views social location as a function of the intersection of a range of factors such as class, ethnicity, gender, age, and immigrant status, and is typically associated with Weberian and feminist perspectives. These explanations acknowledge the influence of both class and ethnicity, and attempt to examine the complex interrelationships between these variables, as well as how the relationship differs among various subgroups or individuals (for example, migrant women, the ethnic aged, second-generation youth, or refugees). Importantly these explanations examine each of these factors as both a cultural and structural phenomenon. For example, they recognise that class, ethnicity, and gender determine both social location (and thus access to health and health care services) and cultural orientation (and thus the meaning of health and illness, as well as views of culturally appropriate health care). These more sophisticated structuralist accounts thereby incorporate the influence of culture; they do not reify culture, and they acknowledge difference within ethnic categories. They therefore avoid the problems of stereotyping inherent in most culturalist explanations.

Health care services

assimilation/ assimilationism
A policy term referring to the expectation that Indigenous people and migrants will 'shed' their culture and become indistinguishable from the Anglo-Australian majority.

Multiculturalism is a policy that emerged in the 1970s as the government began to recognise the failure of **assimilationism**. The assimilationist policy regarded immigrants as having no special needs. One consequence was that the needs of a large number of people were not being met. Demands on service providers led to the perception that migrants were 'people with problems', many of which were health related (Martin 1978).

Multiculturalism was introduced in an effort to redress many of the problems brought about by expectations of rapid assimilation. It was based on the recognition that some ethnic groups had distinct cultures and special needs. Since multiculturalism began, along with changes in its meaning, there have been significant changes in its institutional structure. In the 1970s, the emphasis was on the value of cultural diversity and on the view that migrant welfare was predominantly the responsibility of ethnic groups and 'was based on the notion that the main determinant of social relations and identity was culture, defined in static terms as the language, customs, traditions and behavioural practices which migrants brought with them as "cultural baggage"' (Castles 1992, pp. 195–6). Much criticism was aimed at this version of multiculturalism. In particular, it was argued that it did little, if anything, to address issues of structural inequality in Australian society or, more particularly, the disadvantages experienced by immigrants and ethnic minorities. As Laksiri Jayasuriya (1992) argues, the policy focused on issues to do with lifestyle rather than life chances. It emphasised the need for cultural tolerance while deflecting attention from issues of social inequality.

During the 1980s and 1990s the meaning of multiculturalism changed. The *National Agenda for Multicultural Australia* (1989) placed emphasis on 'removing structural barriers (defined ... as those based on race, ethnicity, culture, religion, language, gender or place of birth) to participation in Australian society' (Castles 1992, p. 196). This was recognised as a key component of meeting equity goals and was reaffirmed by the government in 2002 (DIMIA 2002). Significantly, there is evidence of a shift away from support for multicultural policies (Castles & Davidson 2000) at both community and government levels (Jupp 2002; Hodge & O'Carroll 2006; HREOC 2007).

Despite the experience of almost four decades of multiculturalism, the major institutions in Australian society are still based on a British model: '[t]his suggests that the political task of changing central institutions to truly reflect a multicultural society has yet to be undertaken' (Castles 1992, p. 198). Despite improvements in the overall responsiveness of health care services to the needs of patients from diverse cultural and language backgrounds (Johnstone & Kanitsaki 2008), this is still as true of the health care system as it is of other key institutions in Australian society (Allotey 2003).

The health care system

Discussions about appropriate health care services have traditionally been couched in terms of the debate between **ethnospecific services** and **mainstreaming**. Support for ethnospecific programs is based on the fact that linguistic and cultural barriers significantly affect access to health care for Australia's ethnic minorities. Such services are often viewed as temporary measures. Today, governments typically support mainstreaming for reasons of cost-effectiveness.

ethnospecific services
Services established to meet the needs of specific ethnic groups or a number of ethnic groups. Members of the ethnic group(s) are the targeted clientele, so that these services are distinct from, and often run parallel with, mainstream services.

mainstreaming
A policy term that refers to the provision of services to all members of the community through the same institutional structure. In Australia, it refers to a structure of service provision that is contrasted with that of ethnospecific services.

Critics of mainstreaming argue that its attraction 'seems to lie with the short-term cost savings rather than any long-term policy focusing on the best interest of migrants' (Collins 1991, p. 243). Such a view led Stephen Castles and others (1986, p. 10) to argue that mainstreaming may be the beginning of the end of multiculturalism: '[a]lthough mainstreaming aims to strengthen multiculturalism—and, if sensitively handled, would have that effect—it could become a pretext for dismantling the capacity of services and programs to meet special needs'. As he argues, 'basing service delivery on ethnicity tends to segregate and marginalise migrants, but ignoring ethnicity and catering for migrants only within general services can mean neglecting special needs and perpetuating structural discrimination' (1992, p. 197).

To address this challenge, we must move beyond the narrow confines of the debate as it has been couched in the past. In recent years the concept of **cultural competence** has been suggested as an effective approach to address the quality of health care provided to ethnic communities (Betancourt et al. 2005). Cultural competence has been defined as:

> a set of congruent behaviours, attitudes, policies, and structures that come together in a system or agency or among professionals and enables the system, agency, or professionals to work effectively in cross cultural situations. (Flaskerud 2007, p. 121)

Joseph Betancourt and his colleagues (2005) argue that '[t]he goal of cultural competence is to create a health care system and workforce that are capable of delivering the highest quality care to every patient regardless of race, ethnicity, culture, or language proficiency' (p. 499). For them, cultural competence in health care has the potential to produce radical structural changes in the system because it entails:

- understanding the importance of social and cultural influences on patients' health beliefs and practices;
- considering how these factors interact at multiple levels of the health care delivery system (i.e. organisational, structural, and clinical decision-making levels); and
- devising interventions that take these issues into account to assure quality health care delivery to diverse patient populations (Betancourt et al. 2003).

The strengths of the cultural competence model are clearly evident from the discussion above. Like most 'solutions', it needs to be embraced with caution. Advocates of the model have emphasised the benefits it has for training health care professionals who are more attentive to cross-cultural issues (Nursing Council of New Zealand 2002). Critics note that if it is not thoughtfully executed, it can reinforce the simplistic culturalist approaches it is attempting to replace. Lundy Braun and his colleagues (2007) warn that it 'could produce poor health outcomes if the clinician is more attentive to what he or she *thinks* they know about this "type" of patient than to the individual before them' (p. 1426).

cultural competence
A set of behaviours, attitudes, policies, and structures that enables the health care system to deliver the highest quality care to patients regardless of race, ethnicity, culture, or language proficiency.

BOX 9.1 Doing health sociology: culture and childbearing

The Royal Hospital for Women in Sydney undertook research on the cultural aspects of childbearing that are important to Bangladeshi women and their families. This formed the basis for developing culturally competent staff and culturally appropriate services. The project coordinator was a community-based Bangladeshi woman who was fluent in both English and Bengali. Initially, key community leaders were invited to provide advice about the study. This was followed by focus groups with women and with men who discussed beliefs, practices, rituals, taboos, and appropriate interaction throughout childbearing. The discussion revealed a diversity of views between families, regions, religions, and generations. The research and community participation provided a bridge between the practices at the Royal Hospital for Women and the beliefs and behaviours in childbearing of Bangladeshi women. It resulted in space for daily prayers, the availability of halal meat, and the availability of family space if required (Centre for Culture, Ethnicity and Health 2005).

Conclusion

The review of research on the ethnic patterning of health in Australia indicates the need to move beyond 'either/or' debates about the relative significance of class and ethnicity and to address the 'key analytical question, namely the nature of the relationship between ethnicity, socioeconomic status and health' (Smaje 1996, p. 158; see also Nazroo 1998; Anand 1999). Such research should focus not only on immigrants and minority ethnic groups, but should recognise ethnicity as a significant factor in the lives of all Australians.

The same logic can be applied to a discussion of future directions for the Australian health care system. This chapter has argued that our current health care system is structured to meet the 'ethnic' needs of its Anglo-Australian population but creates barriers for those whose appearance, speech, behaviours, or values reflect cultural difference (Correa-Velez et al. 2005; Sheikh-Mohammed et al. 2006). Efforts to encourage cultural tolerance, while beneficial in their own right, will do little to achieve a socially just health system (Hage 1998; Hodge & O'Carroll 2006). Structural change in the health care system is the key, and this should not be limited to addressing cultural difference among Australia's ethnic minorities. More pervasive structural changes are required. These will be based on the recognition of structural and cultural diversity within the Australian community as a whole and on 'the development of data collection systems that are conceptually sound and useful for the monitoring of ethnic minority health in general, and potential discrimination in particular' (Sundararajan et al. 2007, p. 21). Only then will we begin to see the emergence of a truly multicultural society and a health care system that can adequately begin to address the health needs of all Australians.

Roberta Julian

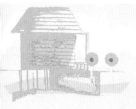

Summary of main points

» Health and illness are social constructions. Definitions of health and illness, and understandings of appropriate health care, vary over time and between cultures.

» Ethnic groups in Australia (both the dominant Anglo-Australian group and ethnic minorities) have different cultural understandings of health and illness, and different expectations of appropriate treatment.

» Ethnicity and class are often interrelated.

» The ethnic patterning of health and illness in Australia is the outcome of a series of socio-historical processes.

» In general, levels of mortality and morbidity for immigrants tend to be lower than those for the Australian-born population. With length of residence, these tend to converge with the Australian rates.

» There are two broad types of explanation for the ethnic patterning of health: culturalist and structuralist (materialist). Culturalist explanations emphasise the problems that arise from cultural misunderstandings and poor communication; they tend to reify culture. Structuralist explanations stress the significance of social location and view health as a product of the intersection of a range of factors, such as class, ethnicity, gender, age, and immigrant status.

» Multiculturalism was introduced to redress many of the problems brought about by assimilationism. Early versions of multiculturalism were criticised for focusing on cultural tolerance and deflecting attention from issues of social inequality.

» The equitable provision of health care in a culturally diverse society requires structural changes that go beyond the debate over ethnospecific versus mainstream services. In recent years 'cultural competence' has emerged as a positive step forward in the provision of culturally and linguistically appropriate health care to all Australians.

Sociological reflection: what is your ethnicity?

We often think of ethnicity as something that immigrants possess, noting how 'they' are different from 'us'. Yet we all have an ethnic identity that reflects the culture in which we have been socialised. Being conscious of your own ethnicity can help you to understand cultural differences and avoid ethnocentrism (judging the beliefs and practices of different cultures from the perspective of one's own culture).

» How would you describe your ethnic background?

» What are some distinctive features of your ethnicity?

» Why might some people be labelled as 'ethnic' in Australia and others not?

» In what ways might ethnocentrism affect the quality, accessibility, and appropriateness of health care delivery?

Discussion questions

1 Discuss either immigrant women, the ethnic aged, or refugees. In what ways would their health concerns be similar to and/or different from those of the Australian-born population?

2 Discuss the ways in which class, ethnicity, and gender might affect the health of the following categories: migrant women, the ethnic aged, second-generation ethnic youth, and refugees.

3 What does 'multiculturalism' mean to you? Compare your views with those of your class members.

4 In what ways has multiculturalism as a social policy had an impact on health services in contemporary Australia?

5 Stephen Castles (1992) states that contemporary multiculturalism 'is about equality of access to government services, rather than about the quality of the services offered'. With respect to health care, do you agree or disagree with this statement?

6 Debate the 'pros' and 'cons' of providing ethnospecific health care services. How would you move beyond the 'either/or' debate with respect to ethnospecific services and mainstreaming? Is 'cultural competence' the answer?

Further investigation

1 Critically assess the relative significance of pre-migration and post-migration factors on the health of immigrants in Australia. What patterns (if any) are apparent?

2 *The Spirit Catches You and You Fall Down* (Fadiman 1997) is a fascinating account of the difficulties that arise when the members of an ethnic minority with a non-Western view of health and illness (in this case the Hmong in the USA) interact with the Western health care system and its experts. Read this book and (a) identify the key factors contributing to the 'problems' that arose, and (b) suggest possible changes to the Australian health care system that would increase the likelihood of positive health outcomes. (Note: You will need to consider who is defining the 'problem' and who is defining the 'positive health outcomes'.)

3 Find out the ethnic composition of the population in your area (if possible, you might also get an age and gender breakdown). What changes would you make to current services in your area in order to meet the needs of the whole community?

Roberta Julian

Further reading

Allotey, P. (ed.) 2003, *The Health of Refugees: Public Health Perspectives from Crisis to Settlement*, Oxford University Press, Melbourne.

Johnstone, M. & Kanitsaki, O. 2008, 'The Problem of Failing to Provide Culturally and Linguistically Appropriate Healthcare', in S. Barraclough & H. Gardner (eds) *Analysing Health Policy: A Problem-oriented Approach*, Elsevier, Sydney, pp. 176–87.

Kai, J. (ed.) 2003, *Ethnicity, Health and Primary Care*, Oxford University Press, Oxford.

Minas, H., Klimidis, S. & Kokanovic, R. 2007, 'Depression in Multicultural Australia: Policies, Research and Services', *Australia and New Zealand Health Policy*, vol. 4, no. 16. Available online: <http://www.anzhealthpolicy.com/content/4/1/16>

Singh, M. & de Looper, M. 2002, *Australian Health Inequalities: 1 Birthplace*, Bulletin no.2, AIHW Cat. no. AUS 27, AIHW, Canberra.

Web resources

Australian Department of Immigration and Citizenship (DIAC): <http://www.immi.gov.au/>

Centre for Culture Ethnicity and Health: <http://www.ceh.org.au>

Diversity Health Institute Clearinghouse: <http://www.dhi.gov.au/clearinghouse/>

Ethnic Health: <http://www.australiahealth.com/Community%20Health/ethnic.htm>

Victorian Transcultural Psychiatry Unit: <http://www.vtpu.org.au/>

World Health Organization: <http://who.int/en/>

● ● **Online case study**
Visit the Second Opinion website to access relevant case studies.

Documentaries/films

Dangerous Ground (2008): 45 minutes. Four Corners, ABC TV. Explores anti-Muslim sentiment in Australia. Available online: <http://www.abc.net.au/4corners/content/2008/s2181743.htm>

Having a Baby in Australia. Centre for Women's Health Nursing, Royal Hospital for Women, Sydney. This video provides information about pregnancy, labour and delivery, and post-partum care and is available in Bengali and English.

Riot and Revenge (2006): 45 Minutes. Four Corners, ABC TV. Examines the tension between ethnic groups that led to the Cronulla riot and its aftermath. Available online: <http://www.abc.net.au/4corners/content/2006/s1588360.htm>

Working Effectively with Interpreters in a Mental Health Setting (Piu, M., Miletic, T. & Minas, I. H., Victorian Transcultural Psychiatry Unit, Melbourne. A DVD resource for educators in mental health settings, for self-directed learning.

References

Adler, S. R. 1996, 'Refugee Stress and Folk Belief: Among Sudden Deaths', *Social Science & Medicine*, vol. 40, no. 12, pp. 1623–9.

Allotey, P. 1998, 'Travelling with "Excess Baggage": Health Problems of Refugee Women in Western Australia', *Women and Health*, vol. 28, no. 1, pp. 63–81.

Allotey, P. (ed.) 2003, *The Health of Refugees: Public Health Perspectives from Crisis to Settlement*, Oxford University Press, Melbourne.

Allotey, P., Manderson, L. & Reidpath, D. 2002, 'Addressing Cultural Diversity in Australian Health Services', *Health Promotion Journal of Australia*, vol. 13, no. 2, pp. 29–33.

Anand, S. S. 1999, 'Using Ethnicity as a Classification Variable in Health Research: Perpetuating the Myth of Biological Determinism, Serving Socio-political Agendas, or Making Valuable Contributions to Medical Sciences?', *Ethnicity and Health*, vol. 4, no. 4, pp. 241–5.

Australian Bureau of Statistics 2004, *Labour Force Status and Other Characteristics of Migrants*, Cat. no. 6250.0, Commonwealth of Australia, Canberra.

Australian Bureau of Statistics 2004–05, *Migration, Australia*, Cat. no. 3307.0, ABS, Canberra.

Australian Bureau of Statistics 2005, *Australian Standard Classification of Cultural and Ethnic Groups (ASCCEG)*, 2nd edn, Cat. no. 1249.0, ABS, Canberra.

Australian Institute of Health and Welfare 2006, *Australia's Health 2006*, Cat. no. AUS 73, AIHW, Canberra.

Australian Institute of Health and Welfare 2004, *Australia's Health 2004*, Cat. no. AUS 99, AIHW, Canberra.

Australian Institute of Health and Welfare 2008, *Australia's Health 2008*, Cat. no. AUS 99, AIHW, Canberra.

Beiser, M. & Hou, F. 2001, 'Language Acquisition, Unemployment and Depressive Disorder among Southeast Asian Refugees: A 10-year Study', *Social Science & Medicine*, vol. 53, no. 10, pp. 1321–34.

Betancourt, J. R., Green, A. R., Carrillo, J. E. & Ananeh-Firempong, O. 2003, 'Defining Cultural Competence: A Practical Framework for Addressing Racial/Ethnic Disparities in Health and Health Care', *Public Health Reports*, vol. 118, pp. 293–302.

Betancourt, J. R., Green, A. R., Carrillo, J. E. & Park, E. R. 2005, 'Cultural Competence and Health Care Disparities: Key Perspectives and Trends', *Health Affairs*, vol. 24, no. 2, pp. 499–505.

Braun, L., Fausto-Sterling, A., Fullwiley, D., Hammonds, E. M., Nelson, A., Quivers, W., Reverby, S. M. & Shields. A. E. 2007, 'Racial Categories in Medical Practice: How Useful Are They?', *PLoS Medicine*, vol. 4, issue 9, e271, pp. 1423–8.

Castles, S. 1992, 'Australian Multiculturalism: Social Policy and Identity in a Changing Society', in G. Freeman & J. Jupp (eds), *Nations of Immigrants: Australia, the United States, and International Migration*, Oxford University Press, Melbourne, ch. 11, pp. 184–201.

Castles, S. & Davidson, A. 2000, *Citizenship and Migration*, Macmillan, London.

Castles, S. & Miller, M. 1998, *The Age of Migration*, 2nd edn, Macmillan, London.

Castles, S., Kalantzis, M., & Cope, B. 1986, 'W(h)ither Multiculturalism?', *Australian Society*, October, pp. 15–18.

Centre for Culture Ethnicity and Health 2005, *Consumer Participation and Culturally and Linguistically Diverse Communities*, Centre for Culture Ethnicity and Health, Melbourne.

Colic-Peisker, V. & Tilbury, F. 2006, 'Employment Niches for Recent Refugees: Segmented Labour Market in Twenty-first Century Australia', *Journal of Refugee Studies*, vol. 19, pp. 203–29.

Colic-Peisker, V. & Tilbury, F. 2007, *Refugees and Employment: The Effect of Visible Difference in Discrimination,* Final Report, Centre for Social and Community Research, Murdoch University, Perth.

Collins, F. S. 2004, 'What We Do and Don't Know About "Race", "Ethnicity", Genetics and Health at the Dawn of the Genome Era', *Nature Genetics Supplement,* vol. 36, no. 11, pp. S13–S15.

Collins, J. 1991, *Migrant Hands in a Distant Land*, 2nd edn, Pluto Press, Sydney.

Collins, J. 1996, 'The Changing Political Economy of Australian Racism', in E. Vasta & S. Castles (eds), *The Teeth are Smiling: The Persistence of Racism in Multicultural Australia*, Allen & Unwin, Sydney, pp. 73–96.

Collins, J., Noble, G., Poynting, S. & Tabar, P. 2000, *Kebabs, Kids, Cops and Crime: Youth, Ethnicity and Crime*, Pluto Press, Sydney.

Correa-Velez, I., Gifford, S. M. & Bice, S. J. 2005, 'Australian Health Policy on Access to Medical Care for Refugees and Asylum Seekers', *Australia and New Zealand Health Policy*. Available online: <http://www.anzhealthpolicy.com/content/2/1/23>

Costa, D. & Williams, J. 2002, 'New Arrival Refugee Women, Health and Well-being Project', *Synergy*, Autumn, Australian Transcultural Mental Health Network, vol. 9, pp. 16–18.

Davis, R. 2000, 'Refugee Experiences and Southeast Asian Women's Mental Health', *Western Journal of Nursing Research*, vol. 22, no. 2, pp. 144–68.

Department of Immigration, Multicultural and Indigenous Affairs 2002, *Annual Report 2001–02*, DIMIA, Canberra. Available online: <http://www.immi.gov.au/about/reports/annual/2001-02/index.htm>

Department of Immigration and Multicultural Affairs 2006, *Annual Report 2005–06*, DIMIA, Canberra. Available online: <http://www.immi.gov.au/about/reports/annual/2005-06/DIMA_AR/default.html>

Department of the Prime Minister and Cabinet 1989, *National Agenda for a Multicultural Australia: Sharing our Future*, Office of Multicultural Affairs, AGPS, Canberra.

Fadiman, A. 1997, *The Spirit Catches You and You Fall Down*, Farrar, Straus and Giroux, New York.

Flaskerud, J. H. 2007, 'Cultural Competence: What Is It?', *Issues in Mental Health Nursing*, vol. 28, pp. 121–3.

Guerin, B., Guerin, P. B., Diiriye, R. O. & Yates, S. 2004, 'Somali Conceptions and Expectations Concerning Mental Health: Some Guidelines for Mental Health Professionals', *New Zealand Journal of Psychology*, vol. 33, pp. 59–67.

Hage, G. 1998, *White Nation: Fantasies of White Supremacy in a Multicultural Society*, Pluto Press, Sydney.

Healey, E. 1996, 'Welfare Benefits and Residential Concentrations amongst Recently Arrived Migrant Communities', *People and Place*, vol. 4, no. 2, pp. 20–31.

Ho, C. & Alcorso, C. 2004, 'Migrants and Employment: Challenging the Success Story', *Journal of Sociology*, vol. 40, pp. 237–59.

Hodge, A. M., English D. R., O'Dea K. & Giles, G. G. 2004, 'Increased Diabetes Incidence in Greek and Italian Migrants to Australia: How Much Can Be Explained by Known Risk Factors?' *Diabetes Care*, vol. 27, pp. 2330–4.

Hodge, B. & O'Carroll, J. 2006, *Borderwork in Multicultural Australia*, Allen & Unwin, Sydney.

Holdenson, Z., Catanzariti, L., Phillips G. & Waters A.M. 2003, *A Picture of Diabetes in Overseas-born Australians*, AIHW Bulletin no. 9, AIHW, Canberra.

Holloway, G. 1994, 'Susto and the Career Path of the Victim of an Industrial Accident: A Sociological Case Study', *Social Science & Medicine*, vol. 38, no. 7, pp. 989–97.

Human Rights and Equal Opportunity Commission 2007, *Multiculturalism: A Position Paper by the Acting Race Discrimination Commissioner*, HREOC, Sydney.

Jamrozik, A., Boland, C. & Urquhart, R. 1995, *Social Change and Cultural Transformation in Australia*, Cambridge University Press, Melbourne.

Jayasuriya, L. 1992, 'The Facts, Policies and Rhetoric of Multiculturalism', in T. Jagtenberg and P. D'Alton (eds), *Four Dimensional Social Space: Class, Gender, Ethnicity and Nature*, 2nd edn, Harper Educational, Sydney, pp. 215–20.

Jayasuriya, L., Sang, D. & Fielding, A. 1992, *Ethnicity, Immigration and Mental Illness: A Critical Review of Australian Research*, AGPS, Canberra.

Johnstone, M. & Kanitsaki, O. 2008, 'The Problem of Failing to Provide Culturally and Linguistically Appropriate Healthcare' in S. Barraclough & H. Gardner (eds) *Analysing Health Policy: A Problem-oriented Approach*, Elsevier, Sydney, pp. 176–87.

Julian, R. & Easthope, G. 1996, 'Migrant Health', in C. Grbich (ed.), *Health in Australia: Sociological Concepts and Issues*, Prentice Hall, Sydney, ch. 6, pp. 103–25.

Jupp, J. 1999, *Immigration*, 2nd edn, Oxford University Press, Melbourne.

Jupp, J. (ed.) 2001, *The Australian People: An Encyclopedia of the Nation, Its People and Their Origins*, Cambridge University Press, Cambridge.

Jupp, J. 2002, *From White Australia to Woomera: The Story of Australian Immigration*, Cambridge University Press, Cambridge.

Kai, J. (ed.) 2003, *Ethnicity, Health and Primary Care*, Oxford University Press, Oxford.

Karantzas-Savva, E. & Kirwan, A. 2004, 'Ethnic Community Stakeholders as Partners in Primary and Secondary Diabetes Prevention', *Australian Journal of Primary Health*, vol. 10, no. 3, pp. 61–6.

Karasz, A. 2005, 'Cultural Differences in Conceptual Models of Depression', *Social Science & Medicine*, vol. 60, pp. 1625–35.

Khoo, S. E., McDonald, P., Giorgas, D. & Birrell, B. 2002, 'Second Generation Australians', *Report for the Department of Immigration and Multicultural and Indigenous Affairs*, Commonwealth of Australia, Canberra.

Kleinman, A. 1980, *Patients and Healers in the Context of Culture*, University of California Press, Berkeley, CA.

Kleinman, A. 1988, *The Illness Narrative: Suffering, Healing and the Human Condition*, Basic Books, New York.

Kleinman, A. & Good, B. (eds) 1985, *Culture and Depression: Studies in the Anthropology and Cross-cultural Psychiatry of Affect and Disorder*, University of California Press, Berkeley, CA.

Langer, B. 1998, 'Globalisation and the Myth of Ethnic Community: Salvadoran Refugees in Multicultural States', in D. Bennett (ed.), *Multicultural States: Rethinking Difference and Identity*, Routledge, London, pp. 163–77.

Lien, O. 1992, 'The Experience of Working with Vietnamese Patients Attending a Psychiatric Service', *Journal of Vietnamese Studies*, vol. 5, pp. 95–105.

Macintyre, M. 1994, 'Migrant Women from El Salvador and Vietnam in Australian Hospitals', in C. Waddell & A. R. Petersen (eds), *Just Health: Inequality in Illness, Care and Prevention*, Churchill Livingstone, Melbourne, ch. 10, pp. 159–68.

Manderson, L. & Allotey, P. 2003, 'Cultural Politics and Clinical Competence in Australian Health Services', *Anthropology and Medicine*, vol. 10, no. 1, pp. 71–85.

Manderson, L. & Reid, J. C. 1994, 'What's Culture Got to Do with It?', in C. Waddell & A. R. Petersen (eds), *Just Health: Inequality in Illness, Care and Prevention*, Churchill Livingstone, Melbourne, ch. 1, pp. 7–25.

Martin, J. 1978, *The Migrant Presence: Australian Responses 1847–1977*, Allen & Unwin, Sydney.

Minas, H., Klimidis, S. & Kokanovic, R. 2007, 'Depression in Multicultural Australia: Policies, Research and Services', *Australia and New Zealand Health Policy*, vol. 4, no. 16. Available online: <http://www.anzhealthpolicy.com/content/4/1/16>

Minas, I. H. 1990, 'Mental Health in a Culturally Diverse Society', in J. Reid & P. Trompf (eds), *The Health of Immigrant Australia: A Social Perspective*, Harcourt Brace Jovanovich, Sydney, pp. 250–87.

Multicultural Mental Health Australia 2004, *Reality Check: Culturally Diverse Mental Health Consumers Speak Out*, Multicultural Mental Health Australia, Sydney.

Nazroo, J. Y. 1998, 'Genetic, Cultural or Socio-economic Vulnerability? Explaining Ethnic Inequalities in Health', *Sociology of Health and Illness*, vol. 20, no. 5, pp. 710–30.

National Health Strategy 1993, *Removing Cultural and Language Barriers to Health*, Issues paper no. 6, AGPS, Canberra.

Nursing Council of New Zealand 2002, *Guidelines for Cultural Safety, the Treaty of Waitangi, and Maori Health in Nursing and Midwifery Education and Practice*, Nursing Council of New Zealand, Wellington.

Nyagua, J. Q. & Harris, A. J. 2008, 'West African Refugee Health in Rural Australia: Complex Cultural Factors that Influence Mental Health', *Rural and Remote Health*, vol. 8, pp. 1–9. Available online: <http://www.rrh.org.au>

Rice, P. L. (ed.) 1994, *Asian Mothers, Australian Birth—Pregnancy, Childbirth and Child-rearing: The Asian Experience in an English-speaking Country*, Ausmed Publications, Melbourne.

Romios, P., McBride, T. & Mansourian, J. 2007, *Consumer Participation and Culturally and Linguistically Diverse Communities: A Discussion Paper*, Health Issues Centre, La Trobe University, Melbourne.

Sheikh-Mohammed, M., MacIntyre, C. R., Wood, N. J., Leask, J. & Issacs, D. 2006 'Barriers to Access to Health Care for Newly Resettled Sub-Saharan Refugees in Australia', *Medical Journal of Australia*, vol. 185, no. 11/12, pp. 594–7.

Singh, M. & de Looper, M. 2002, *Health Inequalities in Australia: 1 Birthplace*, Bulletin no. 2. AIHW Cat. no. AUS 27, AIHW, Canberra.

Smaje, C. 1996, 'The Ethnic Patterning of Health: New Directions for Theory and Research', *Sociology of Health and Illness*, vol. 18, no. 2, pp. 139–71.

Stevens, C. A. 2001, 'Perspectives on the Meanings of Symptoms among Cambodian Refugees', *Journal of Sociology*, vol. 37, pp. 81–98.

Sundararajan, V., Reidpath, D. & Allotey, P. 2007, 'Ethnicity, Discrimination and Health Outcomes: A Secondary Analysis of Hospital Data from Victoria, Australia', *Diversity in Health and Social Care*, vol. 4, no. 1, pp. 21–32.

Sydney Morning Herald 2006a, 'Refugee Baby Triple-000 Tragedy', 13 Feb 2006. Available online: <http://www.smh.com.au/news/national/refugee-baby-triple000-tragedy/2006/02/13/1139679511391.html>

Sydney Morning Herald 2006b, 'The Amputee Who Was Told to Take the Stairs', 13 Feb 2006. Available online: <http://www.smh.com.au/news/national/the-amputee-who-was-told-to-take-the-stairs/2006/02/12/1139679480775.html>

Tran, H. 1994, 'Antenatal and Postnatal Maternity Care for Vietnamese Women', in P. L. Rice (ed.), *Asian Mothers, Australian Birth—Pregnancy, Childbirth and Child-rearing: The Asian Experience in an English-speaking Country*, Ausmed Publications, Melbourne, ch. 5, pp. 61–76.

Vasta, E. & Castles, S. (eds) 1996, *The Teeth are Smiling: The Persistence of Racism in Multicultural Australia*, Allen & Unwin, Sydney.

Viviani, N., Coughlan, J. & Rowland, T. 1993, *Indochinese in Australia: The Issues of Unemployment and Residential Concentration*, AGPS, Canberra.

White, K., Greig, A. & Lewins, F. W. 2003, *Inequality in Australia*, Cambridge University Press, Melbourne.

Windle, J. 2004, 'The Ethnic (Dis)advantage Debate Revisited: Turkish Background Students in Australia', *Journal of Intercultural Studies*, vol. 25, no. 3, pp. 271–86.

Wooden, M., Holton, R., Hugo, G. & Sloan, J. 1994, *Australian Immigration: A Survey of the Issues*, 2nd edn, AGPS, Canberra.

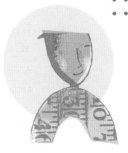

CHAPTER 10

Rural Health

CLARISSA
HUGHES

Overview

- What is the health status of people living outside the major Australian cities?
- Are Australia's health services and workforce evenly distributed between urban and rural areas?
- What challenges are faced by rurally based patients and health professionals when accessing and providing health care services?

RURAL LIFE AND PREGNANCY

Anna is 28 weeks pregnant with her first child. She and her husband James are on holiday on Thursday Island in the Torres Strait. For the first few days of the trip, the weather is beautiful and the couple enjoy the sightseeing. Anna is feeling well, but has noticed a few gentle contractions. She mentions them to James but they agree that it is probably nothing to worry about.

One morning the couple overhear a conversation about the arrival of bad weather. They return to their room, intending to read novels to pass the time until the sunny weather returns. Unfortunately the contractions intensify and so they decide to go to the local hospital. James is worried, and he hardly notices the heavy rain and strong winds during the trip. The situation becomes more worrisome when they learn that the doctor's preference is to transfer Anna to Cairns Base Hospital immediately, as it is better equipped to deal with neonatal intensive care cases.

There are no flights directly from Thursday Island to Cairns. Passengers normally catch a ferry from Thursday Island to Horn Island, a bus from the ferry terminal to the airstrip, then a plane to Cairns. The trip can take up to five hours. Sometimes helicopters transfer patients, but only in calm conditions. Thursday Island is not a particularly remote or isolated place, but transport to and from the island presents logistical difficulties. Under ordinary circumstances this might simply be inconvenient, but on this occasion the health of a mother and baby are at risk.

Introduction

A century ago, only around 13 per cent of the world's population lived in urban areas. By 1950 this figure had increased to 29 per cent (UN 2005). Globally, the process of urbanisation is continuing apace, but rural people still constitute nearly half of the world's population. Urban environments seem, intuitively at least, 'less healthy' than rural environments due to higher levels of overcrowding, air pollution from vehicles, and stress associated with being part of the 'rat-race'. Yet, the available evidence suggests that urban dwellers are in fact healthier than their rurally based counterparts across a range of relevant indicators.

Australia is reflective of global urban–rural health differentials. Over 6 million people—about one third of the population—live in regional and remote Australia (AIHW 2007b). Generally speaking, health status decreases with increasing distance from urban areas. People living in small isolated communities do not only suffer from higher rates of mortality (death) and morbidity (disease), they may also have little choice when it comes to health care providers. Furthermore, accessing preventative or curative services may necessitate time-consuming, costly, and inconvenient travel.

There is no single 'rural Australia'. It runs the gamut from Indigenous out-stations, small country towns, and major provincial centres, to isolated mining communities, and lush wine-producing regions (Humphreys 1998). The first of these is particularly important. Across virtually every indicator, the health status of Indigenous Australians is significantly worse than that of the non-Indigenous population (Dixon & Welch 2000). Given that the more remote Australian regions tend to have higher proportions of Indigenous people, there is considerable over-lap between the issues of 'rural health' and 'Indigenous health' (see Chapter 8). However, neither one is explained by, or reducible to, the other.

Despite a lack of homogeneity among rural and remote populations, there are several issues that unite non-metropolitan communities, and enough commonalities to enable us to speak of 'rural health' in a meaningful way. This chapter, which is divided into four parts, will address and explore a number of those issues. The first section addresses some contextual issues, namely the emergence of 'Rural Health' and the issue of classification. It also situates the issues within a wider sociological context by briefly discussing the nature of social ties and the concept of **community**. The second section presents mortality and morbidity data relating to metropolitan and non-metropolitan Australia, drawing attention to the enduring 'rural–urban health differential', before taking a closer look at the distinctive disease and injury profile of Australia's farming population. The third section explores the geographic (mal)distribution of health care providers in Australia and introduces the range of programs seeking to remedy this problem. It then explores some key challenges faced by health care providers and their patients in rural and remote settings. The fourth and final section presents some ideas on possible ways forward for addressing

community
A society where people's relations with each other are direct and personal and where a complex web of ties links people in mutual bonds of emotion and obligation.

inequities in rural health, and emphasises the key role that sociology and sociologists can play in this endeavour.

The rural health 'landscape'

Rural health emerged in the 1990s as an identifiable field of activity 'focusing on improving the health status and meeting the specific health needs of people living "outback" of metropolitan areas' (Wakerman & Humphreys 2002, p. 457). The governments of many nations, including Australia, formally identified the health of their non-urban populations as a priority. There are three key national rural health policy documents essential to understanding the Australian rural health 'landscape': the Rural Health Strategy (1994), the National Rural Health Strategy Update (1996), and Healthy Horizons 1999–2003 (1999). Australia has been particularly energetic in its efforts to address rural health issues and is now considered a world leader in implementing policy frameworks that encompass governments at the local, state, and national level (McLean et al. 2007).

Rural health is not an academic discipline in as straightforward a manner as sociology or chemistry or other long-established fields of intellectual enquiry. As Lisa Bourke points out, most rural health academics were not trained in rural health *per se* but in a specific health discipline (such as nursing or social work) (Bourke 2007, p. 9). Consequently, rural health research is informed by an eclectic mix of theoretical traditions associated with sociology, psychology, geography, anthropology, epidemiology, and economics as well as clinical and biomedical sciences.

Before delving into the intricacies of rural health, it is important to clarify what is meant by rural Australia. It is a more complex issue than it first appears. Efforts to develop systems of classification have continued for many years. They matter because they influence, or even determine, differences in the patterns of morbidity and mortality (Humphreys 1998). The three major rurality/remoteness classifications currently used in this country are:

- the RRMA (Rural, Remote and Metropolitan Areas) classification;
- the ARIA (Accessibility/Remoteness Index of Australia) classification (based on ARIA index values); and
- the ASGC (Australian Standard Geographical Classification) Remoteness Areas (based on ARIA+ index values—an enhanced version of the ARIA index values) (AIHW 2004c).

Using the ARIA, for example, Hobart, Ballarat, and Goulburn are classified as 'Inner Regional', Darwin, Cairns, and Dubbo are 'Outer Regional', and Alice Springs and Mount Isa are 'Remote'. Later in the chapter we will review some health statistics that utilise these classifications.

Regardless of which classification system is used, rural populations have poorer health status than urban residents. Why should this be the case? Are rural dwellers exposed to particular disease-causing substances? Do they take more risks or live unhealthier lifestyles than people in cities? Unfortunately, the various factors are notoriously difficult to disentangle. For instance, some rural communities have relatively high proportions of unemployed residents and/or people on a low income, and it is often those people who have poorer nutritional status, live in substandard accommodation, and have limited access to transport—factors all of which have implications for health.

social determinants of health
The economic, social, and cultural factors that directly and indirectly influence individual and population health.

A field of enquiry known as the **social determinants of health** is undergoing a rapid increase in interest, as efforts are made to develop more holistic understandings of how health status results from the interaction of a large number of complex factors. The social determinants are 'the economic, social and cultural factors that influence individual and population health both directly and indirectly, through their impact on psychosocial factors and biophysiological responses' (Dixon & Welch 2000, p. 254). This approach is beneficial for rural health research, since the contexts in which rural people 'live, work, and play' can radically contrast with their city-based counterparts.

globalisation
Political, social, economic, and cultural developments—such as the spread of multinational companies, information technology, and the role of international agencies—that result in people's lives being increasingly influenced by global, rather than national or local, factors.

The following section paints a picture of rural Australia in broad brush strokes, noting the ways in which 'climatic vagaries, market fluctuations and the process of deregulation and economic restructuring' (Humphreys 1998, p. 11) have resulted in financial and social hardship for many rural and remote communities. It also touches on the nature of social connectedness and the concept of 'community'. From that vantage point we will gain a more sociological understanding of the issues relating to rural health status and service provision which are addressed in sections three and four.

Rural communities: hardship and resilience

Since the 1980s, many of Australia's rural communities have experienced profound economic and social change. Although the impacts have not been uniformly negative, phrases such as 'the rural decline' and the 'downward spiral of rural communities' abound. Certainly, the resilience and resourcefulness of rural communities have been put to the test. Much of the upheaval experienced by rural communities is attributable to processes/forces at the international level (such as **globalisation** and climate change) and changes in the major rural industries (such as agriculture, forestry, and mining). Primary industries are being increasingly mechanised, so less 'human effort' is required to produce the same outputs. In towns where large proportions of people work in the same industry, the closure of a single mine or sawmill can have significant and long-lasting effects on communities, families, and individuals.

The agricultural sector, which has traditionally been the backbone of rural Australia, is facing problems such as 'declining farm incomes, farm amalgamation and enlargement, and the outmigration of the agricultural population' (Lockie 2000, p. 52). A downturn in agricultural vitality can have a serious domino effect: diminishing farm incomes can increase local unemployment, which can prompt people to leave in search of work, resulting in depopulation which can prompt the closure of hospitals, schools, banks, and other services, which further diminishes the viability and appeal of the community. Changes in infrastructure, such as rail system closures and highway bypasses, can also have a negative impact. The resultant issues of socio-spatial equity are not easily addressed, particularly when the philosophy of economic rationalism underpins much governmental decision-making.

The news is not all bad, though. Not all small towns are in decline, and even some with heavy reliance on primary industries are managing to thrive. Aspects of rural culture, such as resilience and self-reliance, undoubtedly contribute to communities' ability to soldier on under difficult conditions.

Social ties and the nature of 'community'

The nature of social interaction sets rural life apart from urban life. The tendency for 'everybody to know everybody' is intensified when families live in a region for multiple generations. Although rural and urban residents have similar numbers of 'strong ties' or close personal relationships, rural residents have fewer acquaintances resulting in a smaller proportion of so-called 'weak ties' (Bourke et al. 2004, p. 182). This density of social connection is salient here since it affects the experience of rural health care professionals, the nature of the relationships they have with patients, and decision-making regarding services use. The implications of such visibility and interconnectedness will be further explored later in the chapter.

There is a feeling in rural communities that they have special qualities not found in the cities (Strasser 2003). Such 'special qualities' are notoriously difficult to define, but are captured to some degree by the sociological concepts of **Gemeinschaft** and **Gesellschaft** (Tönnies 1957). These concepts are **ideal types** in that they refer to the abstract or pure features of a social phenomenon rather than accurate descriptions of what occurs empirically. Rural relationships are more aligned with *Gemeinschaft* in that they are more often face-to-face and ongoing, and are 'imbued with a strong sense of loyalty not only to friends and relatives, but to the community' (Strasser 2003, p. 458). Urban relationships, by contrast, are more likely to be short-lived, impersonal, and instrumentally or contractually-based, and thereby more closely aligned with *Gesellschaft* (see also Mellow 2005).

The very notion of 'community' sits rather more comfortably in a rural rather than urban framework. One does not often hear the term 'urban community'. Some

Gemeinschaft
A German term referring to a traditional society in which social relationships are based on personal bonds of friendship and kinship and on intergenerational stability.

Gesellschaft
A German term referring to an urban society, in which social bonds are based on impersonal and specialised relationships, with little long-term commitment to the group or consensus on values.

ideal type
A concept originally devised by Max Weber to refer to the abstract or pure features of any social phenomenon.

scholars (Wellman 2001, p. 231) emphasise the ability of communities to provide 'sociability, support, information, a sense of belonging and social identity'. This may be true for some communities, but they can also be sites of violence, prejudice, and **social exclusion**. Rural life can be exceedingly difficult. As the following two sections will demonstrate, despite comparatively high levels of ill health, rural residents can find it very difficult to access health care.

social exclusion
A broad term used to encompass individuals and groups who experience persistent social disadvantage from a range of causes (poverty, unemployment, poor housing, social isolation etc.), preventing participation in social institutions and political processes.

Rurality and health outcomes

As mentioned previously, despite increased investment by governments and the efforts of many organisations and individuals, a significant rural–urban health differential persists in Australia (see also Willis & Elmer 2007). It is characterised by higher mortality and/or morbidity rates for some diseases (such as asthma, diabetes, and coronary heart disease), coupled with increased rates of hospitalisation for many conditions. Living and working in the country, is itself 'a health hazard'. As mentioned earlier, Indigenous people make up a sizeable proportion of the population in many rural and remote regions, and they have much poorer health status than non-Indigenous Australians. This applies across the life-course, with lower birth weights, higher levels of infant mortality, higher levels of chronic illness, infectious disease and mental illness, higher rates of injury and suicide, and shorter life expectancy than non-Indigenous Australians (Bourke et al. 2004).

Mortality rates are a useful indicator of the underlying health status of a population (AIHW 2007b). In 2004, Australia had one of the lowest mortality rates of developed countries. However, given Australia's geographic and demographic diversity, it is useful to look at how these rates differ across urban, regional, and remote regions. Compared with major cities, death rates in regional areas in the 2002–04 period were 10–15 per cent higher for males and 5–10 per cent higher for females. Death rates for all people in remote and very remote areas were, respectively, 20 per cent and 70 per cent higher than in major cities (AIHW 2007b). Data collections indicate that rates of death by suicide and injury, road vehicle accidents, asthma, diabetes, and infant mortality in rural and remote areas are notably higher than those experienced in metropolitan areas (Dixon & Welch 2000, p. 255).

Comparative morbidity statistics give a more comprehensive overview of the rural–urban health differential. This section will present data on the Australian National Health Priority Areas (NHPAs), to provide a broad picture of the health status of rural people. The NHPA initiative is a collaborative effort involving the Commonwealth, state, and territory governments and is Australia's response to the World Health Organization's global strategy *Health for All by the Year 2000*. The initial set of NHPAs included cardiovascular health, cancer control, injury prevention and control, and mental health. Diabetes was added in 1997, followed by asthma in 1999, and arthritis and musculoskeletal conditions in 2002.

Table 10.1 shows how 'Rural and Remote' Australians compare to 'All Australians' across the seven current National Health Priority areas.

Table 10.1 Comparison of rural and remote Australians against the National Health Priority areas

Priority area	All Australians	Rural and remote Australians
Arthritis and musculoskeletal conditions	The most common form of arthritis, osteoarthritis, affects nearly 1.4 million Australians. Almost 1.2 million Australians are reported to have disability associated with arthritis and related disorders (AIHW 2005a)	The self-reported prevalence of arthritis in both 2001 and 1995 was 1.17–1.24 times as high for males, and 1.08–1.13 times as high for regional females as their counterparts in major cities (AIHW 2005a)
Asthma	Asthma affects 14–16% of children and 10–12% of adults (AIHW 2005b). In 2002 it led to over 40,000 hospitalisations and 397 deaths (AIHW 2004a)	The incidence of asthma in rural and remote areas is about the same as in metropolitan areas, but the death rate from asthma in remote areras is much higher (AIHW 2005b)
Cancer control	At the incidence rates prevailing in 2000, it would be expected that 1 in 3 men and 1 in 4 women would be diagnosed with a malignant cancer in the first 75 years of life (AIHW 2003)	Melanoma, lung cancer, and cervical cancer are among the main cancers with significantly higher incidence rates in regional and remote areas in 2001–03 compared with major cities (AIHW 2007a)
Cardiovascular health	Around 20% of the Australian population has a current cardiovascular condition. Cardiovascular disease kills more Australians than any other disease (accounting for 39% of all deaths in 2000) (AIHW 2004b)	Rural people experience higher levels of cardiovascular disease. More rural and remote people smoke, are inactive, overweight, and have high blood pressure (hypertension) than their metropolitan counterparts (AIHW 2002)
Diabetes mellitus	It is estimated that almost a million Australians aged 25 years or over have diabetes, yet half of these people are unaware of it. In 2000, diabetes was the underlying cause of 2.3% of deaths (AIHW 2002)	Rural and remote people experience almost 3 times the incidence of diabetes and twice the hospitalisations and death rates (Strong et al. 1998). Central Australia reports the highest incidence of diabetes in the world (AIHW 2002)
Injury prevention and control	Unintentional injury related to transport, suicide, and falls accounted for nearly three quarters of injury deaths in Australia in 2002 (NPHP 2004)	Death rates from all causes of injury increase with rurality and almost double again with remoteness (Smith 2004). Rates of hospitalisation due to injury are higher for rural/remote populations than for the general population (Pointer et al. 2003)
Mental health	1 in 10 Australians (around 2 million) report a long-term mental or behavioural problem. Around half that many were estimated to have a disabling psychiatric condition in 2003 (AIHW 2006)	Suicide rates for 15–24-year-old Australian men have doubled in metropolitan areas since the 1960s, but they have increased up to 12-fold in towns with fewer than 4000 people (Dudley et al. 1998)

Source: Adapted from Smith 2004

Clarissa Hughes

As noted earlier, there exists 'a worldwide disparity in health status in favour of urban populations' (McLean et al. 2007, p. 2). The preceding table provides an overview of this disparity in the Australian context. We will now take a more focused look at mortality and morbidity associated with a particular rural setting— the farm.

Down on the farm: illness and injury in the Australian farming population

The popular image of 'rural Australia' is inextricably entwined with agriculture and 'life on the farm'. Television soap operas such as *McLeod's Daughters* convey appealing, but not particularly accurate, images of rural life in this country (Botterill 2006). In spite of its sometimes glamorised image, farming is a dangerous occupation. Agriculture has a fatality rate of 19.5 per 100,000 employees, compared to the national rate of only 5.5 deaths per 100,000 employees (Mather & Lower 2001). In New South Wales alone, over 1100 people are admitted to hospital each year as a result of farm injury and illness (Franklin & Davies 2003).

The current rates of farm injury are of grave concern. Unintentional injuries are associated with tractors, motorcycles, animals (mostly horses), and tools and machinery, whereas the fatalities (among the adult population at least) tend to be associated with tractors and farm machinery (Fragar & Coleman 1996). Tractors have been labelled 'the most dangerous machine with which people work'—only 5 per cent of the Australian population work with them, and yet they are associated with 40 per cent of work injuries (Strasser 2003, p. 458). The farming population has a distinct injury profile: the majority of victims are adult males (Franklin & Davies 2003) who suffer from lacerations, puncture wounds, crush injuries, sprains, and fractures (Mather & Lower 2001).

The fact that most victims of farm injury are adult males should not lead us to ignore children and women. Farms can be particularly hazardous environments for children. Not surprisingly, children of different ages suffer different types of harm. There are three main groupings of rural child accidents:

- Babies and preschool children (Birth–5 years)—ingestion and drowning.
- Primary school children (6–10 years)—falls and vehicles.
- Secondary school children (11–15 years)—vehicles and machinery.

This injury profile is reflective of developmental stages. Babies and toddlers tend to be curious, and fond of putting things in their mouths—the latter of which puts them at risk of poisoning from toxic substances commonly used on farms. Preschool children have a higher incidence of farm fatalities than do babies and toddlers, but they sustain more injuries—perhaps as a result of their eagerness to learn and explore. Secondary children may be more coordinated, but they may also become overconfident and take unnecessary risks (Preece 1995).

Many measures can reduce the risk of children being harmed on farms, including providing (and insisting on the use of) helmets that meet current Australian Safety Standards, storing chemicals where they cannot be accessed by children, and ensuring that dams are properly fenced off. Injury prevention is a complex, and often costly, matter. Moreover, it can be difficult to 'keep children away'—since the farm is both an industrial workplace and a home (Preece 1995). In some respects, keeping children safe on farms is akin to keeping them safe in a factory, or on a building site which is replete with potentially risky objects, substances, and situations.

The changing role of women on farms is also relevant here, since farmers' wives/partners are increasingly taking on business-oriented roles as well as becoming responsible for tasks that 'hired help' would have undertaken previously. Mothers of young children on remote homesteads may be isolated from their extended families, have few opportunities for social contact, and limited child care options. Such difficulties may be compounded by transport problems and poor road quality, but they may also be improved by the opportunities for networking presented by the internet and other communication technologies.

Research has revealed a dominant culture of 'soldiering on' within many rural communities, and a masking (or ignoring) of symptoms if people are not coping when they believe they 'should be able to cope'. The resultant stress can result in relationship problems, and some people turn to drugs or alcohol for solace (Greenwood & Cheers 2002). Such problems are exacerbated even further when there is the additional burden of racial or cultural **stigmatisation** and prejudice (see for example, Kelaher et al. 2001).

**stigma/
stigmatisation**
A physical or social trait, such as a disability or a criminal record, that results in negative social reactions such as discrimination and exclusion.

Rural health care provision and access

There is a significant, and increasingly well-documented, uneven geographic distribution of the Australian health care workforce. There are fewer doctors per capita in rural and remote areas compared with urban areas. Furthermore, this situation worsened between 1986 and 1996 (Joyce & Wolfe 2005). A recent report on the rural and remote GP workforce noted the following: 37 per cent intend to leave within 5 years; 40 per cent are aged 50 and older; and 61 per cent reported an inadequate workforce in their practices (RDAA 2003).

Although doctors and specialists play an important role in rural health care delivery, the contribution and importance of other health professionals must not be underestimated. Lamenting the attention paid to the medical sector at the expense of the broader primary/allied health sector, Janie Smith claims that there is enough literature on the former to fill a semitrailer, whereas the literature on all the other health professions combined would only fill a Holden ute and still leave 'room for the Esky' (Smith 2004) (see Chapter 22 on allied health).

Figure 10.1 outlines the rates of primary health workforce per 1000 persons, by remoteness area and occupation groups.

Figure 10.1 Primary health workforce per 1000 persons, by remoteness area and occupation

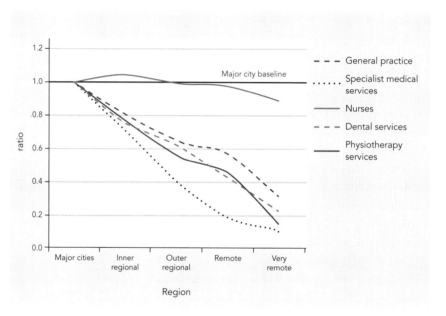

Source: PC 2005

The Australian Government has introduced many initiatives since the early 1990s to maintain and increase the numbers of health professionals in rural areas. The early focus was on the medical workforce, with programs for nursing and allied health coming later (Joyce & Wolfe 2005, p. 129). These initiatives have included, *inter alia*, the:

- Rural Undergraduate Support and Coordination (RUSC)—including increased intake of students of rural origin and establishment of/support for rural placements;
- Creation of University Departments of Rural Health and Rural Clinical Schools to assist with the provision of RUSC initiatives and provide education and training and undertake research relevant to rural health;

- Australian Government Remote and Rural Nursing Scholarships—providing scholarships for rural and remote nurses to undertake postgraduate study, short courses, and upskilling;
- More Allied Health Services (MAHS) Program—employment or contracting of allied health or nursing professionals through the Divisions of General Practice;
- Regional Health Services Program—providing health service programs in small rural communities.

Time (and rigorous evaluation) will tell whether or not these initiatives will be successful in attracting health professionals into non-metropolitan communities. Recruitment is only part of the story, though; longer-term retention is a separate issue. While rural communities can hold a certain appeal, some aspects of rural life can be particularly challenging, as the following section will show.

Rural health care providers: 'living in a fishbowl' and other challenges

> If you get a visit from the police for driving badly ... or playing music loudly until four in the morning, the town will know about it. If you are slow to pay your bills or repay your debts, the town will know about it. If someone sleeps over at your house, the town will probably know about that, too. (Sercombe 2006, p. 12)

This quote captures one rural health care provider's experience of rural life as 'living in a fishbowl'. Empirical research supports this observation of practitioners having a strong sense of 'being known' and lacking privacy. Furthermore, as the title of one recent article accentuates, rural health professionals have to 'face their mistakes in the street' (Allan et al. 2008). On the positive side, sustained social contact may provide the opportunity for more holistic care (Bourke et al. 2004), based on a broader appreciation of a patient's life and circumstances.

The classical sociological literature on the nature of professional–lay relationships emphasises the distinct roles associated with being a provider of care as opposed to a recipient of care (Parsons 1939). The experiences of rural practitioners and patients suggest the need for more sophisticated conceptualisations of these roles since they are inherently more complex than the early formulations suggest. In rural contexts, the nature of the roles themselves and the relationships between them are blurred due to the nature of social relationships within small communities.

The sociological concept of the **dual relationship** (or multiple relationship) is relevant here (see Campbell & Gordon 2003). Examples of dual relationships include: a general practitioner and a patient who is her daughter's school teacher; an ambulance

dual relationship
Refers to two distinct kinds of relationship with the same person (referred to as 'multiple relationship' when more than two aspects are involved).

officer who has been called to attend a car accident involving his cousin. In the health care context, such relationships can present ethical difficulties, and much of the literature on them focuses on the professional's decision-making regarding whether (or not) to enter a dual relationship. As Ruth Endacott correctly points out, such an approach implies that the professional has a choice (Endacott et al. 2006). In some rural and remote communities, practitioners have no choice—the circumstances force them to provide care to their friends, their colleagues, and even their own family members. In the words of one rural social worker:

> We are sole workers. So if I get a call on the weekend, be it a family member of mine, or ... someone I know, I have to respond to it because we have no one else to do it. (cited in Endacott et al. 2006, p. 989)

Rural practitioners also report the frequency with which they are 'consulted' about health issues in settings such as the local supermarket or children's sporting events. Such visibility and the experience of 'always being on call' undoubtedly contribute to stress and burnout among rural practitioners and their families.

Rural practice is also demanding in terms of diversity of skills. There is a strong requirement to be a 'Jack (or Jill) of all trades'—or at least have a level of confidence and competence in dealing with a range of situations and afflictions, particularly when there are few options for referral. Rural practitioners commonly have limited options for training. Even when opportunities are available the scarcity of locum support to enable providers to get away from the job can make taking holidays and continuing professional education difficult. Finally, the relative scarcity of professional colleagues can result in a strong sense of isolation and detract from job satisfaction. On the positive side, health care providers also value the variety associated with their work, the benefits of the rural lifestyle (Green & Lonne 2005), and the personal and professional rewards associated with providing much-needed care in the community setting.

Rural patients: confidentiality and the complexity of 'access'

Confidentiality is a key issue for rural health practice, and the nature of social relations impacts confidentiality for both providers and patients (Bourke et al. 2004). Dual relationships are common, making it more challenging to raise certain topics (sexual or mental health issues, for instance). The perception that 'everyone knows everyone's business' in a small community can prompt people to drive to the next town to have a prescription filled, rather than risk a breach of privacy by going to the local pharmacy. Such issues highlight the complexity of 'access', and prompt us to dig beneath the surface of the 'geographical distribution of services' statistics.

Australia is a vast continent. The 'tyranny of distance' can be acutely felt by rural populations. Simple indicators like 'number of kilometres to the nearest medical centre' overlook a range of issues impacting upon the ease with which rural people are able to access services. For instance, poor road quality (Dixon & Welch 2000), the price of petrol (Bourke 2001), limited public transport, seasonal (and often unpredictable) weather conditions (Panelli et al. 2006) and less regular air services, can all affect rural populations' access to services more significantly than urban ones (Perry & Gesler 2000).

BOX 10.1   Doing health sociology: beyond rural health

Having access to affordable, culturally appropriate, high quality health services is important—but it does not in itself guarantee good health. Access to clean water, nutritious food, and opportunities for exercise and recreation are equally important for the maintenance of good health and the prevention of disease. They, too, may be considered 'rural health issues'. Access to clean drinking water is an ongoing problem for some rural and regional communities (and particularly Indigenous communities) within Australia (Whelan & Willis 2007)—with chemical contamination of water supplies by agricultural herbicides and pesticides posing a risk not present in urban areas (AIHW 2006).

Access to fresh food can be a problem for some rural residents. Unless they grow their own fruits and vegetables, they may be at the mercy of whatever is supplied locally—and prices may be high due to higher transportation costs. Lastly, opportunities for, and facilities to support, exercise and recreation can be problematic. Bike paths, walking tracks, public transport and other infrastructure known to increase incidental exercise are not present in many rural environments. Even sealed footpaths, which are taken-for-granted aspects of urban living, may be absent—thereby posing difficulties for rural people in wheelchairs and those with children in prams.

Conclusion: rural health into the future

This chapter has provided an overview of rural health issues in Australia, including the enduring rural–urban health differential, uneven geographical distribution of health services, problems of access and confidentiality, and the 'tyranny of distance'. It has shown how the physical environment, the nature of social relations in small communities, and various other factors have implications for health and health care. The 'social determinants of health' perspective reminds us to dig beneath the surface of health statistics to see the complexity of both the issues themselves, and what will be required to address them successfully.

Clarissa Hughes

So what is the way forward for rural health? The answer is multifaceted. Collectively, we must ensure that the health of rural and remote populations remains firmly on government agendas at the national, state, and local levels. We also need to acknowledge the progress made thus far, whilst accepting that change takes time. Furthermore, there is a pressing need for rural health researchers and practitioners to utilise, and contribute to, a sound evidence-base for rural health initiatives. Arguably, there are five main priorities that should be focused upon.

First, there is a need to work together to improve rural health. Significant gains are made when the experiences of different regions, states, and countries can be drawn upon and learned from. Furthermore, collaborations should involve rural communities themselves. Community engagement may simply involve consultation or extend to ongoing involvement in rural health initiatives.

Second, innovation and creativity should be further fostered. Flexibility is the key, and alternative forms of delivery such as rural outreach specialists, telehealth initiatives, and multi-purpose services may be as effective in meeting community needs as more conventional models.

Evaluation is the third priority. Rigorous, systematic evaluations of rural health initiatives are essential for building an evidence-base concerning what works and (even more importantly) what does not work in specific community settings. Evaluation should be factored into funding applications, and have a specific allocation within project timelines and budgets, rather than being a poorly planned and underresourced afterthought. Furthermore, a commitment to solid evaluative practices and quality improvement should be present in both academic and health practitioner circles.

A fourth and related priority is that of communication. Too often, project reports gather dust on shelves rather than being disseminated to the various publics who could benefit from them. Communication is essential for the translation of knowledge into both rural health policy and health care practice.

The fifth priority is the need for sophistication. While less self-evident, it relates in part to a need for greater theoretical/conceptual refinement. Rural health research has been theoretically underdeveloped to date—a shortcoming which would be improved by greater social-scientific involvement in the field. More fundamentally, sophistication involves an appreciation of the complexity of rural health issues, combined with a capacity to apply the 'sociological imagination' to the analysis of those issues. Sociology engenders a healthy scepticism towards simplistic explanations, and underscores the importance of relating the lived experiences and choices of rural patients and providers to the wider sociocultural and historical context. The unfortunate reality is that there is no quick fix for rural health problems. Concerted, coordinated, and sustained efforts involving a range of stakeholders will be required to bring about positive impacts and lasting change.

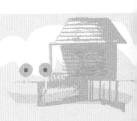

Summary of main points

» Rural health is a relatively new field of academic enquiry and it is influenced by an eclectic mix of social, behavioural, and clinical sciences.

» Internationally, there is a disparity in health status in favour of urban populations. Australia is reflective of this international trend with current mortality and morbidity data showing a significant 'rural–urban health differential'.

» The economic, political, and technological upheaval experienced by rural communities has implications for health and health care.

» The nature of social interaction in rural communities has implications for both the providers and the recipients of health care services. Dual relationships are common and sometimes unavoidable in rural settings.

» Australia's farming population has a distinctive illness/injury profile, characterised by high rates of unintentional injury and fatality.

» Geographically, the health care workforce is unevenly distributed and a range of initiatives are in place to address this inequity. Problems of access extend beyond mere 'distance to services'.

» Flexible and innovative solutions are required to address rural access issues, since traditional urban-based models of health service delivery may not be appropriate or possible in rural settings.

» Rural health would benefit from the increased contribution of a sociological perspective in the formation of a theoretically informed evidence-base for policy and practice.

Sociological reflection: access—more than meets the eye

You are attending a public forum in a small rural community. The forum has been organised so community members can discuss access to health services. Some participants consider the main issues to be the lack of public transport, footpaths, and ramps. Others regard racist attitudes and the absence of translator services as the major barriers to access. At one point the discussion becomes heated when someone insists that those things 'have nothing to do with health care'. Do you agree or disagree? Does your answer change if you imagine yourself to be a recently arrived refugee with limited English, or someone who is confined to a wheelchair? Reflect on other issues which could function as barriers to access for rural residents.

Clarissa Hughes

Discussion questions

1 People living in rural areas should not expect to be as healthy as their urban-based counterparts. Discuss.

2 *Gemeinschaft* is a useful concept for analysing rural communities. In what ways can it be applied to patients and/or health care providers?

3 What are dual relationships and what is their significance in the health care setting?

4 Choose one of the following:

a Type 2 diabetes

b Asthma

c Depression.

How does its prevalence in rural areas compare with metropolitan areas of Australia? Outline the ways in which rurality could present issues for its diagnosis, treatment, and/or management.

5 Explain what is meant by the 'social determinants of health'. Is the approach more or less useful than the biomedical model for explaining the rural–urban health differential and/or other rural health issues?

6 What are the main occupational health and safety issues for people working on farms? Has increased mechanisation resulted in safer work conditions for Australian farmers?

7 'The rural–urban health differential will not be solved simply by improving access to health care services.' Do you agree or disagree with this statement? Support your argument with reference to recent Australian data.

Further investigation

1 Compare and contrast dual relationships in cities and rural communities, with reference to at least one sociological concept or theory about lay–professional interaction in a rural health setting.

2 Familiarise yourself with the Australian Standard Geographical Classification (ASGC) system. Using the ASGC, choose an 'outer regional', 'remote', or 'very remote' town (preferably one that you have lived in, or know reasonably well). Collect information relating to a) the health services available (such as community health centres, allied health practitioners, and hospitals); and b) the region (such as area, topography, transport). In groups, discuss the similarities and differences between the towns in relation to access to health care services.

3 Choose one of the current National Health Priority Areas (see: <http://www.aihw. gov.au/nhpa/index.cfm>). Gather data on this for the Australian rural population. Compare it with equivalent data from one of the following countries: Scotland,

Canada, or New Zealand. To what extent do political, geographical, and socio-cultural similarities/differences between the two countries explain the observed results?

4 Conduct a semi-structured interview with a health professional who has worked in a rural setting. In the interview, explore such issues as community characteristics, referral options, professional role, collegial support, training, and relationships with patients and other community members. Make use of three or more socio-logical concepts or theories when writing up your analysis.

Further reading

Australian Institute of Health and Welfare 2005, *Rural, Regional and Remote Health: Indicators of Health*, Cat. no. PHE 59, AIHW, Canberra.

Hays, R. 1999, 'Common International Themes in Rural Medicine', *Australian Journal of Rural Health*, vol. 7: pp. 1914.

Lockie, S. & Bourke, L. (eds) 2001, *Rurality Bites: The Social and Environmental Transformation of Rural Australia*, Pluto Press, Annandale, NSW.

Ramp, W., Kulig, J., Townsend, I. & McGowan, V. (eds) 1999, *Health in Rural Settings: Contexts for Action*, University of Lethbridge, Lethbridge.

Smith, J. 2004, *Australia's Rural and Remote Health: A Social Justice Perspective*, Tertiary Press, Melbourne.

Wilkinson, D. & Blue, I. (eds) 2002, *The New Rural Health*, Oxford University Press, Melbourne.

Web resources

Australian Rural Health Education Network (ARHEN): <http://www.arhen.org.au>

Institute of Rural Health (IRH): <http://www.rural-health.ac.uk>

National Rural Health Association (NRHA): <http://www.ruralhealthweb.org/>

Rural Sociological Society: <http://ruralsociology.org>

Rural Health Workforce Australia:<http://www.rhwa.org.au/site/index.cfm>

Services for Australian Rural and Remote Allied Health (SARRAH): <http://www.sarrah.org.au>

Online case study • •
Visit the Second Opinion website to access relevant case studies.

Documentaries/films

Big Girls Don't Cry (2002): 26 minutes. A documentary about the strength and resilience of three Indigenous women and their families coping with end-stage renal failure. Available online:<http://australianscreen.com.au/titles/big-girls-dont-cry>

Four Corners (2006): 'Far from Care', shown 5 June, ABC TV. Explores whether rural Australians receive poor quality health services. Program transcripts and links to further resources are available online: <http://www.abc.net.au/4corners/content/2006/s1653599.htm>

Road to Nhill (1997): 95 minutes. A film portraying an affectionate and comical portrait of an Australian rural community. Available online: <http://wwwmcc.murdoch.edu.au/ReadingRoom/film/dbase/2004/road.htm>

Seachange, Treechange, Lifestyle Change (2007): Seven (5 minute) stories of city GPs who have successfully made the transition to work in rural and remote Australia. Available online: <http://www.gplifestylechange.com.au>

References

Allan, J., Ball, P. & Alston, M. 2008, '"You Have to Face Your Mistakes in the Street": The Contextual Keys that Shape Health Service Access and Health Workers' Experiences in Rural Areas', *Rural and Remote Health*, vol. 8, pp. 835.

Australian Institute of Health and Welfare 2002, *Diabetes: Australian Facts 2002*, AIHW, Canberra.

Australian Institute of Health and Welfare 2003, 'Cancer in Australia 2000', in *Cancer Series no. 23*, AIHW & Australasian Association of Cancer Registries, Canberra.

Australian Institute of Health and Welfare 2004a, *Measuring the Impact of Asthma on Quality of Life in the Australian Population*, AIHW & Australian Centre for Asthma Monitoring, Canberra.

Australian Institute of Health and Welfare 2004b, 'The Relationship Between Overweight, Obesity and Cardiovascular Disease', in *Cardiovascular Disease Series no. 23*, AIHW & the National Heart Foundation of Australia, Canberra.

Australian Institute of Health and Welfare 2004c, *Rural, Regional and Remote Health: A Guide to Remoteness*, Classifications, AIHW, Canberra.

Australian Institute of Health and Welfare 2005a, *Arthritis and Musculoskeletal Conditions in Australia 2005*, AIHW, Canberra.

Australian Institute of Health and Welfare 2005b, 'Asthma in Australia 2005', in *AIHW Asthma Series no. 2*, AIHW & Australian Centre for Asthma Monitoring, Canberra.

Australian Institute of Health and Welfare 2005c, *Rural, Regional and Remote Health: Indicators of Health*, AIHW, Canberra.

Australian Institute of Health and Welfare 2006, *Australia's Health 2006*, AIHW, Canberra.

Australian Institute of Health and Welfare 2007a, 'Cancer in Australia: An Overview, 2006', in *Cancer Series no. 37*, AIHW & Australasian Association of Cancer Registries, Canberra.

Australian Institute of Health and Welfare 2007b, *Rural, Regional and Remote Health: A Study on Mortality*, 2nd edn, AIHW, Canberra.

Australian Institute of Health and Welfare 2008, *National Health Priority Areas*, AIHW, Canberra. Available online:<http://www.aihw.gov.au/nhpa/index.cfm>

Botterill, L. 2006, 'Soap Operas, Cenotaphs and Sacred Cows: Countrymindedness and Rural Policy Debate', *Public Policy*, vol. 1, pp. 23–36.

Bourke, L. 2001, 'Australian Rural Health Consumers' Perceptions of Health Issues', *Australian Journal of Rural Health*, vol. 9, pp. 1–6.

Bourke, L. 2007, 'A Supervisor's Perspective of Postgraduate Study in Rural Health', in Q. Le (ed.), *Graduate Research Papers in Rural Health*, University of Tasmania, Launceston, pp. 5–19.

Bourke, L., Sheridan C., Russell U., Jones G., DeWitt, D. & Liaw, S. 2004, 'Developing a Conceptual Understanding of Rural Health Practice', *Australian Journal of Rural Health*, vol. 12, pp. 181–6.

Campbell, C. & Gordon, M. 2003, 'Acknowledging the Inevitable: Understanding Multiple Relationships in Rural Practice', *Professional Psychology: Research and Practice*, vol. 34, pp. 430–4.

Dixon, J. & Welch, N. 2000, 'Researching the Rural–Metropolitan Health Differential Using the "Social Determinants of Health"', *Australian Journal of Rural Health*, vol. 8, pp. 254–60.

Dudley, M., Kelk, N., Florio, T., Howard, J. & Waters, B. 1998, 'Suicide Among Young Australians, 1964–93: An Interstate Comparison of Metropolitan and Rural Trends', vol. 169, pp. 77–80.

Endacott, R., Wood, A., Judd, F., Hulbert, C., Thomas, B. & Grigg, M. 2006, 'Impact and Management of Dual Relationships in Metropolitan, Regional and Rural Mental Health Practice', *Australian & New Zealand Journal of Psychiatry*, vol. 40, pp. 987–94.

Fragar, L. & Coleman R. 1996, *A National Data Collection for Farm Injury Prevention: Final Project Report*, Australian Agricultural Health Unit, Moree, NSW.

Franklin, R. & Davies, J. 2003, 'Farm-related Injury Presenting to an Australian Base Hospital', *Australian Journal of Rural Health*, vol. 11, pp. 292–302.

Green, R. & Lonne, B. 2005, 'Great Lifestyle, Pity about the Job Stress: Occupational Stress in Rural Human Service Practice', *Rural Society*, vol. 15, pp. 254–67.

Greenwood, G. & Cheers, B. 2002, 'Women, Isolation and Bush Babies', *Rural and Remote Health 2*. Available online: <http://www.regional.org.au/au/rrh/2003/greenwood.htm>

Humphreys, J. S. 1998, 'Rural Health and the Health of Rural Communities', Worner Research Lecture, La Trobe University, Bendigo. Available online: <http://www.latrobe.edu.au/worner/assets/downloads/wornerlecture1998.pdf>

Joyce, C. & Wolfe, R. 2005, 'Geographic Distribution of the Australian Primary Health Workforce in 1996 and 2001', *Australian and New Zealand Journal of Public Health*, vol. 29, pp. 129–35.

Kelaher, M., Potts, H. & Manderson, L. 2001, 'Health Issues Among Filipino Women in Remote Queensland', *Australian Journal of Rural Health*, vol. 9, no. 4, pp. 150–7.

Lockie, S. 2000, 'Crisis and Conflict: Shifting Discourses of Rural and Regional Australia', in B. Pritchard and P. McManus (eds), *Land of Discontent: the Dynamics of Change in Rural and Remote Australia,* University of New South Wales Press, Sydney, pp. 14–31.

Mather, C. & Lower, T. 2001, 'Farm Injury in Tasmania', *Australian Journal of Rural Health*, vol. 9, pp. 209–15

McLean, R., Mendis, K., Harris, B. & Canalese, J. 2007, 'Retrospective Bibliometric Review of Rural Health Research: Australia's Contribution and Other Trends', *Rural and Remote Health*, vol. 7, pp. 1–13.

Mellow, M. 2005, 'The Work of Rural Professionals: Doing the Gemeinschaft-Gesellschaft Gavotte', *Rural Sociology*, vol. 70, pp. 50–69.

National Public Health Partnership 2004, *The National Injury Prevention and Safety Promotion Plan: 2004–2014*, NPHP, Canberra.

Panelli, R., Gallagher, L. & Kearns, R. 2006, 'Access to Rural Health Services: Research as Community Action and Policy Critique', *Social Science & Medicine*, vol. 62, pp. 1103–14.

Parsons, T. 1939, 'The Professions and Social Structure', *Social Forces*, vol. 17, pp. 457–67.

Perry, A. & Gesler, W. 2000, 'Physical Access to Primary Health Care in Andean Bolivia', *Social Science & Medicine*, vol. 50, pp. 1177–88.

Pointer, S., Harrison, J. & Bradley, C. 2003, 'National Injury Prevention Plan Priorities for 2004 and Beyond: Discussion Paper', in *Injury Research and Statistics Series Number 18,* AIHW, Canberra.

Preece, J. 1995, 'On the Farm: Children's Safety', *Australian Journal of Rural Health*, vol. 3, pp. 166–70.

Productivity Commission 2005, *Australia's Health Workforce*, Productivity Commission (PC), Canberra.

Rural Doctors Association of Australia (RDAA) 2003, *Viable Models of Rural and Remote Practice, Stage 1 and 2 Reports*, RDAA, Kingston.

Sercombe, H. 2006, 'Going Bush: Youth Work in Rural Settings', *Youth Studies Australia*, vol. 25, pp. 9–16.

Smith, J. D. 2004, *Australia's Rural and Remote Health: A Social Justice Perspective*, Tertiary Press, Melbourne.

Strasser, R. 2003, 'Rural Health Around the World: Challenges and Solutions', *Family Practice*, vol. 20 pp. 457–63.

Strong, K., Trickett, T., Titulaer, I. & Bhatia, K. 1998, *Health in Rural and Remote Australia: The First Report of the Australian Institute of Health and Welfare on Rural Health*, Cat. no. PHE 6, AIHW, Canberra.

Tönnies, F. (ed.) 1957, *Community and Society (Gemeinschaft und Gesellschaft)*, Michigan State University Press, East Lansing.

United Nations 2005, *World Urbanization Prospects: The 2005 Revision*, edited by Department of Economic and Social Affairs, UN.

Wakerman, J. & Humphreys, J. 2002, 'Rural Health: Why it Matters', *Medical Journal of Australia*, vol. 176, pp. 457–8.

Wellman, B. 2001, 'Physical Place and Cyberspace: The Rise of Personalized Networking', *International Journal of Urban and Regional Research*, vol. 25, pp. 227–52.

Whelan, J. & Willis, K. 2007, 'Problems with Provision: Barriers to Drinking Water Quality and Public Health in Rural Tasmania', *Rural and Remote Health*, vol. 7.

Willis, K. & Elmer, S. 2007, *Society, Culture and Health: An Introduction to Sociology for Nurses*, Oxford University Press, Melbourne.

The Social Construction of Health and Illness

The second dimension of the social model of health, and the theme of this part, is the social construction of health and illness. Social construction refers to the socially created characteristics of human life—the way people actively make the societies and communities in which they live, work, and play. The sheer differences in values, traditions, religions, and general ways of life across the globe are manifestations of the social construction of reality. In other words, human life and the way we interact with one another is neither 'natural' nor inevitable, but varies between cultures and over time. In the same way, social construction can be applied to how we view health and illness, revealing that assumptions about normality/abnormality, right/wrong, and healthy/unhealthy reflect the culture of a particular society at a given point in time.

Part 3 consists of seven chapters:

I enjoy convalescence. It is the part that makes illness worth while.

GEORGE BERNARD SHAW

1930, *Back to Methuselah*

CHAPTER 11

The Social Appetite: A Sociological Approach to Food and Nutrition

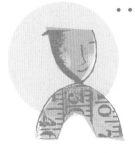

LAUREN
WILLIAMS
and
JOHN
GERMOV

Overview

- What role does food production, distribution, and consumption play in determining health and illness?
- Why is the food supply subject to medicalisation and McDonaldisation, and how do these social trends impact on population health?
- Why is the developed world worried about an obesity epidemic and what are the consequences of this concern?

THE POWER OF GLOBAL SUGAR

Food production and distribution (particularly retail sales) are highly profitable activities, strengthening the political power of these commercial sectors. In 2003, the World Sugar Organization (WSO) and the United States government attacked a World Health Organization (WHO) draft report that advocated restricting sugar intake to be no more than 10 per cent of a healthy diet. The WSO lobbied over forty ambassadors to remove the sugar restriction statement from the guidelines, arguing it could cause significant damage to the economies of both developing and developed countries (Boseley 2003). The sugar industry efforts were successful and the final version of the report, *Global Strategy on Diet, Physical Activity and Health* (WHO 2004) made no mention of the 10 per cent limit. The recommendation was replaced by a more general statement advocating an unspecified reduction in sugar intake.

Introduction: the social appetite

When you don't have any money, the problem is food. When you do have money, it's sex. When you have both, it's health.

J. P. Donleavy, *The Ginger Man* (1955)

This chapter introduces the concept of the social appetite: the sociological approach to understanding the production, distribution, and consumption of food. The social appetite provides a framework for understanding how social factors influence why we eat the way we do which in turn underpins a range of diet-related health problems in contemporary developed societies. The chapter investigates three topical health-related issues: the medicalisation of food; the **McDonaldisation** of the food supply; and the so called obesity epidemic, to examine the role of structure and **agency** around food and eating. First, we will examine the effects of structure and agency on food and nutrition, then we will use three key examples to explore the social influences on the consumption choices people make.

We are all aware that the food we eat impacts on our health. Well-known sayings such as 'an apple a day keeps the doctor away' and 'you are what you eat' are reminders that food influences our health. Health science research has increasingly shown the impact of diet-related illness on population health. (Here the term 'diet' is used to refer to the collection of foods eaten, not an attempt at weight reduction.)

A medical or nutritional science perspective of food and health has tended to obscure the social factors that influence why we eat the way we do. While we all have individual food likes and dislikes, many of our food choices reflect our **social appetite**, that is, the social, cultural, political, religious, and economic factors that affect what we eat. The social appetite can be seen in different national cuisines, for example, Thai, Indian, Italian, and Mexican, and in culturally distinct food practices such as the avoidance of beef among Indian Hindus and pork among orthodox Jews and Muslims (Germov & Williams 2008). Such examples show how our appetites, and indeed what is considered actual food that is acceptable to eat, are **social constructions**, a point long made by anthropologists and sociologists (cf. Murcott 1983, 1998; Mennell et al. 1992; Mennell 1996).

The preparation and consumption of food is an inherently social activity, whether over the family dinner table or eating out with friends at a restaurant. Food can also be used as a means of **social differentiation** between groups of people and as a social marker of identity. For example, people of different social classes tend to choose different foods (Bourdieu 1979/1984; Germov 2008). Food is also a commodity traded across the globe, driving national economies, and the McDonaldisation of food has been the subject of much debate and public concern in terms of chemical additives, food hygiene, and production methods (see Ritzer 2000).

McDonaldisation
A term coined by George Ritzer to expand Max Weber's notion of rationalisation; defined as the standardisation of social life by rules and regulations, such as increased monitoring and evaluation of individual performance, akin to the uniformity and control measures used by fast food chains.

agency
The ability of people, individually and collectively, to influence their own lives and the society in which they live.

social appetite
A term used by John Germov and Lauren Williams to refer to the social patterns of food production, distribution, and consumption.

social construction
Refers to the socially created characteristics of human life based on the idea that people actively construct reality, meaning it is neither 'natural' nor inevitable. Therefore, notions of normality/abnormality, right/wrong, and health/illness are subjective human creations that should not be taken for granted.

The social context of food and the structure–agency debate

Studying the social appetite brings into focus the **structure–agency debate** (discussed in Chapter 1) in terms of the degree to which people's food habits are an outcome of their social environment or the result of personal choice. In the context of food, **social structure** refers to the way in which food is produced and distributed, and includes public policies, government regulation, and the manufacturing and marketing methods of food companies. For example, in countries such as Australia and the USA, the farming sector contributes significantly to the national economy, which makes it important to governments. These governments have adopted policies to protect the sector through subsidies and tariffs, which advantage local producers against imported produce. This has helped to make food (especially meat and dairy produce) both plentiful and cheap for consumption by the population.

Food that is plentiful and cheap potentially encourages over-consumption, particularly when the marketing efforts of food manufacturers are taken into account. The increasing availability and affordability of energy-dense food, exemplified by 'super-sized' or 'up-sized' meals offered by fast food restaurants such as McDonald's, KFC, and Hungry Jack's, have contributed to the rise of obesity in most developed countries. This is an example of how structural changes in the food supply can have an impact on **population health**. A concern for the role played by structural factors should not discount the role of human agency—individuals can choose not to overeat or succumb to the pressure of food advertisements. Furthermore, people have the ability to make food choices that ultimately influence the wider social environment. The public interest inspired by the documentary film *Super Size Me* resulted in McDonald's Australia succumbing to political pressure and axing its super-size meal offers, in addition to expanding its range of low-fat products on their menu.

In considering the role of structure and agency in shaping the social appetite, it is important to bear in mind that they are always linked; an understanding of the social context of food necessitates that both structure and agency are taken into account. It is not a matter of choosing one or the other, but rather of acknowledging their constant tension and interdependence (see Chapter 1).

social differentiation
A trend toward social diversity based on the creation of social distinction and self-identity through particular consumption choices and through group membership.

structure–agency debate
A key debate in sociology over the extent to which human behaviour is determined by social structure.

social structure
The recurring patterns of social interaction through which people are related to each other, such as social institutions and social groups.

population health
The collective health status of a specified population.

The medicalisation of food

> Let food be thy medicine and medicine be thy food.
>
> Hippocrates

There is a long history of humans using food as medicine, and the contemporary application of food in the treatment of disease is a medical nutrition therapy used

Lauren Williams and John Germov

medicalisation
The process by which non-medical problems become defined and treated as medical issues, usually in terms of illnesses, disorders, or syndromes.

by dietitians. In recent decades, technological and industrial changes have occurred in food production methods that have facilitated product development of foods that confer specific health benefits—a process referred to as the **medicalisation** of food. The major agricultural development has been the genetic modification (GM) of plants and animals to produce food more efficiently or to alter the nutrient composition of food in desired directions (see Box 11.1).

BOX 11.1 'Franken-food': the genetic modification of food

Advances in biotechnology and genetic engineering are resulting in the development of a range of genetically modified foods, such as:

» inserting fish genes into tomatoes to delay ripening and increase shelf life

» placing a gene from a chicken into potatoes to increase resistance to bruising

» inserting a gene from the soil bacterium *Bacillus thuringiensis* (Bt) that is toxic to insects, but not humans, into various crops in order to provide inbuilt pest control.

While GM food has potential benefits such as longer shelf life, improved flavour and appearance, greater agricultural efficiency through higher crop yields, and resistance to disease and pests, there are also a significant number of potential disadvantages in terms of environmental, health, and animal-welfare issues. Some critics have termed them 'Frankenstein foods' because of the potential for adverse and uncontrollable side effects, such as the development of super-weeds and pests, the elimination of native species by cross-contamination, and possible allergic reactions to novel components of GM food (Lawrence & Grice 2008).

The food industry has capitalised on increasing public concern over diet and health by producing so-called 'functional foods'. These are food products that deliver a supposed health benefit beyond providing sustenance and nutrients (National Food Authority 1994; American Dietetic Association 1999). They are created by the fortification or addition of components in the food production stage to create modified food products with the alleged therapeutic effect of prescription drugs (Lawrence & Germov 2008). Examples of already available functional foods include yoghurts and fermented milk drinks with acidophilus and bifidus bacteria to aid digestion; breakfast cereals with psyllium fibre; margarines with phytochemicals that may lower cholesterol levels; omega 3 fats (which may help to prevent heart disease); and folate (which may help to prevent neural tube defects (NTDs) in foetuses).

The benefit of functional foods for manufacturers is the ability to make 'health claims' on their food products by stating that consuming a particular food (containing ingredient 'X') will improve health or prevent disease. In Australia, and many other countries, there was a general prohibition on allowing health claims on food products, based on the belief that it is the total diet and lifestyle of individuals that influences their health status. Nonetheless, food manufacturers have effectively lobbied governments to allow health claims. A number of countries, such as the USA, Canada, Sweden, and Japan, have established regulatory frameworks that allow food-related health claims. As of late 2008, Australia moved in the same direction, introducing a new food standard for Nutrition, Health and Related Claims (see Lawrence & Germov 2008). This decision slipped through with little public debate in Australia and occurred despite opposition from many health professionals, who view it as an unnecessary medicalisation of the food supply, despite often unproven benefits of such an approach (see Box 11.2). The food industry once again proved itself to be a powerful political force, using its power to achieve structural change for commercial benefit.

Treating food like a drug reflects an oversimplified, **reductionist**, and **biomedical** view of the causes of health and illness. The implication is that all the individual need do to be healthy is to choose to consume functional foods; therefore, diet-related health problems become a matter of choice (for those who can afford the often premium prices on such products). By oversimplifying the diet–disease link, the medicalisation of food ignores the multi-factorial nature of most illnesses as well as the wider social determinants of health. There is little evidence of the effectiveness of functional foods on population health in countries like the USA where health claims have been allowed since the 1990s. Concerns remain over the substantiation requirements for health claims and the impact these claims will have on population health, especially in terms of dosage effects, and the likelihood of exaggerated claims resulting in defensive eating and public confusion. It is possible to envisage people assuming they are protected from various diseases simply by eating certain functional foods, or that by consuming more of them they will be better protected, ignoring the possibility of side effects or that one food choice may be counteracted by other food and lifestyle choices (Lawrence & Germov 2008). For example, eating margarine that helps reduce cholesterol levels to prevent heart disease may be counteracted by smoking and lack of exercise.

reductionism
The belief that all illnesses can be explained and treated by reducing them to biological and pathological factors.

biomedicine/ biomedical model
The conventional approach to medicine in Western societies, based on the diagnosis and explanation of illness as a malfunction of the body's biological mechanisms. This approach underpins most health professions and health services, which focus on treating individuals, and generally ignores the social origins of illness and its prevention.

BOX 11.2	Doing health sociology: folate and the introduction of functional foods with health claims in Australia

In 1998, a pilot for a new health-claim framework was introduced by trialling the folate fortification of certain products. Folate is a B-group vitamin that has been linked to reduced risks of neural tube defects (NTDs) in foetuses. Manufacturers were granted an

· · ·»

Lauren Williams and John Germov

exemption to the general prohibition on making health claims on foods and allowed to use a specifically worded health claim on how folate reduced the risk of NTDs. An evaluation of the folate health-claims pilot (ANZFA 2001) found the impact of the health claim was inconclusive, noting that it was only likely to affect 5 per cent of women (consciously attempting to have a child). In 2004, a new Health, Nutrition and Related Claims policy framework was drafted by the Food Standards Australia New Zealand (FSANZ) regulatory body, the details of which were still in development in early 2005 following public consultation. The proposed framework consists of 'general-level claims', which are not subject to pre-market approval because they do not refer to a specific or 'serious' disease, and 'high-level claims', which do refer to a 'serious' disease and require pre-

approval and significant substantiation (Lawrence & Germov 2008).

The folate health-claim pilot raises a number of issues about the limitations of health claims on food products. In the case of folate, there is little understanding of the way it helps to prevent NTDs. Furthermore, only a small percentage of women are likely to be predisposed to having low levels of folate; folate fortification unnecessarily exposes a whole population to increased levels of folate intake; dosage effects are unpredictable; and there is little way for consumers to know whether they have consumed enough or too much (Lawrence & Germov 2008). There are possible adverse side effects of folate consumption, with some studies indicating a 40 per cent increased chance of multiple births (Czeizel et al. 1994; Lumley et al. 2001).

The introduction of GM and functional foods into the market is an example of structural changes to the food supply: changes that would not be feasible without government sanction. Despite the public outcry over GM foods in many countries, government food and agricultural policies have supported their development. Australia, along with the European Union, has reacted to public concerns and has mandated stringent labelling requirements to clearly identify GM food, allowing consumers to exercise their agency in terms of whether to buy it, but other countries, such as the USA, have resisted GM labelling altogether.

The McDonaldisation of food: creating an obesogenic environment

agribusiness
The complete operations performed in producing agricultural commodities, including farming, manufacture, handling, storage, processing, and distribution.

A counter-trend to foods promoted for health benefits is the McDonaldisation of food. McDonaldisation of food, a term originally coined by George Ritzer in 1993, refers to the global expansion of **agribusiness** through the standardisation of food production and consumption. Using McDonald's as a modern metaphor for Max

Weber's notion of the increasing rationalisation of social life, Ritzer (2000) argues that by various managerial and technological means, food production is standardised so that more and more food products are uniform, cheap, and readily available. Agribusiness represents one of the largest industries in the world, with global food trade estimated at over US$404 billion per year. In Australia alone, over 47 per cent of all retail sales in 2006–07 were on food and liquor, representing $106 billion in consumer spending (DAFF 2008).

TheoryLink
See Chapter 2 for an overview of Weberianism.

In recent decades there has been a shift away from foods being predominantly prepared and consumed in the home, towards food being prepared outside the home. Findings from the Australian 1995 National Nutrition Survey (NNS) (ABS 1997) indicate that a significant proportion of people's diet consists of meals prepared and consumed outside the home. For adults aged 19 and over, the proportion of energy (kilojoules) and fat from such meals were 24.4 and 34.5 per cent respectively. The rise of fast food occurred at a time of social change, where legislative changes allowed women to enter the paid workforce in large numbers. As Eric Schlosser discusses in *Fast Food Nation* (2001), this change initially had the dual effect of creating a female workforce possessing food-preparation skills, while taking away the time available for women to perform these skills in their own homes. Ironically, over time this reliance on food prepared outside the home has resulted in deskilling the culinary expertise of households.

Fast food continues to increase in popularity, with approximately 2000 new McDonald's restaurants opening each year worldwide (Schlosser 2001). The fast-food industry is promoted by direct advertising (much of it directed to children) backed by huge budgets and indirect initiatives that provide branded toys to children, and larger-than-life characters such as Ronald McDonald, who even has his own charity for children's hospitals. The physical environment of fast-food outlets such as McDonald's is also designed to be appealing to children, with play equipment and organised birthday parties available at most stores. This turns McDonald's into a leisure destination that is fun for the child and a safe haven for parents with children. All of these initiatives are a tacit acknowledgment that the food is insufficient to draw customers to fast-food restaurants on a regular basis.

Yet, we cannot ignore the food itself, because people are consuming it in large quantities. Leaving aside the environmental implications of the agribusiness that supports the industry, fast-food consumption is of concern for its nutritional composition. The food is typically energy dense (that is, contains a high amount of kilojoules or calories for each gram of product), and high in fat, which is a concentrated form of energy. The food is also high in salt and sugar, both of which are flavours that appeal to our taste buds, a fact well understood by the food industry. The more fat, sugar, and salt we consume, the more our taste preferences shift towards foods with high concentrations of these ingredients. Foods low in fat, sugar, and salt, but high in nutrients, such as vegetables, then tend to taste bland in comparison. This is especially problematic if children's palates become habituated to foods high in fat, sugar, and salt, since an extensive body of research by Leann Birch and colleagues (1996) shows that food preferences are formed in childhood. The fast food industry is aware of this, and seeks to capture the childhood market by the variety of strategies mentioned above, in order to establish future lifelong consumers.

The end result of this shift in taste preferences is that the fast food industry, and the broader food industry, has changed the food supply towards products that are high in energy (that is, more fattening). This trend has increased the amount of kilojoules available for consumption and is one of the structural factors contributing to the 'obesogenic' environment in Western countries. While consumers can exert their agency by purchasing low-fat or organically grown versions of products (see Box 11.3), such versions are usually more expensive. As we will see, it is the group of people with the lowest disposable income who experience the highest prevalence of obesity.

BOX 11.3 **The Slow Food revolution: resisting McDonaldisation**

While the McDonaldisation trend has dominated food production and retailing over the past few decades, it has not occurred without critique or resistance. One example of resisting McDonaldisation, which can be considered an opposing social trend to fast food, is the Slow Food Movement (SFM)—a global phenomenon claiming to have over 85,000 members in more than a hundred countries. Slow Food is a reaction against McDonaldisation and the taste-standardisation and cultural homogenisation associated with fast food. Using the emblem of the snail, members support organic produce, traditional cuisines, use of seasonal and regional ingredients, and sustainable agriculture. The SFM blends environmental and political concerns over biodiversity and cultural diversity, with an exaltation of the pleasure of food as a moral imperative of humanity (Petrini 2003).

The detrimental effects on body size and health of the over-consumption of fast food were strikingly illustrated in the documentary *Super Size Me*. Morgan Spurlock gained over 11 kg (25 lb) in just 1 month of consuming three meals per day from McDonald's, weight that it then took over a year to lose. In its defence, the company maintained that their food is not intended to be eaten in this way, yet there are no statements on their products or in their restaurants about eating in moderation (see the sociological reflection at the end of this chapter for more on *Super Size Me*).

The medicalisation and McDonaldisation of food are structural factors that clearly affect the food supply and thus the foods available for people to consume. We turn now to a key issue of public health significance—the case of obesity.

The obesity debate: epidemic or moral panic?

Health authorities across the world are concerned about the 'epidemic' of obesity. Their concern is that social, economic, and health costs will increase as the **prevalence** of obesity rises. A sociological perspective critically examines these assumptions, explores the social factors involved in driving our preoccupation with obesity, and considers the alternative viewpoint that rather than being a health problem, obesity has assumed the characteristics of a **moral panic**, based more on achieving an aesthetic beauty ideal than on a desire to improve public health. Before exploring sociological contributions we first need to define obesity.

What is obesity?

Obesity is defined as an excess of body fat. The most commonly used assessment of obesity on a population level is the Body Mass Index (BMI), which is derived by dividing an individual's weight in kilograms by his or her height in metres squared. The World Health Organization (WHO 1995) has defined weight ranges for women and men as shown in Table 11.1.

prevalence
The rate at which a particular condition occurs in a population.

moral panic
An exaggerated reaction by the mass media, politicians, and community leaders to the actions and beliefs of certain social groups or individuals, concerns which are often minor and inconsequential, but are sensationally represented to create anxiety and outrage among the general public.

Table 11.1 Body Mass Index and weight-range definitions

BMI	Definition
<18.50	Underweight
18.50–24.99	Normal range
25.00–29.99	Grade I overweight
30.00–34.99	Grade IIa overweight
35.00–39.99	Grade IIb overweight
40+	Grade III overweight

Source: WHO 1995

A person with a BMI equal to or above 30 is considered 'obese'. Obesity prevalence is usually reported together with the prevalence of overweight to give the total population of people with a BMI at or above 25. However, BMI should be interpreted with caution since it actually relies on weight rather than fatness. This means that those with a high proportion of lean muscle mass may have a BMI over 25, yet have little body fat, illustrating the limitation of applying a population-based measure to individuals. A further limitation of the international BMI cut-offs is that they are derived for Anglo populations, making them less relevant to other ethnic groups. Despite these limitations, BMI is widely used as a practical measure for estimating the prevalence of overweight in populations.

Obesity is not a peculiarly modern problem, and evidence of high degrees of body fatness dates from antiquity (Bray et al. 1998). However, it is no longer a rare

Lauren Williams and John Germov

pandemic
A worldwide epidemic.

condition. Cross-sectional studies show that the mean weights of developed and developing populations have increased over recent decades, resulting in a worldwide increase in the prevalence of overweight and obesity that the WHO has termed a **pandemic** (WHO 2000). In less developed countries, obesity is associated with rising rates of affluence among the upper classes as nations industrialise and more of the population has access to sufficient income to purchase food. At the same time, industrialisation leads to a decrease in energy requirements as the nature of work shifts from highly labour-intensive practices to sedentary activities involving the use of labour-saving machinery in offices and factories.

Large-scale epidemiological studies and national health surveys have collected measurements or self-reports of weight and height, which enable the calculation of BMI and categorisation according to stages of overweight. In developed countries such as Australia, the proportion of the population above the recommended weight for height is increasing. As shown in Figure 11.1, 17.5 per cent (3.71 million) of Australians were obese based on data using measured BMI (16.5 per cent of men and 18.5 per cent of women). Obesity rates for children aged 2–17 were 10–12 per cent and stable (Access Economics & Diabetes Australia 2008). More recently collected self-reported data, also shown in Table 11.2, place the figures even higher. The incidence of obesity (new cases in a given population) was estimated by *The Australian Diabetes, Obesity and Lifestyle Study*, referred to as AusDiab 2005 (Barr et al. 2006). AusDiab 2005 tracked a cohort of adults over 5 years and found that obesity incidence increased by a rate of 1.9 per cent per year; though the rate was 3.9 per cent per year for those who were already overweight at the start of the study period.

Figure 11.1 Trends in obesity prevalence for adults, 1980–2007

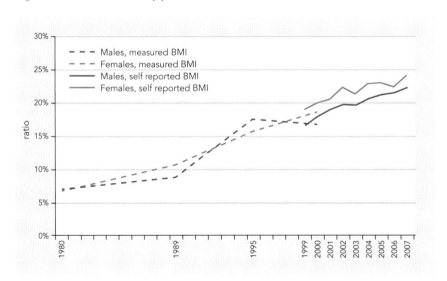

Source: Access Economics & Diabetes Australia 2008, p. ii

The social distribution of obesity

Obesity is the product of complex interactions between social, economic, political, and biological factors. Examining the rates of obesity according to categorisations of gender, class, education, and ethnicity sheds light on the relative influence of these factors.

Recent Australian data shows clear social patterns in overweight and obesity based on socio-demographic factors such as age, gender, socio-economic status (SES), education, indigeneity, and ethnicity (see Table 11.2). A summary of research on the social patterning of overweight and obesity shows that the highest rates are found among those aged 45–64 years, Indigenous Australians (approximately double), and people with low SES, low income, and no post-secondary school qualifications (O'Brien & Webbie 2003; Dixon & Waters 2003). Overseas-born Australians have a lower prevalence of overweight and obesity. The social patterning of obesity indicates that it is not necessarily produced by a person's genetic make up, nor can it be simply explained by a **victim-blaming** approach.

victim-blaming
The process whereby social inequality is explained in terms of individuals being solely responsible for what happens to them in relation to the choices they make and their assumed psychological, cultural, and/or biological inferiority.

Table 11.2 Social patterning of overweight and obesity in Australia, 2001

	Percentage overweight BMI 25–29.9	Percentage obese BMI 30+
Total population	34.4	16.7
Gender differences		
Females	25.8	17.4
Males	42.9	16.0
Socio-economic status		
Least disadvantaged	33.8	12.5
Most disadvantaged	31.3	21.1
Education		
No post-school qualification	33.3	19.0
Post-school qualification	35.5	14.9

Sources: O'Brien & Webbie 2003, Dunstan et al. 2001

The higher prevalence of obesity in those who are most socio-economically disadvantaged illustrates the complexity of the relationship between food and obesity. Household expenditure surveys show that having less money means that a higher proportion of household income is spent on food compared with high-income households. The 1995 NNS found that around 20 per cent of those on welfare or low incomes answered 'yes' to the question, 'In the last twelve months were there any times that you ran out of food and couldn't afford to buy more?' compared with the national average of 5 per cent. This finding indicates the extent of

Lauren Williams and John Germov

**food security/
insecurity**
Food security refers
to the availability of
affordable, nutritious,
and culturally
acceptable food. Food
insecurity is a state of
regular hunger and
fear of starvation.

**stigma/
stigmatisation**
A physical or social
trait, such as a
disability or a criminal
record, that results
in negative social
reactions such as
discrimination and
exclusion.

thin ideal
The dominant
aesthetic ideal of
female beauty in
Western societies,
which refers to the
social desirability of a
thin body shape.

muscular ideal
The social construction
of the male body
that reinforces
the desirability of
a large, muscular
body as epitomising
masculinity.

food insecurity, even in a country as affluent as Australia, where an abundance of food is produced.

The relative poverty experienced by the least affluent Australians leads to a complicated relationship with food, with experiences of hunger superimposed on a background of obesity for one in five people in this group. In the next section we will see how the obese are discriminated against in the workplace, limiting their ability to break the poverty cycle.

The social construction of obesity and stigmatisation

Obesity is a social construction, and notions of how it is perceived have changed over time and vary between different cultures. In times of food scarcity, it is not uncommon to find cultural ideals that value a large body size (Mennell 1996). When this has been the case, fatness has often been viewed as a symbol of affluence, good health, and high social status, reflecting people's ability to avoid manual labour and literally consume more than they need. When food is plentiful, cultural ideals tend to change towards valuing a thin body, which symbolises people's ability to discipline their appetites and restrain themselves from overeating. In many ways, such an ideal reflects the residual effects of the Christian 'sins' of sloth and gluttony, whereby, according to monastic religious orders, the soul could be purified by denying the body worldly pleasures through abstinence and penance (Turner 1992).

Those who are overweight and obese are subject to being **stigmatised** for being different to the social norms. In Western society, the dominant aesthetic is for women to conform to a **thin ideal** and for men to conform to a **muscular ideal**. A thin body is considered the epitome of beauty and sexual attractiveness, and has been linked to social status, health, and even moral worth (Williams & Germov 2008). Those who fail to conform are stigmatised as being at fault for their condition (unlike those with other medical conditions) and are discriminated against in the educational sphere and the workplace. While there have recently been gains against discrimination on the basis of religion, ethnicity, and sexual orientation, systemic discrimination against the obese continues and is often viewed as being socially acceptable (Sobal 2008).

The extent to which society has reproduced the stigmatisation of obesity is evident in the television program entitled *The Biggest Loser*. On the show, overweight people are subjected to humiliation in front of a national audience, to be allowed to stay at the retreat where they hope to lose weight through diet and exercise. Once a week, they have to strip down to body-hugging gym clothes and stand on a scale that clearly displays their weight for the audience. The language of the show's title reinforces the social belief that those who do not conform to a certain size are 'losers' (even if they 'win' the competition in the process). The fact that these people participate voluntarily illustrates the desperation of those considered overweight in Western society.

Responses to obesity

Attempts to deal with obesity distinguish between treating the existing condition in those already overweight or obese, and taking a population-based approach to prevent adult weight gain in those of normal weight. Treatment for overweight is problematic, because the body vigorously defends the newly established level of (over) weight (WHO 2000). This makes it more difficult to lose excess weight and maintain that loss than it is to maintain a desirable body weight initially. Weight-loss treatment for those already obese can be hazardous (Pi-Sunyer 1993; Brownell & Rodin 1994), and a high proportion of the obese regain weight when treatment is withdrawn in the clinical or community setting (Brownell 1993).

This means that people already unfortunate enough to suffer the social stigma of obesity are frequently confronted with failure, or at best only short-term success, in response to their considerable efforts to lose weight. This provides the lucrative commercial weight-loss industry with an almost perpetual market, as the overweight repeat their ill-fated attempts. An alternative to the cycle of yo-yo dieting and weight cycling for the obese is size acceptance, which has become a social movement advocating 'fat rights' (Sobal 1999). For example, in the USA, the National Association to Advance Fat Acceptance (NAAFA) publicly lobbies against obesity stigmatisation and discrimination, and promotes the acceptance of body diversity.

Another seemingly more efficient way to halt the rising prevalence of obesity is to direct those with a BMI under 25 towards the prevention of weight gain. There is evidence to suggest that population-based programs to prevent weight gain may have more success than treating those already obese (Scottish Intercollegiate Guidelines Network 1996; WHO 2000). Yet, despite the concerns of health-professional organisations over several decades, in Australia at least, the federal and state governments have failed to dedicate funds to population-based efforts aimed at halting the problem. It is only recently that the issue of obesity has been portrayed as a **public health** problem in the Australian media, and that only occurred with the realisation that rates of obesity in children were also increasing. This has provoked a moral panic, with childhood obesity becoming *the* health issue dominating the health and political agendas (though there is still little interest in adult obesity).

In response to this perceived problem, the New South Wales state government in Australia convened a three-day summit on childhood obesity in September 2002, following the same format as a previously successful drug summit. Stakeholders included nutrition and physical activity experts, health promoters, primary and secondary school educators, representatives of the food industry, the media, parents, children, and politicians. A series of recommendations were negotiated and documented on the final day of the summit, and the government has prepared a response to the summit (available for download from the New South Wales Health website: <http://www.health.nsw.gov.au/index.html>). The momentum of the summit has created an environment conducive to the development of public health strategies,

public health
Public policies and infrastructure to prevent the onset and transmission of disease among the population, with a particular focus on sanitation and hygiene such as clean air, water and food, and immunisation. Public health infrastructure refers specifically to the buildings, installations, and equipment necessary to ensure healthy living conditions for the population.

the most notable being the Fresh Tastes @ School initiative. This program requires the canteens of all primary and secondary schools managed by the state to conform with a strict set of nutrition recommendations by the commencement of the 2005 school year (with Catholic and independent schools to follow later). There are no comparable public health strategies aimed at adult obesity, where the responsibility appears to be directed at the individuals to pay for and manage their weight problem, despite an obesogenic food supply.

The obesity 'myth' debate

Despite the concern over obesity, and the billions of dollars spent by individuals in the pursuit of thinness, a debate has emerged that questions the extent to which obesity really is a public health problem. The views of those concerned about the extraordinary focus on obesity have recently been summarised in *The Obesity Myth* by Paul Campos (2004). Sociologists and others have claimed for decades that the public hysteria about obesity is based on our hatred of a body type that fails to conform to an aesthetic ideal, rather than a desire for health. Health authorities continue to advocate for weight loss in the obese, while, as Campos points out, they lack an effective formula for achieving weight loss and have failed even to prove that such weight loss will confer health benefits. In fact, he argues that there is evidence that the pursuit of weight loss is linked to the rise of the prevalence of obesity. For example, the rise in obesity rates has been paralleled with a rise in consumption of so-called 'low fat' or 'light' foods (Allred 1995).

Thus, health authorities are unwittingly fuelling the persecution of those who have committed the sin of storing more fat under their skin than is socially desirable. The health authorities also serve to legitimise the role of the dieting and pharmaceutical industries, groups driven to achieve economic profit, not the health of the nation. The ability of these industries to continue to be profitable is evidence of the extent to which the Western world has internalised the ideal of slenderness. Some health professionals are critical of equating thinness with health and have adopted an anti-dieting stance, advocating that overweight people can be fit and healthy through appropriate food choices and moderate exercise (Parham 1999; Ikeda 2000). The sociological perspective encourages us to examine the social, cultural, political, and economic factors that drive the obesity obsession.

Conclusion

The social appetite plays a significant role in population health. The social production, distribution, and consumption of food are determinants of diet-related health problems. This chapter has shown how the issues of medicalisation, McDonaldisation, and obesity affect the structure of the food supply and people's agency regarding the food they eat. A sociological approach to food and nutrition is essential in understanding why we eat the way we do and the implications this has for population health in contemporary societies.

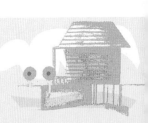

Summary of main points

» The social appetite refers to the social patterning of the production, distribution, and consumption of food, and how these social factors impact on population health.

» Eating habits are an outcome of both structure and agency, reflecting the influence of the social environment on the food choices people make.

» The medicalisation of food through functional food products is likely to have a significant impact on the food supply and people's food choices, though there is no evidence that it will lead to improvements in population health.

» The McDonaldisation of food has helped to create an obesogenic social environment that is partly responsible for the rise in obesity rates across the world.

» Obesity is socially constructed and distributed. Its prevalence varies according to age, gender, SES, education, indigeneity, and ethnicity.

» The debate over obesity highlights the stigma of obesity in contemporary Western society. Effective public health policies will need to address the food supply in order to make healthier choices easier for people.

Sociological reflection: *Super Size Me* and the 'cheeseburger bill': playing the 'blame game'

In 2004, Morgan Spurlock released the satirical documentary *Super Size Me* based on his experience of eating McDonald's for breakfast, lunch, and dinner for one month. He only took the option to super size a meal when it was specifically offered. During that time he gained considerable weight and his health substantially declined, to the extent that doctors warned him to quit his McDonald's diet long before the month had passed (see <http://www.supersizeme.com>). Shortly after the release of the movie in Australia, McDonald's discontinued 'super-size' serves and expanded its 'new taste' menu of meals, which are lower in fat. During the same year in the USA, a Republican Party-initiated law, often referred to as the 'cheeseburger bill', was introduced to protect the fast food industry from being sued by people with weight-related health problems—the only industry to be protected in such a way. Proponents of the legislation claimed that individuals should be responsible for what they eat and that 'society', or the fast-food industry at least, should not be blamed for increasing obesity rates (Teather 2004).

Lauren Williams and John Germov

» Reflect on some of the reasons you think obesity rates are rising across the world. Is the issue solely about individual responsibility over food choice, or should food producers also shoulder responsibility?

» Given that there are more energy-dense foods on the market and that food manufacturers actively advertise them to the public, should food producers be held accountable for the impact of their products in a similar way to the tobacco industry?

» Some have suggested that a 'fat tax' be introduced to make processed energy-dense foods more expensive so as to encourage healthier food choices among the public. What is your view?

Discussion questions

1 In what way is food consumption an important factor in determining health and illness?

2 In what ways is food being medicalised and what effects will this have on eating?

3 What social factors have led to the dominance of the fast-food industry in the production and consumption of food?

4 Why are the least affluent sections of society (who have the highest degree of food insecurity) also likely to be the most obese?

5 Why has there been a strong response to childhood obesity on the part of the public and the authorities, when a response to adult obesity has been lacking for decades?

6 How could the promotion of size acceptance affect the health of those who are overweight?

Further investigation

1 The medicalisation of obesity has both positive and negative implications. Discuss.

2 In what ways might the medicalisation of food be detrimental to population health?

3 Examine the ways in which the McDonaldisation of food has helped to create an obesogenic social environment.

4 Examine the arguments for and against a 'fat tax' on certain foods.

Further reading

Belasco, W. 2006, *Meals to Come: A History of the Future of Food*, University of California Press, Berkeley, CA.

Campos, P. 2004, *The Obesity Myth: Why our Obsession with Weight is Hazardous to our Health*, Viking, Camberwell.

Germov, J. & Williams, L. (eds) 2008, *A Sociology of Food and Nutrition: The Social Appetite*, 3rd edn, Oxford University Press, Melbourne.

Lang, T. & Heasman, M. 2004, *Food Wars: The Global Battle for Mouths, Minds, and Markets*, Earthscan Publications, London.

Nestle, M. 2007, *Food Politics: How the Food Industry Influences Nutrition and Health*, revised edn, University of California Press, Berkeley, CA.

Nestle, M. 2003, *Safe Food: Bacteria, Biotechnology, and Bioterrorism*, University of California Press, Berkeley, CA.

Pollan, M. 2006, *The Omnivore's Dilemma: The Search for a Perfect Meal in a Fast-food World*, Bloomsbury, London.

Schlosser, E. 2001, *Fast Food Nation*, Penguin, London.

Singer, P. & Mason, J. 2006, *The Ethics of What We Eat*, Text, Melbourne.

World Health Organization 2004, *Global Strategy on Diet, Physical Activity and Health*, WHO, Geneva. Available online: <http://www.who.int/dietphysicalactivity/goals/en/>

Web resources

Agriculture, Food, and Human Values Society: <http://www.afhvs.org/>

Agri-food Research Network: <http://www.csafe.org.nz/afrn/index.htm>

Association for the Study of Food and Society: <http://food-culture.org/>

Food and Agriculture Organization: <http://www.fao.org>

Food Standards Australia New Zealand: <http://www.foodstandards.gov.au>

International Journal of Sociology of Agriculture and Food: <http://www.ijsaf.org/>

New South Wales Centre for Public Health Nutrition: <http://www.cphn.biochem.usyd.edu.au>

Social Appetite website: <http://www.oup.com.au/titles/higher_ed/social_science/sociology /9780195551501>

State of Food Insecurity in the World (UN reports): <http://www.fao.org/sof/sofi/index_en.htm>

Super Size Me website: <http://www.supersizeme.com>

Online case study • •
Visit the Second Opinion website to access relevant case studies.

Lauren Williams and John Germov

Documentaries/films

Bad Seed: The Truth About Our Food (2006): 58 minutes. A documentary examining the risks of genetically modified food.

Fast Food Nation (2006): 116 minutes. A movie about the fast food industry that explores how profiteering and industrialisation of the food industry can be detrimental to public health.

The Future of Food (2004): A documentary on the political and corporate power holders that shape the food system, focusing on genetically modified food. Available online: <http://www.thefutureoffood.com>

The Global Banquet: Politics of Food (2000): 56 minutes. A documentary examining the links between globalisation and world hunger. Available online: <http://www.olddog documentaries.com/vid_gb.html>

McLibel: Two Worlds Collide (1997): 58 minutes. A documentary about the long-running legal dispute between McDonald's and anti-fast food campaigners.

Seeds of Change: Farmers, Biotechnology, & the New Face of Agriculture (2002): 70 minutes. A critical investigation of genetically modified food. Available online: <http://www. seedsofchangefilm.org>

Super Size Me (2004): 100 minutes. A documentary that examines the role fast food plays in rising obesity rates, as shown by film maker Morgan Spurlock's 30 day diet of consuming only McDonald's food.

References

Access Economics & Diabetes Australia 2008, *The Growing Cost of Obesity in 2008*, Access Economics, Canberra.

Allred, J. 1995, 'Too Much of a Good Thing?', *Journal of the American Dietetic Association*, vol. 95, pp. 417–18.

American Dietetic Association 1999, 'Position Statement of the American Dietetic Association: Functional Foods', *Journal of the American Dietetic Association*, vol. 99, p. 1278.

Australian Bureau of Statistics 1997, *National Nutrition Survey Selected Highlights, Australia 1995*, Cat. no. 4802.0, Australian Bureau of Statistics (ABS), Canberra.

Australia New Zealand Food Authority (ANZFA) 2001, *Inquiry Report—Proposal P153: Review of Health and Related Claims*, Australia and New Zealand Food Authority, Canberra.

Barr, E. L. M., Magliano, D. J., Zimmet, P. J., Polkinghorne, K. R., Atkins, R. C., Dunstan, D. W., Murray, S. G. & Shaw, J. E. 2006, *AusDiab 2005: The Australian Diabetes, Obesity and Lifestyle Study. Tracking the Accelerating Epidemic: Its Causes and Outcomes*, International Diabetes Institute, Caulfield.

Birch, L. L., Fisher, J. O. & Grimm-Thomas, K. 1996, 'The Development of Children's Eating Habits', in H. L. Meiselman and H. J. H. MacFie (eds), *Food Choice, Acceptance and Consumption*, Blackie Academic and Professional, London.

Boseley, S. 2003, 'Sugar Industry Threatens to Scupper WHO', *Guardian Unlimited*. Available online: <http://www.guardian.co.uk/society/2003/apr/21/usnews.food>

Bourdieu, P. 1979/1984, *Distinction: A Social Critique of the Judgement of Taste*, Routledge & Kegan Paul, London.

Bray, G. A., Bouchard, C. & James, W. P. T. 1998, 'Definitions and Proposed Current Classification of Obesity', in G. A. Bray, C. Bouchard & W. P. T. James (eds), *Handbook of Obesity*, Marcel Dekker, New York, pp. 31–40.

Brownell, K. D. 1993, 'Whether Obesity Should be Treated', *Health Psychology*, vol. 12, no. 5, pp. 339–41.

Brownell, K. D. & Rodin, J. 1994, 'The Dieting Maelstrom: Is it Possible and Advisable to Lose Weight?', *American Psychologist*, vol. 49, no. 9, pp. 781–91.

Campos, P. 2004, *The Obesity Myth: Why our Obsession with Weight is Hazardous to our Health*, Viking, Camberwell.

Czeizel, A., Metneki, J. & Dudas, I. 1994, 'Higher Rate of Multiple Births after Periconceptional Vitamin Supplementation', *New England Journal of Medicine*, vol. 330, no. 23, pp. 1687–8.

Department of Agriculture, Fisheries and Forestry 2008, *Australian Food Statistics 2007*, Department of Agriculture, Fisheries and Forestry (DAFF), Canberra.

Dixon, T. & Waters, A.-M. 2003, *A Growing Problem: Trends and Patterns in Overweight and Obesity among Adults in Australia, 1980 to 2001*, Bulletin no. 8, AIHW Cat. no. AUS 36, AIHW, Canberra.

Donleavy, J. P. 1955, *The Ginger Man*, Neville Spearman, London.

Dunstan, D., Zimmet, P., Welborn, T., Sicree, R., Armstrong, T., Atkins, R., Cameron, A., Shaw, J. & Chadban, S. 2001, *Diabetes and Associated Disorders in Australia, 2000: the Australian Diabetes, Obesity and Lifestyle Study (AusDiab)*, International Diabetes Institute, Melbourne.

Germov, J. 2008, 'Food, Class and Identity', in J. Germov & L. Williams (eds), *A Sociology of Food and Nutrition: The Social Appetite*, 3rd edn, Oxford University Press, Melbourne, pp. 264–80.

Germov, J. & Williams, L. (eds) 2008, *A Sociology of Food and Nutrition: The Social Appetite*, 3rd edn, Oxford University Press, Melbourne.

Ikeda, J. 2000, 'Health Promotion: A Size Acceptance Approach', *Healthy Weight Journal*, January/February, pp. 10–12.

Lawrence, G. & Grice, J. 2008, 'Agribusiness, Genetic Engineering and the Corporatisation of Food', in J. Germov & L. Williams (eds), *A Sociology of Food and Nutrition: The Social Appetite*, 3rd edn, Oxford University Press, Melbourne, pp. 78–99.

Lawrence, M. & Germov, J. 2008, 'Future Food: The Politics of Functional Foods and Health Claims', in J. Germov & L. Williams (eds), *A Sociology of Food and Nutrition: The Social Appetite*, 3rd edn, Oxford University Press, Melbourne, pp. 147–75.

Lumley, J., Watson, L., Watson, M. & Bower, C. 2001, 'Periconceptional Supplementation with Folate and/or Multivitamins for Preventing Neural Tube Defects', *Cochrane Database of Systematic Reviews*, Issue 1.

Mennell, S. 1996, *All Manners of Food: Eating and Taste in England and France from the Middle Ages to the Present*, 2nd edn, University of Illinois Press, Chicago.

Mennell, S., Murcott, A. & van Otterloo, A. H. 1992, *The Sociology of Food: Eating, Diet, and Culture*, Sage, London.

Murcott. A. (ed.) 1983, *The Sociology of Food and Eating*, Gower, Aldershot, UK.

Murcott. A. (ed.) 1998, *'The Nation's Diet': The Social Science of Food Choice*, Longman, London.

National Food Authority 1994, *Discussion Paper on Functional Foods*, AGPS, Canberra.

O'Brien, K. & Webbie, K. 2003, *Are all Australians Gaining Weight? Differentials in Overweight and Obesity among Adults, 1989–90 to 2001*, Bulletin no. 11, AIHW Cat. no. AUS 39, AIHW, Canberra.

Parham, E. S. 1999, 'Promoting Body Size Acceptance in Weight Management Counselling', *Journal of the American Dietetic Association*, vol. 99, no. 8, pp. 920–5.

Petrini, C. 2003, *Slow Food: The Case for Taste*, Columbia University Press, New York.

Pi-Sunyer, F. X. 1993, 'Short-term Medical Benefits and Adverse Effects of Weight Loss', *Annals of Internal Medicine*, vol. 119, pp. 722–6.

Ritzer, G. 2000, *The McDonaldization of Society*, 3rd edition, Pine Forge Press, Thousand Oaks, CA.

Schlosser, E. 2001, *Fast Food Nation*, Penguin, London.

Scottish Intercollegiate Guidelines Network 1996, *Obesity in Scotland: Integrating Prevention with Weight Management*, Scottish Intercollegiate Guidelines Network, Edinburgh.

Sobal, J. 1999, 'The Size Acceptance Movement and the Social Construction of Body Weight', in J. Sobal & D. Maurer (eds), *Weighty Issues: Fatness and Thinness as Social Problems*, Aldine de Gruyter, New York.

Sobal, J. 2008, 'Sociological Analysis of the Stigmatisation of Obesity', in J. Germov & L. Williams, (eds), *A Sociology of Food and Nutrition: The Social Appetite*, 3rd edn, Oxford University Press, Melbourne.

Teather, D. 2004, 'Scales of Justice', *Guardian Unlimited*. Available online:, <http://www.guardian.co.uk/society/2004/mar/12/food.worlddispatch>

Turner, B. S. 1992, *Regulating Bodies: Essays in Medical Sociology*, Routledge, London.

Williams, L. & Germov, J. 2008, 'Constructing the Female Body: Dieting, the Thin Ideal and Body Acceptance', in J. Germov & L. Williams (eds), *A Sociology of Food and Nutrition: The Social Appetite*, 3rd edn, Oxford University Press, Melbourne, pp. 329–62.

World Health Organization 1995, *Physical Status: The Use and Interpretation of Anthropometry: Report of a WHO Expert Committee*, WHO, Geneva.

World Health Organization 2000, *Obesity: Preventing and Managing the Global Epidemic*, WHO, Geneva.

World Health Organization 2004, *Global Strategy on Diet, Physical Activity and Health*, WHO, Geneva. Available online: <http://www.who.int/dietphysicalactivity/goals/en/>

CHAPTER 12

The Medicalisation
of Deviance

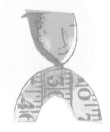

SHARYN
L. ROACH
ANLEU

Overview

- What causes someone to deviate from social expectations?
- Who defines what those expectations are?
- When someone is identified as deviating from social expectations,
  to what extent is that person viewed as sick (requiring a therapeutic
  response) or as a criminal (requiring a legal response)?

PRESCRIPTION DRUGS, THE MEDIA, AND THE DEATH OF A CELEBRITY

Heath Ledger's sudden death in early 2008 sparked widespread media attention. Stories claimed the actor had been 'battling an addiction to heroin', or more broadly, 'battling drugs, alcohol, and depression', that 'he suffered from insomnia', was 'dealing with terrible mood swings', had 'became a recluse', and it was reported that police found 'anti-anxiety and sleeping pills' (Dunn & Balogh 2008) in his apartment. These descriptions paint a picture of a psychologically troubled individual experiencing a number of emotions capable of fitting several different psychiatric diagnostic categories— for example, substance abuse, depressive disorders, sleep disorders, social phobia, and social anxiety disorder—concluding that he was 'too late in getting help'. The kind of help implied in this context is medical intervention: rehabilitation, therapy, and counselling. Though few reports offered a 'cohesive narrative' (Norris 2008, p. 27), the mass media seems to be fascinated by the failures, idiosyncrasies, 'bad' behaviour, and unusual lives of many celebrities. We could take a step further and suggest that the way in which their lives are reported becomes an arena for the articulation of social norms and moral boundaries regarding appropriate and deviant behaviour. Even so, explanations for their aberrations are often highly individualised and sometimes use the language of mental illness. It seems easy to explain unusual or errant behaviour by labelling the individual as suffering from a mental illness, directing our attention to problems restricted to that individual and their life and distracting attention from wider social issues. Almost 50 years ago Thomas Szasz coined the term 'the myth of mental illness' (1960, 1961) to draw attention to the way in which mental illness was being used as a 'catch-all' label applied to a wide range of behaviours that did not have a clearly identifiable biological cause. His claim that many of the conditions and complaints subsumed under the label mental illness are not biomedical in origin but are caused by 'problems in living' that stem from the complexities of modern life is no less true today.

Introduction

This chapter examines the ways in which deviation from some social **norms** and expectations becomes defined and treated as illness, or as a medical phenomenon, requiring intervention and treatment by medical personnel. The **medicalisation** of **deviance** is a historical and social process, and is the outcome of professional and social-movement activity. The dominance of the medical model in explaining certain types of behaviour or conditions means that the emphasis is on the individual, who must be treated in some way in order to restore conformity or health. The chapter first outlines the concepts of deviance and **social control**, and then examines the relationship between medicalisation and social control. It focuses on the role of psychiatry in identifying and regulating deviance, including criminal deviance.

Deviance and social control

Deviance can be defined as behaviour that violates social norms. Types of norms range from implicit expectations to criminal laws. The emergence of social norms is shaped by political and historical factors, and by specific social structures and situations (Parsons 1951a; Meier 1982). **Labelling theorists** shift attention away from the person who deviates from social norms to the social audience that defines, reacts to, labels, and punishes behaviour and individuals as deviant. Social movements, interest groups, and individuals affect the shape and application of social norms. Howard Becker terms those engaged in the creation and application of social rules 'moral entrepreneurs'—that is, actors who seek general acceptance of their particular values and perspectives, and who often adopt a self-righteous or crusading stance (Becker 1963, pp. 147–63).

norms
Shared expectations about how people ought to act or behave.

medicalisation
The process by which non-medical problems become defined and treated as medical issues, usually in terms of illnesses, disorders, or syndromes.

deviance
Behaviour or activities that violate social expectations about what is normal.

social control
Mechanisms that aim to induce conformity, or at least to manage or minimise deviant behaviour.

labelling theory
Focuses on the effect that social institutions and professions (such as the police, the courts, and psychiatry) have in labelling (defining and socially constructing) behaviour and activities as deviant.

● ● **TheoryLink**
● ● See Chapter 2 for an
● ● overview of symbolic
● ● interactionism.

Several kinds of questions can be asked regarding the concept of deviance. What causes or motivates someone to deviate from social expectations? Who defines what those expectations are? To what extent are such expectations shared or imposed on some people or groups by others? Does deviance necessarily invoke sanctions? What kinds of sanctions are invoked and under what conditions? What is the relationship between various forms of social control (for example, between legal regulation and medical intervention)? To what extent does the type of deviance or societal reaction depend on gender, age, socio-economic status, ethnicity, sexual identity, or other social attributes and structural inequalities? Medicine is one kind of social audience; it is concerned with identifying various conditions as deviations from a model of health and well-being that makes assumptions and values about normality.

Figure 12.1 The moral entrepreneur

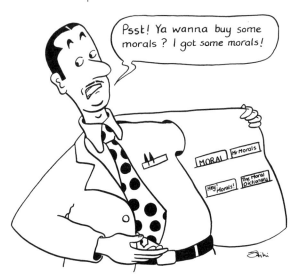

Medicalisation and social control

sick role
A concept used by
Talcott Parsons to
describe the social
expectations of how sick
people are expected to
act and of how they are
meant to be treated.

Medicalisation describes the process whereby non-medical problems or phenomena become defined and treated as medical issues, usually in terms of illnesses, disorders, or syndromes (Conrad 1992). Successful medicalisation means that the dominant form of social control is therapeutic, and that individuals diagnosed as deviating from a model of health confront a new set of normative expectations stemming from the **sick role**. Talcott Parsons (1951a, 1951b) first specified the connections between deviance and illness in his conception of the sick role. In addition to the constraints of physiological conditions, the sick role itself exempts people from fulfilling their normal social duties as long as they seek medical assistance. By entering into a relationship with medical personnel, the sick person becomes a patient with attendant expectations and requirements.

● ● **TheoryLink**
● ● See Chapter 2 for an
● ● overview of the sick role
● ● and functionalism.

While the sick role legitimates some kinds of deviance and imposes a new set of social norms (and social control), access to this status is not automatic. The manifestation of certain physiological conditions is not the only, or indeed necessary, prerequisite for contact with institutionalised medicine. Social groups deemed 'at risk' due to prevailing medical and social norms may be targeted in public health programs. For example, Indigenous people, female-headed households, gay men, or young people may be the subject for early intervention or education in order to prevent drug addiction, child abuse, suicide, or crime.

The medicalisation thesis posits that physical conditions do not, by their nature, constitute illness; rather, they require identification and classification, which entail subjective and value-laden considerations—that is, they are socially constructed. **Social constructionism** counters medicine's claims to be scientific, objective, and disinterested. Eliot Freidson (1988) argues that medicine actively constructs illness, and therefore determines how people must act in order to be treated. Rather than disinterestedly detecting symptoms and physiological causes, and administering scientifically validated therapeutic techniques, medical practice involves interpretation and judgment about what is normal and abnormal—about which circumstances are suitable for medical intervention and which are not. The symptoms do not speak for themselves; their interpretation and categorisation are informed by social values and assumptions about what constitutes health (normal) and illness (deviant). Illness and disease are human constructions: they do not exist without someone proposing, describing, and recognising them as abnormal. The central question becomes: how is it that certain areas of human life come to be defined, or not, as medical issues under certain conditions? The success of the medical profession in monopolising definitions of health and illness provides it with considerable authority and scope for social control (Freidson 1988).

Within this context, **empirical** research identifies the social conditions under which certain illnesses emerge, and it analyses the effect of medical practitioners' claims on the development of conceptions of illness. The medicalisation of infertility is a recent example. Traditionally, involuntary childlessness was considered a personal and private issue, but now it is viewed as a condition warranting medical attention and intervention. The experience of infertility also causes many people, especially women, to feel as though they are deviating from gender norms, which specify motherhood as essential to womanhood, even when their male partners are infertile but they are not (Roach Anleu 2006).

Discussions of medicalisation often refer to psychiatry as the primary example or prototype of medical social control. Such discussions tend to emphasise the negative and coercive aspects of social control, in contrast to medical **discourses** that focus on medical intervention as positive and necessary for health and well-being. The concept of medicalisation—and of social constructionism in general—has been subject to considerable critique regarding the relativity of its proponents' own position (Bury 1986). Critics point out that these theorists tend to view medicalisation as wholly

social constructionism
Refers to the socially created characteristics of human life based on the idea that people actively construct reality, meaning it is neither 'natural' nor inevitable. Therefore, notions of normality/abnormality, right/wrong, and health/illness are subjective human creations that should not be taken for granted.

empirical
Describes observations or research that is based on evidence drawn from experience. It is therefore distinguished from something based only on theoretical knowledge or on some other kind of abstract thinking process.

discourse
A domain of language-use that is characterised by common ways of talking and thinking about an issue (for example, the discourses of medicine, madness, or sexuality).

Sharyn L. Roach Anleu

negative and coercive—as something bad that should be averted. They also suggest that arguments about medical imperialism—and about medicine's displacement of religion and law as a source of social control—are exaggerated and not borne out in practice (Strong 1979). On the other hand, medicalisation can also confer certain benefits, including legitimating the conditions as real rather than imaginary; access to the sick role; and access to health insurance. The extent to which medicalisation has detrimental or beneficial consequences is an empirical, not a definitional, question.

Historical analyses and case studies identify the ways in which various phenomena come to be defined in medical terms and to be viewed as warranting medical intervention. Medicalisation is not necessarily fuelled solely by the efforts of the medical profession: developments in biotechnology, social movements and market forces—especially profit-driven pharmaceutical and insurance companies—can successfully advance the emergence of new medical categories (Conrad 2005; Furedi 2006). Medicalisation occurs on several levels, namely at the:

- *conceptual level*, at which medical vocabulary is used to describe or define a problem, but where medical professionals and treatments may not be involved. For example, alcohol abuse may be defined as evidence of sickness or mental impairment, but its management—although it may be viewed as therapeutic—does not necessarily entail medical intervention.
- *institutional level*, at which organisations may adopt a medical approach to particular problems, and medical personnel may be gatekeepers for the organisation, but the everyday routine work is performed by non-medical personnel. Access to some workers' compensation schemes requires a referral from a medical practitioner, even when human services personnel such as psychologists, counsellors, or social workers implement the rehabilitation program.
- *interactional level*, at which medicalisation occurs as part of doctor–patient interaction, with the former medically defining and/or treating the latter's problem. The doctor provides a medical diagnosis and prescribes a medical treatment. (Conrad 1992, p. 211)

The practices and processes that result in greater medicalisation at these different levels are diverse. Individual medical practitioners might claim that a problem or set of issues should be in the domain of medicine; however, successful medicalisation usually involves collective action and coalitions between different groups (Halpern 1992; Brown 1995). Patients and support groups may lobby with medical practitioners to have a condition recognised as a medical problem and thus gain access to the benefits that medicalisation may entail. Peter Conrad and Deborah Potter (2000) show how the combined (collective and parallel) efforts of the largest attention deficit [hyperactivity] disorder (AD[H]D) support group in the USA, a giant pharmaceutical firm, medical professionals, as well as the media, successfully extended the diagnosis of AD[H]D to adults in the 1990s. Similarly, post-traumatic stress disorder (PTSD), which originally applied to Vietnam War veterans to diagnose anxiety, sleep problems, and flashbacks emanating from their combat experience, has been extended to survivors or witnesses of horrendous accidents and crimes (Smith 2006).

Medicalisation can involve defining non-medical problems, or natural biological processes, as sickness or disease requiring pharmaceutical, surgical, or therapeutic intervention. For example, the inevitable process of ageing can be perceived as entailing deviation from social norms regarding youth, vitality, performance, and appearance. Julia Szymczak and Peter Conrad (2006) describe the emerging discourse around male menopause, known as andropause, and the increased availability of medical treatment for hair loss as evidence of the medicalisation of masculinity. Anthony Elliott (2008) suggests that cosmetic surgery is becoming increasingly popular among men who wish to conform to appearance norms as their bodies age and as workplaces require flexibility, the capacity for reinvention, and personal makeover. Research on the widespread marketing of the pharmaceutical drug Viagra points to the underlying social norms regarding masculinity and fertility (Loe 2006; Wienke 2006).

Medicalisation also includes the extension of pre-existing medical categories to include more potential sufferers and situations. The process is dynamic; not simply a case of 'doctors colonizing new problems or labeling feckless patients' (Conrad & Potter 2000, p. 560). Attempts to medicalise a problem or expand a medical category vary in their levels of success. The support and agreement of individual medical practitioners or professional medical associations often bolster claims for biomedical explanations and intervention. However, sometimes medical practitioners or segments of the medical profession resist, or at least are ambivalent towards, claims for medicalisation as is the case with what is termed fibromyalgia syndrome, a term used to describe such diverse symptoms as pain, fatigue, sleeplessness, and digestive disorders. The absence of visible or objective indicators of an underlying specific condition was part of medical practitioners' reticence to accept these symptoms as a medical illness (Barker 2002). Successful medicalisation does not necessarily mean that doctors are the key gatekeepers to some treatments, given the diversity of over-the-counter and over-the-internet drugs and medications available without a doctor's prescription.

The rise of psychiatry

Psychiatry, a sub-field of the medical profession, has always been involved in the identification and regulation of deviance. The emergence and dominance of a medical approach to madness (later to be redefined as mental illness) began in the late eighteenth century. Despite the lack of cures or explanatory theories of madness, physicians assumed a small but central role as gatekeepers of the asylums: from 1774, a physician's certificate was required for a patient to be committed to a British asylum. As Michel Foucault observes:

> The physician ... played no part in the life of confinement. Now he becomes the essential figure of the asylum. He is in charge of entry ... the doctor's intervention is not made by virtue of a medical skill or power that he possesses in himself and that would be justified by a body of objective knowledge. It is not as a scientist that *homo medicus* has authority in the asylum, but as wise man. (Foucault 1988, p. 270)

The decline of the Church, the scientific discoveries of the Enlightenment, and the humanitarianism of the Renaissance all aided physicians' 'professional dominance' in this area and fostered a unitary conception of mental illness—that is, a single illness category to encompass diverse conditions and symptoms. The Enlightenment, an eighteenth-century philosophical movement, questioned traditional, especially religious, values and doctrines; it emphasised **individualism**, rational thought, and the empirical method in science, and was oriented to human progress. Similarly, the Renaissance, which occurred between the fourteenth and seventeenth centuries, had heralded the transition from medieval to modern society, the latter being distinguished by the power and influence of rational science, which displaced some of the authority of religious expertise and its concern for the sacred. At the close of the eighteenth century, the notion of mental illness as a disease and as a topic of medical and scientific intervention was becoming the dominant conception of madness, and the influence of religious or supernatural explanations was waning (Conrad & Schneider 1992).

By the end of the eighteenth century, reformers sought to eliminate the physically punitive aspects of life in the insane asylum and to reinforce the benefits of moral treatment. They emphasised training, obedience, and work. Dr Philippe Pinel in France developed one of the first typologies of madness by distinguishing melancholia, mania, dementia, and idiocy. Physicians argued that as both moral and medical responses were appropriate to the management of these conditions, they should have a monopoly on dispensing both. Physicians' successful bid to provide moral assistance was especially important since they were unable to show the physiological causes of mental illness and had not demonstrated any cures. The asylum emerged during the nineteenth century as the state's solution to the increasing numbers of people identified as insane, and the history of psychiatry and its authority is inextricably intertwined with this development. Even so, there was considerable optimism and hope that new scientific advances in medicine would be able to solve problems associated with mental illness (Conrad & Schneider 1992).

The separation of those people identified as deviant was an essential precondition for the development of a medical specialty (the forerunner of psychiatry) that claimed to possess specific expertise in dealing with madness. This, in turn, further

individualism
A belief or process supporting the primacy of individual choice, freedom, and self-responsibility.

legitimised the concept of mental illness as a distinct phenomenon (caused by an underlying pathology), rather than the widespread cultural view of insanity that had previously prevailed and that had emphasised demonological and non-human influences (Scull 1975). During the nineteenth century, psychiatrists identified ill health, religious anxiety, disappointed love, financial embarrassment, acid inhalation, suppressed menstruation, and general poor health as causes of mental illness. Their interventions included physical restraints, cold baths, tooth extractions, and surgery of the brain and reproductive systems (Sutton 1991).

By the close of the nineteenth century, a whole range of new personal problems paralleled enormous social changes, especially in the USA. Everyday problems became defined as nervous diseases, providing a focus for new professional groups. One of the forebears of psychiatry—neurology—dealt with an ill-defined and diverse range of residual conditions that conventional medicine was unable to cure or manage. Up to a third of the neurologists' patients in the USA were diagnosed as suffering from 'general nervousness' and complained of conditions that would now be described as depression, anxiety, and insomnia. Discussions about general nervousness included complex theories of psychic and organic aetiology (causes), with treatments ranging from 'rest cure' to electrotherapy and psychotherapy (Abbott 1988).

The growth of asylums consolidated the professional development of psychiatrists; however, psychiatry was not approved as a medical specialty until 1934 (Neff et al. 1987). The number of patients in mental hospitals increased more than sixfold between 1880 and the mid-1920s, making them the largest of all custodial institutions in the USA. Similar patterns existed in the United Kingdom and France (Ingleby 1985). Psychiatrists had successfully monopolised the treatment of insanity by officially defining it as a medical condition with identifiable causes, but moral judgments and lay concerns still influenced diagnosis. Insanity was an elastic concept—a category of residual deviance—that could be applied to a variety of individuals whose deviance stemmed from poverty, homelessness, or physical disability. Unlike confinement in other custodial institutions, commitment to an insane asylum entailed neither a trial, a fixed term of internment, nor the legal protection associated with criminal proceedings (Sutton 1991).

It is clear that close links exist between mental hospitalisation and social control. Erving Goffman's classic study of a state mental hospital shows that very few of the everyday activities of the institution are devoted to therapy or treatment; most activities are oriented to maintaining the organisation, performing routine tasks, and maintaining social control among the patients. The psychiatrist's presence is brief and the input non-specific (Goffman 1961). Mental institutions also play a role in wider social policy and in the regulation of sub-populations that are identified as problematic. The increasing numbers of people confined to mental hospitals in the USA between 1880 and the 1920s did not indicate an epidemic of mental illness. Rather, the pattern stemmed from the government's incapacity systematically to address and solve poverty, especially among the aged; from the closure of the almshouses (charitable housing), combined with flexibility in the medical concept of insanity; and from the relatively simple commitment procedures (Sutton 1991).

Case studies of psychiatric hospitals illustrate the power of psychiatric diagnosis, the pervasiveness of psychiatric discourse, and the high status of psychiatrists (Goffman 1961). A stark example is provided in David L. Rosenhan's article 'Being Sane in Insane Places'. He describes an experiment in which eight sane people gained secret admission to psychiatric institutions (Rosenhan 1973). The pseudo-patients claimed that they had been hearing voices but, upon admission to the hospital ward, ceased simulating any symptoms of abnormality. The only people who detected that they were not suffering from a psychiatric condition were the other patients, not the medical staff. Indeed, the label 'schizophrenic'—that is, the diagnosis—determined psychiatrists' and nurses' perceptions and interpretations of the pseudo-patients' behaviour, even when it was completely 'normal' (Rosenhan 1973, p. 253).

Psychiatry and norm-breaking

As an emergent occupation and as a segment of the medical profession, psychiatry has developed notions of normal behaviour in areas such as sexual behaviour and identity, mental health, gambling, alcohol and drug use, eating, reproduction, and child development. Psychiatry seeks to locate a pathological basis within the individual for such 'deviance' and views certain types of behaviour as evidence of addiction, syndromes, conditions, personality disorders, or other mental illnesses. It attempts to attribute causes to—or perhaps, more accurately, to identify sites of intervention on the basis of—individual rather than to social or definitional factors. Conditions that psychiatrists view as warranting their intervention include deviations from moral or religious norms (for example, gambling or alcohol use, which may be 'diagnosed' as evidence of addictive behaviour, personality disorder, or depression), or from legal norms (for example, child abuse, juvenile delinquency, rape, or homicide).

Other significant developments in the history of psychiatry include the rise of psychoanalysis, which enabled psychiatrists to help people who were anxious and depressed, and who experienced problems with everyday life, as well as to treat the insane. Sigmund Freud, a physician and a neurologist, provided a new approach to understanding personal problems. He replaced a biological model with a psychogenic explanation and intervention that was based on free discussion (by the patient) in the context of a relationship with the therapist (Conrad & Schneider 1992). Parallels between this therapeutic relationship and the Christian confessional are obvious: the penitent/patient confesses his or her sins/deviance to a priest/psychiatrist, who has the power to specify and require remedial action. The one who receives confessions is able to exert social control—that is, instruct penitents/patients how to atone for their sins or manage their deviance in order to become conforming, normal people (Hepworth & Turner 1982). The popularity of psychoanalysis also provided psychiatry with competition from psychology, which led to a re-biologising of personal problems in the late 1970s (Abbott 1988).

A second important development in the 1950s was the availability of new psychotropic (mood-altering) drugs, which were used in mental hospitals as well as to enable more people to be discharged and treated outside the hospital. However, the use of prescription drugs raised questions of compliance and self-medication. While drug treatment reinforced the medical model of mental illness, the curative effect was contested, and critics argued (and continue to argue) that the drugs merely sedated, and thereby regulated, the behaviour of people identified as mentally ill. In the 1960s, criticisms of psychiatry, of the unitary conception of mental illness, and of the social control functions of mental hospitals and the 'therapeutic' relationship became more evident. Proponents of the labelling perspective doubted that diverse symptoms, behaviours, and conditions constituted a single classification of mental illness. Thomas Scheff (1966), for example, argues that mental illness became almost a label of convenience for a range of norm-breaking behaviour that could not be accommodated within other types of deviance. He termed this behaviour 'residual deviance' to include crime, alcoholism, and illness. Commentators identified enforced drug therapy—which violated patients' rights by denying them due process and the capacity to make informed consent—as an unacceptable outcome of the influence of psychiatry in the mental health and criminal-justice systems (Kittrie 1971).

A contemporary example of a controversial psychiatric classification, and associated diagnosis and treatment, is that of Personality Disorder. The past 20 years have seen a rapid elaboration of this category in the *Diagnostic and Statistical Manual of Mental Disorders* (*DSM*).[1] The *DSM-IV-TR* defines personality disorder as: 'an enduring pattern of inner experience and behavior that deviates markedly from the expectations of the individual's culture ... and leads to distress or impairment' (American Psychiatric Association 2000, p. 685). It identifies ten specific personality disorders. Nonetheless, personality disorders do not include obvious organic or psychological impairment but are identified through their interpersonal effects, including chaotic and distressing relationships, instability of identity, or criminal records incurred (Manning 2000). The *DSM* distinguishes personality disorders according to such descriptive terms as 'odd and eccentric' and 'anxious and fearful' (Nuckolls 1997, p. 52), thus attesting to the classification's broad scope.

Another, more ambiguous, but wide-ranging, psychiatric or psychological classification is depression, or more specifically 'depressive disorders'. Some suggest that the recent and continued popularity of Prozac—the anti-depressant drug—can be explained to some extent by the increasing tendency of individuals to redefine life's problems, stresses, and disappointments as evidence of depression. Prozac is not only prescribed to people suffering serious disturbances. Its application is more ordinary: 'a formulation that could improve the lives of people with minor disturbances and distresses' (Conrad & Potter 2000, p. 571). In contrast to the more frequent negative portrayals of mental illness in the daily press, a content analysis of two Australian newspapers in 2000 suggests that depression is presented more ambiguously. It is rarely associated with violent behaviour directed towards others, though there is some discussion of self-harm (Rowe et al. 2003). The research also shows an almost equal coverage of biomedical and psycho-social explanations for depression, suggesting that the representation of depression is not entirely medicalised, but more 'normal' and ordinary.

One interesting example of the increasing scope of psychiatry is the medicalisation of shyness (Scott 2006). In a society where assertion, communication, self-expression, ambition, and social interaction in public settings are valued and rewarded highly, caution, inhibition, social withdrawal, and timidity become viewed as problematic. Shyness can be perceived as interrupting the flow of social interaction and the expectations contained therein, and defined as deviant and sanctioned negatively. The categories used in the *DSM* are Social Phobia, Social Anxiety, and Avoidant Personality Disorder which, for diagnosis, require high levels of anxiety in relation to social performance and can be treated by cognitive-behavioural and other therapies. 'The essential feature of Social Phobia is a marked and persistent fear of social or performance situations in which embarrassment may occur' (American Psychiatric Association 2000, p. 450). The distinctions between the psychiatric labels and ordinary or normal shyness can be impossible to make in practice (Scott 2006).

Despite the influence of psychiatry, attempts to medicalise a field of behaviour are not always successful. Different medical specialties may compete with one another for jurisdiction over a problem, or aspects of it, and medical personnel are not the only ones to advocate the process of medicalisation. Other occupational groups may adopt a medical frame of reference, and individuals who experience a condition may seek to have it legitimated medically. The history of psychiatry, its interrelationships with allied occupations and other segments of the medical profession, and the influence of wider social changes all illustrate unevenness in the process of medicalisation along with great shifts in psychiatric knowledge and treatments.

deinstitutionalisation
A trend in mental health treatment whereby individuals are admitted for short periods of time rather than undergoing lifetime hospitalisation. In theory, such policies are meant to be supported by extensive community resources, to 'break down the barriers' and integrate the mentally ill into the community. However, in practice, this has not occurred on a wide scale because of the lack of funding of community services.

Deinstitutionalisation

Widespread criticism and research demonstrates the coercive dimensions of state mental hospitals and their failure to cure or treat mental illness. This, along with a renewed community interest in the management of all kinds of social problems, legitimates the process of **deinstitutionalisation**: the emptying of publicly funded mental hospitals (also prisons and juvenile detention centres), the closure of many facilities, and a trend whereby individuals may be admitted for short periods of time (often on many occasions) rather than undergo lifetime hospitalisation. Combined with the continual winding back of the welfare state, which began in most Western industrial nations in the 1970s, such criticisms have been used to justify the closure of state-run mental hospitals and have led to massive changes in mental health policy. In 1992 the health ministers of the Commonwealth, states, and territories of Australia established the National Mental Health Policy which advocates a shift away from reliance on separate psychiatric hospitals, an increased emphasis on community-based care, and the integration of mental health care with other types of health and community care (Australian Health Ministers 1995). Mental health issues remain a focus of considerable government policy formulation. A recent statement of government approaches, priorities, expenditure, and expected outcomes is the National Action Plan on Mental Health 2006–11 (Council of Australian Governments 2006).

The scope of psychiatric influence

As a profession, psychiatry has never been completely successful. As its authority stems in large part from its institutional base within mental hospitals, governmental policy directly affects psychiatrists' access to patients and resources. Moreover, psychiatrists' ability to identify, diagnose, and treat mental illness is contested by other disciplines that are concerned with human relations or personal problems, such as psychology, social work, and counselling, as well as by other medical specialties. Its claims to provide precise and exact explanations are questioned, and its ability to demonstrate aetiology difficult, making psychiatry particularly vulnerable to the criticism that its knowledge base is socially constructed and historically contingent. Indeed, psychiatry continues to be one of the most contested areas of medicine. Discussion about the causes of mental illness—genetic, physiological, psychological, and social—is far from conclusive, and psychiatrists' ability to predict the potential for mental illness in patients is highly questionable (Cocozza & Steadman 1978).

Psychiatry's jurisdiction over certain conditions and patients stems from its own self-interested quest to achieve and maintain professional status. The failure to provide an uncontested scientific rationale for mental illness has led psychiatry to develop a greater interest in prevention, thereby widening its potential for intervention (Abbott 1988). Current research—as part of the human genome project to map the genes that (allegedly) determine mental illness, alcoholism, Alzheimer's disease, and even depression—will renew psychiatrists' claims that they offer scientific explanations, diagnoses, and treatments that are not socially constructed (see Chapter 16). Nonetheless, psychiatry remains a dominant and institutionally recognised profession, with psychiatric treatment being covered by national health schemes (for example, Medicare), unlike the services of many other human services personnel.

Sharyn L. Roach Anleu

Psychiatry is not the only medical specialty or type of medical knowledge engaged in designating and normalising deviance. Other segments of medicine (as well as other social movements, occupational groups, and individuals) are involved in normative work—that is, identifying problematic behaviour and proposing medical, including psychiatric, intervention to achieve normality. In other words, psychiatry may dominate current discourses and approaches to problems or issues, even though psychiatrists do not. For example, Alcoholics Anonymous (AA) is a hybrid organisation that combines elements of the disease model of alcoholism with a spiritual program emphasising individual change and recovery and the achievement of inner peace (Valverde & White-Mair 1999). Another example, the National Alliance for the Mentally Ill (NAMI), one of the most influential mental health organisations in the USA, grew from the concern that the families of the mentally ill had insufficient input into the management of their afflicted relatives. NAMI adopts the medical model, viewing schizophrenia and manic depression as diseases caused by chemical imbalances in the brain. This organisation focuses on the mental patient's inability to hold and exercise rights, and criticises the legal extension of rights to individuals involuntarily committed to mental institutions. It maintains that psychotherapeutic approaches—which may view family dynamics, rather than a chemical imbalance, as responsible for the disease—stigmatise care givers, and that the patient's legal right to refuse medication establishes an inappropriate adversarial relationship between patients and their families (Milner 1989).

Other research shows that family members have been particularly influential in the construction of hyperactivity in children as evidence of a psychiatric disorder, namely attention deficit [hyperactivity] disorder (AD[H]D) (Lloyd & Norris 1999). In Britain, as elsewhere, active parents' organisations articulated their 'rights' and the right of their children to be classified as having a medically defined disorder requiring prescribed medication, thus rejecting a more social model of the deviantisation of certain childhood behaviours. Parents' claims for medicalisation have been met by resistance and disagreement from segments of the medical profession. Conrad and Potter (2000) detail how the activities of the support group Children and Adults with Attention Deficit Disorder, comprising medical professionals, adults who diagnosed themselves as suffering from AD[H]D, the manufacturer of Ritalin (the major treatment for hyperactivity), and the media, were successful in extending this medical category to include adult sufferers. Conversely, others have questioned the medicalisation of behaviour via a diagnosis of AD[H]D, instead focusing on ineffective or deviant parenting (Singh 2004; Hart 2006).

Some women have been active participants in the construction of premenstrual syndrome (PMS) as a disorder, and seek its inclusion in the *DSM*. It is significant that the original term was 'premenstrual tension'; the use of the term 'syndrome' indicates increased medicalisation. *DSM-IV-TR* proposes premenstrual dysphoric disorder (PDD) as an official category for possible inclusion in later editions following further research. The discussion of PDD in the appendix of *DSM-IV-TR* refers to criteria for research on the disorder rather than diagnostic criteria. It identifies symptoms such as markedly depressed mood, feelings of hopelessness or self-deprecating thoughts, marked anxiety, affective lability interspersed with frequent tearfulness, and decreased interest in usual activities as the essential features of the disorder (see American Psychiatric Association 2000, pp. 771–3). *DSM-IV-TR* distinguishes PMS (which it specifies as far more common) from PDD in terms of the symptoms' severity and distinctiveness, and resulting impairment. It notes: '[t]he transient mood changes that many women experience around the time of their period should not be considered a mental disorder' (American Psychiatric Association 2000, p. 773).

Both medical and everyday literatures tend to emphasise the negative, debilitating symptoms of PMS. An analysis of popular magazines and self-help books shows that PMS is portrayed in a generally negative tone, which effectively defines how a normal woman should feel or behave in contrast to an 'abnormal' woman who experiences PMS. Popular discourse identifies the causes as physiological and focuses on women's hormones as the source of the problems. Intervention and alleviation of the symptoms identified—ranging from dizziness, backache, and lack of concentration to decreased school or work performance, mood swings, and irritability—include drug therapy and management of individual lifestyles, through diet, exercise, and rest, rather than considering the relevance of social, structural, or cultural factors (Martin 1987; Markens 1996).

The medicalisation of PMS presents a dilemma for women: on the one hand, it legitimises the experiences of premenstrual symptoms as real and worthy of medical and public attention, but on the other it reasserts the pathology of women's bodies, especially their reproductive systems, and views women's actions and thoughts as being determined by biology (in this case, their hormones). Opponents worry that medicalisation could lead to stigmatisation and result in sex discrimination. This is an example of a situation in which some medicalisation, but not necessarily 'psychiatrisation', may be helpful in order to have complaints taken seriously by medical practitioners, and for strategies to be adopted for the alleviation or management of symptoms. Research on chronic fatigue syndrome finds that diagnosis—that is, medicalising a condition during consultation—can enable patients to explain their symptoms and to feel more in control of their situations; they are not dismissed as having imagined their symptoms or as being malingerers. On the other hand, medicalisation that reflects **medical dominance** and preconceived notions about gender-specific behaviour—for example, that women are naturally emotional, hysterical, or prone to depression or hypochondria—is unhelpful (Broom & Woodward 1996).

Some **epidemiological** surveys indicate that depressive and some anxiety disorders are more frequent among women, while antisocial personalities, and alcohol and drug abuse or dependence, are more common among men (Aneshensel et al.

medical dominance
A general term used to describe the power of the medical profession in terms of its control over its own work, over the work of other health workers, and over health resource allocation, health policy, and the way that hospitals are run.

epidemiology/social epidemiology
The statistical study of patterns of disease in the population. Originally focused on epidemics, or infectious diseases, it now covers non-infectious conditions such as stroke and cancer. Social epidemiology is a sub-field aligned with sociology that focuses on the social determinants of illness.

1991). Some mental illnesses may not be independent of gender, as they relate to perceptions of 'normal' male and female behaviour (Busfield 1988). Using data from the National (US) Survey of Families and Households, Robin Simon concludes: '[r]egardless of marital status, women report more depression than men and men report more alcohol abuse than women' (2002, p. 1079). He explains the enduring differences between men's and women's mental illness as stemming from different gendered expectations about appropriate emotions: sadness is more appropriate for women and anger for men (Simon 2002). Sadness is related to affective and anxiety disorders, including depression, which is more common among women, whereas anger is more related to antisocial behaviour and drug/alcohol dependence and is more common among men. Such observed differences may result from the greater likelihood that women will report illness: it is more culturally acceptable for women to be ill and more appropriate for them to express their psychological problems and symptoms, whereas men (or at least those conforming to dominant forms of masculinity) are more reluctant to admit certain unpleasant feelings and sensations (Phillips & Segal 1969). Alternatively, women may actually experience more mental illness than men as a result of their social status (rather than their biology); the stresses and tensions that many women experience in the context of their families and workplaces, and the connections between these areas of their lives, may lead to depression, neurosis, and other mental health problems (Busfield 1989).

Women's deviation from criminal laws has also been interpreted in terms of mental instability or illness, rather than as a result of rational action, or environmental or social structural forces. For example, kleptomania became an explanation for shop-stealing, with the 'normal' kleptomaniac being female (Smart 1976).

Psychiatry, law, and criminal deviance

Psychiatry has greater input into the criminal justice system when the criminal law and the sentencing policy move away from emphasising punishment for past illegal activities and towards examining the causes of the behaviour, the offender's motivations, and ways of preventing future criminal activity. Violators of the criminal law may be defined as requiring treatment or rehabilitation, which implies that they are sick, that they are not entirely responsible for their actions, and that they require psychiatric intervention. This type of definition is especially common in the area of juvenile delinquency, where there is a particular concern to prevent subsequent offending and the perceived risk of developing criminal careers (Abbott 1988).

Multiple crimes or crimes that are especially unusual or particularly violent or cruel are often identified by psychiatrists as being both caused by, and evidence of, psychoses. The mass media and members of the public also tend to equate 'abnormal' crimes with mental illness on the part of the perpetrator. The opposite is also true. A common theme in media depictions of mental illness is the assumed close association between the illness and crime. The media often portrays the activities and behaviour of people diagnosed with a mental illness as random, irrational, and potentially violent. Some representations go further, claiming such people are devils, possessed by evil, and not in control of bizarre impulses (Olstead 2002).

In Western legal systems, the central example of psychiatry's legal role is the 'insanity defence' for murder, formulated in the nineteenth century and still used, albeit rarely, in contemporary criminal trials. To establish a defence on the ground of insanity, the legal test requires that 'it must be clearly proved that, at the time of the committing of the act, the party accused was labouring under such a defect of reason, from disease of the mind, as not to know the nature and quality of the act he [or she] was doing; or, if he [or she] did know it, that he [or she] did not know he [or she] was doing what was wrong' (as cited in Bronit & McSherry 2001, p. 201).

With the defence of insanity, the court relies on psychiatric opinion to determine whether or not the accused person was insane at the time of the alleged offence. The psychiatrist does not assess whether or not the defendant's actions violated the law; indeed, if the defence succeeds, that issue disappears altogether: the defendant is acquitted of murder and is usually hospitalised for a period of time. As Michel Foucault notes, 'the gravity of the act was not altered by the fact that its author was insane, nor the punishment reduced as a consequence; the crime itself disappeared. It was impossible, therefore, to declare that someone was both guilty and mad' (1978, pp. 17–18).

The therapeutic approach to crime and its control reached a high point during the 1950s. Various personality tests were developed to identify the differences of emotionality, temperament, and character between criminals and non-criminals, and as a basis for early intervention to prevent criminal behaviour. However, the inaccuracy of such tests, their inability directly to link personality with criminality, and the fact that they were usually performed on prison populations, undermined their validity (Schuessler & Cressey 1950).

Another example of the intertwining realms of criminal justice and mental health relates to juvenile justice. An examination of the closure of state-run detention centres for young people in Massachusetts from the 1970s, shows that private providers with a mental health service orientation gained the contracts to provide community programs for young offenders (Armstrong 2002). The dominant model of offender treatment became cognitive behaviour therapy—a psychological approach—emphasising self-reflection regarding the offending and programs to encourage behavioural modification, which might include interventions with other family members. The individuals are held responsible and accountable for their actions while the mental health strategies are oriented to behavioural change or management. This allows the juvenile justice system to grapple with its ambivalence regarding whether young offenders 'are criminals or children in need' and to respond

Sharyn L. Roach Anleu

to wider demands that young people (and adults) be punished for their criminal offending while simultaneously having access to helpful programs and services (Armstrong 2002, p. 616).

therapeutic justice
Specialised courts (such as drug courts) based on a philosophy that some crimes are the result of illness and require a focus on the rehabilitation of offenders.

Recently, in Australia and overseas, **therapeutic justice** has returned to the courts in several jurisdictions, in the context of problem-oriented or specialist courts often heralded within the specific philosophy of 'therapeutic jurisprudence' (McMahon & Wexler 2002). These courts represent a shift away from a focus on individuals and their criminal conduct to offenders' problems and their solutions, following frustration among the courts and the public with traditional, adversarial approaches to case processing (Freiberg 2001). A proliferation of these courts has been established to deal with specific groups of people or certain types of offenders. Drug courts and mental health courts have a specifically therapeutic aim (Skrzypiec et al. 2004). In the case of drug courts, certain criminal offences (such as property crimes) are viewed as related to, even caused by, an individual's addiction to illicit drugs. The treatment or cure of this addiction (therefore the prevention/reduction of crime) requires both legal and therapeutic intervention from the judge as well as the 'psy' (psychiatry, psychology, and social work) professionals who constitute the drug treatment team attached to the drug court (Burns & Peyrot 2003; Moore 2007). A Canadian study of two drug treatment courts shows the ways in which judges rely on 'psy' knowledge to justify various legal decisions and outcomes. The opposite also occurs with the 'psy' professionals drawing on legal discourse and knowledge in offering advice and making assessments. Punishment, including imprisonment, can be redefined as therapeutic and essential for the treatment of the defendant's addiction (Moore 2007).

Towards demedicalisation?

Just as segments of the medical profession gain exclusive or partial jurisdiction over managing certain behaviour or individuals whom they define as sick, they also lose jurisdiction. The term 'demedicalisation', the reverse of medicalisation, denotes that an issue is no longer defined in medical terms and that medical intervention is no longer thought to be appropriate. Demedicalisation does not necessarily indicate that the behaviour in question ceases to be subject to normative evaluation and social control. An example is homosexuality, which arguably has been demedicalised. In 1973, as a result of social activism and the work of individual psychiatrists, the American Psychiatric Association agreed that homosexuality was not an illness and voted to exclude it from the *DSM* (Conrad & Schneider 1992). This change did not mean that gay men were no longer subject to discrimination or were no longer viewed as 'deviant'. The readiness with which many people have associated gay men and AIDS in Western societies attests to gay men's lack of integration and acceptance. Because of the increasing prevalence of the human immunodeficiency virus (HIV), gay men (as well as intravenous drug users, prostitutes, and others) are subject to increasing medical scrutiny, albeit in a different form.

The rise of epidemiology has been central in identifying **risk factors** for a range of illnesses, which in turn has resulted in greater public concern and surveillance in relation to various activities, behaviours, and lifestyles (Petersen 1996). Early epidemiological studies in the 1950s found strong relationships between socio-economic status (SES) and mental illness (Hollingshead & Redlich 1958). However, the nature of the relationship is the source of much disagreement about whether low SES is a cause of mental illness, given the stresses and strains poverty can entail, or whether individuals who suffer from a mental illness drift into lower socio-economic circumstances, because, for example, of an incapacity to sustain employment in well-paying jobs. Part of the confusion seems to be a frequent failure to disentangle the kinds of mental illness being examined. The terms 'mental illness' or 'psychological disturbance/distress' are non-specific and potentially encompass an array of disorders. A recent study using New Zealand data on adolescents confirms the relationship between low SES and relatively high rates of mental disorders (Miech et al. 1999).

risk factors
Conditions, such as alcohol misuse, smoking, and poor diet, that are thought to increase an individual's susceptibility to illness or disease.

BOX 12.1 Doing health sociology: questioning the *DSM*

One way of doing health sociology is to investigate any social values or assumptions that underpin medical categories. These can also change over time or vary across different societies. Look at the ways in which the *DSM* sets out diagnostic criteria for various mental illnesses and conditions. Consider whether some of these behaviours constitute, or are evidence of, an illness, whether they are examples of social deviance, or simply 'natural and inevitable features of human existence' (Scott 2006, p. 144) or difference, and ask yourself whose norms are being offended by the particular behaviour, and who defines the behaviour as problematic and why.

» To what extent are social values implicit in identifying some of these behaviours or phenomena as mental illness?

» Do the diagnostic categories make implicit or explicit expectations about normal and deviant behaviour?

» Are there examples of social issues or problems cast as individual failings, weaknesses, or mental deficiencies?

An interesting example of research which identifies the moral underpinnings of the definitions of pathological gambling in the *DSM*, is a 2007 article by Bo J. Bernhard, 'The Voices of Vices: Sociological Perspectives on the Pathological Gambling Entry in the Diagnostic and Statistical Manual of Mental Disorders', *American Behavioral Scientist*, vol. 51, no. 1, pp. 8–32.

Sharyn L. Roach Anleu

Conclusion

This chapter demonstrates how, over the past century, psychiatry has been engaged in the regulation of deviance. Psychiatrists seek to locate the source of deviation—from moral or sexual norms, or from legal norms, for example, within the individual. According to the therapeutic model, the deviant individual suffers from a syndrome, illness, or personality disorder, or experiences 'adjustment' problems, thus requiring psychiatric intervention. There is little attention to social factors, cultural differences, or disagreements about what constitutes deviance and normality. The influence of psychiatry is diffuse: the therapeutic model has been applied to manage or regulate such diverse activities, behaviours, and conditions as gambling, sexuality, drug and alcohol use, criminal offending (especially with young and female offenders, and those convicted of serious and violent crimes), mental disorders, premenstrual tension, and child development.

Despite its power and influence, psychiatry has never achieved complete juris-diction over certain patients, conditions, or resources. It is a medical specialty that has been particularly dependent on government practices and mental health policies, which currently emphasise deinstitutionalisation. Psychiatry's authority has historically been derived from its central role as a gatekeeper for publicly funded mental hospitals, which are currently being closed or reduced in size. The movement towards community-based mental health facilities also highlights the competition that psychiatrists are facing from other human services personnel, who themselves may adopt a medical model of deviance. The role and influence of psychiatry in the criminal justice system is also changing: there is widespread discontent with the therapeutic and rehabilitative approach to corrections, and renewed emphasis on punishment of offences rather than the treatment of offenders. Nonetheless, the criminal law remains interested in the defendant's motivations or intentions in committing an alleged crime most recently in the problem-oriented courts. It often seeks expert evidence from psychiatrists to provide information on various syndromes that might support a related defence.

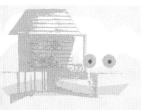

Summary of main points

» Medicalisation is the process whereby non-medical problems or phenomena become defined and treated as illnesses, disorders, syndromes, or problems of adjustment. Medicalisation can occur on at least three levels: the conceptual, the institutional, and the interactional.

» Deviance can be defined as behaviour or activities that violate social expectations about what is normal.

» The medicalisation of deviance is a historical and social process, and the outcome of professional, and social-movement activity, as well as developments in biotechnology and market forces, especially regarding the insurance and pharmaceutical industries.

» The term 'social control' refers to the mechanisms that aim to induce conformity, or at least to manage or minimise deviant behaviour and to reaffirm social norms. Therapeutic, surgical, or other medical interventions can be used to increase compliance with social norms, or conformity.

» Successful medicalisation means that 'therapy' becomes the dominant form of social control and that individuals diagnosed as deviating from a model of health must confront normative expectations stemming from the sick role.

» The late eighteenth century was the beginning of the critical period for the emergence and dominance of a medical approach to madness, which was redefined as mental illness.

Sociological reflection: the labelling process

Think of some examples from everyday life, perhaps directly familiar to you, where someone (or a group or people) is identified or labelled as breaking social norms and the behaviour is viewed as evidence of mental illness. This might include situations where individuals or their actions are labelled crazy, mad, mental, lunatic, insane, maniac, disturbed, unbalanced, demented, psychopathic, psychotic, or perhaps more colloquially, nutty, wacko, loony, batty, off one's rocker, or round the bend.

» Are these labels or terms attempts to medicalise or individualise understandings of social deviance?

» Discuss whether and why medical categories or diagnoses are used by laypeople to explain behaviour defined as inappropriate, inconvenient, disruptive, or unacceptable.

Discussion questions

1 What is the role of psychiatry in the medicalisation of deviance?

2 What are the implications of deinstitutionalisation for the professional status and autonomy of psychiatry?

3 Outline the intersections between law and psychiatry as institutions of social control.

4 Has deinstitutionalisation brought about the demedicalisation of various problems? Explain.

Sharyn L. Roach Anleu

5 Discuss the existence of gender differences in relation to mental illness and deviance.

6 Critically examine the proposition that everyday stresses and strains of life are becoming medicalised or that some mental illnesses are becoming normalised.

Further investigation

1 Critically analyse the proposition that psychiatry is one of the most powerful institutions of social control in contemporary societies.

2 Discuss the relationship between one of the following social problems: crime, juvenile delinquency, homelessness, drug use, poverty—and mental health. To what extent do policy makers and others view social problems as caused by mental illness or individual deficiency?

3 The decline of the welfare state runs parallel with an increasing emphasis on individuals to take responsibility for their own well-being. What role, if any, does psychiatry play in contemporary cultures that increasingly emphasise the individual?

4 Discuss the interrelationships between government policy on mental health and the interests of psychiatry as a profession.

5 With examples, investigate the various groups that seek to have a problem or set of issues defined as a medical condition. Why do groups or individuals consciously seek medicalisation?

6 Examine the intersections between the criminal justice system and the mental health system.

7 Provide examples of the ways in which daily newspapers present mental illness. Explain if and how connections are made with criminal offending.

Further reading

Busfield, J. (ed.) 2000, 'Sociology of Health & Illness, Special Issue', *Rethinking the Sociology of Mental Health*, vol. 22, pp. 543–719.

Conrad, P. 1992, 'Medicalization and Social Control', *Annual Review of Sociology*, vol. 18, pp. 209–32.

Conrad, P. 2005, 'The Shifting Engines of Medicalization', *Journal of Health and Social Behavior*, vol. 46 (March), pp. 3–14.

Conrad, P. & Schneider, J.W. 1992, *Deviance and Medicalization: From Badness to Sickness*, expanded edn, Temple University Press, Philadelphia.

Freidson, E. 1988, *Profession of Medicine: A Study of the Sociology of Applied Knowledge*, University of Chicago Press, Chicago.

Roach Anleu, S. L. 2006, *Deviance, Conformity and Control*, 4th edn, Pearson Education Australia, Frenchs Forest.

Web resources

Australian Institute of Criminology: <http://www.aic.gov.au>

The Australian Sociological Association (TASA): <http://www.tasa.org.au>

Mental Health Thematic Group: <http://www.tasa.org.au/thematic-group/mental-health. php>

Crime and Governance Thematic Group: <http://www.tasa.org.au/thematic-group/crime-governance.php>

Crime, Law & Deviance Section of the American Sociological Association: <http://www2. asanet.org/sectioncld/>

Mental Health Foundation: <http://www.mentalhealth.org.uk>

National Institute of Mental Health: <http://www.nimh.nih.gov>

Society for the Study of Social Problems: <http://www.sssp1.org>

SocioSite—Crime and Social Deviance: <http://www.sociosite.net/topics/right.php#CRIMI>

Online case study
Visit the Second Opinion website to access relevant case studies.

Documentaries/films

The Ellis/Szasz Debate: Mental Illness—Fact or Myth. Available online: <http://www. wesassoc.com/>

One Flew over the Cuckoo's Nest (1975): 133 minutes. Film adaptation of the 1962 novel of the same name by Ken Kesey.

The Psychology of Criminal Behavior (2001): 25 minutes. Explores societal influences on crime. Available online: <www.insight-media.com>

Born Bad (1994): 45 minutes. Explores the cause of criminal behaviour from biological, psychological and sociological viewpoints. Available online: <www.insight-media.com>

References

Abbott, A. 1988, *The System of Professions: An Essay on the Division of Expert Labor*, University of Chicago Press, Chicago.

American Psychiatric Association 2000, *Diagnostic and Statistical Manual of Mental Disorders*, 4th edn, text revision, American Psychiatric Association, Washington, DC.

Aneshensel, C. S., Rutter, C. & Lachenbruch, P. A. 1991, 'Social Structure, Stress, and Mental Health: Competing Conceptual and Analytic Models', *American Sociological Review*, vol. 56, pp. 166–78.

Armstrong, S. 2002, 'The Emergence and Implications of a Mental Health Ethos in Juvenile Justice', *Sociology of Health & Illness*, vol. 24, pp. 599–620.

Australian Health Ministers 1995, *National Mental Health Policy*, AGPS, Canberra.

Barker, K. 2002, 'Self-Help Literature and the Making of an Illness Identity: The Case of Fibromyalgia Syndrome (FMS)', *Social Problems*, vol. 49, pp. 279–300.

Becker, H. S. 1963, *Outsiders: Studies in the Sociology of Deviance*, Free Press, New York.

Bernhard, B. J. 2007, 'The Voices of Vices: Sociological Perspectives on the Pathological Gambling Entry in the Diagnostic and Statistical Manual of Mental Disorders', *American Behavioral Scientist*, vol. 51, no. 1, pp. 8–32.

Bronit, S. & McSherry, B. 2001, *Principles of Criminal Law*, Law Book Company, Sydney.

Broom, D. H. & Woodward, R. V. 1996, 'Medicalisation Reconsidered: Toward a Collaborative Approach to Care', *Sociology of Health and Illness*, vol. 18, no. 3, pp. 57–78.

Brown, P. 1995, 'Naming and Framing: The Social Construction of Diagnosis and Illness', *Journal of Health and Social Behavior* (extra issue), pp. 34–52.

Burns, S. L. & Peyrot, M. 2003, 'Tough Love: Nurturing and Coercing Responsibility and Recovery in California Drug Courts', *Social Problems*, vol. 50, pp. 416–38.

Bury, M. R. 1986, 'Social Constructionism and the Development of Medical Sociology', *Sociology of Health and Illness*, vol. 8, no. 3, pp. 137–69.

Busfield, J. 1988, 'Mental Illness as Social Product or Social Construct: A Contradiction in Feminists' Arguments?', *Sociology of Health and Illness*, vol. 10, no. 4, pp. 521–42.

Busfield, J. 1989, 'Sexism and Psychiatry', *Sociology*, vol. 23, pp. 343–64.

Cocozza, J. J. & Steadman, H. J. 1978, 'Prediction in Psychiatry: An Example of Misplaced Confidence in Experts', *Social Problems*, vol. 25, pp. 265–76.

Conrad, P. 1992, 'Medicalization and Social Control', *Annual Review of Sociology*, vol. 18, pp. 209–32.

Conrad, P. 2005, 'The Shifting Engines of Medicalization', *Journal of Health and Social Behavior*, vol. 46 (March), pp. 3–14.

Conrad, P. & Potter, D. 2000, 'From Hyperactive Children to ADHD Adults: Observations on the Expansion of Medical Categories', *Social Problems*, vol. 47, pp. 559–82.

Conrad, P. & Schneider, J. 1992, *Deviance and Medicalization: From Badness to Sickness*, 2nd edn, Temple University Press, Philadelphia.

Council of Australian Governments (COAG) 2006, *National Action Plan on Mental Health 2006–2011*. Available online: <http://www.coag.gov.au/search.cfm>

Dunn, M. & Balogh, S. 2008, 'Heath Ledger Dies Battling Drugs and Depression', *The Herald Sun*, 24 January. Available online: <http://www.news.com.au/heraldsun/story/0,21985,23099380-661,00.html>

Elliott, A. 2008, *Making the Cut: How Cosmetic Surgery is Transforming our Lives*. Reaktion Books, London.

Foucault, M. 1978, 'About the Concept of the "Dangerous Individual" in 19th Century Legal Psychiatry', trans. A. Baudot & J. Couchman, *International Journal of Law and Psychiatry*, vol. 1, pp. 1–18.

Foucault, M. 1988, *Madness and Civilization: A History of Insanity in the Age of Reason*, trans. R. Howard, Vintage Books, New York.

Freiberg, A. 2001, 'Problem-oriented Courts: Innovative Solutions to Intractable Problems?', *Journal of Judicial Administration*, vol. 11, pp. 8–27.

Freidson, E. 1988, *Profession of Medicine: A Study of the Sociology of Applied Knowledge*, University of Chicago Press, Chicago.

Furedi, F. 2006, 'The End of Professional Dominance', *Society*, vol. 43, no. 6, pp. 14–18.

Goffman, E. 1961, *Asylums: Essays on the Social Situation of Mental Patients and Other Inmates*, Penguin, Harmondsworth.

Halpern, S. A. 1992, 'Dynamics of Professional Control: Internal Coalitions and Cross-professional Boundaries', *American Journal of Sociology*, vol. 97, pp. 994–1021.

Hart, N. with Grand, N. & Riley, K. 2006, 'Making the Grade: The Gender Gap, ADHD, and the Medicalization of Boyhood', in D. Rosenfeld & C. A. Faircloth (eds) *Medicalized Masculinities*, Temple University Press, Philadelphia, pp. 132–64.

Hepworth, M. & Turner, B. S. 1982, *Confession: Studies in Deviance and Religion*, Routledge & Kegan Paul, London.

Hollingshead, A. B. & Redlich, F. C. 1958, *Social Class and Mental Illness: A Community Study*, John Wiley & Sons, New York.

Ingleby, D. 1985, 'Mental Health and Social Order', in S. Cohen & A. Scull (eds), *Social Control and the State*, Basil Blackwell, Oxford, pp. 52–75.

Kittrie, N. N. 1971, *The Right to be Different: Deviance and Enforced Therapy*, Penguin, Baltimore.

Lloyd, G. & Norris, C. 1999, 'Including ADHD?', *Disability and Society*, vol 14, pp. 505–17.

Loe, M. 2006, 'The Viagra Blues: Embracing or Resisting the Viagra Body', in D. Rosenfeld & C. A. Faircloth (eds) *Medicalized Masculinities*, Temple University Press, Philadelphia, pp. 21–44.

Manning, N. 2000, 'Psychiatric Diagnosis Under Conditions of Uncertainty: Personality Disorder, Science and Professional Legitimacy', *Sociology of Health & Illness*, vol. 22, pp. 621–39.

Markens, S. 1996, 'The Problematic of "Experience": A Political and Cultural Critique of PMS', *Gender and Society*, vol. 10, pp. 42–58.

Martin, E. 1987, *The Woman in the Body: A Cultural Analysis of Reproduction*, Beacon Press, Boston.

McMahon, M. & Wexler, D. 2002, 'Therapeutic Jurisprudence: Developments and Applications in Australia and New Zealand', *Law and Context*, vol. 20, pp. 1–23.

Meier, R. F. 1982, 'Perspectives on the Concept of Social Control', *Annual Review of Sociology*, vol. 8, pp. 35–55.

Miech, R. A., Caspi, A., Moffitt, T. E., Wright, B. R. E. & Silva, P. A. 1999, 'Low Socio-economic Status and Mental Disorders: A Longitudinal Study of Selection and Causation during Young Adulthood', *American Journal of Sociology*, vol. 104, pp. 1096–131.

Milner, N. 1989, 'The Denigration of Rights and the Persistence of Rights Talk: A Cultural Portrait', *Law and Social Inquiry*, vol. 14, pp. 631–75.

Moore, D. 2007, 'Translating Justice and Therapy: The Drug Treatment Court Networks', *British Journal of Criminology*, vol. 47, pp. 42–60.

Neff, J. A., McFall, S. L. & Cleaveland, T. D. 1987, 'Psychiatry and Medicine in the US: Interpreting Trends in Medical Specialty Choice', *Sociology of Health and Illness*, vol. 9, no. 1, pp. 45–61.

Norris, C. 2008, 'There Were 24,267 Stories About Heath Ledger in the Three Weeks After his Death. Some of Them May Have Been True', *The Weekend Australian Magazine*, 8–9 March, pp. 26–28, 30.

Nuckolls, C. 1997, 'Allocating Value to Gender in Official American Psychiatry, Part I: The Cultural Construction of the Personality Disorder Classification System', *Anthropology & Medicine*, vol. 4, pp. 45–66.

Olstead, R. 2002, 'Contesting the Text: Canadian Media Depictions of the Conflation of Mental Illess and Criminality', *Sociology of Health & Illness*, vol. 24, pp. 621–43.

Parsons, T. 1951a, *The Social System*, Free Press, New York.

Parsons, T. 1951b, 'Illness and the Role of the Physician: A Sociological Perspective', *American Journal of Orthopsychiatry*, vol. 21, pp. 452–66.

Petersen, A. 1996, 'Risk and the Regulated Self: The Discourse of Health Promotion as Politics of Uncertainty', *Australian and New Zealand Journal of Sociology*, vol. 32, pp. 44–57.

Phillips, D. L. & Segal, B. E. 1969, 'Sexual Status and Psychiatric Symptoms', *American Sociological Review*, vol. 34, pp. 58–72.

Roach Anleu, S. L. 2006, *Deviance, Conformity and Control*, 4th edn, Pearson Education Australia, Frenchs Forest.

Rosenhan, D. L. 1973, 'Being Sane in Insane Places', *Science*, no. 179, pp. 250–8.

Rowe, R., Tilbury, F., Rapley, M. & O'Farrell, I. 2003, '"About a Year Before the Breakdown I was Having the Symptoms": Sadness, Pathology and the Australian Newspaper Media', *Sociology of Health & Illness*, vol. 25, pp. 680–96.

Scheff, T. J. 1966, *Being Mentally Ill: A Sociological Theory*, Aldine de Gruyter, Chicago.

Schuessler, K. F. & Cressey, D. R. 1950, 'Personality Characteristics of Criminals', *American Journal of Sociology*, vol. 55, pp. 476–84.

Scott, S. 2006, 'The Medicalisation of Shyness: From Social Misfits to Social Fitness', *Sociology of Health & Illness,* vol. 28, no. 2, pp. 133–53.

Scull, A. T. 1975, 'From Madness to Mental Illness: Medical Men as Moral Entrepreneurs', *Archives Européennes de Sociologie*, vol. 16, pp. 218–61.

Scull, A. T. 1977, 'Madness and Segregative Control: The Role of the Insane Asylum', *Social Problems*, vol. 24, pp. 337–51.

Simon, R. W. 2002, 'Revisiting the Relationships among Gender, Marital Status and Mental Health', *American Journal of Sociology*, vol. 107, pp. 1065–96.

Singh, I, 2004, 'Doing Their Jobs: Mothering With Ritalin in a Culture of Mother-blame', *Social Science & Medicine*, vol. 59, no. 6, pp. 1193–205.

Skrzypiec, G., Wundersitz, J. & McRostie, H. 2004, *Magistrates Court Diversion Program: An Analysis of Post-Program Offending*, Office of Crime Statistics and Research, Adelaide.

Smart, C. 1976, *Women, Crime and Criminology: A Feminist Critique*, Routledge & Kegan Paul, London.

Smith, M. M. 2006, 'Medicalizing Military Masculinity: Reconstructing the War Veteran in PTSD Therapy', in D. Rosenfeld & C. A. Faircloth (eds), *Medicalized Masculinities*, Temple University Press, Philadelphia, pp. 183–202.

Strong, P. M. 1979, 'Sociological Imperialism and the Profession of Medicine: A Critical Examination of the Thesis of Medical Imperialism', *Social Science & Medicine*, vol. 13A, no. 2, pp. 199–215.

Sutton, J. R. 1991, 'The Political Economy of Madness: The Expansion of the Asylum in Progressive America', *American Sociological Review*, vol. 56, pp. 665–78.

Szasz, T. S. 1960, 'The Myth of Mental Illness', *The American Psychologist*, vol. 15, pp. 113–18.

Szasz, T. S. 1961, *The Myth of Mental Illness*, Holber-Harper, New York.

Szymczak, J. E. & Conrad, P. 2006, 'Medicalizing the Aging Male Body: Andropause and Baldness', in D. Rosenfeld & C. A. Faircloth (eds), *Medicalized Masculinities*, Temple University Press, Philadelphia, pp. 89–111.

Valverde, M. & White-Mair, K. 1999, '"One Day at a Time" and Other Slogans for Everyday Life: The Ethical Practices of Alcoholics Anonymous', *Sociology*, vol. 33, pp. 393–410.

Wienke, C. 2006, 'Sex the Natural Way: The Marketing of Cialis and Levitra', in D. Rosenfeld & C. A. Faircloth (eds), *Medicalized Masculinities*, Temple University Press, Philadelphia, pp. 45–64.

ACKNOWLEDGMENT

I gratefully acknowledge the valuable research assistance provided by Carolyn Corkindale.

NOTES

1   The Diagnostic and Statistical Manual of Mental Disorders is the widely used and standard classification of mental illnesses or disorders first published by the American Psychiatric Association in 1952. There have been four editions of the *DSM*. The most recent edition is the *DSM-IV*, published in 1994, the text of which was revised to become the *DSM-IV Text Revision* (*TR*), published in 2000. The introduction to this edition provides a valuable overview of the aims, historical background, and revisions to the *DSM*. It also acknowledges some of its limitations: '[a]lthough this manual provides a classification of mental disorders, it must be admitted that no definition adequately specifies precise boundaries for the concept of "mental disorder"' (American Psychiatric Association 2000, p. xxx).

CHAPTER 13

Mental Illness: Understandings, Experience, and Service Provision

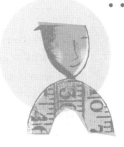

PAULINE
SAVY
and
ANNE-MAREE
SAWYER

Overview

- Who becomes mentally ill?
- What are the societal responses to mental illness?
- What are people's experiences of mental illness?

DRUG-RELATED PSYCHOSIS IN YOUNG PEOPLE

Seventeen-year-old Josh is under pressure. His high school exams are only two months away and he wants good marks to get into an accounting course at university. In his family's home in a prosperous Melbourne suburb, Josh has his own study and a computer and he has worked hard until now.

Since he was thirteen, Josh has occasionally been using marijuana with his mates. Recently, his use has increased and at the last few parties, he has tried amphetamines. Josh and his friends see these drugs as 'recreational' and 'harmless' but he knows his parents would see things differently.

Over the last month, Josh has found it hard to concentrate on study. Some days he skips school. He stays in bed wanting to be

alone. His appetite has plummeted and he has lost at least two kilograms in weight. Strange and frightening ideas grow in his mind: his thoughts seem to float out of his head. At night, the light bulbs in his room take on a special intensity and seem to grow into cameras. Josh begins to suspect that someone is spying on him. He feels confused but has no idea what he should do.

One afternoon, on learning of Josh's increasing absenteeism, his mother, Jenny, comes home to find him still in bed. He appears preoccupied; he is unable to answer her questions. Jenny contacts Orygen Youth Health, a public mental health service specifically for young people. The service responds quickly. That evening, a psychiatric

... »

nurse and a social worker visit Josh, assess his mental state, and arrange for him to see the team's psychiatrist the following day. Josh is diagnosed with 'drug-induced psychosis' and prescribed a low dose of anti-psychotic medication. He receives counselling and education about drug use and mental illness. The Orygen Team visits him regularly at home over the next four weeks. Josh recovers well and resumes his studies.

Introduction

mental illness
Definitions of mental illness differ over time and across cultures. In contemporary Western societies mental illness is formally defined via an elaborate system known as the *DSM-IV-TR*, which describes 374 categories of illness.

mental health
Allows individuals to make sense of the world around them, and their inner experiences. Mentally healthy individuals are able appropriately to fulfil their social roles, conduct relationships with others, and attend to their own basic bodily and psychological needs.

psychosis
A group of symptoms characterised by gross impairment of perception and thought, which manifests in misapprehension and misinterpretation of the nature of reality, but which is not caused by a physical illness. Hallucinations and delusions are often central to a diagnosis of psychosis.

Mental illness is usually thought of as a problem of an individual's mind, sometimes even more narrowly as 'all in the mind'. Sociologists expand this view by exploring the ways that mental illness may be produced within environmental and social circumstances, and the means available for individuals to regain **mental health**. Sociologists trace the changing prevalence and definitions of mental illness over time and across cultures, and research the personal worlds of afflicted individuals as these are constituted by experiences and meanings.

Following this approach, we commence this chapter by asking 'who becomes mentally ill?' We then identify societal responses to mental illness as exemplified in policy and service provision. Referring particularly to **psychosis**, we go on to focus on its alienating and disorienting effects on an individual's self-identity and capacity for social involvement. We note that **social exclusion** may be both cause and consequence of mental illness and that some groups are more excluded than others. Throughout the chapter we refer to the central theme of our case study: drug-related psychosis in young people. This growing social problem demonstrates the relationship between social conditions, individual actions, biology, psychiatric pathology, and illness.

Who becomes mentally ill?

Cultural and professional interpretations of mental illness define who is mentally ill and who is not. Influential theories offered by medical science and noted individuals such as Sigmund Freud, Emile Kraepelin, Eugen Bleuler, and Hans Selye provide language and frameworks for understanding mental illness as the result of genetic, neurological, metabolic, and psychological causes. Their explanations have contributed to the expansion of diagnostic categories over the last 200 years. In this time, the labels lunacy, idiocy, and insanity have been replaced by an elaborate system known as the *Diagnostic and Statistical Manual of Mental Disorders* (*DSM*). The *DSM-IV-TR* classifies some 374 disorders within diagnostic groupings such as psychotic disorders, adjustment disorders, sexual disorders, impulse control disorders, and personality disorders (*DSM-IV 2000*).

Social scientists (notably Goffman 1961; Scheff 1966; Foucault 1967) examine the broad sociocultural and situational contexts in which mental illnesses occur and how they are defined, researched, and experienced. For example, the 'epidemic' of anxiety and depressive disorders currently sweeping Australia and other Western countries can be linked to commonplace circumstances and stressors such as financial strain, drought, unemployment, overwork, pressure to achieve, and relationship breakdown. Sociologists associate prevalent stresses and fears with the particular conditions of late Western **modernity**, namely individualism, the decline in traditional sources of social support, and mediated worries about environmental threats and terrorism (Orr 2006; Sennett 2006).

In the 2004–05 National Health Survey (NHS), 3.8 per cent of Australian respondents reported suffering high psychological distress, an increase of 1.6 per cent since 1997 (ABS 2006). Of this percentage, children under 15 years constituted 6.7 per cent and teenagers aged 15–17 years 9.5 per cent. Long-term mental health problems also increased with age. In the 15–17 age group, 9.4 per cent of respondents reported long term conditions and for the 18–64 age group, this percentage increased to 12.3 per cent. These age-related findings may be considered in the context of increasing social responsibilities and aspirations to achieve scholastically, join the workforce, establish a clear sense of self, and settle into intimate relationships.

Anxiety and depressive conditions are currently described as **high prevalence disorders**. In the 2004–05 NHS, approximately 5 per cent of surveyed Australians reported anxiety disorders and the same number reported depressive disorders (ABS 2006). To understand the construction of this 'epidemic', sociologists might start by examining the methods used to estimate it. Methods include obtaining self-report data, identifying numbers of formally diagnosed individuals, and counting prescriptions written for anti-depressant, anxiolytic (anxiety-related drug treatments), and anti-psychotic medication. In the NHS statistics, considerably more women than men report anxiety-related conditions and use of medication to relieve symptoms (ABS 2006). Could this mean that women are more biologically susceptible to high levels of distress? Or does it mean that women are more likely to admit to high levels of distress and inability to cope? Sociolinguistic studies suggest that men and women use different language to describe similar subjectivities, that women's socialisation entails learning to admit to and talk about worries and hardships. Thus, we may assume that women are more likely to report symptoms of anxiety and depression to their doctors and to be prescribed medication.

Our opening vignette depicts stress during adolescence, a critical, transitional stage of life. Josh is overwhelmed by his need to do well in his exams and to please his parents. At the same time, he is especially sensitive to peer pressure and to persuasive ideas. Josh and his friends regard 'getting high' as an ordinary part of being young

social exclusion
A broad term used to encompass individuals and groups who experience persistent social disadvantage from a range of causes (poverty, unemployment, poor housing, social isolation…), preventing participation in social institutions and political processes.

modernity/ modernism
A view of social life that is founded upon rational thought and a belief that truth and morality exist as objective realities that can be discovered and understood through scientific means. See *reflexive modernity* and *postmodernism*.

high prevalence disorders
This term refers to the most commonly diagnosed mental disorders of anxiety, depression, and substance abuse.

Pauline Savy and Anne-Maree Sawyer

schizophrenia
A long-term mental disorder characterised by a breakdown in the relation between thought, feeling, and behaviour, which results in impaired perception, socially inappropriate behaviours and feelings, and social withdrawal. Both the subjective experiences and observable behaviours involved in this illness are highly variable. In acute stages, delusions and hallucinations are often experienced, whilst chronic symptoms often manifest as lethargy, apathy, and loss of motivation and drive.

delusion
A persistent, idiosyncratic belief, unusual in the person's cultural context and which is held onto despite arguments and evidence to the contrary. In psychiatric terminology, delusions may be described as 'grandiose', 'paranoid', 'persecutory', 'hypochondriacal', and 'nihilistic'.

dual diagnosis
The presence of a mental health disorder and substance abuse in the same person. Treatment is often problematic as services tend to cater to one diagnostic group, and the symptoms of one disorder may intensify the effects and experiences of the other.

and daring. The following account exemplifies this attitude as it tells of its author's regular use of marijuana and other drugs with his university friends:

> Steve has some mull. We excitedly take tokes from a small pipe he's hidden in his pocket. We run to get the train—across a vacant field, up and over the overpass, down the ramp—and just make it. It's creepy gear and when the train takes off I feel I am floating. I can't contain my laughter, life is good… We are young, naïve and invincible. (McLean 2003)

This kind of anecdote is hardly a revelation; illicit drug use is common in our times and cannabis is the drug most widely used by youth in Western societies (Lynskey et al. 1999). Cannabis use is likely to start around 16–17 years of age and up to 50 per cent of Australians aged 16–24 years have tried this drug at least once (Hamilton et al. 2004). You may view the anecdote as a lark, no more than what is expected of young people in liberal Westernised cultures such as Australia. This interpretation fits with the idea that the use of 'soft' drugs such as marijuana has been normalised (Gourley 2004). Normalisation can be associated with prevailing realities and discourses. Illicit drugs are relatively easy to obtain. Persuasive voices calling for the legalisation of some illicit drugs and decrying the social control inherent in zero-tolerance and harm minimisation programs permeate parts of the community and the virtual world (Zjadow 2005).

This relaxed view conflicts with growing scientific evidence of the harm inflicted on young brain tissue and subsequent onset of depression and **schizophrenia** by even the 'soft' drug, marijuana (Arsenault et al. 2002; Raphael et al. 2005). Amphetamines too are linked with psychotic episodes characterised by paranoid **delusions** and hallucinations and in some cases, usage may precipitate schizophrenia. The use of amphetamines by individuals aged 14 years and over doubled between 1995 and 2001 (Drug and Alcohol Office, Government of Western Australia 2006). The co-occurrence of a mental illness related to prescribed or illicit drug use is a growing problem and is referred to as **dual diagnosis**.

Changing approaches to mental health policy and treatment

The 'epidemic' of high prevalence disorders, notably depression and anxiety, has caught political attention around the globe. Depression is said to be the fourth leading contributor to the 'global burden of disease' (WHO 2008). Locally, the Australian Institute of Health and Welfare (AIHW 2006, p. xii) reports mental ill health as the 'leading cause' of non-fatal disease and injury. When examining the specific causes of disease and injury, rather than broad disease categories, we find that ischaemic heart disease is the principal cause, followed by anxiety and depression, Type 2 diabetes, and stroke (AIHW 2006). Over the last decade, mental health has become a National Health Priority Area (AIHW 2006, p. 97) with a view to decrease this burden as it impacts on individuals, service provision, and society more generally.

Since the early 1990s, several national inquiries have also raised the profile of mental health in Australia (Human Rights and Equal Opportunity Commission 1993; Groom et al. 2003; Mental Health Council of Australia and the Brain and Mind Research Institute 2005; Senate Select Committee on Mental Health 2006). These inquiries consulted widely with mentally ill individuals, their families and carers, and mental health professionals, and reported frequent difficulties in accessing inpatient care and early intervention services, poor integration amongst services, and an urgent need for more mental health services to meet increasing demand (see Hickie et al. 2005).

Service reform—contemporary social arrangements for managing the 'problem' of mental illness

Community care has become the prominent form of mental health service delivery, at least nominally, across all the Australian states and territories. Deinstitutionalisation (see Chapter 12) has taken place at different rates across the states and even within states themselves, largely as a consequence of particular local conditions (see Meadows et al. 2007).

Traditionally, the states have taken responsibility for mental health services, but since the beginnings of asylum closure in the early 1990s, the Federal Government has overseen policy development through a series of National Mental Health Plans, implemented every 5 years. For example, the *First National Mental Health Plan* (1993–98) articulated strong commitment to deinstitutionalisation through 'mainstreaming' (establishing small psychiatric inpatient units in general hospitals) and 'integration' between hospital and community-based services, and prioritised care for individuals with serious, **low prevalence disorders**, such as psychosis. The *Second National Mental Health Plan* (1998–2003) continued this emphasis whilst prioritising the high prevalence disorders of depression and anxiety and focusing on such strategies as mental health promotion, early intervention, and service integration, particularly with the primary care sector. Again, the *Third Mental Health Plan* (2003–08) emphasised integration and coordination across and within different service sectors, along with mental health promotion, prevention and early intervention, and the development of accommodation options and workforce capacity (see also Council of Australian Governments 2006). Still, poor integration persists among mental health services and broader health care services, particularly in drug and alcohol programs, and the legal system (Singh & Castle 2007).

low prevalence disorders
This term refers to psychotic disorders, including schizophrenia, which occur significantly less frequently in the population than 'high prevalence' mental disorders.

These Federal Government initiatives were driven in large part by the UN's *Principles for the Protection of Persons with Mental Illness and the Improvement of Mental Health Care*, (in place since 1992). This code of 'best practice' focuses on the rights of the mentally ill to be treated with dignity and compassion; to 'be free from exploitation, abuse and degrading treatment; ... to exercise their civil, political and economic rights ... and be entitled to care and treatment at the same standard as other people who are ill' (Zifcak 1996, p. 2; see also Healy & Renouf 2005).

Each Australian state has its own Mental Health Act, a set of statutory laws that govern and regulate the way public mental health services are to be delivered. All states and territories have passed new mental health legislation that takes into account the UN's *Principles for Care and Treatment of Mentally Ill People*. These new Acts articulate a discourse of individual rights, community care and treatment in the least restrictive environment (for example, see the Victorian *Mental Health Act 1986*, available at: <http://www.legislation.vic.gov.au>). Importantly, they also specify the criteria under which a person can be treated against his or her will, either in hospital or in the community via a **Community Treatment Order**.

Since the 1990s, the community (rather than the hospital) has become the more usual setting for the delivery of mental health care. Our vignette provides an example of community-based treatment. In 1993, 29 per cent of state mental health resources were directed to community-based care; by 2002 this figure had risen to 51 per cent (Whiteford & Buckingham 2005, p. 397). As a consequence of the shift to community-based care, the average length of stay in a psychiatric inpatient unit decreased from 21.7 days in 1998–99 (AIHW 2001, p. xxi) to 9.2 days in 2003–04 (AIHW 2006, p. 103).

Service types

Mental health care in Australia falls into three main categories: primary care, **specialist mental health services**, and disability rehabilitation and support services (an example of the latter is the Richmond Fellowship, now known as 'MIND'). Primary care refers in the main to general practitioners and community health centres, which are utilised most frequently as the first point of contact for those seeking mental health services. Ten per cent of consultations with general practitioners in 2004–05 were for mental health problems and depression is the fourth most commonly managed problem in general practice (AIHW 2006, p. 104). The Federal Government's *Better Outcomes in Mental Health Care* initiative was established in 2001 to facilitate the care and treatment of mental health problems through the primary care sector (see Hickie & Groom 2002; Meadows 2007, pp. 91–2). This initiative includes education and training in mental health assessment and counselling for general practitioners, and access to allied health services

Community Treatment Order
A legal order made on behalf of individuals by their psychiatrists to enforce treatment outside the confines of the hospital. Conditions of an Order include regular attendance at a nominated public community mental health centre, and adherence to a prescribed medication regimen. Failure to comply with such conditions results in involuntary admission to a psychiatric inpatient unit.

specialist mental health services
These services, located in both public and private sectors, focus on providing mental health care. They employ professionals who specialise in assessing and treating mental health problems—psychiatrists, psychiatric nurses, and allied health professionals. The specialist sector tends to treat the individuals with the most severe mental health problems, and is usually accessed via a primary care practitioner.

(e.g. psychologists and social workers) for support and early short-term intervention in mental health problems.

Specialist mental health services are provided in both the public and private sectors. Private psychiatric services operate as small businesses and charge a fee for service (see Fielding 2007, p. 89). The private psychiatric sector has expanded since the advent of asylum closure. In 1993, 14 per cent of all psychiatric beds were in private hospitals; by 2002, this figure had climbed to 23 per cent (Whiteford & Buckingham 2005, p. 397). An increasing proportion of psychiatrists work across the private and public systems; 'private psychiatrists are more likely to provide psychotherapeutic approaches, whereas public mental health services are more likely to provide biological and social treatment approaches' (Fielding 2007, p. 90). Despite the express emphasis in the *Second National Mental Health Plan* on addressing the burden of depression, public mental health services continue to focus on the spectrum of severe psychotic disorders.

Specialist mental health services in the public sector encompass acute mental health inpatient units in general hospitals (as well as a number of old-style psychiatric hospitals yet to close), and continuing care teams, which provide ongoing case management in the community (Dowling et al. 2007), along with a range of other very highly specialised teams. The latter may include assertive outreach or crisis teams, which provide short-term home-based intensive case management to a small number of clients with very high needs; and mobile support teams, which provide high levels of support to clients with severe psychiatric disabilities who would have spent long periods in hospital in the past (Healy & Renouf 2005; Lester & Glasby 2006). The team from Orygen Youth Health that provided treatment for Josh in our vignette is an example of a highly specialised short-term home-based intensive service (see <http://www.orygen.org.au>). Specialist teams are generally multidisciplinary, made up of clinicians such as medical officers, psychiatric registrars and consultant psychiatrists, psychiatric nurses, social workers, psychologists, and occupational therapists.

Asylum closure has reduced available beds for psychiatric inpatients. This factor, along with the trend toward shorter admission periods, means that hospitalisation is an option of last resort. Hospital wards are now only available to patients with the most severe psychiatric symptoms and high levels of risk to self or others (Lelliott & Quirk 2004; Quirk et al. 2005; Lester & Glasby 2006). Thus, community mental health workers must now deal with higher levels of acuity and need in their caseloads. In some programs, demand has increased to such an extent that collaborative work with clients is barely possible; thus the propensity 'to retreat to a narrow definition of "core business"—case-managing the illness, by means of the monitoring of symptoms and medication' (Healy & Renouf 2005, p. 45). To a large extent, then, the tension between care and social control has come to characterise the moral and professional dilemmas involved in contemporary community mental health work.

Pauline Savy and Anne-Maree Sawyer

Social control and the rise of risk discourse

Mental health policy is distinctive from other forms of health policy in that it encompasses specific mental health laws that define and regulate the conditions under which people with an identified (or suspected) mental illness may be detained and treated against their will. Enforced treatment entails notions of protection and the 'commonplace use of compulsion' (Rogers & Pilgrim 2005, p. 199)—whether for the best interests of the person or the community. Anne Rogers and David Pilgrim (2005, p. 189) argue that the old asylum model of managing mental illness fulfilled 'three interweaving functions of care, control and accommodation'. While all three functions are necessary in maintaining social order, the new context of community care means that each function has to be considered as a separate policy area (Rogers & Pilgrim 2005). During the asylum era, social control was exercised via confinement in a hospital; a number of social scientists and mental health clinicians have suggested that technologies of 'risk assessment' and 'risk management' have become the new form of social control in the era of community care (see Rose 1998; Foster 2005; Sawyer 2005).

Over the past two decades, in Australia and most Western countries mental health work has become increasingly focused on 'managing' the risks posed by service users (Godin 2004). Indeed, 'risk' has become the central criterion for prioritising and rationalising mental health services (Foster 2005, p. 26). This has occurred in the broader context of neo-liberal reforms in the provision of health and welfare services, greater regulatory control via audits and external reviews, and public concern over apparent 'failures' in community care, along with increasing demand on mental health services (Singh & Castle 2007, p. 400). As a result of the growing prominence of risk management, mental health service users are increasingly viewed in terms of their riskiness to self and others, rather than their needs. Moreover, the ascendancy of risk discourse masks a narrowing of service to the client and, in particular, a sidelining of such established approaches as short-term counselling and support (Healy & Renouf 2005; Sawyer 2005).

Clients classified as 'high risk' become the focus for service provision, and Hazel Kemshall (2002, p. 93) argues that public sector mental health services are 'now dominated by concerns with low-frequency/high-impact risks of homicide and suicide, with the high-frequency/low-impact risks faced by users in their daily lives largely neglected'. This creates new forms of exclusion. In a system that prioritises 'risk' and rationalises intervention on its basis, clients classified as 'low risk' are disadvantaged, often provided with only minimal support, rejected outright, or left to their own devices, or to the goodwill of family and carers (Green 2007).

In addition, some clients are excluded from service because of increasingly stringent intake criteria, especially within specialist programs, which in turn is also related to increased demand. In some cases, increased sensitivity to risk by particular programs means that clients are seen as not 'risky enough' for the service, particularly in relation to acute crisis care, and may thus be rejected on that basis. 'Low risk' clients and those with dual diagnosis (typically co-morbidity of a mental health diagnosis and a substance abuse problem) 'fall between the gaps'. Ironically, the exclusion of 'low risk' clients from service may be risk-producing in itself through thwarting efforts toward early intervention and prevention.

Experiencing mental illness

The *DSM-IV-TR* classifications guide practitioners' assessment of clients' clinical presentations. Sociological analyses of consultations and diagnostic processes show how practitioners transform clients' stories of illness, often muddled narratives of feelings, events, ideas, perceptions, habits, and so on, into discrete categories of illness types. The interpretive work of diagnosis imparts a sense of certainty and implies treatability often by reducing or sidelining experience that does not fit neatly within medical determinations of disease (Brown 1987).

In contrast, social science researchers seek to learn of and retain the subjective, disorderly dimensions that constitute sufferers' daily lives and their suffering. The researchers describe the personal and social worlds of mentally ill people, their idio-syncratic explanations of illness and treatment, their relations with others, and their place in a society that turns on norms for rationality, mood, appropriate behaviour, and social contribution. This kind of work involves gathering first-hand data through interviews and conversations with and observations of informants in settings such as their homes, clinics, hospitals, and, in the case of homeless individuals, on the streets (Lovell 1997; van Dongen 2003; Savy 2008). Such research requires meticulous ethical attention to ensure that impaired and vulnerable informants and their accounts are treated respectfully. It is also methodologically demanding as researchers must find ways to grasp and re-present the meanings of illness as these appear in 'unruly' data, whilst staying within the accepted practices and idioms of their disciplines.

In research on individuals with schizophrenic illness, a central aim is to understand the experiences of psychosis through concepts other than schizophrenia and irrationality. This intention is more than a semantic exercise: researchers who employ narrative methods make the point that woven through a person's symptoms of disorder are ordinary emotions and attachments to the same culture from which 'sane' others draw meanings (van Dongen 2003). From this perspective, we are more able to follow what at first seem to be chaotic experiences and accounts of illness.

The self in severe mental illness

Autobiographical accounts offer secondary data for sociological analysis of the impact of psychiatric symptoms on a person's relationship with self and with others. Richard McLean's story, for example, offers rich insights into the social context of the development of drug-related schizophrenia during young adulthood. McLean's anecdotes describe the insidious development of frightening delusions and auditory hallucinations which permeated every dimension of his mental, physical and social life.

> I am crouching in an alleyway. They can't see me here, so for the moment I am safe. There must be hundreds of loudspeakers projecting secret messages, and umpteen video cameras tracking every move I make ... The stone wall in front of me is a microcosm of conspiracies: lines, connections, synchronicities. (McLean 2003)

Increasingly, ideas and voices suggested a 'real' conspiracy against him. These became so elaborately entrenched in all dimensions of McLean's experience that he could only know them as truth; his capacity for insight and logic was disabled by the hold these symptoms had over him. As McLean's story shows, not only was his self ill but his illness was self. His efforts to water down delusions made him feel that he was robbing himself of something. Of his symptoms and his attempts to be rid of them, he says: '[y]ou are me, I don't want to kill you' (McLean 2003, p. 79).

The self in schizophrenia loses its capacity reflexively to check for reality, to organise ideas and actions logically, and to present itself coherently in culturally expected ways. Within the theory of **symbolic interactionism**, these impairments are understood in terms of the ill individual's difficulties in engaging in the nuanced process of interacting and maintaining positive relationships with others. From this perspective, presentations, which include bizarre ideas and unconventional or 'off-the-wall' behaviours, impede the work of others to understand and share meanings and to affirm the ill person's selfhood (Rosenberg 1984).

Ordinary sociability is an obvious casualty of psychotic disturbance as the capacity to observe norms for mood, encounters, conversation, dress, and intimacy unravels. The ability to form and sustain close relationships is hampered when **affect** is 'flattened' by illness, that is, when a person loses the inability to feel and express ordinarily robust emotions such as joy. Paranoid interpretations of others' meanings and motives may lead to fear of and withdrawal from company. The pronounced lethargy that accompanies schizophrenia, often occurring as a side effect of anti-psychotic medication, stifles energy for participating in ordinary social events. All up, these and many other symptoms lead to social isolation and decreased opportunities for reality testing.

For their part, witnesses to the illness may be wary, afraid, and at a loss to know how they might understand and help. Loved and trustworthy others may be seen as part of a paranoid conspiracy regardless of whether or not they support the 'truth' of delusions and 'voices'. For the same reason, their suggestions of seeking psychiatric help are likely to be ignored by the ill person. Even when help and treatment are sought, the prescription of a medication regimen may be viewed with suspicion and in some cases, ignored. Consultations with health care practitioners may be depersonalising occasions especially when patients, already mistrustful, perceive that they are constructed as 'cases', as 'selves-on-file' (Holstein & Gubrium 2000, p. 206).

symbolic interactionism
This theory focuses on the micro-worlds of people as these are constructed by individuals themselves. It positions individuals, including those with mental illness, as social actors who draw from wider cultural meanings to describe their lives and circumstances.

affect
The expression of feeling or emotion as it influences a person's behaviour; in psychiatric terminology a person suffering from depression may present as 'restricted' or 'flat' in affect.

Stigma and social exclusion

Many sociologists have written about the **stigma** attached to being mentally ill, especially when symptoms lead to unconventional behaviours that flout norms for mood and emotion (see Goffman 1963; Karp 1996). Understanding stigma in mental illness is a complex matter. Feelings of being less worthy than 'sane' others may be an inherent part of the experience of some mental illnesses. Such feelings may be bound up in delusions and hallucinations, especially those characterised by persecutory and abusive messages. Additionally, others may stigmatise sufferers by avoiding contact with them, refusing them employment, and by generally 'looking down' on them as incompetent, recipient, or dangerous members of society.

Mental illness is frequently a marginalising experience; because of its personal and social implications, it leads to social exclusion. For some individuals, social exclusion in the form of unemployment, sparse social networks, and poverty, is both a cause and consequence of mental illness. Liz Sayce (2001, p. 122) defines social exclusion as 'the interlocking and mutually compounding problems of impairment, discrimination, diminished social role, lack of economic and social participation and disability'. People with mental health problems and illnesses tend to have fewer social contacts than other people; a large proportion of their social interaction takes place with health and welfare workers, rather than within and through sporting groups, employment, educational institutions, family relationships, and friendships. Unemployment is a highly significant issue for people suffering from mental illnesses, often leading to long-term financial hardship. Loss of employment opportunities, however, is not simply economic—work provides 'latent benefits such as social identity and status, social contacts and support, a means of occupying and structuring time and a sense of personal achievement' (Lester & Glasby 2006, p. 89). Groups such as some Indigenous communities, prisoners, and refugees face these problems (see Chapter 8; Brough et al. 2003; White & Whiteford 2006; Savy & Sawyer 2008), to the extent that their exclusion means having no place in mainstream society.

> **stigma/ stigmatisation**
> A physical or social trait, such as a disability or a criminal record, that results in negative social reactions such as discrimination and exclusion.

BOX 13.1 Doing health sociology: 'out of the institution'

Patients discharged from long-stay wards of psychiatric institutions need housing and support services to enable them to live independently in the community. To prepare for deinstitutionalisation in Victoria, a model of housing and support was established in 1995 to assist long-stay patients in making the transition back to the community. This program involved three components: housing, clinical support, and psychiatric disability rehabilitation support (PDRS). In 2005, a similar program was established in South Australia, as part of a plan to downsize a large stand-alone psychiatric hospital in that state. 'Out of the Institution' is a sociological study that explores the implementation of these programs in Victoria

. . . »

Pauline Savy and Anne-Maree Sawyer

and South Australia.[1] Implementation in South Australia has been slow and problematic compared to the Victorian experience. In South Australia there was little public discussion of the program when it was established, and no policy statement about it. Interviews with different participants, including managers and staff in hospital and community-based clinical services, PDRS and housing services, showed how the low-profile approach to implementation adopted in SA contributed to the development of disparate understandings about the program among those responsible for implementing it (Carter 2007). Where policy initiatives are contentious, 'multiple perspectives' methodology is especially useful for identifying shortcomings in program implementation and in suggesting improvements to these processes.

Conclusion

Mental illness can be understood as a complex psychological, social, and biological response to environmental stressors, individual predispositions, and organic pathologies. The sociology of mental illness directs attention to societal and cultural factors which are inseparable from the prevalence of some types of mental disorder and from the illness experiences of individuals. As members of society, individuals are expected to relate to others in mutually understandable ways and to fulfil their day-to-day obligations and roles. At times, these expectations exceed individuals' physical and psychological capacities to present themselves conventionally and to act as they want and ought.

Stress may become distress and, in turn, lead to short- or long-term mental illness. Sometimes, individuals employ strategies, such as drinking alcohol and taking illicit drugs, to 'remove' themselves from stressful situations. These measures may make matters worse by causing neurological damage and further isolation from the ordinary flow of social life, and by inhibiting more therapeutic ways of restoring health and function. Societal responses to mentally ill individuals in terms of service provision change over time as new understandings and treatments of illness develop. Whilst these changes have generally become more reflective of individual rights, some individuals are more advantaged by services than others.

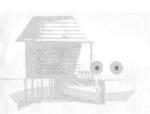

Summary of main points

» Mental illness has its causes inside and outside the individual. To understand the experiences and prevalence of mental illness, sociologists examine a wide range of societal factors, the methods used to estimate rates of illness, and the personal worlds of individuals.

» Anxiety and depressive disorders are estimated to be epidemic in Australia and other Western countries. Similarly, substance abuse is regarded as an increasing social problem and the use of some drugs is linked to the development of psychosis in young people.

» Since widespread asylum closure in the early 1990s, community-based services comprise the main form of care offered in Australia and are in high demand.

» Service provision is shaped by the concept of 'risk management' which together with increasing program specialisation may lead to the exclusion of some individuals from services.

» Some groups are more excluded from services than others because of their marginal circumstances and status, and multiple or dual diagnoses.

» Experiences of mental illness are fundamentally bound up with the inner experience of selfhood and relationships with others.

Sociological reflection: mental illness and the media

How are individuals suffering mental illness constructed in media reports? Reflect on your response to these portrayals in terms of:

» How social markers such as gender, class, and ethnicity appear to influence the report.

» How empathetic you feel towards the individuals in the account. Why might some 'cases' arouse sympathy and others blame?

» The kinds of formal services you think should be available and for whom.

» The social factors that impact on your own experience of mental health and illness.

Discussion questions

1   In your experience, how is drug and alcohol use 'normalised'?

2   What social reasons help explain the so-called 'epidemic' of depression and anxiety?

3   Why are women over-represented in statistics concerning 'high prevalence disorders' and prescriptions for medication?

4   Suggest how family life might be affected when a member is severely mentally ill. What kinds of support would be helpful?

Pauline Savy and Anne-Maree Sawyer

5   What mental health services are available in your locality? Which groups are not catered for?

6   What is the significance of marginal status for the experience of mental illness and treatment?

Further investigation

1   The number of mental illness diagnoses in Western societies has exploded in the last two centuries. Does this mean we are more and differently insane than our forebears? As part of your consideration, locate a copy of your state's mental health act and critique the way it defines mental illness.

2   Discuss the relationship between drug use and mental health problems in young people. Identify key studies that show Australian statistics concerning the use of illicit drugs by school students. Consider the personal and societal implications for regular use of marijuana and amphetamines.

3   Consider the social situation of a marginal group (e.g. Indigenous communities, refugees, prisoners) and identify the kinds of social factors that contribute to members' mental ill health. How might contributing factors be reduced?

Further reading

Bell, G. 2005, 'The Worried Well: The Depression Epidemic and the Medicalisation of our Sorrows', *Quarterly Essay*, issue 18, Black Inc., Melbourne.

Gattuso, S., Fullagar, S. & Young, I. 2005, 'Speaking of Women's "Nameless Misery": The Everyday Construction of Depression in Australian Women's Magazines', *Social Science and Medicine*, vol. 61, pp. 1640–8.

Healy, B. & Renouf, N. 2005, 'Contextualised Social Policy: An Australian Perspective' in S. Ramon & J. E. Williams (eds) *Mental Health at the Crossroads: The Promise of the Psychosocial Approach*, Ashgate Publishing, Aldershot, Hants, England & Burlington, VT, pp. 39–50.

Karp, D. 1996, *Speaking of Sadness*, Oxford University Press, New York.

Lester, H. & Glasby, J. 2006, *Mental Health Policy and Practice*, Palgrave Macmillan, Houndmills (England) & New York.

McLean, R. 2003, *Recovered Not Cured: A Journey Through Schizophrenia*, Allen & Unwin, Crows Nest.

Rogers, A. & Pilgrim, D. 2005, *A Sociology of Mental Health and Illness*, 3rd edn, Open University Press, Maidenhead.

Web resources

ABC Radio National, *All in the Mind:* <http://www.abc.net.au/rn/allinthemind/default.htm>

Australia's Health 2008: < http://www.aihw.gov.au/publications/index.cfm/title/10585>

AIHW's Mental Health Services in Australia publication series: <http://www.aihw.gov.au/mentalhealth/index.cfm>

Beyond Blue: the National Depression Initiative: <http://www.beyondblue.org.au/index.aspx>

Diagnostic and Statistical Manual of Mental Disorders, Fourth Edition (*DSM-IV-TR*): <http://www.dsmivtr.org/index.cfm>

Mental Health Act 1986 (Vic.): <http://legislation.vic.gov.au>

Mental Health Council of Australia: <http://www.mhca.org.au/>

Sane Australia: <http://www.sane.org/>

Senate Select Committee on Mental Health, 2006, *A National Approach to Mental Health: From Crisis to Community*: <http://www.aph.gov.au/Senate/committee/mentalhealth_ctte/report/>

Online case study • • •
Visit the Second Opinion website to access relevant case studies.

Documentaries/films

A Beautiful Mind (2001): 135 minutes. A film directed by Ron Howard and starring Russell Crowe that explores the life of mathematician John Nash who suffered from schizophrenia.

Enough Rope with Andrew Denton (2008): 'Angels and Demons', shown 7 April, ABC TV. Streaming video of the program is available online: <http://www.abc.net.au/tv/enoughrope/interactive/angelsanddemons/>

Four Corners (2006): 'The Ice Age', shown 20 March, ABC TV. This is a close-up study of the increasing use and effects of the illicit drug 'ice' or crystal methamphetamine. Program video, extended interviews and transcripts are available online: <http://www.abc.net.au/4corners/content/2006/s1593168.htm>

Four Corners (2005): 'Messing with Heads', shown 7 March, ABC TV. In this program, young cannabis users in treatment for psychosis discuss their experiences, and doctors and researchers reveal the latest findings concerning the link between cannabis use and psychosis. It features the Orygen Youth Health Service. Program video, extended interviews and transcripts are available online: <http://www.abc.net.au/4corners/content/2005/s1315274.htm>

Four Corners (2005): 'Out of Mind', shown 19 September, ABC TV. This program investigates the plight of homelessness and mental illness in Sydney and includes interviews with homeless people and service providers. Program transcripts and links to further resources are available online: <http://www.abc.net.au/4corners/content/2005/s1460924.htm>

References

Arsenault, L., Cannon, M., Poulton, R., Murray, R., Caspi, A. & Moffitt, T., 2002, 'Cannabis Use in Adolescence and Risk for Adult Psychosis: A Longitudinal Prospective Study', *British Medical Journal*, vol. 325, 23 November, pp. 1212–13.

Australian Bureau of Statistics 2006, *National Health Survey: Summary of Results, 2004–05*, Cat. no. 4364.0, ABS, Canberra. Available online: <http://www.abs.gov.au/AUSSTATS/abs@.nsf/DetailsPage/4364.02004-05?OpenDocument>

Australian Institute of Health and Welfare 2001, *Mental Health Services in Australia 1998–1999: National Minimum Data Sets—Mental Health Care*, Cat. no. HSE 15, Mental Health Series no. 2, AIHW, Canberra.

Australian Institute of Health and Welfare 2006, *Australia's Health 2006*, Cat. no. AUS 73, AIHW, Canberra.

Brough, M., Gorman, D, Ramirez, E. & Westoby, P. 2003, 'Young Refugees Talk About Well-Being: A Qualitative Analysis of Refugee Youth Mental Health from Three States', *Australian Journal of Social Issues*, vol. 38, no. 2, pp. 193–208.

Brown, P., 1987, 'Diagnostic Conflict and Contradiction in Psychiatry' *Journal of Health and Social Behaviour*, vol. 28, no. 1, pp. 37–50.

Carter, M. 2007, '"Death By a Thousand Cuts": Perspectives on Deinstitutionalisation', in B. Curtis, S. Matthewman & T. McIntosh (eds), *Public Sociologies: Lessons and Trans-Tasman Comparisons: TASA/ SAANZ Joint Refereed Conference Proceedings*, Department of Sociology, The University of Auckland, Auckland.

Council of Australian Governments (COAG) 2006, *National Action Plan on Mental Health 2006–2011*. Available online: <http://www.coag.gov.au/search.cfm>

Diagnostic and Statistical Manual of Mental Disorders (*DSM-IV*), 4th edn. Available online: <http://allpsych.com/disorders/dsm.html>

Dowling, R., Fossey, E., Meadows, G., Minas, H. & Purtell, C. 2007, 'Case Management' in G. Meadows, B. Singh & M. Grigg (eds), *Mental Health in Australia: Collaborative Community Practice*, 2nd edn, Oxford University Press, Melbourne, pp. 341–62.

Drug and Alcohol Office, Government of Western Australia 2006, *Clinical Guidelines: Management of Acute Amphetamine Related Problems*. Available online:, <http://www.mental.health.wa.gov.au/one/resources_view.asp?ResourcesID=107>

Fielding, J. 2007, 'Private Psychiatric Services Practice' in G. Meadows, B. Singh & M. Grigg (eds) *Mental Health in Australia: Collaborative Community Practice*, 2nd edn, Oxford University Press, Melbourne, pp. 87–91.

Foster, N. 2005, 'Control, Citizenship and "Risk" in Mental Health: Perspectives from UK, USA and Australia', in S. Ramon & J. E. Williams (eds), *Mental Health at the Crossroads: The Promise of the Psychosocial Approach*, Ashgate Publishing, Aldershot, Hants, England & Burlington, VT, pp. 25–37.

Foucault, M. 1967, *Madness and Civilisation: A History of Insanity in the Age of Reason*, Tavistock, London.

Godin, P. M. 2004, '"You Don't Tick Boxes on a Form": A Study of How Community Mental Health Nurses Assess and Manage Risk', *Health, Risk and Society*, vol. 6, no. 4, pp. 347–60.

Goffman, E. 1961, *Asylums: Essays on the Social Situation of Mental Patients and Other Inmates*, Penguin, London.

Goffman E. 1963, *Stigma: Notes on the Management of Spoiled Identity*, Prentice-Hall, New Jersey, Englewood Cliffs.

Gourley, M. 2004, 'A Subcultural Study of Recreational Ecstasy Use', *Journal of Sociology*, vol. 40, no. 1, pp. 59–73.

Green, D. 2007, 'Risk and Social Work Practice', *Australian Social Work*, vol. 60, no. 4, pp. 395–409.

Groom, G., Hickie, I. & Davenport, T. 2003, *Out of Hospital, Out of Mind!*, Mental Health Council of Australia, Canberra.

Hamilton, M., King, T. & Ritter, A., 2004, *Drug Use in Australia: Preventing Harm*, Oxford University Press, Melbourne.

Healy, B. & Renouf, N. 2005, 'Contextualised Social Policy: An Australian Perspective' in S. Ramon & J. E. Williams (eds), *Mental Health at the Crossroads: The Promise of the Psychosocial Approach*, Ashgate Publishing, Aldershot, Hants, England & Burlington, VT, pp. 39–50.

Hickie, I. & Groom, G. 2002, 'Primary Care-led Mental Health Service Reform: An Outline of the *Better Outcomes in Mental Health Care* Initiative', *Australasian Psychiatry*, vol. 10, no. 4, pp. 376–82.

Hickie, I., Groom, G. L., McGorry, P. D., Davenport, T. A. & Luscombe, G. M. 2005, 'Australian Mental Health Reform: Time for Real Outcomes', *Medical Journal of Australia*, vol. 182, no. 8, pp. 401–6.

Holstein, J. & Gubrium, J. 2000, *The Self We Live By: Narrative Identity in a Postmodern World*, Oxford University Press, New York.

Human Rights and Equal Opportunity Commission, 1993, *Human Rights and Mental Illness: Report of the National Inquiry into the Human Rights of People with Mental Illness*, AGPS, Canberra.

Karp, D. 1996, *Speaking of Sadness*, Oxford University Press, New York.

Kemshall, H. 2002, *Risk, Social Policy and Welfare*, Open University Press, Buckingham.

Lelliott, P. & Quirk, A. 2004, 'What is Life Like on Acute Psychiatric Wards?', *Current Opinion in Psychiatry*, vol. 17, no. 4, pp. 297–310.

Lester, H. & Glasby, J. 2006, *Mental Health Policy and Practice*, Palgrave Macmillan, Houndmills (England) & New York.

Lovell, A. 1997, '"This City is My Mother": Narratives of Schizophrenia and Homelessness', *American Anthropologist*, vol. 99, no. 2, pp. 355–68.

Lynskey, M., White, V., Hill, D., Letcher, T. & Hall, W. 1999, 'Prevalence of Illicit Drug Use Among Youth: Results From the Australian School Students' Alcohol and Drugs Survey', *Australian and New Zealand Journal of Public Health*, vol. 23, October, pp. 519–24.

McLean, R. 2003, *Recovered Not Cured: A Journey Through Schizophrenia*, Allen & Unwin, Crows Nest.

Meadows, G. 2007, 'Better Outcomes in Mental Health Care' in G. Meadows, B. Singh & M. Grigg (eds), *Mental Health in Australia: Collaborative Community Practice*, 2nd edn, Oxford University Press, Melbourne, pp. 91–2.

Meadows, G., Singh, B. & Grigg, M. 2007, *Mental Health in Australia: Collaborative Community Practice*, 2nd edn, Oxford University Press, Melbourne.

Mental Health Council of Australia and the Brain and Mind Research Institute, 2005, *Not for Service: Experiences of Injustice and Despair in Mental Health Care in Australia*, Mental Health Council of Australia, Canberra.

Orr, J. 2006, *Panic Diaries*, Duke University Press, Durham.

Quirk, A., Lelliott, P. & Seale, C. 2005, 'Risk Management by Patients on Psychiatric Wards in London: An Ethnographic Study', *Health, Risk and Society*, vol. 7, no. 1, pp. 85–91.

Raphael, B., Wooding, S., Stevens, G. & Connor, J. 2005, 'Comorbidity: Cannabis and Complexity', *Journal of Psychiatric Practice*, vol. 11, no. 3, pp. 161–76.

Rogers, A. & Pilgrim, D. 2005, *A Sociology of Mental Health and Illness*, 3rd edn, Open University Press, Maidenhead.

Rose, N. 1998, 'Governing Risky Individuals: The Role of Psychiatry in New Regimes of Control', *Psychiatry, Psychology and Law*, vol. 5, no. 2, pp. 177–95.

Rosenberg, M. 1984, 'A Symbolic Interactionist View of Psychosis', *Journal of Health and Social Behavior*, vol. 25, September, pp. 289–302.

Savy, P. 2008, 'Witness and Duty: Answering the Call to Speak for Dementia Sufferers in Advanced Illness', in E. Denny and S. Earl (eds), *Long-term Conditions and Nursing Practice*, Palgrave, London.

Savy, P. & Sawyer, A. 2008, 'Risk, Suffering and Competing Narratives in the Psychiatric Assessment of an Iraqi Refugee', *Culture, Medicine and Psychiatry*, vol. 32, no. 1, pp. 84–101.

Sawyer, A. 2005, 'From Therapy to Administration: Deinstitutionalisation and the Ascendancy of Psychiatric "Risk Thinking"', *Health Sociology Review*, vol. 14, no. 3, pp. 283–96.

Sayce, L. 2001, 'Social Inclusion and Mental Health', *Psychiatric Bulletin*, vol. 25, pp. 121–3.

Scheff, T. 1966, *Being Mentally Ill: A Sociological Theory*, Aldine de Gruyter, New York.

Senate Select Committee on Mental Health 2006. Available online: <http://www.mhfa.com.au/documents/SenateSelectCommitteeFinalReport.pdf>

Senate Select Committee on Mental Health 2006, *A National Approach to Mental Health: From Crisis to Community*. Available online: <http://www.aph.gov.au/Senate/committee/mentalhealth_ctte/report/>

Sennett, R. 2006, *The Culture of the New Capitalism*, Yale University Press, New Haven.

Singh, B. S. & Castle, D. J. 2007, 'Why Are Community Psychiatry Services in Australia Doing It So Hard?', *Medical Journal of Australia*, vol. 187, no. 7, pp. 410–12.

van Dongen, E. 2003, 'Walking Stories: Narratives of Mental Patients as Magic', *Anthropology and Medicine*, vol. 10, no. 2, pp. 208–22.

White, P. & Whiteford, H. 2006, 'Prisons: Mental Health Institutions of the 21st Century?', *Medical Journal of Australia*, vol. 185, no. 6, pp. 302–3.

Whiteford, H. A. & Buckingham, W. J. 2005, 'Ten Years of Mental Health Service Reform in Australia: Are We Getting it Right?', *Medical Journal of Australia*, vol. 182, no. 8, pp. 396–400.

World Health Organization (WHO) 2008, *Depression*. Available online: <http://www.who.int/mental_health/management/depression/definition/en/print/html>

Zifcak, S. 1996, 'The United Nations Principles for the Protection of People with Mental Illness: Applications and Limitations', *Psychiatry, Psychology and Law*, vol. 3, no. 1, pp. 1–9.

Zjadow, G. 2005, 'What Are We Scared of? The Absence of Sociology in Current Debates about Drug Treatments', *Journal of Sociology*, vol. 41, no. 2, pp. 185–200.

NOTES

1 'Out of the Institution' is an Australian Research Council Linkage Project conducted by the Institute for Social Research at Swinburne University of Technology. Two non-government organisations, Neami and Supported Housing Limited, are industry partners in the project. Additional funding was provided by the South Australian Department of Health.

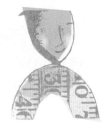

CHAPTER 14

The Illness Experience: Lay Perspectives, Disability, and Chronic Illness

DAPHNE HABIBIS

Overview

- How is illness understood and experienced by individuals?
- What are the strategies used by individuals to cope with the experience of illness?
- How does the experience of illness influence interactions with health professionals and health care systems?

THE ABC BREAST CANCER CLUSTER

In 2002, Nadia Farha was working at the ABC's Brisbane office when she noticed a small lump in her breast. Her GP was willing to wait for a couple of months before further investigation because there was no history of breast cancer in her family but she asked for it to be checked out straight away.

The lump turned out to be breast cancer that required surgery and six months of chemotherapy. Nadia was only 35 at the time and had two young children. When she was first diagnosed, Nadia put it down to a bit of 'bad luck' but over the next few years a number of her colleagues in the building were also diagnosed with breast cancer. As more women became sick Nadia began to

wonder if there could be something about the work site that was causing the cancer. All the women who were diagnosed with breast cancer were young and fit and most had had children in their 20s. This profile did not fit her understanding of the norm of the breast cancer sufferer. She and her colleagues demanded that management investigate the issue.

By 2006, despite promises of an inquiry, nothing had happened. When a ninth woman was diagnosed with breast cancer in June of that year, the staff went on strike, demanding they be relocated. By the end of the year an independent investigation had confirmed the existence of a cancer cluster at the Brisbane

ABC office, with an incidence rate up to 11 times higher than the national rate and up to 20 times higher than the normal incidence for young women. The building was closed and all 305 staff members were relocated. By 2008, seventeen women who had worked at the Brisbane site had been diagnosed with breast cancer and a nationwide investigation was established into the incidence of breast cancer amongst all staff working at ABC facilities (ABC 2007; 2008).

Introduction

Biomedical constructions of health focus on disease as a deviation from a biological norm. **Social constructions** explore the interaction between the self, society, and the body. Understanding how illness is subjectively experienced and interpreted provides valuable insights into this interaction. This chapter examines the illness experience by first considering lay understandings of health and illness and aspects of **chronic illness** and **disability**. These foundational ideas are then used to examine how people experience chronic illness and the coping strategies they develop. The chapter concludes with a review of the contribution these understandings make to improvements in health care provision.

A sociological approach to the understanding of health involves drawing a distinction between disease and illness. Disease is the theoretical construction of a condition by a specialist. Illness is the way individuals experience and make sense of bodily conditions (Kleinman 1988). How patients understand illness is influenced by cultural and interpersonal factors derived from a wide range of sources. This includes the expert knowledge of health professionals as well as popular accounts. Social variables such as gender, age, and ethnicity contribute to the patterning of these understandings within the general population. This is reflected in the saying: 'women get sicker but men die quicker'. This observation is based on perceptions that women visit their GPs frequently and that men are generally reluctant to pay attention to signs of bodily dysfunction. This saying also reveals the close association that exists between the experience of illness and patient interactions with the health care system.

Disease does not exist in a social vacuum, but is deeply intertwined with self-understandings about the meaning of embodied experience and the social relationships that surround this. Interactions with friends and family, with work colleagues and health professionals, as well as broader cultural constructions through the media and other sources, shape responses to illness. The manner in which symptoms are perceived, and the meanings given to illness, influence coping strategies and responses to treatment. In traditional Chinese medicine, for example,

biomedicine/ biomedical model
The conventional approach to medicine in Western societies, based on the diagnosis and explanation of illness as a malfunction of the body's biological mechanisms. This approach underpins most health professions and health services, which focus on treating individuals, and generally ignores the social origins of illness and its prevention.

social construction/ constructionism
Refers to the socially created characteristics of human life based on the idea that people actively construct reality, meaning it is neither 'natural' nor inevitable. Therefore, notions of normality/abnormality, right/wrong, and health/ illness are subjective human creations that should not be taken for granted.

chronic illness
A long-term or permanent illness condition that has no known cure (for example, diabetes).

and between ca...
that broadly refers to
physical and/or mental
limitations, restrictions,
or impairments that
can be chronic or last
for a sustained period
of time.

**lay concepts of
health and illness**
Refers to personal
and non-expert
explanations of
health attainment and
illness causation and
treatment.

onchial asthma in children is understood to result from an imbalance between
ιe life forces of *yin* and *yang*, which may be caused by the mother taking too much
:old' food during pregnancy. Treatment with inhalers is seen as undesirable because
эf the belief that children get addicted to them. Instead, cures involve avoiding
fruits, vegetables, and icy water (Arif & Beng 2006).

Health promotion initiatives are based on models about how people will respond
to guidance about self-care and self-monitoring. Understanding how different groups
receive health messages is essential to their success. In the USA, the unsubstantiated
belief among some African Americans that HIV/AIDS was deliberately created
by the Federal Government to kill and wipe out Black people has been found to
be associated with negative condom attitudes and inconsistent condom use. If
governments and public health organisations are to achieve their goal of reducing the
incidence of HIV/AIDS, they need to understand how and why these beliefs exist.
Research suggests that these concerns are based on the USA's long history of racial
discrimination so that an effective campaign can only be established if trust within
Black communities is first addressed by reducing current discrimination within the
American health care system (Bogart & Thorburn 2005).

Lay concepts of health and illness

While expert conceptualisations of health undoubtedly form the dominant paradigm for understanding health and illness within Western cultures, they are
not the only paradigms. How people actually experience and interpret illness is
usually influenced by these understandings, but they do not preclude alternative
interpretations which overlap, contradict, and supplement them. The meanings
people give to experiences of illness, referred to as **lay concepts of health and illness**,
are derived from multiple sources, including their individual experience of their
own and others' illness, and knowledge that is passed down within families. Both
mainstream and alternative understandings of health exist within the broader culture. The plurality of interpretations is especially prevalent in a globalised culture
where multiculturalism and the mass media expose people to many different frameworks for explaining bodily experiences.

The terms 'lay' and 'expert' models of illness denote the distinction between
the popular models of illness employed by ordinary people and the expert models
employed by health professionals. The term 'lay expert' is also used to signal the
overlap between these two models that results from the incorporation of expert
interpretations into lay models of illness. It also points to the development of a well-
informed public as a result of widespread access to 'previously obscure and inaccessible
medical information' through the internet and the creation of a new struggle over
expertise in health that is transforming the relationship between health professionals

and their clients (Hardey 1999). Nonetheless, it appears that while patients actively seek out information to help them understand and manage symptoms, the primary relationship continues to be that between doctor and patient, so that knowledge derived from the internet complements rather than contradicts the expert knowledge of health professionals (Kivits 2006).

Lay models of health influence many aspects of health behaviour including compliance and help seeking. The term **lay epidemiology** refers to the processes by which people understand and interpret health risks. These understandings are important for public health because they influence how health messages are received and the likelihood of their acceptance. These understandings are shaped by the campaigns themselves but they are also mediated by existing frameworks. This mix can produce undesirable effects. A study of a prominent health education campaign directed at reducing the incidence of heart disease in the UK found that the way in which people talked about illness and death influenced the explanations they derived about its causes, sometimes producing contradictory effects (Davison et al. 1991). The campaign sought to encourage a rational approach to health management but because people observed that who did and did not get sick did not always fit the model, it had the undesirable effect of supporting fatalistic views about health risks.

lay epidemiology
Refers to people's everyday understanding of health risks, which may or may not be supported by the research evidence.

Chronic illness

Much of the work on the illness experience has been conducted in relation to chronic diseases. Chronic illness is the most common form of illness in the Western world and accounts for the bulk of the burden of disease. In Australia, chronic diseases and conditions are estimated to be responsible for around 80 per cent of the total burden of disease (including mental illness, and injury) (AIHW 2002). This figure is based on disability adjusted life years (DALY) which combines years of healthy life lost due to disability and premature mortality to arrive at a single indicator of disease burden. As infectious diseases are now far less threatening in mass terms than in the past, chronic illnesses have become more significant, so that 'sickness has become a way of life, not a way of dying' (Stacey cited in Gregory 2005, p. 373). In the past, people would either die or recover from their illness, but current medical knowledge enables their survival, although not necessarily their cure. Within the health profession, the rise in chronic disease and conditions has led to its conceptualisation within the health profession as an 'epidemic'. Arthritis alone affects 15 per cent of the population, high blood pressure affects 10 per cent, and diseases such as chronic obstructive pulmonary disease and angina are also commonly reported (AIHW 2002).

Chronic diseases can be defined as 'conditions that are prolonged, which do not often resolve spontaneously, and which are rarely cured completely' (AIHW 2002). A wide diversity of conditions is covered by the term. Chronic diseases cross the spectrum of physical and mental disease as well as injury-related conditions. They include asthma, arthritis, high blood pressure, depression, kidney disorders, and lung cancer as well as acquired brain injury. Their symptomatology, prognosis, and impact on social and physical functioning, are therefore equally wide ranging. For example, chronic fatigue syndrome is a far more contested condition than diabetes, less easily diagnosed and managed, affecting different population groups, and with a different risk of premature mortality. The uncertainty surrounding chronic fatigue syndrome is also associated with a degree of **stigma** that is absent from diabetes.

Despite this diversity, the concept is important, providing an important distinction from the characteristics of **acute illness** on which medical models of treatment are based. In acute illness, the individual progresses from illness to wellness, but in chronic illness the condition is prolonged and characterised by constant or intermittent ill health. The uncertainty of recovery means that the idea of progression is also absent. People can have a chronic illness and still live a relatively normal life, but it is also true that chronic diseases and conditions are the leading cause of premature mortality.

The onset of chronic illness is often slow and insidious and people often have little understanding that their experience represents an ongoing condition. What appears at first as an everyday problem, requiring a commonsense solution, is gradually reframed as a health issue that requires expert help and medical investigation. The effects of chronic illness are often long term and involve suffering and enduring functional limitations. Catherine Garrett describes chronic illness as 'a type of constant and ongoing suffering, like an unhealed wound' (2005, p. 5). While chronic illness may be popularly understood as a static condition, change is a key characteristic, often in an undesirable direction (AIHW 2002).

When people initially seek medical help for a condition that turns out to be chronic, they often have no idea that it will be a semi-permanent state and may not even have identified that they have an illness. Diagnosis is often lengthy and lacking in clarity and certainty. The stress of the illness is therefore compounded by poor interaction with health professionals and uncertainty of diagnosis and prospects of recovery. Further, patients may not always be provided with adequate information about what is known about their illness.

Disability

Although most people living with chronic illness function very well, chronic diseases such as asthma and arthritis make up a significant proportion of disability groups (AIHW 2002). Long years of living with an impairment or restriction can be a common feature of chronic illness. According to the Australian Bureau of Statistics (ABS), disability refers to any person with a limitation, restriction or impairment, which has lasted, or is likely to last, for at least six months and restricts everyday

---

stigma/ stigmatisation
A physical or social trait, such as a disability or a criminal record, that results in negative social reactions such as discrimination and exclusion.

acute illness
Illness with a rapid onset, short duration, and needing urgent attention.

activities. Nearly 4 million Australians, that is 20 per cent of the population, fit this description with 2.6 million aged less than 65 years (Begg et al. 2007, p. 153).

Measures of the extent of disability depend on how the term is operationalised. An ABS survey of disability in Australia in 2003 showed that there were 1.2 million individuals with a severe or profound core activity limitation. This means that they sometimes or always required help or supervision with self-care, mobility, or communication. Of these, 0.7 million are under the age of 65 years (Begg et al. 2007, p. 153). In 2003, there were over one million people who needed assistance with at least one of the following activities: self-care, mobility, communication, health care, housework, property maintenance, paperwork, meal preparation, transport, and cognition.

As with chronic illness, increased life expectancy and medical advances are changing the extent and significance of disability within the nation, creating new health system challenges as the age and number of people living with a disability increases. Women are disproportionately affected because their greater life expectancy translates to increased years of disability. Current estimates suggest that while men can expect to have five years of living with a disability, the figure for women is eight years (Begg et al. 2007).

The widespread nature of disability means that most people can expect to experience it, either directly or indirectly, as carers. Despite this, disability continues to be socially constructed as an out-of-the-ordinary experience. People whose physical or mental abilities challenge normative expectations have historically experienced discrimination and abuse, often behind locked doors. Until relatively recently, disabled groups in Western nations were segregated from mainstream society, treated in special institutions, and subjected to techniques of control with little opportunity to control their own lives.

The disempowerment and marginalisation of disability groups form the historical context for understanding contemporary models for disability treatment and care. These stress the normality of disability and the extent to which the social environ-ment shapes the degree to which a physical or mental condition is disabling. The **social model of disability** distinguishes between impairment and disability. Impairment refers to the physical or mental condition that affects functioning, while disability 'is what society makes of someone's impairment' (Goggin & Newell 2005, p. 28). If the environment is designed to provide for wheelchairs, for example, then the disabling aspects of mobility limitations may be minimal. The impact of cerebral palsy on a person's capacity to live a fulfilled life is similarly mediated by social factors such as the availability of support, opportunities for carer respite, accessible education and work opportunities, and the level of discrimination within the community.

The social model of disability is located within a human rights framework arguing that different physical or mental capability and functioning does not justify different

social model of disability
An approach that views society as 'disabling' and thus focuses on the rights of disabled people so as to address cultural and structural discrimination and ensure similar treatment and opportunities afforded to able-bodied people.

deinstitutionalisation
A trend in mental health treatment whereby individuals are admitted for short periods of time, rather than undergoing lifetime hospitalisation. In theory, such policies are meant to be supported by extensive community resources, to 'break down the barriers' and integrate the mentally ill into the community. However, in practice, this has not occurred on a wide scale because of the lack of funding of community services.

social exclusion
A broad term used to encompass individuals and groups who experience persistent social disadvantage from a range of causes (poverty, unemployment, poor housing, social isolation etc.), preventing participation in social institutions and political processes.

illness trajectory
Refers to the changing nature of a person's experience of illness over time and how this is influenced by the actions of the patients and their interactions with health professionals, family, and friends.

treatment. People living with impairment are as entitled as the rest of the population to a fulfilled life and the opportunity to contribute to society. This model has been associated with the **deinstitutionalisation** of disability services and the closure of the large institutions which provided treatment and care. Yet, while the mainstreaming of disability services has been in existence for over two decades, disability advocates argue that a form of 'social apartheid' remains even though people with disabilities are no longer physically segregated from the rest of the population. There remain many symbolic, physical, and social barriers that create isolation and **social exclusion**, preventing a normal existence. This is reflected in a range of negative outcomes, including low incomes, poor health, difficulties in establishing intimate relationships and friendships, and weak labour market participation. Despite the willingness of many people with a disability to enter the paid workforce, for example, their levels of employment are 53 per cent compared with 81 per cent for people with no disability. For people with severe or profound limitation the figure is only 30 per cent (Begg et al. 2007, p. 197).

Experiencing illness

The experience of serious illness can have life-changing effects on how patients see the world and their place within it. It often challenges taken-for-granted certainties and creates new dynamics in interpersonal relationships. Experiences of weakness, pain, and dependence lead to questions about the self and interpersonal relationships. It can also provide opportunities for new insights. This is especially the case with chronic illness due to its prolonged nature, its effects on daily functioning, and association with impairment. Accounts of the subjective aspects of illness focus on how the experience of illness influences self-identity and the implications of this for relationships with family members, health professionals, and the broader health system.

The illness trajectory

Sociologist Anselm Strauss and nursing academic Juliet Corbin (1988) interviewed patients and carers about how they managed the changing course of illness. They saw that managing diseases such as Alzheimer's, stroke, and kidney disease involves the establishment of management regimes that affect social interaction. The changing course of illness, often in a deteriorating direction, also affects self-identity and this requires biographical adjustment. They employed the idea of the **illness trajectory** to analyse the biographical work associated with this as patients made efforts to control and adjust to their changing health status and the new requirements and arrangements associated with this. This involved both inner reflection and negotiations with friends, families, and professionals. This idea was further developed by sociologist Michael Bury's (1982) concept of illness as **biographical disruption**.

Illness as biographical disruption

In his writings on self-identity, Anthony Giddens (1991) points out that our sense of who we are is not automatically given but involves an ongoing, creative act of reflexive self-awareness. Through this act we establish a sense of safety, or ontological security, the taken-for-granted nature of which shields us from the reality of the uncertainty of existence. It establishes a feeling of living in a stable world in which the contours are familiar and which we know how to negotiate. This anchoring of the self is assisted by the predictable nature of our world and the fit between anticipation and experience. The experience of serious illness ruptures this predictability because it places a question mark over the future, threatens relationships, and dislocates existing arrangements. Certainty is replaced by uncertainty and feelings of risk, presenting a profound challenge to ontological security.

This understanding of the effects of chronic illness on individual subjectivities is captured by Bury's notion of biographical disruption. This concept highlights how chronic illness 'disrupts the structures of everyday life and the forms of knowledge which underpin them' (Bury 1982, p. 169). Using semi-structured interviews with thirty rheumatoid arthritis patients in England, Bury explores how chronic illness raises questions about 'what is going on here?' that challenge plans and expectations for the future, disrupts routine explanatory systems, and has wider implications for the 'normal rules of reciprocity and mutual support' on which individuals normally depend (Bury 1982, p. 169). He describes how what at first appears to be an everyday pain is slowly understood as a serious, long-term, and disabling condition. This recognition involves a biographical shift from a perceived normal trajectory to one fundamentally abnormal and inwardly damaging (Bury 1982). The limited medical knowledge that commonly characterises chronic illness means that diagnosis is often followed by a prolonged feeling of uncertainty further adding to the shock of the experience. As people search for answers to the questions 'Why me? Why now?' they may draw on medical knowledge, but the uncertain nature of their health status means they also draw on their personal biography, finding meaning in past incidents or family history in order to adjust to the new reality. Adjustment also involves the mobilisation of material resources. Access to strong friendship networks or wealth assist with this, so some groups, such as women and the middle and upper classes, are better placed than others to respond to the challenges of illness. The disruptive effects of illness are therefore mediated by social variables such as gender, age, and **class**, as well as the seriousness of the illness.

biographical disruption
Refers to the effect of chronic illness on a person's self-identity, such as loss of control and certainty, that influences how the person deals with the illness experience.

class (or social class)
A position in a system of structured inequality based on the unequal distribution of power, wealth, income, and status. People who share a class position typically share similar life chances.

Daphne Habibis

Moral dimensions of illness: shame, stigma, and discrimination

Historically, chronic illness and disability have been associated with discrimination and rejection within the broader community; research suggests that stigmatisation continues to be associated with some physical and mental conditions. Illness, by definition, involves the departure from some socially constructed ideal or expectation of bodily appearance or function, and its association with a judgment of moral worth is therefore unsurprising. In *Stigma: Notes on the Management of Spoiled Identity* (1963), sociologist Erving Goffman suggests that when people deviate from established social expectations it often leads to the imposition of a spoiled identity because possession of the undesirable characteristic is seen as a mark of moral failure. The existence of a single imperfection becomes associated with a range of other features so that the whole person is judged as morally problematic. In this way, the person is no longer perceived by others as an individual but becomes the illness. The stigmatised individual then becomes vulnerable to social condemnation and categorisation as somehow 'less than human' (1963, p. 5). This tainted identity can become the basis of prejudice and formal and informal discrimination including the withholding of legal privileges.

While Goffman (1963) recognises the internalisation of stigma, he sees it as an imposed identity of which the origins lie in the negative reaction of others. This has been described as 'enacted stigma' (Scambler & Hopkins 1986). Yet self-stigmatisation, or felt stigma (Scambler & Hopkins 1986), can also occur among people experiencing debilitating mental and physical conditions such as epilepsy, multiple sclerosis, or Parkinson's disease. Feelings of inadequacy or shame as a result of an embarrassing condition or appearance, or limited mobility, for example, can lead to people questioning their self-worth regardless of whether their situation is visible to others or not. Such judgments can make it even more difficult to participate in normal social activities, thereby further deepening the sense of social isolation. This may be especially acute in contested medical conditions such as chronic fatigue syndrome or post-traumatic stress disorders where there exist perceptions that personal inadequacy, incompetence, or psychological weakness are implicated in the aetiology. It may also extend beyond the ill individual to caregivers and other family members in a ripple effect that has repercussions in many areas of life (Wasow 1995).

The HIV/AIDS pandemic provides an illustration of the kind of moral panic that can be associated with a stigmatised disease. Researchers Jeffrey Huber and Mary Gillaspy argue that those population groups associated with HIV and AIDS were subjected to extreme rejection, prejudice, and formal and informal discrimination (1998). The stigmatised status of the disease was associated with a range of biomedical and non-biomedical factors including physical aspects of the illness, its

association with homosexuality and intravenous drug use, and fear of its transmission through everyday contact. The imposition of shame on those directly and
indirectly affected by HIV and AIDS was so extreme that denial of its occurrence
was common and it was sometimes not acknowledged as a cause of death. Fear
of the disease was closely tied to misinformation about the science surrounding
the condition. It became associated with metaphors such as the 'body turns nasty
on itself', which linked it with notions of pollution and contamination (Alonza &
Reynolds 1995). False ideas about its causes, transmission, and effects were common
and formed a further source of popular anxiety, which fuelled negative stereotypes
about the kind of person likely to get it.

While the idea of stigma has been valuable in drawing attention to the delegit-
imating effects of embarrassment at, and fear of, bodily difference, it has also been
critiqued. Theoretically the concept is so general that it can apply to any process of
negative labelling and therefore has limited analytical value. It also tends to deny
the extent to which people resist labels and redefine situations to their advantage.
Neville Millen and Christine Walker, for example, found that people experiencing
chronic illness actively seek to influence the health agenda in their favour through
the formation of consumer and self-help groups (2003). By this means they exchange
their illness status for 'political activist status'.

Coping with chronic illness

Adjusting to the disruptions to bodily and social integrity created by chronic illness
generates a need for practical and emotional coping strategies designed to re-establish
a sense of normality and control. External aspects of coping involve questions about
how to complete essential tasks and obtain necessary support while internal aspects
involve dealing with the disturbances to self-identity. Questions such as how to
manage informing people about the illness ('Whom and what do I tell?') and how
to behave when bodily conditions are out of control generate social tensions as well
as risks to identity and self-esteem. Adjusting to chronic illness therefore involves
establishing strategies that mediate this tension between the public social identity
and the private personal self (Kelly cited in Pierret 2003).

Much of the work relating to the practical strategies for coping takes place
within the home, where family relationships are critical. The demands of care may
impact on other family members in ways that are as disruptive to them as they are
to the patient themselves (Bernardes cited in Gregory 2005). Women carry much
of this responsibility, as part of normative expectations about their nurturing role.
Health researcher Susan Gregory (2005) points out that as well as contributing to
the monitoring and maintenance of health, domestic work is central to the illness

experience because it establishes the routine activities around which normality and ontological security are established for family members. Illness is an unwelcome intrusion into family life, disturbing domestic routines in ways that can test family relationships. Gregory found that it sometimes required a reversal of traditional gender roles and new relationships of dependence. In her analysis of how family members manage tasks and activities around food and meals when having to deal with a diet-related illness, she discovered that it was through simple family tasks such as meal preparation that these changes were negotiated. The routine activities of domestic life provided a language and opportunity around which individual and social identities could be reconstructed and reinterpreted.

How people respond to chronic illness also involves cognitive strategies such as optimising the situation by saying it could be worse, reordering priorities and values, seeking information that validates personal experience, and minimising the struggles and adjustments made (Royer 1998). In managing social relationships the question of how much information to provide about the illness becomes a central issue, mediated by factors such as its visibility. Goffman (1963) identifies two adaptive techniques for establishing normality in the face of the tensions created by difference. 'Passing' is when strategies to disguise signs of abnormality are employed, while 'covering' involves strategies to reduce the social obtrusiveness of the embarrassing condition. In covering the aim is to reduce the tensions created by knowledge of the condition. In passing the aim is to deny the existence of the condition, by for example, engaging in normal activities despite physical limitations or making extraordinary efforts to maintain a normal appearance (Royer 1995). However, research by Millen and Walker (2003) found that most respondents made little attempt to deny their situation and instead were more likely to express a desire to acknowledge it in order to seek government support for all people with chronic illnesses.

Social psychologists Alan Radley and Ruth Green (1987) propose a four-type model of adjustment to chronic illness. 'Accommodation' involves the integration of the illness into the person's life through the pursuit of modified goals. 'Secondary gain' occurs when other rewarding activities are established which compensate for the areas of inactivity imposed by the illness. 'Active denial' involves an attempt to ignore the illness and its implications by minimising symptoms and the retention of social activities. 'Resignation' is characterised by a feeling of being overwhelmed by the illness and associated loss of activities.

Nursing academic Clare Williams (2002) studied how adolescents with either Type 1 diabetes or asthma managed disease. She found that young boys were far more likely than young girls to attempt to 'pass' as healthy because of the risk represented by illness to their masculine identity. Girls took more responsibility for self-management while boys' denial of it was paradoxically associated with greater dependence on their mothers. Yet while the girls' adherence to treatment regimes was greater than that of the boys, this did not necessarily improve their health.

Making meaning of illness: narrative approaches

The reorientation of the self that is involved in adjusting to chronic illness has been widely conceptualised as a process of self-storying. In *The Illness Narratives* (1988) medical anthropologist Arthur Kleinman points out that making meaning of the experience of illness takes a narrative form that links life history with the chronic course, providing answers to the question about who one is, and how one came to be in the present situation. Through **narrative reconstruction** biographical integrity is reasserted in the context of the ruptures between body, self, and the world that illness represents (Pierret 2003). As well as helping self-understanding and adjustment, story-telling is performative; it enables communication with others about what is happening and the practical and emotional effects of this (Williams 2000).

A framework for analysing illness narratives in terms of three types of narrative form is offered by Bury (2001). Contingent narratives address beliefs about the origins of the disease, its initial causes, and immediate effects. Ideas that it was caused by an especially stressful event or some predisposing medical condition fit within this type. Contingent narratives also involve how people story their attempts at normalisation, either through passing strategies or through the reframing of what it means to be normal in light of the changed lifestyle and circumstances that serious illness may bring.

Moral narratives are stories that help to establish the moral status of the patient in the context of the changes to person and identity that follow from illness. They introduce an evaluative element into the illness experience as part of an attempt to answer the questions 'Why me? Why now?' They bring together moral considerations, such as fatalism or self-discovery, as a way of connecting diverse aspects of the illness such as family history, coincidences of symptoms, biographical events, and the particular social contexts in which these have occurred (Bury 2001).

Core narratives form the last of Bury's narrative typologies. These connect experiences of illness with deeper cultural forms such as 'heroic, tragic, ironic and comic and regressive/progressive narratives' (2001, p. 263). These narratives provide a temporal ordering of illness experiences, which 'give expression to the changed relationship between body, self and society' (2001, p. 278).

In his analysis of people living with a diagnosis of HIV/AIDS, Douglas Ezzy (2000) argues that the narratives people use to make sense of their lives need to be understood as an ongoing process of self-understanding that changes over time as new conditions arise, such as the appearance of new forms of treatment.

narrative reconstruction
Refers to individuals' beliefs about the causes and implications of their illness and how this shapes a redeveloped sense of self-identity.

Daphne Habibis

BOX 14.1	Doing health sociology: discourses of tragedy

Katrina Breaden's (2003) study of the experiences of women with advanced breast cancer explored how they make sense of an incurable illness and the unhelpful way in which they are positioned by a 'discourse of tragedy' in both media representations and the 'expert' literature.

Through critical textual analysis and interviews with twelve young mothers with advanced breast cancer, Breaden shows how the media tends to sensationalise this condition, focusing, for example, on its implications for young women's ability to have children and form relationships. These accounts of the 'tragedy' of breast cancer make no distinction between the different experiences associated with different stages of the illness, nor the reality of the profound challenge of dealing with the possibility that young children will grow up without their mothers, nor that these women have a partner who will be left behind.

A similar contrast is present in the expert literature which 'alienates and sanitises the awful lived realities of the disease' (Breaden 2003, p. 125). In focusing on survival rates or the latest drug it draws attention away from the reality of a lack of a cure or the experiences of suffering that treatment entails. Breaden links this to other studies that argue public discourses of breast cancer often contain hidden messages of blame, linking the disease to poor early detection or to late childbearing in ways that suggest the women who get breast cancer somehow failed to act responsibly.

Breaden argues that these discourses provide little cultural space for women with advanced breast cancer to make sense of the multi-layered nature of the difficult experiences they must deal with. These do not only involve an uncertain future and painful treatments, but also experiences of enormous loss extending well beyond that of their own lives. Such analyses show how limited and limiting popular and professional representations of illness can be and the importance of locating patients within the reality of their lived illness experiences.

Conclusion: health care systems and the patient experience

Illness experiences are situated within the institutional framework of health care systems and are profoundly shaped by this. Features such as how symptoms are understood within current disease paradigms, access to alternative sources of care, and relationships with local health care professionals impact both positively and negatively on patients and their health outcomes. The rise in the predominance of chronic illness over the last century has meant that management and care have become as, if not more, important to health care than treatment and cure (Bury 2001). With this has come a focus on the everyday experiences of illness and recognition of the need to account for lay understandings of health and illness and their practical and emotional effects. This shifts the health care model away from a biomedical approach to a more social model of the body, which locates it within a holistic framework of self and society. Understanding how illness impacts on home and work and how disabling conditions can be better managed necessitates a multidimensional approach to care, which takes account of where the patient sits in relation to such things as social networks and self-understanding.

An understanding of patient experiences also offers insights into the symbolic meanings of illness, especially in relation to its moral dimensions. The tendency to impose negative meanings on disease and related conditions, which extend to the personal character of the individual, has harmful consequences for patient self-esteem and coping. Understanding this is especially important for health professionals whose interactions with patients can sometimes be a contributing factor to patient experiences of stigmatisation and whose assumptions about the moral worth of patients can interfere with objective assessment.

The concern with patient subjectivities, which has accompanied the shift from acute to chronic illness, has to some degree changed the role of health professionals from one of 'medical dominance' (Willis 1989) to one of being a 'witness to suffering' and a source of practical advice and guidance (Bury 2001, p. 267). Performing this role necessitates a deeper and more empathetic understanding of patient and family stories. It reduces the authoritarian power of medicine by providing an alternative strand which acknowledges the self as well as the body as an object of medical investigation. In an information-rich age it also has potential to change the role of the patient from passive recipient of expert knowledge to that of lay expert and empowered consumer. The willingness of health care systems to pay attention to the voices of patients fits within a broader shift of the democratisation of society (Bury 2001). Patients no longer have to rely on the advice provided by a very limited number of professionals, but can research and investigate from a virtually unlimited source of knowledge and alternative perspectives.

There is also an alternative interpretation of how the emergence of the 'expert patient' might be used by health systems. Rather than opening the door to improved relationships between health care providers and patients, it may instead contribute to the reconstruction of the relationship between the state and its citizens. In this dystopian scenario the state divests itself of its responsibilities for care for its citizens. Instead its patients and their families are expected to be active in monitoring and interpreting their health needs. From this perspective, the expert patient provides an opportunity for the state to reduce the costs of health care by increasing expectations that individuals will meet their own health needs.

Daphne Habibis

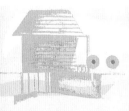

Summary of main points

» Understanding the meaning people give to illness is important for health professionals because of its influence on patient coping and interaction with health care systems.

» Lay concepts of health and illness are the common sense understandings used by people to explain bodily conditions and their interaction with the social environment. This knowledge is derived from multiple sources including individual experience, family traditions, cultural norms, and biomedical constructs.

» Acute and chronic forms of illness differ in their longevity and the presence or absence of a cure. People experiencing chronic illness often have poor interactions with health professionals due to lengthy diagnoses and uncertainty of treatment and outcome.

» Chronic illness makes up a significant proportion of disability groups. Contemporary frameworks for understanding disability stress the role of the environment in shaping the degree to which a physical or mental condition is disabling.

» The experience of chronic illness may include negative moral judgments by others about the illness. These may extend to encompass the whole person. Patients may also experience self-generated feelings of failure and low self-esteem. Disability is especially associated with experiences of discrimination and exclusion.

» Chronic illness often has disruptive effects on individual biographies, necessitating coping strategies to deal with its practical effects and risks to personal and social identity. Narrative approaches shed light on how patients make sense of these experiences through stories which link personal biography with the changing experiences of illness and the social environment.

Sociological reflection: the GP encounter

Think about the last time you went to see a GP. Were there some things that you failed to disclose even though they might have been relevant to your health? What were the reasons for this? How might disclosure have assisted diagnosis or treatment? What could the GP have done to encourage you to provide this information? Alternatively, think about what kinds of situations or conditions might lead to reluctance to provide all potentially relevant information in a medical interaction?

Discussion questions

1   Identify six ways in which an improved understanding of the experience of illness is important for health professionals.

2   Explain the meaning of the following terms: lay concepts of health and illness; biographical disruption; stigmatisation of illness.

3   What impact is the internet having on the relationship between patients and the health system in terms of how illness is understood and experienced? How is this connected to broader changes within society?

4   What is narrative reconstruction and what aspects of the illness experience does it shed light on?

5   Review the introductory vignette at the start of the chapter. What aspects of the chapter does it highlight?

6   How do disability and chronic illness differ from acute illness? What is their impact on the health system?

Further investigation

1   What is stigma and why is it relevant to an understanding of experiences of health? Answer this question in relation to one of the following diseases: HIV/AIDS; chronic fatigue syndrome; intellectual disability.

2   What is the social model of disability? How does it differ from earlier models of disability and what are its implications for treatment and care?

Further reading

Anderson, R. & Bury, M. 1988, *Living with Chronic Illness: The Experience of Patients and their Families*, Unwin Hyman, London.

Barnes, C. & Mercer, G. 2003, *Disability*, Polity Press, Cambridge.

Corbin, J. & Strauss, A. 1988, *Unending Work and Care: Managing Chronic Illness at Home*, Jossey-Bass, San Francisco.

Ezzy, D. 2000, 'Illness Narratives: Time, Hope & HIV', *Social Science and Medicine* vol. 50, pp. 387–96.

Kleinman, A. 1988, *The Illness Narratives: Suffering, Healing and the Human Condition*, Basic Books, New York.

Pierret, J. 2003, 'The Illness Experience: State of Knowledge and Perspectives for Research', *Sociology of Health and Illness*, vol. 25, pp. 4–22.

Shakespeare, T. 2006, *Disability Rights and Wrongs*, Routledge, London.

Williams, C. 2002, *Mothers, Young People and Chronic Illness*, Ashgate, Hampshire.

Reader bonus
Available on the Second Opinion website: Lupton, D. 2005, 'The Body, Medicine, and Society', in J. Germov (ed.), *Second Opinion: An Introduction to Health Sociology*, 3rd edition, Oxford University Press, Melbourne.

Daphne Habibis

Web resources

Chronic Illness Alliance: <http://www.chronicillness.org.au/>

DIPEx: <http://www.dipex.org>

Sociology of Health and Illness (journal): <http://www.blackwellpublishing.com/shil_enhanced/>

Expressions of Suffering: <http://medanthro.kaapeli.fi/>

Documentaries/films

The Money or the Gun (1990): 'The International Year of the Patronising Bastard', 47 minutes, ABC TV. An amusing award winning documentary by Andrew Denton on the experience of disability.

Philadelphia (1993): 125 minutes. A film starring Tom Hanks and Denzel Washington that explores the prevalence of discrimination against homosexuals, particularly those suffering HIV/AIDS.

References

Alonza, A. A. & Reynolds, N. R. 1995, 'Stigma, HIV and AIDS: An Exploration and Elaboration of a Stigma Trajectory', *Social Science and Medicine,* vol. 41, no. 3, pp. 303–15.

Arif, K. M. & Beng, K. S. 2006, 'Cultural Health Beliefs in a Rural Family Practice: A Malaysian Perspective', *Australian Journal of Rural Health*, vol. 14, no. 1, pp. 2–8.

Australian Broadcasting Corporation (ABC) 2007, *The Inside Story: Breast Cancer at the ABC's Brisbane Offices*, The Health Report, 5 February 2007. Available online: <http://www.abc.net.au/rn/healthreport/stories/2007/1838331.htm>

Australian Broadcasting Corporation (ABC) 2008, *ABC Probes Breast Cancer Pesticide Link*, ABC online, 22 February 2008. Available online: <http://www.abc.net.au/news/stories/2008/02/22/2169576.htm>

Australian Institute of Health and Welfare 2002, *Chronic Diseases and Associated Risk Factors in Australia, 2001*, AIHW, Canberra.

Arif, K. M. & Beng, K. S. 2006, 'Cultural Health Beliefs in a Rural Family Practice: A Malaysian Perspective' *Australian Journal of Rural Health,* vol. 14, no. 1, pp. 2–8.

Begg, S., Vos, T., Barker, B., Stevenson, C., Stanley, L. & Lopez, A. 2007, *The Burden of Disease and Injury in Australia 2003*, Australian Institute of Health and Welfare, Canberra.

Bogart, L. & Thorburn, S. 2005, 'Are HIV/AIDS Conspiracy Beliefs a Barrier to HIV Prevention Among African Americans', *Journal of Acquired Immune Deficiency Syndromes,* vol. 38, no. 2, pp. 213–18.

Breaden, K. 2003, 'You'll Never Hear Them Say "You're Cured": The Language of Tragedy in Cancer Care', *Health Sociology Review*, vol. 12, no. 2, pp. 120–8.

Bury, M. 1982, 'Chronic Illness as Biographical Disruption', *Sociology of Health and Illness*, vol. 4, no. 2, pp. 167–82.

Bury, M. 2001, 'Illness Narratives: Fact or Fictions?', *Sociology of Health and Illness*, vol. 23, pp. 263–85.

Corbin, J. & Strauss, A. 1988, *Unending Work and Care: Managing Chronic Illness at Home*, Jossey-Bass, San Francisco.

Davison, C., Davey Smith, G. & Frankel, S. 1991, 'Lay Epidemiology and the Prevention Paradox: The Implications of Coronary Candidacy for Health Education', *Sociology of Health and Illness*, vol. 13, pp. 1–20.

Ezzy, D. 2000, 'Illness Narratives: Time, Hope and HIV', *Social Science & Medicine*, vol. 50, pp. 605–17.

Garrett, C. 2005, *Gut Feelings: Chronic Illness and the Search for Healing*, Rodopi, Amsterdam.

Giddens, A. 1991, *Modernity and Self-identity: Self and Society in the Late Modern Age*, Stanford University Press, Stanford CA.

Goffman, E. 1963, *Stigma: Notes on the Management of Spoiled Identity*, Simon & Schuster, New York.

Goggin, C. & Newell, C. 2005, *Disability in Australia: Exposing a Social Apartheid*, University of New South Wales Press, Sydney.

Gregory, S. 2005, 'Living with Chronic Illness in the Family Setting', *Sociology of Health & Illness*, vol. 27, no. 3, pp. 372–92.

Hardey, M. 1999, 'Doctor in the House: The Internet as a Source of Lay Health Knowledge and the Challenge to Expertise', *Sociology of Health and Illness*, vol. 21, no. 6, pp. 820–35.

Huber, J. T. & Gillaspy, M. L. 1998, 'Social Constructs and Disease: Implications for a Controlled Vocabulary for HIV/AIDS', *Library Trends*, vol. 47, no. 2, pp.190–208.

Kivits, J. 2006, 'Informed Patients and the Internet: A Mediated Context for Consultations with Health Professionals', *Journal of Health Psychology*, vol. 11, no. 2, pp. 269–82.

Kleinman, A. 1988, *The Illness Narratives: Suffering, Healing and the Human Condition*, Basic Books, New York.

Millen, N. & Walker, C. 2003, 'Overcoming the Stigma of Chronic Illness: Strategies for Normalisation of a "Spoiled Identity"', *Health Sociology Review*, vol. 10, no. 2, pp. 89–97.

Pierret, J. 2003, 'The Illness Experience: State of Knowledge and Perspectives for Research', *Sociology of Health and Illness*, vol. 25, pp. 4–22.

Radley, A. & Green, R. 1987, 'Illness as Adjustment: A Methodology and Conceptual Framework', *Sociology of Health and Illness*, vol. 9, pp. 179–207.

Royer, A. 1995, 'Living with Chronic Illness', *Research in Sociology of Health Care*, vol. 12, pp. 25–48.

Royer, A. 1998, *A Life with Chronic Illness: Social and Psychological Dimensions*, Praeger, Westport, CT, London.

Scambler G. & Hopkins A, 1986, 'Being Epileptic, Coming to Terms with Stigma', *Sociology of Health and Illness*, vol. 8, pp. 26–43

Wasow, M. 1995, *The Skipping Stone: Ripple Effects of Mental Illness on the Family*, Science and Behavior, Palo Alto.

Williams, C. 2002, *Mothers, Young People and Chronic Illness*, Ashgate, Hampshire.

Williams, G. 2000, 'Knowledge Narratives', *Anthropology and Medicine*, vol. 7, no. 1, pp. 135–40.

Willis, E. 1989, *Medical Dominance: The Division of Labour in Australian Health Care*, Allen & Unwin, Sydney.

CHAPTER 15

Ageing, Health, and the Demographic Revolution

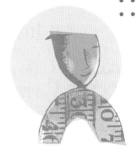

MARILYN
POOLE

Overview

- What are the social and health implications of Australians living longer?
- In what ways does ageing affect health and health service delivery?
- What role can social policy play in addressing the needs of an ageing population?

ISOLATED AND LONELY

Muriel, an 85-year-old widow, lived alone. She had no close relatives and few visitors. Her friends had grown old and become less mobile, or moved away, or died. The neighbourhood changed, and no one noticed that Muriel had many bruises due to falls, or that her house was no longer immaculate. One day Bob, her nephew, was called by the hospital as Muriel had had a bad fall in the street. After a second more serious fall in her bathroom where she lay naked for hours before help arrived, Bob was informed that she could no longer live alone given the likelihood of falls and also due to the signs of dementia which she displayed. Bob and his wife Mary were then faced with a major problem. No one else offered to lend a hand so they had to clean up Muriel's house getting it ready for sale, dispose of her

furniture, and settle Muriel in a residential aged-care facility near their home.

Bob and Mary visited Muriel as often as they could. She had many falls while in care and was confined to a wheelchair. Muriel became more and more withdrawn and vague and did not seem to know Bob and Mary; she did not communicate with people in the aged-care accommodation. Almost two years later Muriel died.

Norbert Elias (1985) was one of the first sociologists to recognise the social isolation of older people. Australian sociologist Allan Kellehear in *The Social History of Dying* (2007, p. 224) writes that loneliness is not simply a matter of physical isolation, or of being institutionalised, rather, it is 'the loneliness of being in the midst of many people for whom one is without social significance'.

Introduction

The **social exclusion** of older people happens in many different ways. This chapter explores the ageing process and the resulting changes to the self-identity of older people. Many people are fit and well in their 60s and 70s and lead productive lives. However, in the last years of life, frailty and dependency may preclude people from taking charge of their own lives. In this situation, loneliness, isolation, and institutionalisation may lead to an uneasy death. Improved living conditions and medical advances have enabled us to live longer than ever before; now health providers, policy makers, and social scientists need to provide solutions to ensure the last years are worth living.

The Demographic Revolution: the Silver Tsunami

> Since 1901, the Australian population has undergone a significant demographic transition. Two major features of this have been declining fertility and declining mortality. A decline in fertility since the 1950s has led to slow growth of the population at younger ages, whereas declining mortality has contributed to large growth in the number of people in the older age groups. (AIHW 2008, p. 19)

In previous centuries, life tended to be short. Many babies and children died, as did people in their prime, and so questions of ageing and aged people were something of a rarity. The common forms of death were infections, violence, accidents, and death during childbirth (Brown 2007). The improvement in life expectancy was due to changing social conditions such as improved living standards (housing and diet), improved sanitation, sewerage, provision of a clean water supply, and medical advances such as mass vaccinations and the use of antibiotics. In developed countries today people tend to die of degenerative diseases, such as cancer and heart disease, which are associated with ageing. More recently, medical advances dealing with heart disease and strokes have improved life expectancy further. Health services are faced with increasing problems concerning the health and well-being of the elderly. In fact, to some extent, medicine has become a victim of its own success (Schilling 1993).

People aged 65 or over represent 13 per cent of the total Australian population (up from 12 per cent in 1996), with the proportion of people aged 85 years at 1.6 per cent as of 2006. According to the June 2006 Census, an estimated 2.7 million Australians were 65 years and older; more than half of these were aged between 65 and 74 years. Women account for 55 per cent of the older population, and are an even higher share of those aged over 85 years (ABS 2006b; AIHW 2007b). A global demographic transformation is taking place due to significant changes to fertility and mortality (death) rates that affect all aspects of society. The number of older people in the world is expected to double in the next twenty years (Kalache et al. 2005). Australian estimates indicate that by 2047, 25 per cent of the population is likely to be aged 65 and over (see Figure 15.1).

Figure 15.1 Age distribution of the Australian population, real and projected

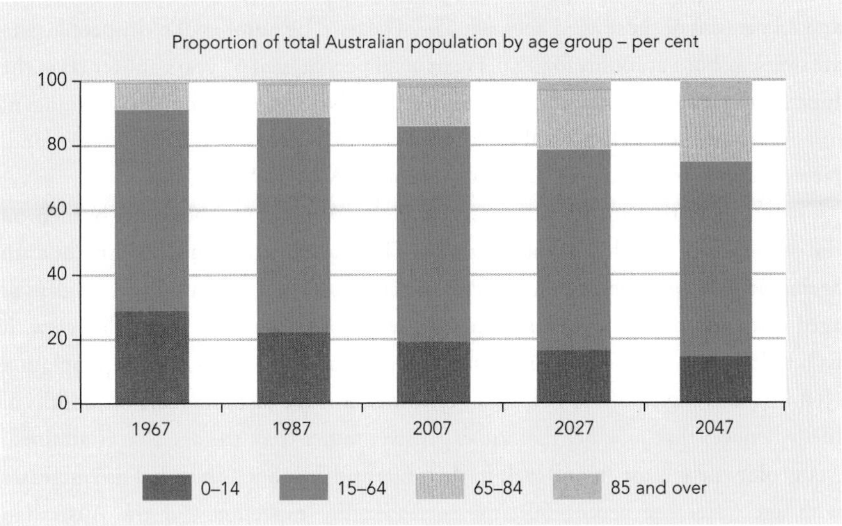

Source: Commonwealth of Australia 2007, p. 4
Copyright Commonwealth of Australia, reproduced with permission

The median age of Australia's population is 36.8—the point at which half are older and half younger—a figure that increased by 5.5 years over the two decades (AIHW 2008). As Figure 15.1 shows, the biggest changes occurred in the older age groups, with a consequent decline in the proportion of children in the population (aged 0–14 years) over the same period. This changing **demographic** is likely to become even more pronounced. Using 2006 census data it is estimated that 18 per cent of the population is aged between 50–64 years (AIHW 2007c, p. 2). What some demographers have referred to as the 'silver tsunami' is close at hand—that is the time when the baby boomers (those born between 1946 and 1964) reach retirement age (Goldenberg 2007). This will occur around 2010 when the first of the baby boomer generation reach the age of 65 (AIHW 2007b). It is estimated that the baby boomers, as a large section of the population, will drive Australian policies 'in relation to retirement incomes, health costs and aged care' (Quine et al. 2006, p. 145).

The extent of population ageing varies among immigrant and Indigenous groups, reflecting differing mortality and fertility rates. For example, Australian Aboriginal people have a lower life expectancy than non-Aboriginal people and a relatively high fertility rate, resulting in a younger age profile compared with the

**demography/
demographic**
The statistical study of populations (demography) that identifies selected characteristics of a population (demographics), such as age profile, sex, income, education, and employment.

rest of the population (Weston et al. 2003). Some immigrant groups also have different age profiles largely depending on the patterns of immigration. For example, immigrants are often fairly young on arrival, and so the older and younger age groups are differentially expressed depending on the timing of the main sources of immigration (Weston et al. 2003). People from non-English-speaking backgrounds (NESBs) currently make up a small proportion (15 per cent) of the very old (85+ years), but a significant proportion (21 per cent) of those aged between 75–84 years and 23 per cent of those aged between 65–74 years. The number of older people who are overseas-born accounts for 35 per cent of all people aged 65 years or over (as at the June 2006 census date), with the majority from NESBs, even though a significant minority are from English-speaking countries such as the United Kingdom, Ireland, New Zealand, South Africa, Canada, and the USA (AIHW 2007b).

It is argued that increased life expectancy will place an enormous burden on the provision of health care in Australia. These arguments render ageing and an ageing population problematic in terms of the pressure on hospital beds, residential aged care, and home support services but recent research contradicts this view. It is 'proximity to death' that drives health costs rather than an ageing population (Johnson & Yong 2006, p. 74). In other words, it is the last few years or months of life (whenever that may be) that are expensive, rather than the age that is attained. Many older people are fit and well in their 60s and 70s, but as hospital use increases with age (after the age of 50), the increased life expectancy of the Australian population will affect both the demand and provision for hospital services (AIHW 2007a). This may be summarised as follows:

- Older people are greater users of hospitals than younger people, with 53 per cent of people in hospitals on the night of 30 June 2004 being aged 65 and over
- Older men have higher rates of hospital use than older women
- On average, older people have longer stays in hospital than younger people, particularly for acute care episodes
- Falls are a common cause of injury for many older people and hospitalisation due to a fall increases with age
- On discharge, older patients are less likely than younger patients to return to their usual residence and are thus more likely to go into residential care (AIHW 2007a, 2007c).

When do you become 'old'?

Guy Brown (2007) considers concepts of 'old' and 'old age' to be outdated. Nor is it useful, in his opinion, to categorise people aged between 60–80 years as 'old', those between 80–100 as 'very old', and those over 100 as 'extremely old'. Centenarians used to be very rare, but they are no longer so and this trend is likely to continue

(Brown 2007). People in the more affluent societies are 'living longer, healthier and more productive lives than ever before' (Giddens 2006, p. 179).

For much of the twentieth century, the legal age of retirement of employees from the workforce was the marker for 'old age'. Chancellor Bismarck first granted regular payments by the state when people reached a specific age in the late 1880s in Germany. New South Wales adopted a means-tested age pension in 1900 (followed very quickly by Victoria and Queensland), and in 1908 the Commonwealth of Australia passed the *Invalid and Old Age Pensions Act 1908*. Eligibility was limited according to character, 'race', age, residency, and means, and the pension was paid to eligible men and women at the age of 65. In 1910, the age for eligible women was reduced to 60 (Nielson & Harris 2008).

In the late twentieth century, the meanings given to old age and retirement began to be viewed rather differently. Nowadays, the definition of old age no longer depends on someone retiring from paid work. Whereas in the past retirement meant the sudden cessation of paid employment, today some workers phase out from full-time paid work to part-time, others withdraw from the workforce and re-enter in another occupation, or work fewer hours, or on a casual basis. The Commonwealth *Age Discrimination Act 2004* gave older workers protection from discrimination in the workplace and allowed them to continue working past what was formerly the compulsory retirement age of 65.

The most common reason for retirement given by people is their eligibility to receive superannuation or pension payments and this is ranked higher than health or physical disability, though other factors such as lifestyle, job satisfaction, and retrenchment are also factors (AIHW 2007c). The connection between retirement and old age has applied mostly to male workers. In previous generations, the pattern for most women was to work prior to marriage or having children, then re-enter the workforce as the children grew older. The age pension for women was payable originally at age 60, perhaps in recognition of the fact that women tended to marry men older than they were and the life expectancy of men is shorter than that of women. In 2004 Australia raised the pension age of women to 65 to match that of men.

Changing notions of retirement

Andrew Blaikie (1999, p. 58) comments that retirement has been a useful vehicle 'to separate older people from the sphere of production'. He suggests that as traditional values were eroded and outmoded, older people were excluded from the workforce through statutory retirement age and thus rendered obsolete to the production process. Just as 'childhood' was an invention of an earlier era, so 'retirement' became a **social construct**, the invention of the late nineteenth and early twentieth centuries. Retirement became the vehicle for segregating people using chronological markers

social construction/ constructionism
Refers to the socially created characteristics of human life based on the idea that people actively construct reality, meaning it is neither 'natural' nor inevitable. Therefore, notions of normality/abnormality, right/wrong, and health/ illness are subjective human creations that should not be taken for granted.

(Blaikie 1999). Older people were marginalised and relied on welfare provisions such as old age pensions and other social support mechanisms. The classification of people as 'old' has marginalised them and given rise to apocalyptic notions of the heavy burden of old people on the rest of the population with their demands and needs. Exclusion from paid work led to other forms of social exclusion and inequalities.

Since the age pension was introduced in 1908, the majority of Australians depended on it for their retirement income. Unlike many other countries, Australia has a non-contributory pension scheme. This is in contrast to some European countries which have compulsory, contributory pension schemes or like the United States that has a social security system that is a contributory, earnings-related scheme (Nielson & Harris 2008). The retirement income system in Australia today is based on three 'pillars' (AIHW 2007b), these are:

1   the age pension and war veterans service pension
2   compulsory employer superannuation contributions often topped up by employee voluntary contributions
3   home equity, bank savings and other assets.

By June 2006, 1.9 million people received either the age pension or a part-pension. An additional 338,600 people over the age of 60 received a pension from the Department of Veterans Affairs (DVA). Around 75 per cent of all Australians of qualifying age received a pension—either an age pension or one similar from DVA (AIHW 2007b).

The retirement income system is changing. In 1992, the Hawke Labor Government introduced a new compulsory superannuation system known as the Superannuation Guarantee (SG) in which employers were required to contribute to their employees' superannuation. Initially, this contribution was 3 per cent of income and has since risen to 9 per cent. It is anticipated to rise further. By 2006, 90 per cent of employed persons had employer-paid superannuation (Nielson & Harris 2008). The 2006 Federal Budget introduced further changes to superannuation that increased its preferential tax treatment and thus made it an attractive investment option (particularly for those able to make voluntary contributions). One of the outcomes of the SG is that highly paid workers not only enjoy the benefits of high salaries but their retirement incomes are likely to be considerably higher than that of lower paid workers.

The implications of compulsory superannuation are that people will rely less on government financial support and look after themselves in their old age. Both the young and the middle-aged are reminded of this and encouraged to make voluntary contributions to superannuation as the age pension is increasingly seen as a 'safety net' than the main provision of financial support for older people. The growth of the financial planning industry has ensured that people of all ages are encouraged to 'take stock' and 'plan ahead'. Newspapers and magazines are full of advice from financial 'experts' telling people how to best manage their finances. Taking responsibility for oneself and taking control of one's own life has become a persistent message since the latter part of the twentieth century.

Drawing on the work of Anthony Giddens (1991), in late **modernity** (present day), individuals write their own biographies because the old certainties, traditions, and norms no longer apply. We are in an era of what is termed **individualism**. In this social environment people are expected to take control of their own lives and lifestyle (Howarth 2007). Giddens (1991, p. 5) claims that '[r]eflexively organized life planning, which normally presumes consideration of risks as filtered through contact with expert knowledge, becomes a central feature of structuring self-identity'. Taking responsibility for financial matters in later life is now part of our personal biographies.

There remain great disparities in wages and retirement income of men and women. Given there are gender differences in work and care-giving patterns, women tend to suffer a cumulative disadvantage in economic status as they age. The benefits from pensions and superannuation schemes are usually based on years of paid employment and level of earnings. Older women who never married, or are divorced or separated tend to have lower incomes and fewer assets. The financial disadvantages they have suffered all their lives continue into retirement (Weston et al. 2003, p. 11).

One of the great challenges of ageing populations is how to sustain public pension/social security systems as a bigger percentage of people reach retirement and live longer to enjoy it. Not only is there likely to be a strain on governments to finance pensions, the other major concern is the strain on the health care system to service ever-increasing numbers of older people. Given that a nation's prosperity is in part dependent on tax collection from workers and from industry, another commonly expressed concern about an ageing population relates to future labour supply. Although there is no statutory retirement age at 65, workforce participation of people aged 65 and over is low (AIHW 2007b).

More recent data indicates that people over the age of 65 are staying on in the workforce. More people in their late 50s still have children to support and mortgages to pay; their employers are fully aware of labour and skills shortages and are not pushing them to leave (Colebatch 2008). Given the fact that fewer younger people will enter the workforce and the current skills shortage in Australia, encouragement is given to mature-aged workers to continue working either on a part-time or full-time basis. A further source of anxiety has been the prospect of the retirement of the baby boomers over the next 20 or so years. The first of the baby boomers have now turned 60, and, if current trends continue, this group may well stay in employment albeit on a part-time or flexible basis.

The prospect of a smaller workforce in the future has focused attention on the dependency ratio. The dependency ratio is the comparison of those who are

modernity/ modernism
A view of social life that is founded upon rational thought and a belief that truth and morality exist as objective realities that can be discovered and understood through scientific means. See *reflexive modernity* and *postmodernism*.

individualism
A belief or process supporting the primacy of individual choice, freedom, and self-responsibility.

considered economically active (that is, in paid employment) with those who are dependent (that is, those not employed, including children and retired people). The 'doom and gloom' scenario is that Australia will sink under the economic burden of a small workforce trying to support a large cohort of older people. Yet, the dependency ratio is a flawed concept as it ignores the social and economic contributions of older people through various forms of volunteer work, which are essential to the operation of many families and community and welfare organisations.

BOX 15.1 Doing health sociology: confronting ageism and 'social death'

In a youth-obsessed society, where health, beauty, sexual prowess, and vitality are valued, it is little surprise that ageing is viewed negatively. The 'anti-ageing' industry—replete with age-defying cosmetics, injections (e.g. botox), drugs (for example, Viagra and hormone replacement therapy), and cosmetic surgery—is a clear sign of the social value placed on youth and avoiding the signs of ageing. Old age stereotypes and **ageism** are commonplace (Hepworth 1995), such as targeting workers in their 40s and 50s for redundancy because they are allegedly more prone to memory loss, too slow to learn new skills and adapt to new technologies, or are argumentative because they are 'set in their ways'. Such stereotypes and prejudices oversimplify the diversity of older people and devalue the varied contributions they make. They also precipitate older people's social exclusion, marginalisation, and isolation, a **social death** that may occur long before biological death (Mulkay 1993).

---

ageism
A term that denotes discrimination based on age.

social death
The marginalisation and exclusion of elderly people from everyday life, resulting in social isolation.

The hidden contribution of older people

For many people retirement has become a time of opportunity. The strict boundary between the 'worker' and the 'retired' is now much more fluid. One cannot assume that all retired people are over the age of 65 nor can one assume that they do no work (paid or unpaid). Retirement offers older people many opportunities to give their time and energy to their families and communities as well as personal interests (AIHW 2007b).

Although it is sometimes argued that older people are a burden on society, the reality is rather different. There have been a number of studies that indicate that older people make substantial contributions to society. In particular, people in their 60s and early 70s tend to be in good health and lead productive lives. They are likely to provide more support to their families than they receive from them (Weston et al. 2003). Grandparents make a large contribution to childcare so that parents can work or study, with a 2005 Australian Bureau of Statistics (ABS) survey finding that they provided 60 per cent of informal care for children (AIHW 2007c). Some grandparents take responsibility for raising their grandchildren when parents are no longer able to do so.

Older people are the mainstay of many community and civic organisations (see Table 15.1). Of people over the age of 65, 27 per cent participated in voluntary work in 2006. Older people are more likely to volunteer for community or welfare organisations than in sport and recreation (ABS 2006). The activities undertaken by older people as volunteers were 'fundraising and sales, preparing and serving food, administration, clerical, recruitment and information management' (AIHW 2007c, p. 28).

Table 15.1 Community and civic participation in last 12 months by age and sex, 2006

	Active involvement in governance and citizenship groups	Active involvement in community organisation	Engagement in civic activity
	%	%	%
Males			
55–64	25.4	24.3	47.7
65–74	18.6	26.4	41.0
75–84	15.2	20.3	32.9
85+	2.3	20.8	17.7
Total males 65+	16.3	23.9	36.5
Females			
55–64	19.9	32.0	53.9
65–74	12.5	30.8	42.9
75–84	9.6	24.0	28.9
85+	5.8	15.4	17.8
Total females 65+	10.7	26.7	35.1

Source: Adapted from AIHW 2007c, p. 31

The Third Age

This is the first time in the history of Australia and other developed countries that a large segment of the population is no longer fully involved in education or paid work. Peter Laslett's (1989) model of the Third Age as a time when older people are engaged and fulfilled in a range of voluntary and rewarding leisure activities is a useful one. Laslett (1989) suggests that there are four 'ages', the first being characterised by socialisation and dependence in childhood; the second age is characterised by maturity and independence yet circumscribed by the demands of paid work, having families and responsibilities; the third age is one of independence from responsibility and opportunities for self-fulfilment; and the fourth age is when frailty and dependency curtail opportunities. As these 'ages' are socially constructed segments of the lifespan, individual transitions may vary considerably. For example, the second age could continue for a considerable time, given the number of re-marriages following divorce and separation, where people in their 50s and early 60s may still carry family responsibilities and mortgages.

While health education and promotion models have tended to stress the benefits of exercise and diet to promote healthy ageing, Laslett believed that older people also need cognitive challenges and learning opportunities. He was one of the early proponents of the University of the Third Age (U3A) set up in Britain in the 1980s (following the *'universités du troisième age'* model established first in Toulouse, France) and now a global success story. The first U3A in Australia was established in Melbourne in 1984 (U3A Network Victoria 2008). There are of course flaws in Laslett's concept of the Third Age where healthy and fit older people pursue a variety of activities seeking enjoyment and fulfilment. It is essentially a middle-class aspirational model and not one possible for those living in poverty or difficult circumstances (Mann 2001).

Throughout Australia there are many clubs and organisations for older people such as the U3A, Probus clubs, and Life Activities Clubs (LAC) as well as the more traditional bowling or RSL (Returned and Services League) clubs. Advertisements for retirement communities now stress 'lifestyle' and 'resort style' living. Popular perceptions of ageing have changed, the 'chronological bonds', which once manipu-lated people into behaving in age-appropriate ways, have gone and now older people 'are encouraged to have sex, diet, take holidays, and socialise in ways indistinguish-able from those of their children's generation' (Blaikie 1999, p. 74). The reasons for this, according to Blaikie (1999), lie with the emergence of **consumerism**. The 'grey' dollar is now a target for niche marketing. Specials for 'seniors' abound: hotels and clubs offer 'seniors' lunches at reduced prices; tour groups take 'seniors' to the outback or on cruises overseas; and hotels and motels offer 'seniors' discounts mid-week and off-season.

'Healthy ageing' is seen as a means of older people having a good quality of life; for many people this goes hand in hand with feeling useful and productive and needed. When older people were excluded from the workforce they were regarded as an economic burden and classified as dependent. With the emergence of active Third Agers, the question of intergenerational conflict has surfaced with claims that an affluent older generation is holding onto or spending their assets whereas young people are unable to afford housing and are burdened with debt.

consumerism
The processes and institutions by which individuals satisfy their needs by purchasing goods and services in a market. Mass consumerism refers to post-Second World War consumer practices, whereby the reduction of the cost of goods and the extensive use of advertising and new credit arrangements created a mass market. It is often argued that consumerism has less to do with the satisfaction of wants than with the desire to be different and distinctive.

Ageing brains and ageing bodies

Ageing brains

It is well known that the mature brain cannot learn as well as the immature brain; for instance, this accounts for the inability of adults in general to learn to speak a new language without an accent. Children under the age of 12, on the other hand, can completely master this skill (Gordon 2000). As the brain ages further, a broader range of deficits are gradually manifested. Not only is learning new material more difficult, but recalling past memories, especially of names and numbers, becomes harder. People make light of their 'senior moments' when they forget something, but memory loss is a very real fear for older people. According to Stephen Bondy, the reasons for this loss of plasticity are unclear but are likely to involve reduced proliferation or ramification of nerve cells in the main centre of the brain involved in new learning—the hippocampus. Another feature that may underlie impeded performance of the aged brain is the tendency of the nervous system to keep reacting to insults incurred in the past. The defences of the body in general respond rapidly to injury or infection, with enhanced activity, but this rapidly returns to normal after the disorder is dealt with, but the brain seems to stay in a reactive state for extended periods. Thus, the aged brain appears to be chronically inflamed even in the absence of an external provocative stimulus. This is especially the case in a variety of neurodegenerative disorders such as **Alzheimer's disease**. Irrelevant and prolonged immune activation can be injurious to nerve cell function (Bondy 2008).

Age-related deficits of performance are especially pronounced in a very common disease associated with brain ageing: Alzheimer's disease. This serious disorder is characterised by the presence of amyloid plaques within the brain. Alzheimer's disease appears qualitatively different than normal brain ageing but may in fact merely be an exaggeration of processes that are already under way during senescence (the state of old age). Again there is evidence of inflammation, perhaps representing a futile attempt by the body to clear the amyloid plaques found in the Alzheimer brain. The prevalence of Alzheimer's disease rises with age. It is suggested that 25 per cent of people over 85 years are affected, rising to 35 per cent of those over 95 years (Kellehear 2007, p. 203).

The best possibility of prolonging brain function may lie in using exercise and dietary regimens resembling those recommended for optimising heart performance and overall well-being. A good mix of antioxidant and anti-inflammatory agents can protect against age-related oxidative damage, and from the consequences of excess inflammatory responses that characterise several aged tissues. For example, a diet high in fruits and vegetables has been shown beneficial in animal models of human brain ageing. The beneficial constituents of plants are especially concentrated in berries and fruits of red and blue colour and in dark green leafy vegetables. Rather

Alzheimer's disease
An incurable and terminal type of dementia indicated by significant memory loss and degenerative mental and physical abilities, resulting in confusion, language decline, loss of bodily functions, and ultimately in death.

Marilyn Poole

surprisingly, exercise has also shown to benefit the responses of the ageing brain directly. Exploitation of these findings need not await a complete explanation of their mechanism of action (Bondy 2008). As far as exercises for the mind are concerned, the debate continues; however, few would dispute the value of continued social interaction and the pursuit of hobbies and interests.

Ageing bodies

We age at different rates. This is easily discerned at reunions or catching up with friends we have not seen for some time. Body composition changes, as does physical function and performance. Chris Schilling (1993) argues that through the life course some bodily postures and facial expressions become literally inscribed on the flesh. As we age, the ravages of time are physically represented on our bodies, our faces, our hands, and upon our sense of self. So important a value has appearance become in a contemporary consumer culture that the body has become a signifier of social identity. As a consequence, ageing has become a sensitive social and personal issue (Blaikie 1999).

While notions of age often invoked decay, frailty, and loss of independence in the past, a deconstruction of the life-course is occurring in a postmodern and consumer culture (Poole 1999, p. 88). As Bryan Turner (1995, p. 256) points out, in contemporary societies 'the body has become a site of regulative practices and as a consequence of these regulative practices the body has become a project'. Mike Featherstone and Mike Hepworth (1995, p. 31) argue that since the 1960s the 'construction of positive ageing' has spread and that discourses on ageing 'have become a significant feature of popular and consumer culture', an important force behind these being the emergence of the 'ageing industry' (Poole 1999, p. 88). The body is now a legitimate site for rejuvenation and cosmetic practices and a great deal of effort is now put into managing the ageing process (Blaikie 1999). In *The Presentation of Self in Everyday Life*, Erving Goffman (1959) describes people as actors who stage appropriate performances. The 'presentation of self' is now seen as signifying the real character of people. Chris Schilling (1993, p. 34) comments that in a contemporary consumer culture people *become* their bodies: '[t]he management and moulding of the body has become increasingly central to the presentation of self image and this has been backed up by a growing industry catering for keep-fit, dieting and general body care' (Schilling 1993, p. 92). The discourses on taking responsibility for one's own health are powerful. Many health promotion and health education schemes urge people to watch their diets and to exercise; many imply that through these regimens the scourges of old age, such as heart disease and cancer, might be prevented. The health promotion model stresses individual responsibility or **agency** and tends to ignore structural factors, which might inhibit or prevent individual participation, such as living in poverty or a neighbourhood lacking sporting or recreational facilities, or factors such as ethnic and social class differences

agency
The ability of people, individually and collectively, to influence their own lives and the society in which they live.

(Howarth 2007). The normal processes of ageing cannot be avoided forever. Sagging skin, wrinkles, muscles that have lost their strength and tone, and inflexible limbs are all physical manifestations of ageing. Older people are reminded of their own ageing when they see photographs of themselves in earlier years and when they look in a mirror. They may feel young inside, but the outward appearance is that of an old person. Turner (1995, p. 252) comments that the photograph has 'become an essential feature, therefore, not only of individual images of ageing, but of collective, generational ageing'.

The last scene of all

Although people everywhere die at different ages, those in Western, developed countries can reasonably expect to get close to (or reach) their 80s and 90s (Kellehear 2007). In fact there is now some debate as to what might be considered the natural life span of human beings.

Caring for older people

It was estimated that in 2006, 94 per cent of older people (65 years and older) lived in private dwellings (family groups, couple, or single person households). Although a relatively small percentage of older people live in care accommodation, the situation changes for those of 85 years and over with 31 per cent in care (AIHW 2007b). People from NESBs use permanent residential care at a lower rate compared with the rest of the Australian population (AIHW 2007c). As women tend to outlive men, many older women are living alone. Not only do many of these women require assistance of some kind, but they also face isolation, reduced social participation, and loneliness.

About half of all people over the age of 65 suffer some kind of disability that restricts their daily activities (AIHW 2007b). People with profound and severe limitations to their mobility may require considerable assistance but well-designed home environments and access to aids are beneficial not only to the disabled but also their carers; however, 'poor housing conditions, low income and lack of transport services, low levels of community information and lack of community services' impede the functioning of older people with disabilities (AIHW 2007b, p. 85). 'Functional limitation is strongly associated with depressive symptoms in older people' and 'perceived inability in meeting basic needs predicts depression in older adults' (AIHW 2007b, p. 85). In 2002, the National Aboriginal and Torres Strait Islander Social Survey (NATSISS) revealed higher rates of disability and poor health across all age groups compared to non-Indigenous people; with 72 per cent of Indigenous people aged 65 years having a disability or long-term health condition (AIHW 2007c, p. 142).

Marilyn Poole

Older people with major disabilities living in the community are likely to have a primary carer. Spouses and adult children (mainly daughters) make up approximately equal proportions of all primary carers of older people. Of these carers, many are themselves in older age groups. Of the assistance provided by primary carers, some care is considered core such as help with bathing, dressing, eating, and managing incontinence, while non-core activities include help with mobility assistance (AIHW 2007b). People with dementia are considered as needing a high level of long-term care, given they may not be able to carry out core activities and live without assistance (AIHW 2006).

The continuing supply of informal carers is a matter of concern for policy makers. As women's workforce participation has risen, women find themselves in a 'double bind' in terms of caring for a frail elderly relative and continuing paid employment. International studies indicate that the 'nature of the association between employment and care giving depends on the support available from community services' (AIHW 2007b, p. 101). It is interesting to note that frail, older people receive more assistance from informal providers than from any government-funded aged-care program (AIHW 2007b). The wider implications of demographic ageing are profound; there will be fewer children and fewer grandchildren available to care for the increasing numbers of older people. If this is the case, how will governments cope to meet the rising demands for care? There has been a shift in Australia from long-term care in nursing homes and residential care to community-based care allowing people to remain in their own homes. Currently, there are a range of programs funded by Australian state and local governments that offer care for older people. Among the national programs that deliver care in residential and community settings are the Home and Community Care program (HACC), Community Aged Care Packages (CACPs), and programs for Department of Veterans' Affairs (DVA) clients and residential aged care (respite and permanent). The Australian Government is the largest source of funding for the aged-care system mainly due to funding for residential aged care. Although residential aged-care accounts for the largest proportion of expenditure on older people, the HACC program was the second largest (AIHW 2007b). As people grow increasingly frail and old, it is sometimes impossible for them to live independently even with help from family members and aged-care support services such as meals on wheels, or assistance with shopping, housework, or personal care arranged by local councils and social support programs in community centres. In these situations a decision may be made for the older person to enter residential care accommodation. This is traumatic in terms of abandoning an independent life in one's own home, disposing of all but a few belongings and moving away from family and friends. Allan Kellehear (2007, p. 221) writes passionately that residents in aged care are patronised, denigrated, and that their 'former lives are all but ignored'. In his view it is no accident that old people fear abandonment in such places, as they are segregated and devalued. Many older people end up dying in nursing homes, which are sometimes referred to as 'God's waiting room'. Nursing homes have suffered a great deal of criticism both in Australia and overseas. Critics argue that they are impersonal institutions with poor staffing levels and insufficient funding where old people are treated like children, suffer from bed sores and infections, have restraints on their mobility, sometimes suffer abuse, and ultimately experience an 'uneasy death'.

Dying and death

Death is a certainty for all of us. A less recognised feature of the demographic revolution is the age of death. At the beginning of the twentieth century, death occurred at any age. Babies died at birth, young children died of infectious diseases, poverty, unsanitary conditions, or accidents, adult males died from hazardous working conditions, whereas women's mortality was associated with pregnancy, childbirth, or abortion. Since the mid-twentieth century, this pattern of mortality declined in all age groups. For the first time in Australia's history (with the exception of Indigenous people) death now tends to be 'the preserve of old age' (Kellehear 2007). Despite medical advances and the achievements of public health many of us will end our lives dying of an assortment of diseases that will not provide us with a clear death bed scene for ourselves or our families (Kellehear 2007). Given increased life expectancy, it is likely that the process of dying will also be prolonged. Kellehear writes that 'arthritis, organ failure or dementia, and sudden body system failures such as strokes, pneumonia or accidental falls will deny most of us a good death or even a well-managed one' (Kellehear 2007, p. 213).

Death is a biological event but it is also a social process. The meanings of dying and death are constructed differently in different cultural and social contexts (McNamara 1998). For dying people, it matters where, when, and how life will end. Their experiences will be influenced by how much they can participate in the decision-making process and by the degree of control they have over their dying, such as input on pain medication or life-prolonging medical treatments. Although the message of empowerment of the dying person has informed the palliative care and hospice movement it is clear that there is still great community dissatisfaction with the manner of dying and the unnecessary delay of death through medical interventions.

euthanasia
Meaning 'gentle death', the term is used to describe voluntary death, often medically assisted, as a result of incurable and painful disease.

BOX 15.2 Voluntary euthanasia

With the exception of the Netherlands, voluntary **euthanasia** and physician-assisted suicide is illegal in most countries; though between July 1996 and March 1997, it was legalised in the Northern Territory before being overturned by the Federal Government.

Proponents of voluntary euthanasia maintain that individuals should have the right to control

... »

Marilyn Poole

their own bodies, and particularly choose the timing and nature of their death. They point out that passive forms of euthanasia already exist as part of the treatment regimen for terminally ill patients, when medical treatment is withdrawn and pain management ultimately leads to death. Opponents argue that assisting in the ending of any life is morally repugnant, and that legislation of such a right would eventually lead to non-voluntary euthanasia. The fear is that those with the power to decide may expand to include the state, medical experts, or relatives giving rise to the concept of a 'duty to die', particularly in the context of an ageing population and prevailing notions of the aged as a social burden.

Conclusion

The consequences of population ageing have profound social implications and challenge governments, policy makers, and health care providers. Although public debate tends to focus on the negative stereotypes of ageing such as dependency, illness, and frailty, the reality is that many people in their 60s and 70s are fit and well and contribute to society and their families in a myriad of ways. There is a downside however; our increased lifespan has not necessarily been matched by extra years of healthy life (Brown 2007). Making them worth living constitutes one of the great challenges of this century.

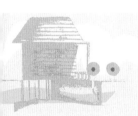

Summary of main points

» Low fertility, low mortality rates, and higher life expectancy have contributed to population ageing throughout the world.
» Retirement from paid employment was formerly a social marker for the beginning of old age.
» The ageing of the population has led to debates about the cost and provision of health services for older people.
» It is possible to divide older people into third and fourth ages that are not specific chronological markers.
» The normal processes of ageing cannot be avoided forever but many people remain fit and healthy well into old age.
» Only in the final years of life do older people require considerable support to maintain their independence.
» The process of dying and death, in developed countries at least, is now predominantly associated with old age.

Sociological reflection 1: living to over 100

Jeanne Louise Calment (1875–1997), born in Arles, France, was the oldest recorded living person with her 122 years and 164 days. She outlived her husband, daughter, and grandson; she lived independently until the age of 110 and smoked until she was 117.

» Research the life of Jeanne Calment and other people who have lived longer than 100 years. Have they anything in common?

» Do you think there are limits to human ageing? What social consequences would occur if centenarians became more commonplace?

Sociological reflection 2: dead alone

An elderly man was found in his public housing unit in Sydney about a year after he had died. Neighbours noticed increasing piles of uncollected mail, but did nothing. This is not an isolated case. According to an article in *The Age*, coroner's reports for 2007 indicate that in Victoria 454 people were not discovered for at least two weeks after death and 43 for more than three months. Similarly, in New South Wales, it was at least seven days before the bodies of 283 residents were found (Stafford 2008).

» What do you think are some of the solutions to prevent this kind of occurrence?

» What programs exist to prevent it?

Discussion questions

1 How does the state contribute to the marginalisation of old people?

2 Do you believe we are heading for a 'demographic time bomb' or that society will change and successfully adjust to ever-increasing numbers of older people?

3 When do you think people become old? Give your reasons.

4 How is age constructed as a social problem?

5 How has Giddens' concept of individualisation contributed to our understanding of ageing in the twenty-first century?

6 How would you distinguish between the Third Age (young–old) and the fourth age (old–old)?

Further investigation

1 Old age is a social construction. Discuss.

2 Compare the factors underpinning healthy and unhealthy ageing.

3 Examine recent policies and related debates about funding the health and social services required for an ageing population.

Marilyn Poole

4 Explore the different viewpoints of proponents and opponents to voluntary euthanasia and physician-assisted suicide.

Further reading

Australian Government 2007, *Intergenerational Report 2007*, The Treasury, Common-wealth of Australia, Canberra. Available online: <http://www.treasury.gov.au/igr/IGR 2007.asp>

Department of Families, Housing, Community Services and Indigenous Affairs 2008, *Pension Review: Background Paper*, Commonwealth of Australia, Canberra. Available online: <http://www.facsia.gov.au/internet/facsinternet.nsf/seniors/pension_review.htm>

Foos, P. W. & Clark, M. C. 2008, *Human Aging*, 2nd edn, Allyn and Bacon, Boston.

House of Representatives Standing Committee on Health and Ageing 2005, *Future Ageing: Inquiry into Long-term Strategies to Address the Ageing of the Australian Population Over the Next 40 Years*, Commonwealth of Australia, Canberra. Available online: <http://www.aph.gov.au/House/committee/haa/strategies/report.htm>

Howarth, G. 2007, *Death and Dying: A Sociological Introduction*, Polity Press, Cambridge.

Johnson, M. L. (ed.) in association with V. L. Bengtson, P. G. Coleman & T. B. L. Kirkwood 2005, *The Cambridge Handbook of Age and Ageing*, Cambridge University Press, Cambridge.

Kellehear, A. 2007, *A Social History of Dying*, Cambridge University Press, Cambridge.

Productivity Commission 2005, *Economic Implications of an Ageing Australia*, Research Report, Commonwealth of Australia, Canberra. Available online: <http://www.pc.gov.au/projects/study/ageing/docs/finalreport>

Reader bonus

Available on the Second Opinion website: Strazzari, M. 2005, 'Ageing, Dying, and Death in the Twenty-first Century', in J. Germov (ed.), *Second Opinion: An Introduction to Health Sociology*, 3rd edition, Oxford University Press, Melbourne.

Online case study

Visit the Second Opinion website to access relevant case studies.

Web resources

Australian Department of Health and Ageing (DOHA): <http://www.health.gov.au/>

Australian Institute of Health and Welfare: <http://www.aihw.gov.au/>

Death-related Weblinks: Michael Kearl's website on the sociology of death, dying and bereavement: <http://www.geocities.com/ajarnmike/deathweb.html>

SocioSite—Sociology of Ageing: <http://www.sociosite.net/topics/aging.php>

Documentaries/films

As Good as it Gets (1997): 139 minutes. A film directed by James L. Brooks starring Jack Nicholson and Helen Hunt, that explores ageing and gender issues through the relationships of the characters.

Away from Her (2006): 110 minutes. A film about a man coping with a wife suffering Alzheimer's disease, who not only forgets him, but develops affection for another man in the nursing home in which they reside.

The Bucket List (2007): 97 minutes. A film directed by Rob Reiner starring Jack Nicholson and Morgan Freeman about two terminally ill men who escape from a cancer ward and head off on a road trip with a wish list of to-dos before they die.

Cocoon (1985): 117 minutes. A film directed by Ron Howard about senior citizens who develop youthful energy after swimming in a pool with alien cocoons.

Difference of Opinion (2007): 'How Can we Turn the Ageing Population Problem into an Opportunity?', Broadcast 29 November, ABC TV. Available online: <http://www.abc.net.au/tv/differenceofopinion/content/2007/s2101402.htm>

The Picture of Dorian Gray (1945): 110 minutes. Based on the famous novel by Oscar Wilde about a handsome young man who sells his soul for eternal youth.

References

Australian Bureau of Statistics 2006a, *Voluntary Work, Australia 2006*, Cat. no. 4441.0, ABS, Canberra.

Australian Bureau of Statistics 2006b, *Population by Age and Sex, Australia*, Cat. no. 3235.0, ABS, Canberra.

Australian Institute of Health and Welfare 2006, *Australia's Health 2006*, AIHW, Cat. no. AUS 73, AIHW, Canberra.

Australian Institute of Health and Welfare 2007a, Karmel, R., Lloyd, J. & Hales C., *Older Australians in Hospital*, Bulletin no. 53, Cat. no. AUS92, AIHW, Canberra.

Australian Institute of Health and Welfare 2007b, *Australia's Welfare 2007*, Cat. no. AUS93, AIHW, Canberra.

Australian Institute of Health and Welfare 2007c, *Older Australia at a Glance*, 4th edn., Cat. no. AGE52, AIHW, Canberra.

Australian Institute of Health and Welfare 2008, *Australia's Health 2008*, Cat. no. AUS 99, AIHW, Canberra.

Blaikie, A. 1999, *Ageing & Popular Culture*, Cambridge University Press, Cambridge.

Bondy, S. C. 2008, March, personal communication.

Brown, G. 2007, 'We Have Invested in Prolonging Our Agony', *Comment & Debate, The Guardian Weekly*, 23 November 2007, p. 22.

Colebatch, T. 2008, 'Older Workers Postpone Retirement, *The Age News* Wednesday, 26 March 2008, p. 2.

Commonwealth of Australia 2007, *Intergenerational Report 2007: Overview*, The Treasury, Commonwealth of Australia, Canberra. Available online: <http://www.treasury.gov.au/igr/IGR2007.asp>

Elias, N. 1985, *The Loneliness of Dying,* Basil Blackwell, Oxford.

Featherstone, M. & Hepworth, M. 1995, 'Images of Positive Ageing: A Case Study of Retirement Choice Magazine', in M. Featherstone & A. Wernick (eds), *Images of Aging: Cultural Representations of Later Life*, Routledge, London, pp. 27–46.

Giddens, A. 1991, *Modernity and Self-identity: Self and Society in the Late Modern Age*, Stanford University Press, Stanford, CA.

Giddens, A. 2006, *Sociology* (5th edn), Polity Press, Cambridge.

Goffman, E. 1959, *The Presentation of Self in Everyday Life*, Doubleday, New York.

Goldenberg, S. 2007, '"Silver Tsunami" Threatens to Swamp America's Social Security System', International News, *The Guardian Weekly*, 30 November 2007, p. 9.

Gordon N. 2000, 'The Acquisition of a Second Language', *European Journal of Paediatric Neurology*, vol 4, no. 1, pp. 3–7. Review.

Hepworth, M. 1995, 'Positive Ageing: What is the Message?', in R. Bunton, S. Nettleton & R. Burrow (eds), *The Sociology of Health Promotion*, Routledge, London.

Howarth, G. 2007, *Death & Dying: A Sociological Introduction,* Polity Press, Cambridge.

Johnson, D. & Yong, J. 2006, 'Costly Ageing or Costly Deaths: Understanding Health Care Expenditure Using Australian Medicare Payments Data', *Australian Economic Papers*, vol. 45, no. 1, pp. 33–7.

Kalache, A., Barreto, S. M. & Ketter, I. 2005, 'Global Ageing: The Demographic Revolution in All Cultures and Societies' in M. L. Johnson (ed.), in association with V. L. Bengtson, P. G. Coleman & T. B. L. Kirkwood, *The Cambridge Handbook of Age and Ageing*, Cambridge University Press, Cambridge, pp. 30–46.

Kellehear, A. 2007, *A Social History of Dying*, Cambridge University Press, Cambridge.

Laslett, A. 1989, 'The Demographic Scene: An Overview', in J. Eekelaar & D. Pearl (eds), *An Aging World*, The Clarendon Press, Oxford, pp. 1–10.

Mann, K. 2001, *Approaching Retirement: Social Divisions, Welfare and Exclusion*, The Policy Press, Bristol.

McNamara, B. 1998, 'A Good Enough Death?' in A. Petersen & C. Waddell (eds.) *Health Matters: A Sociology of Illness, Prevention and Care*, Allen & Unwin, Sydney, pp. 169–84.

Mulkay, M. 1993, 'Social Death in Britain', in D. Clark (ed.), *The Sociology of Death*, Blackwell, Cambridge, pp. 31–49.

Nielson, L. & Harris B. 2008, '*Chronology of Superannuation and Retirement Income in Australia,*' Parliamentary Library, Parliament of Australia. Available online:<http://www.aph.gov.au/LIBRARY/pubs/BN/200708/Chron_Superannuation.htm>

Poole, M. 1999, 'It's a Lovely Feeling: Older Women's Fitness Programs', in M. Poole & S. Feldman (eds), *A Certain Age: Women Growing Older,* Allen & Unwin, Sydney, pp. 87–100.

Quine, S., Bernard, D. & Kendig, H. 2006, 'Understanding Baby Boomers' Expectations and Plans for Their Retirement: Findings from a Qualitative Study', *Australasian Journal on Ageing*, vol. 25, no. 3 pp. 145–50.

Schilling, C. 1993, *The Body and Social Theory*, Sage, London.

Stafford, A. 2008, 'Isolated and Lonely, the Unnoticed Deaths of the Elderly', *The Age*, 12 April, p. 7.

Turner, B. S. 1995, 'Ageing and Identity: Some Reflections on the Somatization of the Self' in M. Featherstone et al. (eds), *Cultural Images of Ageing: Cultural Representations of Later Life*, Routledge, London, pp. 245–62.

U3A Network Victoria website 2008, Available online: <http://home.vicnet.net.au/~u3avic/About.htm>

Weston, R., Qu, L. & Soriano, G. 2003, 'Australia's Ageing Yet Diverse Population', *Family Matters*, no. 66, Spring/Summer, pp. 6–13.

CHAPTER 16

The Human Genome Project: A Sociology of Medical Technology

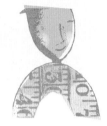

EVAN WILLIS

Overview

- How can we apply the sociological imagination to explain the likely implications of the Human Genome Project for society?
- How might we understand such developments in terms of the treatment of disease from a sociological point of view?
- How will the knowledge and possibilities that such a project provides shape the kind of society in which we live?

DNA TESTING

You are in your late thirties with a young family. A close relative is diagnosed with a genetically caused illness that is expected to be fatal. Looking back through the family genealogy, it is clear that a number of other relatives also died of the same condition. Your doctor suggests that you might consider being genetically tested by having your own DNA analysed. If you do have the particular genetic defect, the chances are quite high (but not certain) that your own life will be shortened. There is no treatment that is known to prevent or delay the onset. Would you want to know? Is it time to take out the life insurance policy you have been contemplating but not got around to? Life insurance companies are understandably wary of people taking out policies when there is a high chance the companies will have to pay out (what is called 'adverse selection'). Indeed their profitability depends on it.

Introduction: the Human Genome Project

The International Human Genome Consortium today announced the successful
completion of the Human Genome Project more than two years ahead of schedule.
(The Sanger Institute, press release, 4 April 2003)

With such a triumphant announcement, the 'Genomic Age' was ushered into
human history and societies, almost fifty years to the day after James Watson and
Francis Crick announced they had identified the double helix structure of DNA (see
Lorentz et al. 2002). These rapid developments in molecular genetics, which have
collectively become known as the Human Genome Project (HGP), have resulted in
the completion of the task of mapping the human genetic code—sometimes referred
to as 'the book of life'. How can a sociological perspective help us to understand, even
predict, what will be the implications of the HGP? How do sociologists study aspects
of health and illness in society and what sorts of features do they concentrate on and
analyse? These questions are addressed in this chapter in the context of a sociology
of medical technology, using the HGP as a case study. This chapter considers the
question of how the knowledge and possibilities that such a project provides might
shape the kind of society in which we live. Analysing the sociological and related
social policy implications of the project involves considering the tension between the
individual and collective uses to which emerging genetic biotechnologies are put.

The HGP is an international research program in molecular biology (based in
the USA) to identify and map the 30,000–35,000 genes on the 23 different human
chromosomes, and sequence the approximately three billion nucleotide bases from
which these genes are composed. The project was initially funded through the
United States Department of Energy; some US$3 billion is involved, making it the
largest scientific project since the Moon landing. The HGP has been a joint effort
between the US National Institutes of Health, the US Department of Energy, the
Wellcome Trust in the UK, US venture-capitalist **biotechnology** company Celera,
and universities around the world (including ones in Australia). Beginning in
1988, rapid progress was made with a first draft announced with much fanfare at
the White House in late June 2000, before its completion in 2003. Since 2003,
the focus has turned to applying the discoveries and knowledge gained not only
to human genetic disease generally but also to a search for monetary profits from
patenting those discoveries. Although some of the genetic discoveries predated the
formal establishment of the project, two directions of research have arisen out of this
basic mapping expedition. The first direction is what could broadly be called 'disease
genetics'. This is the search for specific gene mutations thought to cause particular
ill health conditions: on the one hand, single gene disorders such as Huntington's
disease, and on the other, a predisposition to common diseases such as, for example,
certain types of breast and ovarian cancer. The second and much more controversial

biotechnology
The use of molecular
biology and genetic
engineering to modify
plants and animals,
including humans, at the
molecular level.

Evan Willis

direction has been in the area of 'behavioural genetics'. This has involved a search for genes that are thought to be likely to affect behaviours that some define as socially undesirable and therefore potentially amenable to 'alteration' such as depression, alcoholism, homosexuality, obesity, and the 'holy grail': intelligence.

All the social sciences are concerned with studying the relationship between the individual and society, but arguably it is to sociology that this relationship is most central. The relationship between the individual and the group is often in tension. How can maximum individual liberty be reconciled with the need for people to get along together in the interests of social harmony? The HGP has resulted in rapid discoveries in the genetic basis of disease; however, understanding of the social (including the legal, ethical, and political) impact of these findings lags far behind. By way of analogy, if we think of the project as a 400-metre race, the molecular biology aspect—that is, the basic sequencing of the human genome—having streaked away, has already finished. Working out what is the basic map and using it to reduce the burden of illness and disease that is part of the human condition, by developing medical (bio)technologies based on that understanding, however, is only part-way down the back straight. The understanding of the social implications, including the legal and ethical ramifications, has only just left the starting blocks. This is despite the fact that 5 per cent of the project's funds have been committed to what has become known as the ELSI (ethical, legal, and social implications) part of the project. Central to these more social implications is the tension between the individual and collective uses of the biotechnologies that are resulting from the project. One illustration of this tension is the example reported at a recent genetics conference. An airline pilot has consistently refused to be tested for Huntington's disease, even though, on the basis of family genetic history, he has a fifty-fifty chance of having inherited the genetic mutation, and irrational psychotic behaviour is a known symptom of the disease. The question here is how a balance can be found between individual and collective uses of the biotechnologies.

There are both sociological and social policy aspects to be investigated here. The study of sociology, as Anthony Giddens (1986) has argued, is the search for alternative futures—the study not only of what is, but of what might be. So a concern with social policy, or 'what is to be done', is an important part of the sociological enterprise. In other words, we are interested in social phenomena not only for their own sake, but also for their social policy implications. The social policy question that arises out of the sociological analysis is 'how can the benefits be maximised and the drawbacks be minimised?' For instance, do we need social policies to ensure that the benefits of the HGP will be available to all (not just the wealthy) within first-world countries let alone in the rest of the world?

In the case of the HGP, it should be noted from the outset (lest this chapter be considered hostile to the attempts to reduce the individual and community toll of genetically caused illness) that benefits will flow from the project to lessen the human burden of suffering (morbidity) and death (mortality) that result from genetically caused illness. In some cases, the benefits are relatively clear: for instance where there is the possibility of intervention to delay the development of clinical disease, as with polycystic kidney disease. With other cases, such as myotonic dystrophy, intervention can avoid life-threatening complications. Or in other cases—such as familial colonic polyposis, a syndrome that runs in families—surgery can be curative. Where screening for the presence of genetically caused conditions can be done prenatally (of the foetus *in utero*), then the possibility exists (at least for those whose values and beliefs support abortion) to terminate the pregnancy. It can be seen then that there are some benefits for individuals that should be maximised. Still, it is evident already that there are drawbacks to be minimised, which are more the subject of this chapter.

After a slow start, a specifically sociological literature analysing the HGP and the 'new genetics' has begun to appear, some of it Australian. Most of the effort has been in a few areas: an overview of the main issues for social scientists (e.g. Davison et al. 1992; Conrad 1997; Rothman 1998; Conrad & Gabe 1999); an analysis of how the project has been reported in the media (e.g. Henderson & Kitzinger 1999; Petersen 2001, 2002; Smart 2003); and the implications for other areas of health care such as public health (Petersen 1998; Willis 1998). There is also the beginning of a literature on the sociological issues surrounding particular genetic illness be it Huntington's disease (Cox & McKellin 1999; Taylor 2004) or breast cancer (Hallowell 1999; Hallowell et al. 2003). There are also some book-length treatises that effectively explore sociological issues in much more depth (Petersen & Bunton 2002; Pilnick 2002), and a specialist journal, *Genetics and Society*, devoted to the social aspects. In more recent times as **biobanks** have emerged, a sociological literature has begun to emerge (e.g. Corrigan & Tutton 2004; Gottweis & Petersen 2008). Finally, the **social control** uses, to which DNA testing is being put, has begun to be investigated, for example, by Lyn Turney (2004; see also Gilding & Turney 2006), on the complex social issues surrounding paternity testing. The sociological analysis in this chapter follows the general framework established for this book—a framework that takes account of the four sensibilities: historical, cultural, structural, and critical. How does an understanding of each of these elements improve our understanding of the opportunities and dangers of a project as important as the HGP? And how does its analysis reveal what a sociological explanation has to offer?

There is one other important proviso. The relationship between technology and society—which this chapter deals with in the context of biotechnologies resulting from the HGP—is what is called a dialectical relationship; that is to say, each influences the other. Most studies of new technologies focus upon their impact on society—how the introduction of a particular technology (say, mobile phones) has an impact on the society into which it is introduced. But that is only half the question. As important to the sociology of technology is the study of the impact of society

biobank
The organised collection of biological samples including DNA. It can range in scope from small collections of samples in academic or hospital settings to large-scale national repositories.

social control
Mechanisms that aim to induce conformity, or at least to manage or minimise deviant behaviour.

Evan Willis

on the technology—that is, how a particular society shapes the technology that it develops and uses (known as the social shaping of technology). As a discussion of the sociology of medical technology, this chapter presents both aspects: the technology's social impact, and how society shapes the technology.

History lessons: genetics and eugenics

As far as the use of genetic information is concerned, what are the 'lessons from history'? An adequate answer to this question would require a much lengthier treatise than is possible here, but a few points can be made. The first concerns **eugenics**. There has been a systematic attempt to avoid the use of this highly controversial term in discourses surrounding the HGP but the shadow of eugenics hangs over the project. Although the Nazis are most often and most obviously associated with the abuses of genetic knowledge, the history of misuse predates them by half a century. The term 'eugenics' (meaning 'well born') was coined by Englishman Francis Galton in 1883 as 'a brief word to express the science of improving the stock' (Galton 1883, p. 24). Eugenics can be understood as an **ideology** in the sense that it is a set of ideas that justifies a course of action. Historically, two types of eugenics-based social engineering programs have been advocated: positive eugenics (to encourage the 'fit' to have more children) and negative eugenics (to exclude the 'unfit' and, through the use of sterilisation, to prevent them from having children). Eugenics has been embraced by 'progressives' from across the political spectrum as holding the promise of human betterment. The Nazis' process of selection and eradication—first of people labelled as having mental and physical disabilities, and then later of other 'inferior types', such as Jews, homosexuals, and 'gypsies'—drew directly on eugenic programs that had been developed in the United Kingdom and the USA (see Caplan 1992). This was especially the case with the United States' *Immigration Restriction Act* of 1924, which was designed to limit immigration into the country of 'defectives' from Southern and Eastern Europe. These ethnic groups were felt to have a much higher proportion of 'mental defectives' than **immigrants** from the United Kingdom and Northern Europe.

After the Second World War, interest in eugenics declined, partially in revulsion from the Nazi practices and partially because advances in genetics changed the understanding of dominant and recessive conditions (Hubbard & Wald 1997). But eugenicist ideology remains, though the word itself is consciously shunned because of its history. Positive eugenicist policies have been in force for some time in the state of Singapore, for instance, where well-educated couples are encouraged to have more children (see Duster 1990). A current example of negative eugenics comes from the People's Republic of China, where Article 38 came into operation on 1 January 1995. It bans the marriage of anyone diagnosed with a serious genetic disease who

---

eugenics
The study of human heredity based on the unproven assumption that selective breeding could improve the intellectual, physical, and cultural traits of a population.

ideology
In a political context, ideology refers to those beliefs and values that relate to the way in which society should be organised, including the appropriate role of the state.

immigrants
A term for those in the population who were born in another country, which is sometimes extended to the descendants of immigrants through the terms 'second-generation' and 'third-generation' immigrants. However, this usage confuses the term and obscures the key fact that those born overseas have a set of immigrant experiences that their descendants do not have.

is considered medically inappropriate for bearing children, unless the couple agrees to be sterilised or undertake permanent contraception. The aim is to prevent the transmission of genetic illnesses from one generation to the next. The classic problem is always how to define what is 'inappropriate'.

This has been the stumbling block for eugenics in the past. There have been two problems: the knowledge basis required to achieve the desired ends, and the value judgments about how to define good and bad genes. What are the positive genes and what are the negative? Arguably what the HGP does is provide a much better knowledge base on which to make decisions, but the issue of what is considered 'defective' remains as problematic as it has ever been (see Duster 1990).

So, although, as Ruth Hubbard and Elijah Wald argue, the earlier forms of eugenics have died out; the root concepts remain, especially:

> the idea that it is more beneficial for certain people to have children than others, and that a vast range of human problems can be cured once we learn how to manipulate our genes ... Testing prospective parents to see if they are carriers of genetic 'defects' leads to the labelling of large groups of people as 'defective' ... Such tests are usually considered to be altogether helpful because they increase people's choices, but it would be a mistake to ignore the ideology that almost inevitably accompanies their use ... Any suggestion that society would be better off if certain kinds of people were not born puts us on a slippery slope. (1997, pp. 24–5)

The second 'lesson of history' relates to the first: that political conservatives have often used biology to explain the social order, including structured forms of social inequality, and thus legitimate their own privileged position in that same social order. A historical example is the disease Pellagra, which reached epidemic proportions in the American South in the early part of this century. Pellagra is a chronic condition involving skin lesions, nervous and muscular disturbances, and eventual mental deterioration, and eugenicists assumed that its causation was hereditary and therefore irremediable by social programs. In 1919, an epidemiologist discovered the condition to be the result of a dietary deficiency of niacin, a member of the vitamin B complex group, which is commonly found in vegetables and grains that were missing from the diet of many sufferers (see Hubbard & Wald 1997, p. 17). Yet consecutive United States' administrations, under the Republicans, resisted the funding of nutrition programs until in 1933 the Democrats introduced the New Deal.

The third lesson is that the unintended consequences of using genetic information cannot be predicted easily in advance. Sickle cell anaemia is a genetic condition that disproportionately affects people of African descent. In the 1970s it was supposed (wrongly as it turned out) that altitude posed a hazard to people who were susceptible to sickle cell anaemia (they were thought less able to withstand the stress of low oxygen at high altitude). This was used as grounds for excluding, for

Evan Willis

instance, African Americans from employment in the US Air Force (see Hubbard & Wald 1997).

The final lesson to be learnt here is that, once developed, a technology can be put to uses not at first envisaged. An example is the development of amniocentesis to predict birth defects in the foetus. This technology could also be used to determine sex, and then could become widely used to practise selected female abortion in cultures (including affluent countries) that traditionally favour male children. Likewise, the genetically engineered human growth hormone (HGH) was first developed to treat pituitary dwarfism (see Hubbard & Wald 1997, pp. 69–70). The number of people who suffer from this condition, and hence the market for the product, is relatively small. In an attempt to improve the market for the product, HGH has been marketed to (wealthy) parents of children who are at the short end of the normal height range but who understand the social advantages of height, especially for men. There is also a black market in body-building circles, where HGH is the latest performance-enhancing substance, replacing anabolic steroids. Because it is naturally occurring, this latest form of cheating could not be detected by any drug test until the eve of the Athens Olympics and so has been attractive to some sportspeople (see Reuters 2004). Another looming consequence is the controversial suggestion that HGH might slow some of the ageing processes (Wilkie 1994).

In the same way, advances in prenatal genetic diagnosis is enabling parents to make decisions in the genetic supermarket, not only about how 'perfect' the child has to be ('Shall we abort this foetus, which has been shown to carry the gene for baldness?'), but also about what sort of child they want to bear (blonde haired? blue eyed?). An example is a couple, in which both people were dwarfs, who chose to abort a foetus because it was expected to be within the normal height distribution (Fisher 1996). The apparent discovery of a gene for obesity (the so-called 'fat gene') and the likelihood of the development of a gene therapy to treat the condition may well have similar consequences. For those in the population who are medically defined as 'obese', the discovery may well have benefits for health and longevity (so long as they can afford the technology), but it is likely also to be used by some who are within the normal weight range who attempt, through self-starvation, to be extremely slender for social reasons.

Gene culture

A cultural sensibility is the second feature of a sociological analysis. It enables a consideration of the social context into which technologies are introduced and through which they are shaped. These technologies are linked to the cultural pre-occupations of those societies. This is seen most clearly in the USA, where the gene has become a cultural icon that:

intersects with important American cultural values. Genetic explanations appear to locate social problems within the individual rather than in society, conforming to the ideology of individualism. They are thus a convenient way to address troubling social issues; the threats implied by the changing roles of women, the perceived decline of the family, the problems of crime, the changes in the racial and ethnic structure of American society and the failure of welfare programs. (Nelkin & Lindee 1995, p. 194)

In the USA, the claim has even been made in the behavioural genetics field that the HGP will provide a 'cure' for much homelessness—a problem in many parts of that country as welfare policy to provide public housing has been wound back. According to Daniel Koshland (1989), one of the staunch advocates of the HGP and editor of the journal *Science*, since many homeless people suffer from mental disorders, which the HGP will show have a genetic basis, then the knowledge gained from the project will lead to a cure or treatment for homelessness (see Beckwith 1991).

In a similar vein, it is asserted that the main potential benefit of screening tests is that they permit the avoidance of transmitting the 'problematic' gene to future generations. The technology used to achieve this benefit is termination of pregnancy following prenatal diagnosis. The politics of abortion in different countries, especially the USA, will affect the social acceptability of benefiting from prenatal diagnosis. Certainly, the social and political process makes for interesting conflict, involving both 'pro-choice' feminist groups and the 'pro-life', anti-abortion lobby. The implications of advances in the genetic understanding of diseases, and therefore of the HGP itself, are inextricably linked with the issue of abortion (Schwartz-Cowan 1992).

Another cultural issue relates to how particular genetic diseases are more commonly associated with particular ethnic groups. Cystic fibrosis is most common among people of Caucasian descent, thalassaemia among those of Mediterranean and South-East Asian descent, Tay-Sachs disease among the Jewish population, and sickle cell anaemia among those of African descent. This raises the possibility of culturally specific solutions to these problems. One such community solution—to combat Tay-Sachs disease in the Jewish communities in New York and Israel—is a mate-selection service called Chevra Dor Yeshorim (the Association of an Upright Generation). Tay-Sachs disease is a particularly unpleasant genetically transmitted disease that causes children to die at an early age. The service operates as a premarital genetic screening agency. When a person begins to date someone from within the community, that person is able to dial up this agency, provide a six-digit code, which will identify the other person, and be told if that other person has genes not only for Tay-Sachs but also for other genetically caused illnesses such as cystic fibrosis and Gaucher's disease. It functions as a sort of genetic roadworthy test and apparently enjoys a high degree of community support as an effective means of avoiding the transmission of major genetic defects. Would such agencies be likely to occur on a wider scale in society as a whole? Is it considered culturally appropriate only because it occurs in a community in which arranged marriage is not unknown? Certainly it raises the possibility of creating 'genetic wallflowers', whom nobody may want to marry because of their genes.

Structural influences on the 'new genetics'

A structural sensibility involves considering the aspects of social organisation that influence both the social impact and the social shaping of emerging biotechnologies. How do different societal contexts affect the ways in which technologies are introduced and used? These biotechnologies result from the differing characteristics of the various societies into which they are introduced. A couple of examples will illustrate this point. In the USA, the lack of a universal health insurance scheme funded through taxation (as exists in most other developed countries) means that there is a greater likelihood that developments in molecular biology will result in abuses of genetic knowledge. Medicare in Australia, as with the National Health Service in the United Kingdom, will shield 'genetically impaired' people from many of the adverse consequences faced by those in the USA who rely on their employment for health insurance. Hence the likelihood of discrimination on the basis of an individual's genetic make-up is a greater fear for Americans than it is for Australians.

A second example involves different attitudes to the patenting of discoveries, which have been a source of conflict between the different countries involved in the HGP (see Cook-Deegan 1994). It has traditionally been thought that scientific activity necessarily involves cooperation between scientists in order to maximise progress. The patenting of individual genes to allow biotechnology companies, funded through venture capital, to 'cash in' on these discoveries has been considered more acceptable within the politico-economic context of the USA than elsewhere. The latter stages of the project indeed became a race to complete the genome sequencing process, characterised by considerable public squabbling. On one side, private venture capitalist firms, notably Celera Genomics, hope to become the Microsoft of the biotechnology industry by selling its information. On the other side, government agencies aim as much as possible to keep the knowledge in the public domain. In other cultural contexts, the response has been different. The European Community has decided not to allow contractors in the HGP to exploit on an exclusive basis any property rights arising from discoveries (Commission of the European Communities 1989, cited in Kevles & Hood 1992, p. 314). It has been suggested that United States investment in the HGP has been directed at giving the USA a competitive edge in the burgeoning biotechnology marketplace (see Rose 1994). Thus, throughout the HGP something of a contradiction has existed between, on the one hand, international cooperation, which has traditionally been one of the norms of scientific activity and, on the other, national interest, in the form of enhancing competitiveness through private control. The challenge is to maintain international competitiveness in the face of high commercial stakes (Kevles & Hood 1992).

The politico-economic context is important in understanding the HGP. The project was conceived under the Reagan administration, during which the causes of disease were held to be based in an individual's genes rather than the wider social context. This is **genetic reductionism**, a form of biological reductionism. According to this view, individuals are the sum of their genes and represent the latest version of the 'biology is destiny' scheme—a sort of 'genes-R-us' approach that represents a new twist to **social Darwinism** and sociobiology. In the past, the search was for 'germs'. The Rockefeller Foundation, for instance, funded research into germs for laziness in the 1930s in the American South (see Brown 1979). Now it is genes. The move from germs to genes focuses attention away from the social environment. As Hilary Rose (1994, p. 173) argues, '[t]his new genetics, a product of an alliance between an aggressively entrepreneurial culture and life sciences, fused the conservatism of biology as destiny with the modernist philosophy of genetic manipulation'. The HGP is a **modernist** project in the sense that it is based on a belief that the problems faced by humanity can be solved by rational applications of science and technology.

Critique: geneism and social control

A critical sensibility involves asking 'how could it be otherwise?' It involves paying attention to the social policy implications of these technological developments. There are a number of biotechnologies that have been mooted as arising out of the HGP. Gene therapies, long anticipated as a technological innovation, are still largely at the potential, 'cautious optimism' stage of development and according to the HGP information website run by the US Department of Energy, have not proven very successful in clinical trials. Little progress has been made since the first gene therapy clinical trial began in 1990. A Norwegian report found that despite several thousand articles published on gene therapy, and between 3000 and 4000 people treated with different gene therapy strategies in more than 400 clinical studies—with the exception of a treatment for eye infections in AIDS patients—gene therapy was not yet an established treatment modality for any disease (Kolberg 2000). Furthermore, in the USA, the Food and Drug Administration (FDA) has, in 2007, not yet approved any human gene therapy product for sale. Indeed, in 1999 the FDA placed a temporary halt on all gene therapy trials in relation to liver disease, one of the main areas being investigated, after the death of a patient receiving gene therapy.

The most widespread technology resulting from the project is genetic screening tests. These are the main commercial products being developed by biotechnology companies on the basis of their patented discoveries. A screening test can tell if the individual has the 'defective gene' and is therefore at a higher than normal risk of

genetic reductionism
An assumption that people are simply the sum of their individual genes, so that the causes of disease are reduced to an individual's genes rather than the social, economic, and political context in which people live.

social Darwinism
The incorrect application of Charles Darwin's theory of animal evolution to explain social inequality by transferring his idea of 'survival of the fittest' among animals to 'explain' human inequality.

modernity/ modernism
A view of social life that is founded upon rational thought and a belief that truth and morality exist as objective realities that can be discovered and understood through scientific means.

developing an ill-health condition. In social policy terms, the crucial question is: under what circumstances is the knowledge gained on the basis of screening likely to be oppressive or liberating for the individual? The relationship between 'oppressive' and 'liberating' should be thought of as a continuum rather than a dichotomy; there are likely to be degrees of each. Whether a person would want to know if they carried the genes for a particular condition would vary from individual to individual. The social policy aim is to maximise benefits and minimise drawbacks. There are likely to be elements of both; there are some conditions that appear to have a heritable basis, for which the benefits of screening are relatively clear. Phenylketonuria (PKU) is an example, for which mandatory screening (using 'the heel-prick test') has operated effectively with community support in many countries. For those with this condition, a course of action is available that benefits the individual. However, with other supposedly genetically caused phenomena, the benefits are questionable. An example is the so-called (hypothetical) gene for homosexuality (see Hubbard & Wald 1997). If homosexuality is genetically determined, then it must be 'natural' (people are 'born that way') so any form of discrimination on the basis of sexual preference would be clearly inappropriate. In that sense its discovery would be liberating. But there are also drawbacks. If homosexuality should turn out to be genetically determined (rather than some combination of genetic and environmental influences, as most researchers believe), then the likelihood of having a homosexual child can also be screened for. It is likely that a significant number of parents would choose to abort such a foetus and try again. This outcome would hardly be liberating for the gay community or for the foetus itself. James Watson, the first director of the HGP, stirred controversy when he was reported as advocating the right of parents to abort the foetus if found to be carrying a hypothetical gene for homosexuality (*Age*, 6 July 2003).

A more basic and immediate problem is that, with many conditions (for which the gene has been located), nothing can be done for the person. Huntington's disease is an example of this: onset of the disease occurs in the mature adult, and people die unpleasantly over a long period of time. In this case, a legitimate question is: why would people want to know? Is knowing that you are likely to develop Huntington's disease in your forties or fifties likely to be liberating or oppressive (see Cox & McKellin 1999; Taylor 2004)?

There appear to be two types of relationship between the presence of genes and the health outcomes that those genes suggest. One is direct, as occurs with the heritable cancers. The presence of the gene brings a considerably enhanced probability of the onset of cancer. The second is more indirect, with the presence of the gene implying only a predisposition to certain diseases—in effect, a recognition of the complex interaction between genotypes and environmental factors.

Similar issues exist, of course, with all screening. It needs to be asked: if screening is the answer, what is the question? For what purpose is screening being done? There is a classic tension in sociological terms between the individual and society. How can the individual ends be reconciled with the collective ends? The collective ends are public health ends, and this tension is, of course, the basis of the controversy surrounding eugenics. What level of coercion of individuals is acceptable in the interests of public health? This has been an issue in terms of managing public health over a very long period of time. Some degree of compulsion is accepted, as in the case of wearing a car seatbelt or bicycle helmet. But what is already occurring is that screening is increasingly being used for the purposes of social control, such as in the surveillance of populations in China as mentioned earlier. Often nothing can be done for the individual concerned, but there are lots of benefits to others in knowing an individual's genetic make-up. Screening may have liberating consequences in the future, but it is already having oppressive consequences. It opens the way for the individual to be discriminated against in various ways. **Geneism** is starting to take its place alongside other forms of discrimination, such as racism, sexism, and ageism. What they have in common is the allocation of social rewards on the basis of ascribed rather than achieved status; on the basis of what an individual is born like rather than what that person achieves in life. This goes against the whole thrust of social policy in recent decades, especially **social justice** policies, according to which social rewards should be allocated on the basis of achievement.

Geneism has become apparent, especially in the USA, as information about people's genes is increasingly being used for the purposes of social control. It is used to deny access to certain socially desired ends, such as life insurance and health insurance, employment, and even a driver's licence (see Billings et al. 1992). In Australia, there has been some evidence of this form of discrimination emerging. David Keays (2000), a law researcher at the University of Melbourne, has uncovered such several cases, including:

- an 18-year-old school-leaver denied a public service job unless he passed a genetic test for Huntington's disease, a severe condition that hits in middle age. He had a fifty-fifty chance of having the gene but, having seen his mother suffer, preferred not to know. At times he threatened to kill himself if he ever found out. On a second appeal, he was offered the job, with reduced superannuation.
- a 37-year-old quality manager refused an increase in a pre-existing income insurance policy after a research project genetic test revealed he had Charcot-Marie-Tooth disease, a physical condition that, even if it progressed from its mild state, would not affect his ability to earn income in his desk-bound work (see also Button 2000).

Thus, geneism can be considered a current phenomenon, not simply something that may occur in the future. Furthermore, in countries such as Australia, it will probably not be very long before immigration authorities propose genetic screening to exclude potential immigrants as a means of avoiding future impost on the country's health system, in the same way that HIV testing has been mandatory for potential immigrants for some time.

geneism
A form of discrimination—such as racism, sexism, and ageism—in which people are judged on their ascribed, rather than achieved, status. In this case, their genetic make-up is used as the basis for determining access to social rewards such as employment or health insurance.

social justice
A belief system that gives high priority to the interests of the least advantaged.

Evan Willis

Moreover, there appears to be a clear political program attached to the HGP, which helps to explain how it is funded, given the blanket influence of neo-conservative economics around the globe and the hegemony of post-Cold War American values. This context is important in relation to the project's role in providing a rationale and a justification for inequality. The emphasis is upon a genetic form of **biological determinism**: people are the way they are because of their genes rather than the sort of society in which they live. Therefore, government programs are not likely to have any impact, as inequality is determined by nature, not by culture. As is occurring in the USA, social justice and welfare programs can 'legitimately' be abolished, and tax cuts can be made that will disproportionately benefit the rich. Social policy considerations of equity issues feature largely here, especially equity of resource allocation. In the USA, these changes are occurring at a time when, in the absence of a universal health insurance scheme, 40 million American citizens have no health insurance at all and major illness can expose these people to financial ruin. The issue is even more apparent on a world scale where many more people die of simple preventable diseases, such as malnutrition and infectious diseases, than of genetic diseases. Individual treatments based on genetic therapies will probably never be affordable by the majority of the world's population. Furthermore, the deterioration in the world environment as a result of climate change is likely to take a greater toll on human health than genetic disease ever will. Access to basic nutrition and basic medical care is likely to remain a greater priority for most people, with the promised benefits of the new genetic medicine remaining out of reach for all but an affluent few in the richest countries (see Beardsley 1996).

biological determinism
An unproven belief that individual and group behaviour and social status are an inevitable result of biology.

BOX 16.1   Doing health sociology: DNA analysis—individual and social impacts

Sociology is the study of the relationship between the individual and society and an important aspect of sociological analysis is the search for alternative futures. The developments in the understanding of the genetic basis of some diseases raise many social and social policy issues—at both the individual and societal level. How do we balance the hoped-for advances in reducing the individual burden of genetically caused disease with the broader social issues at a societal level? If DNA analysis gives powerful information about identity, what balance should we strike between individual and collective uses of that powerful knowledge? At a societal level how do we prevent it being used so that the possibilities of individual achievements are not ascribed on the basis of their genetic makeup but instead are based on whatever achievements those individuals can make? These are important social policy issues to which sociological analysis can contribute.

Conclusion: future directions

The ramifications of the HGP on the sort of society in which we live are likely to be considerable. Understanding these implications from a sociological point of view involves considering the four core sensibilities of sociological explanation: historical, cultural, structural, and critical. These sensibilities illuminate the sociological issues, as well as the related social policy question of how the benefits can be maximised and the drawbacks minimised. How can the tensions between individual and collective uses of the technologies arising from the new genetics be reconciled? If there are to be benefits flowing from widespread genetic testing, then, arguably, considerably more attention will need to be given to the social implications and consequences of this testing for those benefits to be realised.

But there is one other benefit flowing from a sociological awareness of these issues, and it acts as something of an antidote to the daily hype surrounding developments in biotechnology. A sociological perspective with the inherent reflexivity or scepticism, which is a key feature of a sociological imagination, demands that the 'technophoria' with which many developments are reported, be taken with a metaphorical grain (even lump) of salt. It enables, even requires, questions to be asked, such as:

- Who benefits from these developments?
- Is the knowledge generated likely to be oppressive or liberating for the individuals concerned?
- What are the likely societal implications arising out of these developments?
- Are there likely to be drawbacks associated with this knowledge, and if so, what can be done about them?

Articulating questions of this type is what sociology, in its search for alternative futures, seeks to do.

Summary of main points

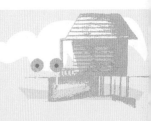

» Rapid developments have occurred in the understanding of the genetic basis to ill health. Understanding the social impact of these findings, though, lags far behind.

» There is an emerging tension between individual and collective uses of the bio-technologies being developed.

» Considering the social impact of new medical technologies is only part of the sociological task; the other part concerns understanding the social shaping of those technologies.

Evan Willis

» In social policy terms, the focus is upon how to maximise any benefits that may flow from these biotechnologies, as well as how to minimise any drawbacks.

» Consideration of the historical, cultural, structural, and critical elements that together comprise a sociological perspective provides something of a balance to the 'technophoria' surrounding many of these developments.

Sociological reflection 1: the genetic sum of us

Imagine that in the near future genetic screening of humans allows the possibility to identify genes that are believed to contribute to various 'behavioural conditions' such as alcoholism, obesity, and homosexuality. If you were given the power to remove such genes from humans through terminating pregnancies or through permanent sterilisation of adults who carry the 'suspect' genes, would you use that power in the case of alcoholism, obesity, and homosexuality?

» Do your answers differ according to the situation? Why?

» Why do sociologists consider behavioural genetics to be highly suspect?

» What would be the likely social implications if such genetic choices were widely available? Who should be responsible for regulating it (private enterprise, the state, individuals)? Why?

Sociological reflection 2: ensuring benefits for humanity

Will humankind as a whole benefit from the advances in the understanding of the genetic basis of disease? Or will some benefit more than others? If an important part of the sociological imagination is the search for alternative futures, how can this new genetic knowledge be applied so that it is not mainly used in the vehicle for private profit making by biotechnology companies for the primary benefit of a wealthy few patients? By what means can any benefits that flow for individuals be made available on a global sense?

Discussion questions

1 What is the difference between the social-shaping and the social-impact aspects of the relationship between (medical) technology and society?

2 In what ways are advances in genetic medicine linked to issues about abortion?

3   What is geneism? How can we as a society prevent genetic testing being used as the basis for discrimination?

4   What are the social implications of theories alleging the genetic basis of human behaviour?

5   What are the social policy considerations that are important to understanding the HGP?

6   In your view, how can any tension between individual and collective uses of genetic biotechnologies be reconciled?

Further investigation

1   What can sociology offer to an understanding of the likely implications of the Human Genome Project for society?

2   'Analysing the relationship between technology and society requires a consideration not only of the impact of new technologies on society, but also of how the technology is shaped by society.' Discuss in relation to the Human Genome Project.

Further reading

Hubbard, R. & Wald, E. 1997, *Exploding the Gene Myth*, revised edn, Beacon Press, Boston.

Nelkin, D. & Lindee, S. 1995, *The DNA Mystique: The Gene as a Cultural Icon*, Freeman & Co., New York.

Petersen, A. & Bunton, R. (eds) 2002, *The New Genetics and the Public's Health*, Routledge, London.

Pilnick, A. 2002, *Genetics and Society: An Introduction*, Open University Press, Buckingham.

Web resources

Centre for Law and Genetics: <www.lawgenecentre.org>

Council for Responsible Genetics: <www.gene-watch.org>

Genome Programs of the US Department of Energy Office of Science: <http://genomics. energy.gov/>

National Human Genome Research Institute: <www.genome.gov>

Online case study • • •
Visit the Second Opinion website to access relevant case studies.

Evan Willis

Documentaries/films

Gattaca (1997): 102 minutes, Columbia Pictures. Written and directed by Andrew Niccol. Borrow the film from the local video store. View it as a means of thinking about the social and ethical issues associated with the new genetics, especially pre-implantation genetic diagnosis from 'the genetic supermarket'. The film's rather negative and sensationalist view has been analysed in an essay by Colin Gavaghan entitled 'Off-the-peg Offspring in the Genetic Supermarket', which can be found at: <http://www.philosophynow.org/archive/articles/22gavaghan.htm>

The Story of A Previvor—a documentary from the *New York Times'* Website at: <http://video.on.nytimes.com/?fr_story=0aff7eb1147f98a41e989541f3fc114c8e71dcd2>

The advent of the genomic era throws up new issues that we, as a society, have to contemplate. In this four-part video, a young woman with a family history of breast cancer but no diagnosis decides she will have a double prophylactic mastectomy (that is to have both her healthy breasts surgically removed as a strategy to prevent her getting breast cancer at some later date); hence the use of the term 'previvor'.

Warning: if you have a history of cancer in your family you may find this video confronting and choose not to watch it. If you do watch it and it raises issues for you that you would like to discuss further, the Cancer Council Helpline can be accessed on: <http://www.cancer.org.au/cancersmartlifestyle/cancercouncilhelpline.htm>

References

The Age, 2003, 'Abortion Justified for "Better Babies"', 6 July 2003. Available online: <http://www.theage.com.au/articles/2003/07/05/1057179206284.html>

Beardsley, T. 1996, 'Trends in Human Genetics', *Scientific American*, March, pp. 25–7.

Beckwith, J. 1991, 'Foreword: The Human Genome Initiative: Genetics', *Lightning Rod American Journal of Law and Medicine*, vol. 17, nos 1–2, pp. 1–13.

Billings, P., Kohn, M., de Cuevas, M., Beckwith, J., Alper, J. & Natowicz, M. 1992, 'Discrimination as a Consequence of Genetic Testing', *American Journal of Human Genetics*, vol. 50, pp. 476–82.

Brown, E. R. 1979, *Rockefeller Medicine Men*, University of California Press, Berkeley, CA.

Button, V. 2000, 'Genetic Testing: Call for Reform', *Age*, 21 July.

Caplan, A. 1992, *When Medicine Went Mad: Bioethics and the Holocaust*, Humana, NJ.

Conrad, P. 1997, 'Public Eyes and Private Genes: Historical Frames, News Constructions and Social Problems', *Social Problems*, vol. 44, no. 2, pp. 139–54.

Conrad, P. & Gabe, J. 1999, 'Introduction: Sociological Perspectives on the New Genetics: An Overview', *Sociology of Health and Illness*, vol. 21, no. 5, pp. 505–16.

Cook-Deegan, R. 1994, *The Gene Wars: Science, Politics and the Human Genome*, Norton, New York.

Corrigan, O. & Tutton, R. 2004, *Genetic Databases: Socio-ethical Issues in the Collection and Use of DNA*, Routledge, London.

Cox, S. & McKellin, S. 1999, 'There's This Thing in Our Family: Predictive Testing and the Construction of Risk for Huntington Disease', *Sociology of Health and Illness*, vol. 21, no. 5, pp. 622–46.

Davison, C., Finkel, S. & Davey Smith, G. D. 1992, '"To Hell with Tomorrow": Coronary Heart Disease Risk and the Ethnography of Fatalism', in S. Scott, G. Williams, S. Platt & H. Thomas (eds), *Private Risks and Public Dangers*, Aldershot, Avebury, pp. 95–111.

Duster, T. 1990, *Backdoor to Eugenics*, Routledge, New York.

Fisher, A. 1996, 'The Brave New World of Genetic Screening: Ethical Issues', in J. Flader (ed.), *Death or Disability?*, University of Tasmania, Hobart, pp. 22–46.

Galton, F. 1883, *Inquiries into Human Faculty*, Macmillan, London.

Giddens, A. 1986, *Sociology: A Brief but Critical Introduction*, 2nd edn, Macmillan, London.

Gilding, M. & Turney, L. 2006, 'Public Opinion on DNA Paternity Testing: The Influence of the Media', *People & Place*, vol. 14, no. 2, pp. 4–13.

Gottweis, H. & Petersen, A. 2008, *Biobanks: Governance in Comparative Perspective*, Routledge, London.

Hallowell, N. 1999, 'Doing the Right Thing: Genetic Risk and Responsibility', *Sociology of Health and Illness*, vol. 21, no. 5, pp. 597–621.

Hallowell, N., Foster, C., Eeles, A., Arden-Jones, M. & Watson, M. 2003, 'Accommodating Risk: Responses to BRCA1/2 Genetic Testing of Women Who Have Had Cancer', *Social Science & Medicine*, vol. 59, pp. 553–66.

Henderson, L. & Kitzinger, J. 1999, 'The Human Drama of Genetics: Hard and Soft Media Representations of Inherited Breast Cancer', *Sociology of Health and Illness*, vol. 21, no. 5, pp. 560–78.

Hubbard, R. & Wald, E. 1997, *Exploding the Gene Myth*, revised edn, Beacon Press, Boston.

Keays, D. 2000, 'Genetic Testing and Insurance: When is Genetic Discrimination Justified?', *Monash Bioethics Review*, vol. 19, no. 4, pp. 79–88.

Kevles, D. & Hood, L. 1992, 'Reflections', in D. Kevles and L. Hood (eds), *The Code of Codes: Scientific and Social Issues in the Human Genome Project*, Harvard University Press, Cambridge, MA, pp. 210–22.

Kolberg, B. 2000, *Gene Therapy: Status and Prospects in Clinical Medicine*, SMM report 1/2000, Norwegian Center for Health Technology Assessment.

Koshland, D. 1989, 'Sequences and Consequences of the Human Genome', *Science*, no. 246, p. 246.

Lorentz, C., Wieben, E., Tefferi, A., Whiteman, D. & Dewald, G. 2002, 'Primer on Medical Genomics: Part I: History of Genetics and Sequencing of the Human Genome', *Mayo Clinical Proceedings*, vol. 77, pp. 773–82. Available online: <http://www.mayoclinicproceedings.com/pdf%2F7708%2F7708mg1.pdf >

Nelkin, D. & Lindee, S. 1995, *The DNA Mystique: The Gene as a Cultural Icon*, Freeman, New York.

Petersen, A. 1998, 'The New Genetics and the Politics of Public Health', *Critical Public Health*, vol. 8, no. 1, pp. 59–71.

Petersen, A. 2001, 'Biofantasies: Genetics and Medicine in the Print News Media', *Social Science & Medicine*, vol. 52, no. 8, pp. 1255–68.

Petersen, A. 2002 'Replicating our Bodies, Losing Our Selves: News Media Portrayals of Human Cloning in the Wake of Dolly', *Body & Society*, vol. 8, no. 4, pp. 71–90.

Petersen, A. & Bunton, R. (eds) 2002, *The New Genetics and the Public's Health*, Routledge, London.

Pilnick, A. 2002, *Genetics and Society: An Introduction*, Open University Press, Buckingham.

Reuters News Agency 2004, 'Olympics Great Success After HGH Testing, WADA Says'.

Rose, H. 1994, *Love, Power and Knowledge: Towards a Feminist Transformation of the Sciences*, Polity Press, Cambridge.

Rothman, B. K. 1998, *Genetic Maps and Human Imaginations*, Norton, New York.

Sanger Institute 2003, 'The Finished Human Genome—Wellcome to the Genomic Age', press release, 14 April 2003. Available online: <http://www.sanger.ac.uk/Info/Press/2003/030414.shtml>

Schwartz-Cowan, R. 1992, 'Genetic Technology and Reproductive Choice', in D. Kevles & L. Hood (eds), *The Code of Codes: Scientific and Social Issues in the Human Genome Project*, Harvard University Press, Cambridge, MA, pp. 244–63.

Smart, A. 2003, 'Reporting the Dawn of the Post-genomic Era: Who Wants to Live Forever?', *Sociology of Health and Illness*, vol. 25, no. 1, pp. 24–49.

Taylor, S. 2004, 'Predictive Genetic Test Decisions for Huntingdon's Disease: Context, Appraisal and New Moral Imperatives', *Social Science & Medicine*, vol. 58, pp. 137–49.

Turney, L. (2004) 'Power, Knowledge and the Discourse of "Paternity Fraud"', *The International Journal of the Humanities*, vol. 2, no. 1, pp. 223–31.

Wilkie, T. 1994, *Perilous Knowledge: The Human Genome Project and Its Implications*, Faber & Faber, London.

Willis, E. 1998, 'Public Health, Private Genes: The Social Context of Genetic Biotechnologies', *Critical Public Health*, vol. 8, no. 2, pp. 131–9.

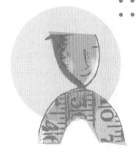

CHAPTER 17

Media and Health:
Moral Panics, Sinners,
and Saviours

JOHN
GERMOV
and
MARIA
FREIJ

Overview

- What role does the mass media play in producing and reproducing our understanding of health and illness?
- How does the mass media influence our perception of health risks and illness experience?
- How influential is the media in shaping public views on health and illness?

MEDIA SENSATION: THE 'EPIDEMIC' OF ERECTILE DYSFUNCTION

We could all be forgiven for thinking there is an epidemic of male erectile dysfunction in the community. On Australian television there are regular adverts promoting the condition and where men can seek help. The most common advert has two tuxedo-clad men standing behind a grand piano, allegedly playing it with their (hidden) erect penises. The adverts have coincided with the availability of prescription drugs such as Viagra and Cialis. In Australia, it is illegal for drug companies to advertise prescription drugs directly to consumers. Much effort and money thus goes into bypassing this restriction through such 'educative' commercials and by influencing journalists to do stories that effectively amount to free publicity. Take for example the following excerpt from *Channel 9 News* (29 April 2008), where newsreader Mark Ferguson and reporter Gabriella Rogers do a story based on a media release by a public relations company working for Eli Lilly, a global pharmaceutical company that makes the erection treatment drug Cialis.

· · · »

Mark Ferguson: There's new hope for thousands of Australian men trying to cope with erectile dysfunction. It works in much the same way as Viagra but adds a welcome dose of spontaneity.

Gabriella Rogers: Many Australian couples struggle with their relationship when all is not right in the bedroom.

Brett McCann: Thirty per cent of men over the age of 40 will have some difficulty with erectile functioning...

Gabriella Rogers: Like Viagra, Cialis promotes erection through increased blood flow but unlike current medications the new tablet is active 24 hours a day. (*Media Watch* 2008a, b)

The news story coincided with the release of Cialis and received widespread coverage on many news and current affairs shows at the time. The story was subsequently followed by regular erectile dysfunction adverts in TV, print, and on billboard media. Some authors have described this process as the corporate construction of disease for profit maximisation (Moynihan et al. 2002).

Introduction: why study media and health?

We are saturated by mass media information on a daily basis and to such an extent that for most people it is the key source of information, understanding, and experience of the world. Therefore, it is crucial to develop a sociological understanding of media content and influence. Health issues feature prominently in news reporting and popular entertainment (see Box 17.1), and thus media representations of health deserve critical attention. As the case of erectile dysfunction discussed above shows, the media can play a major role in how we think about health, illness, and health care. The mass media is the major means through which information and entertainment is transmitted in developed societies. While traditionally defined as being constituted by television, movies, radio, newspapers, and magazines, the rise of information and communication technologies (such as mobile phones and the internet) has led to a convergence of media forms, whereby people can use their mobile phones to watch a movie, read an online newspaper, search the web, update their blog on sites such as Facebook and MySpace, and view or upload content to sites such as YouTube (Marjoribanks 2007). Such a development indicates that the mass media is an increasingly complex and dynamic phenomenon whereby audiences can be interactive and generative of content.

BOX 17.1 Health in the popular media: TV shows

Our inevitable personal preoccupation with health and health care is reflected in the popularity of fictional television shows throughout the decades (listed opposite). While more recent TV shows tend to deal with ethical debates and the frailties of health professionals, the dominant theme remains that of the heroic medical professional who uses high-tech interventions and rare expertise to save lives and alleviate suffering (Bury & Gabe 2006).

» *Australia:* Young Doctors (1976–83), Flying Doctors (1985–91), A Country Practice (1981–94), GP (1989–96), All Saints (1998–)

» *UK:* Casualty (1986–), Peak Practice (1993–2002), Doc Martin (2004–)

» *USA:* Dr Kildare (1961–66), General Hospital (1963–), MASH (1972–83), Marcus Welby M.D. (1969–76), Quincy M.E. (1976–83), St. Elsewhere (1982–88), Dr. Quinn, Medicine Woman (1993–98), Chicago Hope (1994–2000), Crossing Jordan (2001–07), ER (1994–), House M.D. (2004–), Grey's Anatomy (2005–), Scrubs (2001–)

The media conveys explicit and implicit meanings about health, illness, health professionals, and the health system through the language, images, and tones used, and in the way a story is framed, which may influence public understanding. As much sociological analysis has exposed, the popular media can be biased toward particular commercial or political interests, and due to competition and tight deadlines, can present information in a sensationalist, superficial, and misrepresentative way (Lupton 1998). This chapter explores how the media represents matters of health and illness, and how this may affect people's experience of illness and their public expectations of health and health care.

Media templates

Jenny Kitzinger (2000) proposes the notion of 'media templates' as a way of understanding how journalists construct news reports. Templates are based on typical story types, usually drawn from previous stories, and help both the journalist and the audience understand the narrative and the context of the news. Media templates present issues in the form of a pattern, and by doing so tend to marginalise alternative interpretations, as well as oversimplify the issues involved by either distorting or ignoring key details or dissenting accounts. According to Clive Seale (2002, p. 27), media health stories tend to align to a number of templates based on a series of oppositions: 'heroes and villains, pleasure and pain, safety and danger, disaster and repair, life and death, the beautiful and the ugly, the normal and the freak'.

John Germov and Maria Freij

The use of opposition and confrontation is a common feature of media templates to create tension, viewer interest, and 'newsworthiness'. For example, news stories in the 1980s on HIV/AIDS commonly constructed sufferers as 'deserving/guilty' (homosexuals, drug users, and prostitutes) and 'undeserving/innocent' (mothers and babies, people requiring blood transfusions, health professionals contracting the disease via needle-stick accidents). Deborah Lupton (1998a) notes that news stories on HIV/AIDS gradually changed from homophobic notions of the 'gay plague', which had originally been termed by some scientists as GRIDs—gay-related immune deficiency syndrome—towards stories on broader moral concerns about promiscuity compared with the desirability of monogamous marriage. In the case of HIV/AIDS, media templates drew on the themes of **deviance**, **stigma**, and irresponsibility.

The mass media has long been a site for health promotion campaigns, which aim to raise public awareness and promote change in individuals towards health-promoting behaviours or at least limit or avoid health-damaging ones. Such approaches have been criticised for their over-reliance on notions of media consumers as passive, as well as for being ineffective due to the lack of attention to **social determinants of health** (see Chapter 23). Sometimes, such campaigns can have unintended effects, such as the infamous Grim Reaper TV commercial that aired in Australia in 1987. The commercial created a **moral panic** by implying AIDS was plague-like and that all people were susceptible, creating widespread fear in the community and resulting in many people who were not at risk seeking to be unnecessarily tested for HIV status. Nonetheless, the media template used was consistent, with irresponsible sinners cast against innocent victims (Critcher 2003).

Scientism versus Frankenstein science: media representations of genetic research

The cloning of Dolly the sheep sparked fears that humans were next. Concerns that people would 'lose their identity' and that the 'bonds of the family' were at stake were common, as was the risk that scientists were 'going too far' (Petersen 2002, p. 72). Demands for a ban on cloning came from different quarters, including religious ones, as many reports focused on the 'dangers of unregulated cloning research' (Petersen 2002, p. 71). Alan Petersen's studies of media representations of cloning research point out that 'there has been little debate about whether fears about human cloning were justified in light of existing evidence, and what exactly it was that people believed was at stake' (2002, p. 74) but indeed, news media was playing on old fears by alluding to Aldous Huxley's *Brave New World* and Adolf Hitler's genetic experiments, and by asking the question of whether humans were 'playing God'. The perceived threats were phrased as 'against nature', 'threats to human dignity', and 'moral unacceptability', but nowhere were these threats defined and discussed;

---

deviance
Behaviour or activities that violate social expectations about what is normal.

stigma/stigmatisation
A physical or social trait, such as a disability or a criminal record, that results in negative social reactions such as discrimination and exclusion.

social determinants of health
The economic, social, and cultural factors that directly and indirectly influence individual and population health.

moral panic
An exaggerated reaction by the mass media, politicians, and community leaders to the actions and beliefs of certain social groups or individuals, concerns which are often minor and inconsequential, but are sensationally represented to create anxiety and outrage among the general public.

what the 'threat to human dignity' consisted of was not addressed. Several fears were raised in terms of what cloning humans could bring, like 'armies of clones', or a 'Master race'. None of the reports made the distinction between the popular and scientific understandings of cloning; the popular idea that cloning equals making a 'carbon copy' is far from the scientific one (Petersen 2002).

The fearful response to Dolly's arrival 'raises questions about how public perceptions of human cloning are formed and sustained. Where does the lay public derive its information about human cloning from, and what kind of messages and images are communicated?' (Petersen 2002, p. 74). Petersen considers how news reporting may have contributed to shaping public opinion of, and fuelling fears about, cloning by reminding us that the media frames issues 'by reporting some "facts", views and images, and ignoring others' and that in so doing is 'likely to influence public debates in a powerful way' (2002, p. 75). The framing of a story is always selective and will influence what information is being reported and how that information is being reported.

Studies on this model of diffusion of science popularisation 'generally conclude that not enough information was published, and that what was published was not provided in sufficient quantity or detail to have been useful' (Petersen 2001, p. 1256). Simplification, the metaphors and images used, and the language applied decide the way scientists get to popularise their research. Scientists are eager to present a positive image of their work in genetics due to its shared history with **eugenics** and have increasingly used public relations firms to promote this positive message (Petersen 2001).

eugenics
The study of human heredity based on the unproven assumption that selective breeding could improve the intellectual, physical, and cultural traits of a population.

The media, as the interface between scientists and the general public, has a large impact on how research is portrayed and the public's reactions to this information. Lay people's response to news media articles is a complex process also shaped by their pre-existing knowledge and experiences. Genetics are often presented through stories of hope and geneticists as warriors or heroes. The idea that scientists can create life and solve the complicated puzzle of life has long fascinated the public. There is awe and fear alike in the way the public perceives these topics; fascination and optimism can be countered by fears that eugenics will enter the picture. Many remain fearful that genetics will be used for selective reproduction, and the lengths that selective reproduction will go to (Petersen 2001).

Breakthroughs such as Dolly and discoveries arising from the Human Genome Project (see Chapter 16) are popular and highly newsworthy. The media has ways of both personalising and universalising human experience through the telling of 'human interest' stories. Many articles rely heavily on the researchers' own descriptions and positive evaluations and narratives. There is a great lack of independent confirmation of the research and its significance, as journalists often rely on pre-packaged sources or media releases which are invariably influenced by the researchers' interests and sources where the flow of information is controlled by public relations staff. As Petersen notes, '[i]n the face of widespread public fears about human cloning, and efforts to outlaw cloning research in a number of jurisdictions, many scientists began to make extensive use of the media to defend and explain their work' (2001, p. 1265). Distinctions were made between 'good' genetic research and 'bad' genetic research, the latter referring mainly to the cloning of human beings, in order to portray scientists as ethical and responsible.

Many descriptions of genetics in the print news media 'reinforce the perception that our health problems originate inside us and draw attention away from external factors that need to be addressed' (Petersen 2001, p. 1261). The role of the social environment goes largely unmentioned as do multi-factorial notions of disease. Instead, the **reductionist** view that 'once the gene has been found and isolated, there will be a cure' is supported.

reductionism
The belief that all illnesses can be explained and treated by reducing them to biological and pathological factors.

Geneticists often portray themselves, and are often portrayed in the media, as 'saviours' or 'warriors' on a mission to 'solve the mysteries of nature' (Petersen 2001, p. 1261). The researchers are ascribed divine qualities, described as aware of mysteries which only the initiated can fathom. Researchers appear as 'altruistic defenders of the public's health' (Petersen 2001, p. 1264). Genetics research is often portrayed as constantly on the brink of a major breakthrough; drugs and cures will be available in 'a foreseeable future' and support a view that 'technological solutions for even the most intractable medical problems' will eventually be found (Petersen 2001, p. 1264). Such 'medical scientism' (Capra 1982) assumes that only reductionist scientistic approaches can serve to cure humanity of disease.

Amidst positive portrayals of the potential of genetic research, a contrary media template is also used, one that plays on 'fears about scientists, science and its pro-ducts, epitomised in the image of Frankenstein's monster, surfaced in stories about the dangers of unregulated cloning research and "mad scientists" creating new diseases and threatening human diversity' (Petersen 2001, p. 1266). Claiming to be 90 per cent ready to clone a human being, Richard Seed stirred people's greatest fears: that no matter the government regulations, scientists would still clone human beings. The fear that a rogue scientist would play out the fears expressed in Mary Shelley's *Frankenstein* were reignited but died down when Seed dropped off the radar, and further, when Dolly was reported as having aged prematurely. Scientists were not on the brink of cloning human beings after all, and the mass hysteria created in, and by, the media was forgotten (Petersen 2002).

Overweight, obesity, and illness: media representations of responsibility and blame

In a 2004 study, Deborah Lupton examined the reporting of food risks in three metropolitan papers in Sydney. She found that the relationship between food intake and obesity, with a special focus on childhood obesity, was the major topic reported:

47 per cent of the items focused on issues concerning overweight and obesity caused by an unbalanced diet or excessive food consumption. Many of these articles were front-page stories and many were accompanied by large photographs, further adding to the sensationalist qualities of the reporting. In terms of the reporting of overweight and obesity in children, articles 'often used extreme and alarming language' (Lupton 2004, p. 190).

The concept of risk arguably permeates every aspect of our lives as it has become central to late modern thinking. People are becoming increasingly aware of risks and subsequently, of the impacts of these risks on their health and well-being—a trend encapsulated by Ulrich Beck's (1992) concept of a **risk society**. According to Lupton, this heightened awareness is 'nowhere more apparent than in contemporary representations of food and eating' (2005, p. 449).

News media attention to controversies and issues relating to foodstuffs has been significant; reports on genetically modified (GM) foods, bovine spongiform encephalopathy (BSE or 'mad cow' disease), avian bird flu, and bacterial outbreaks are prominent. Food has also become medicalised in its association with health and illness, making it an important player in views of guilt and blame as relating to disease (Lupton 2005). Given that food is both an essential and pleasurable part of the human condition, a common media template drawn upon is the 'hidden dangers' that may lurk within food (Seale 2002).

Lupton's study showed that few Australians were concerned about BSE; very few people worried about bacterial contamination such as food poisoning, and even fewer about GM foods. Instead, food risks, for Australians, were largely associated with a high consumption of fats. Lupton states that 'this demonising of fat reflects several decades in Australia of public health and medical warnings about and mass media coverage of overweight and obesity, heart disease, stroke and some types of cancer' (2005, p. 462).

The issue of blame was given a special focus in the news items. Most items emphasised parental responsibility in controlling the lifestyle of their children. A second emphasis was on the schools' role, and some blame was attributed to advertising and fast-food purveyors. Mainly, news items relating to children's overweight and obesity were portrayed as due to poor diet and lack of exercise, with the assumption being that these were simply 'amenable to change' (Lupton 2004, p. 192), with no discussion of social factors contributing to poor eating habits.

In the reporting of adult overweight, writers acted as prophets of doom. Many visual images and verbal descriptions were startling and grotesque—dwelling on 'the "freak factor" of fatness' (Lupton 2004, p. 192), with blame placed entirely upon adult individuals (Lupton 2004). Occasionally, responsibility was drawn away from the individual and placed upon fast-food purveyors, but no attempt was made to discuss the impact of the structure of society or to engage in a **structure–agency debate**. Instead, the media targeted individuals as entirely responsible. Thus, the

risk society
A term coined by Ulrich Beck to describe the centrality of risk calculations in people's lives in Western society, whereby the key social problems today are unanticipated hazards, such as the risks of pollution, food poisoning, and environmental degradation.

structure–agency debate
A key debate in sociology over the extent to which human behaviour is determined by social structure.

victim-blaming
The process whereby social inequality is explained in terms of individuals being solely responsible for what happens to them in relation to the choices they make and their assumed psychological, cultural, and/or biological inferiority.

biomedicine/ biomedical model
The conventional approach to medicine in Western societies, based on the diagnosis and explanation of illness as a malfunction of the body's biological mechanisms. This approach underpins most health professions and health services, which focus on treating individuals, and generally ignores the social origins of illness and its prevention.

deprofessionalisation
A general theory predicting the decline of medical status and power due to the public's increased education about health issues and diminishing trust in medical practice as a result of media exposés of medical fraud and negligence.

medical dominance
The process by which non-medical problems become defined and treated as medical issues, usually in terms of illnesses, disorders, or syndromes.

media contributes to the culture of **victim-blaming** by identifying the individual as responsible for risk exposure, particularly when concerning obesity and food habits. Rather than producing a balanced report, the media adapts a victim-blaming perspective that does nothing to address the social roots of the problem; instead, it ascribes guilt to the individual and revels in the representations of 'Other' that the overweight body has come to represent in Western society (Lupton 2005; see also Chapter 11).

The medical profession and the media: sinners and saviours

As Deborah Lupton (1998) has noted, media health stories vacillate between depicting health professionals and doctors in particular as either sinners (due to negligence, mistakes, or greed) or as saviours (with saintly dispositions and God-like powers). Despite tales of medical scandals (e.g. medical fraud), media representations predominantly portray doctors as the authority on health matters, with **biomedical** notions of health and illness presented in a taken-for-granted and unproblematic fashion.

It has been argued that 'people at the end of the twentieth century do not unproblematically invest their trust in experts such as doctors, but are more willing to challenge and question them' (Lupton & McLean 1998, p. 948). Some argue that there is a move towards a **deprofessionalisation** of the medical profession and that patients are taking more consumerist approaches leading to a reduction in **medical dominance** (Haug 1988; see Chapter 19). This is a highly contested debate fraught by disagreement, but the medical profession clearly maintains a high level of dominance in the health system. Lupton points out, though, that 'some sociologists have asserted that the mass media have contributed to the diminishing of doctors' social status over the past three decades' (1998, p. 36). In response to the perceived threat to the authority of the medical profession, professional bodies such as the Australian Medical Association (AMA) have run their own promotional campaigns in the media in order to emphasise the importance of traditional Western medicine in order to try to win back patients disillusioned with orthodox medicine who may have sought alternative care.

Lupton and Jane McLean (1998) considered several crucial aspects of representations of health care and health care givers and takers in the media by looking at the language and visual imagery of news texts. By analysing headlines occurring in Australian news media over a period of time, they found that the terms 'doctor(s)', 'health', 'AMA', 'cancer', 'hospital', and 'patient(s)' were used frequently. Cancer ranked highly due to the mysterious aspects of the illness and HIV/AIDS was the only other disease named in the headlines due to its link with sexuality and stigmatised behaviours. The data shows that negative topics featured rather prominently in news media reporting (19 per cent). In photographs used, the archetypal medical practitioner was represented as male. A discourse analysis of the headlines showed that doctors were agents and patients were objects (a doctor-saves-patient structure): 'media discourse tends to legitimise biomedicine and the medical doctors who practice it by representing them as the ultimate authorities, the agents of action, with patients as the recipients of their actions' (Lupton & McLean 1998, p. 956). The results of this study suggest that 'doctors and the medical practice are the source of competing and diverse representations. While medicine may be portrayed as a fraught, conflictual and politicised profession in this forum, it is also represented as offering considerable benefits to patients' (Lupton & McLean 1998, p. 956).

Further, Lupton (1998b) found that doctors' and lay people's interpretations of media coverage differed widely: doctors maintained that the negative coverage was by far more commonly reported even though this is not what the statistics showed (indeed, even though the most frequently recorded topic was about malpractice and medical negligence and/or mistakes, negative topics were, in total, outweighed by reports presenting neutral or positive accounts), and they worried that they were unfairly being measured against the lowest of standards. In contrast, lay people voiced a general distrust of the media; '[p]eople tend to see news accounts as biased and marginalising, even consciously manipulative' (Lupton 1998, p. 41), not a general distrust of doctors. Indeed, as Table 17.1 shows, lay people were arguably as reluctant as doctors to see a shift in authority.

Table 17.1 Opinions on news media coverage: doctors compared to lay people

Doctors	Lay people
Had highly emotive responses and were pessimistic about the coverage	Did not find the coverage nearly as negative as doctors did
Were worried about the social status of the profession	Remembered positive accounts as well as negative ones
Felt that the reporting was unfair and spoke of a 'trial by media'	Acknowledged that 'doctors are only human' and that 'mistakes occur'
Felt that the news media neglects the work of competent doctors	Interpreted media reports based on their already existing doctor–patient relationships and experiences
Were concerned about patients being inappropriately influenced by negative news media coverage	Those with pre-existing negative experiences were more prone to see the negative exposure and those with pre-existing positive experiences discounted negative reporting as sensationalist

Source: Adapted from Lupton 1998b

Lay people can have a strong investment in doctors; trust is an important part of the healing process. Patients are reluctant to give up this faith and doctors are equally eager to keep this trust (Lupton 1998). It is thus in the emotional interest of patients to keep their faith in doctors and in biomedicine. The intense media attention

John Germov and Maria Freij

given to the medical profession in Australia means that doctors come under great scrutiny professionally as well as personally, but the fact that they are subject to such great mass media interest also cements their position as an elite group, ultimately underlining their position as an influential professional group enjoying cultural and social authority (Lupton & McLean 1998).

Indeed, the need is great for the medical profession to be presented in the best possible light in order maintain its social status. Lay people are found to give more credence to stories reporting on 'medical breakthrough; while aware of reports of malpractice, sexual assault charges, and other negative media attention, in general they thought 'highly of doctors' and 'acknowledged that "doctors are only human" and that "mistakes happen"' (Lupton & McLean 1998, p. 957).

BOX 17.2   Doing health sociology: the commodification of body parts and the media

The commodification of body parts has been a major topic in the news media. The commodification of bodies, that is, the making of bodies or body parts into tradeable objects, means a reorganisation of the boundaries of the body implying that the body is a form of merchandise. The commodification of the female body is well known. The debate also concerns the trade in transplant organs and the commodification of DNA.

Clive Seale and colleagues (2006) argue that it is necessary to look outside of biomedicine and science for other agents of commodification; namely into the mass media. In their 2006 study, Seale and colleagues look at media representations of a UK hospital 'scandal', at Alder Hey Children's Hospital, in which it was revealed that the hospital stored children's body parts without parental permission. The organ retention scandal received a great deal of media attention. The language employed borrowed from the horror genre, employing words such as 'gruesome',

'macabre', and 'ghoulish' (Seale et al. 2006, p. 31). The news stories also fetishised some body parts over others by focusing on body parts of great physical and cultural status, such as hearts and brains. The scandal at Alder Hey received widespread media attention, and public interest was great. The government responded by implementing a range of regulatory conditions including a new *Human Tissue Act 2004*.

It was found that media accounts, while criticising the objectified scientific view of body parts, 'made an independent contribution to the commodification of body parts, recruiting them for use in the manufacture of a media scandal. Ironically, this scandal was itself about the objectification of children's body parts by bio-science' (Seale et al. 2006, p. 37). It is clear that the reports were not merely written in the interest of 'public knowledge'; rather, these shocking accounts, in which a new way of commodifying the body was employed, were made to create public interest, and in turn, to sell more newspapers.

Magic pills: disease mongering by drug companies

In recent years, an extreme variant of **medicalisation**—'disease mongering'—has become common. The term refers to media and marketing campaigns that aim to unjustifiably 'widen … the boundaries of treatable illness in order to expand markets for those who sell and deliver treatments' (Moynihan et al. 2002, p. 886). The term was originally used by Lyn Payer (1992), and has been popularised by others (see Moynihan et al. 2002; Moynihan & Cassels 2005; Moynihan & Henry 2006), and attempts to encompass the efforts by pharmaceutical companies to convince basically healthy people that they are unwell (see Angell 2005; Critser 2005).

Alliances between drug companies, doctors, and consumer groups (often funded by drug companies) work together to raise awareness about an allegedly under-diagnosed condition for which they have come up with an effective treatment. Alternative views, such as the debate over the legitimacy of these conditions and alternative non-invasive treatments, become marginalised when these campaigns run by marketing and public relations firms take effect. In recent years, conditions such as 'restless legs syndrome', erectile dysfunction, and female sexual dysfunction (FSD) (with a US campaign claiming up to 45 per cent of women were afflicted) have been heavily promoted as serious health problems for which there are now effective drug therapies (Moynihan & Henry 2006). For example, pharmaceutical giant Eli Lilly promoted premenstrual dysphoric disorder to sell a re-branded version of Prozac for its treatment despite many medical professionals questioning whether the condition actually exists. Female sexual dysfunction was heavily promoted by Pfizer, one of the largest pharmaceutical companies, by attempting to get approval for Viagra—so effectively deployed with men—for use with women, but clinical trials were inconclusive at best and the company eventually ceased further trials. Consequently FSD was no more (Lexchi 2006; Moynihan & Henry 2006).

Disease mongering tends to develop in the following way:

1   A normal life condition is identified, usually a symptom commonly experienced, and defined as a disease suffered by a significant proportion of the population.

2   A new scientific breakthrough treatment is promoted.

3   The news media is targeted with a media release announcing a research study about the prevalence of a new condition and the treatment available.

4   The likely benefits of the treatment are exaggerated so that it appears as virtually 'risk free'.

5   'Independent experts' (usually funded by the drug company making the treatment) are made available to verify the new disease as a real and common condition to shape medical and public opinion and develop demand for the treatment.

6   An independent scientific body is established as a source of information on the condition (a professional-looking website is now essential); their guidelines on how to diagnose and treat the condition are made available.

medicalisation
The process by which non-medical problems become defined and treated as medical issues, usually in terms of illnesses, disorders, or syndromes.

John Germov and Maria Freij

7   Patient support groups based on the alleged disease are funded (again generally by drug companies) to advocate the need for treatment and provide access to individual cases of suffering.

8   An advertising campaign about the condition to coincide with the initial news reports is implemented (McKinlay 1979; Payer 1992; Moynihan et al. 2002).

Disease mongering individualises and privatises health problems and proposes costly biomedical interventions. It effectively targets new drugs at healthy people, with cost to individuals and the health system, as well as the potential for major **iatrogenic** outcomes. Some consumer groups and health professionals are attempting to combat disease mongering, through outlets such as Health Action International (see http://www.haiweb.org) and Media Doctor (see http://www.mediadoctor.org.au). The profitability of disease mongering is likely to be here to stay, and represents another example of the power of the **medical–industrial complex**.

The internet as a source of health information

Increasing accessibility to the internet is one factor explaining why more and more people look for medical advice online—the internet offers a plethora of sites dedicated to health. In a culture that focuses on individuals' responsibility for their health, it is not unusual that the internet becomes an increasingly important contributor to how people gather information and to the choices they make about their health (Lewis 2006).

Individualised technologies mean that people take a greater responsibility, but interestingly, the media coverage is not entirely positive: there is a concern that lay people are unable to handle the processing of online information, unable to separate low-quality from high-quality information. Patients are seen as passive recipients of information and as potential victims of 'cyberchondria' or 'cyberquackery' (Lewis 2006). Indeed, there are concerns about the regulation of the quality of online material, largely because of the idea that the patient needs to be protected from being potentially misinformed. The internet is seen as 'an unruly, unregulated space marked by a plurality of claims to knowledge and authority' (Lewis 2006, p. 528). Tania Lewis argues that the image of the passive, lonely, and isolated health-advice seeker is proved wrong; many users are active participants in email support groups or online forums.

Lewis's study shows that a recurring theme 'that emerged among the young people in the study was anxiety about whether or not the information available on the internet was "trustworthy"' (2006, p. 533). Still, the study showed that the young people interviewed about their health-seeking practices online were 'active and critical users of the internet. From the outset, people were sceptical about the information on the web because "just anyone" can put their opinion out there'

iatrogenesis/ iatrogenic
A concept popularised by Ivan Illich that refers to any adverse outcome or harm as a result of medical treatment.

medical–industrial complex
The growth of profit-oriented medical companies and industries, whereby one company may own a chain of health services, such as hospitals, clinics, and radiology and pathology services.

(Lewis 2006, p. 534). Because of this reason, the people would compare and contrast information. The study showed that young people were aware of the fact that online material is of differing quality and that media audiences can be misled. The users tended to privilege information associated with biomedicine; using the internet for information was not seen as an alternative to visiting a doctor; online health advice was seen as complementary rather than supplementary.

The findings by Lewis are reinforced by a study by Alex Broom and Philip Tovey (2008), who examined how cancer patients used the internet. Rather than supporting a deprofessionalisation or democratisation thesis, whereby patients became so knowledgeable as to challenge the authority of medical professionals, they found conversely that the ability of patients to access a wealth of biomedical information reinforced traditional notions of medical diagnosis and treatment (Broom & Tovey 2008). While some used the internet to seek out alternative therapies, the major theme was one of reasserting the dominance of a biomedical perspective, adding support for medical professionals' expertise rather than undermining it.

Conclusion

Health issues feature prominently in news reporting and the more controversial or conflict-laden, the more newsworthy the story, ranging from the very positive (medical breakthroughs) to the very negative (health risks). The media also tends to use media templates that promote 'magic bullet' and quick-fix medicine, in the form of a pill or surgical intervention, to solve often complex health, personal, and social problems.

The news media is an increasingly important player in how lay people perceive health issues. The exaltation of heroic technological cures marginalises the social determinants of health and preventive alternatives. The focus is placed on the individual and a culture of victim-blaming is encouraged. The media tends to sensationalise reports in order to sell more newspapers or get higher ratings. Many people recognise that the media is biased, but still the media's representations invariably shape our understanding of health and health care delivery. Disease mongering, a process promoted and funded by pharmaceutical companies, is supported by the media due to the 'newsworthiness' of these stories. 'Epidemics' and 'scandals' are frequent.

In the name of 'public interest', the media frames and shapes stories to appeal to the general public. Borrowing from the horror genre, they use words like 'gruesome' and 'shock' to get the public's attention; a news account is rarely objective. Bearing in mind the importance of the news media as a strong influence on the way we perceive the world, we can understand more about the way lay people's opinions and attitudes to health and health care delivery are shaped. We do this by applying the sociological perspective, which is so often ignored by the media, to the media itself.

John Germov and Maria Freij

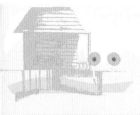

Summary of main points

» The news media influences how we perceive health problems and health care delivery. It reports, but also creates, issues around health and health care delivery through for example, supporting disease mongering due to its sensationalist and 'newsworthy' aspects.

» The framing of reports will affect how medical information is conveyed; some views will be highlighted and others ignored. It is crucial that we keep asking ourselves whose messages are being conveyed and whose interests are being promoted.

» Under the perceived threat of deprofessionalisation, doctors and medical associations are increasingly employing public relations strategies of their own. Patients seem equally reluctant to give up their belief in biomedicine as there are emotional gains of this relationship.

» With increased internet accessibility, more people are seeking health advice online. Studies show that this is a complementary rather than supplementary practice.

» The news media employs a clear focus on individual responsibility for illness, overweight, and obesity, and largely ignores multifactorial, environmental, and sociological reasons, thereby supporting a victim-blaming view.

Sociological reflection: media influence

Watch an episode of a popular television show dealing with health issues and consider the way health care, health issues, and health professionals are represented.

» In what ways are health professionals portrayed?

» What assumptions about health and illness are made, particularly in terms of treatment?

» To what extent do you think that such shows affect public expectations of health care and understandings of health issues?

» Do media representations of health in fictional shows reinforce or undermine the news media reports on health and illness?

Discussion questions

1 Why is it important to study media representations of health sociologically?

2 What are media templates? Give examples in your answer.

3 How influential is the media in the shaping of public views of illness, the health system, and health professionals?

4 What effect does the media have on your views of health and illness?

5 How do you decide what is reliable and trustworthy in the media?

6 What could be done to improve the way the media represents health issues?

Further investigation

1 Examine an illness that is currently the subject of media attention. Research the nature of the condition and also who is behind its promotion. What direct and indirect messages are being conveyed about health and illness?

2 The media is significantly responsible for shaping public understanding of health issues. Discuss.

Further reading

Bury, M. & Gabe, J. 2006, 'Television Medicine: Medical Dominance or Trial by Media?', in D. Kelleher, J. Gabe & G. Williams (eds), *Challenging Medicine*, 2nd edn, Routledge, London, pp. 62–84.

'A Collection of Articles on Disease Mongering' 2006, *PLoS Medicine*, vol. 3, no. 4. Available online: <http://collections.plos.org/plosmedicine/diseasemongering-2006.php>

King, M. & Watson, K. (eds) 2005, *Representing Health: Discourses of Health and Illness in the Media*, Palgrave Macmillan, Basingstoke.

Lupton, D. 1998, 'Medicine and Health Care in Popular Media', in A. Petersen & C. Waddell (eds), *Health Matters: A Sociology of Illness, Prevention and Care*, Allen & Unwin, Sydney, pp. 194–207.

Marjoribanks, T. 2007, 'Media and Popular Culture', in J. Germov & M. Poole (eds), *Public Sociology: An Introduction to Australian Society*, Allen & Unwin, Sydney, pp. 389–405.

Seale, C. (ed.) 2004, *Health and the Media*, Blackwell, Oxford.

Seale, C. 2002, *Media and Health*, Sage, London.

Web resources

Behind the Headlines (UK): <http://www.nhs.uk/news/Pages/NewsIndex.aspx>

Behind the Medical Headlines (Scotland): <http://www.behindthemedicalheadlines.com/>

Center on Media and Child Health (USA): <http://www.cmch.tv/>

Health Action International: <http://www.haiweb.org/01_about_a.htm>

Health News Review (USA): <http://www.healthnewsreview.org/>

Informed Health Online: <http://www.informedhealthonline.org/>

Media Doctor (Australia): <http://www.mediadoctor.org.au/>

Media Doctor Canada: <http://www.mediadoctor.ca>

Media Storm: <http://www.mediastorm.org>

Online case study • •
Visit the Second Opinion website to access relevant case studies.

Documentaries/films

Media Watch 2008, 'Gilding the Lily', and 'Bitter Pill', ABC TV. An examination of the promotion of Cialis as a treatment for erectile dysfunction through the news media. Available online: <http://www.abc.net.au/mediawatch/transcripts/s2249537.htm> and <http://www.abc.net.au/mediawatch/transcripts/s2297042.htm>

References

Angell, M. 2005, *The Truth about Drug Companies*, Scribe, Melbourne.

Beck, U. 1992, *Risk Society: Towards a New Modernity*, Sage, London.

Broom, A. & Tovey, P. 2008, 'The Role of the Internet in Cancer Patients' Engagement with Complementary and Alternative Cancer Treatments', *Health: An Interdisciplinary Journal for the Social Study of Health, Illness and Medicine*, vol. 12, no. 2, pp. 139–56.

Bury, M. & Gabe, J. 2006, 'Television Medicine: Medical Dominance or Trial by Media?', in D. Kelleher, J. Gabe & G. Williams (eds), *Challenging Medicine*, 2nd edn, Routledge, London, pp. 62–84.

Capra, F. 1982, *The Turning Point: Science, Society and the Rising Culture*, Simon & Schuster, New York.

Critcher, C. 2003, *Moral Panics and the Media*, Open University Press, Philadelphia.

Critser, G. 2005, *Generation Rx: How Prescription Drugs are Altering American Lives, Minds, and Bodies*, Houghton Mifflin, Boston.

Haug, M. 1988, 'A Re-examination of the Hypothesis of Deprofessionalisation', *Milbank Quarterly*, vol. 2, (supp.), pp. 58–66.

Kitzinger, J. 2000, 'Media Templates: Patterns of Association and the (Re)construction of Meaning over Time', *Media, Culture & Society*, vol. 22, no. 1, pp. 61–84.

Lewis, T. 2006, 'Seeking Health Information on the Internet: Lifestyle Choice or Bad Attack of Cyberchondria?', *Media, Culture & Society*, vol. 28, pp. 521–39.

Lexchi, J. 2006, 'Bigger and Better: How Pfizer Redefined Erectile Dysfunction', *PLoS Medicine*, vol. 3, no. 4, pp. 1–4. Available online: <http://www.plosmedicine.org>

Lupton, D. 1998a, 'Medicine and Health Care in Popular Media', in A. Petersen & C. Waddell (eds), *Health Matters: A Sociology of Illness, Prevention and Care*, Allen & Unwin, Sydney, pp. 194–207.

Lupton, D. 1998, 'Doctors in the News Media: Lay and Medical Audiences' Responses', *Journal of Sociology*, vol. 34, no. 1, pp. 35–48.

Lupton, D. 2004, 'A Grim Health Future: Food Risks in the Sydney Press', *Health, Risk & Society*, vol. 6, no. 2, pp. 187–200.

Lupton, D. 2005, 'Lay Discourses and Beliefs Related to Food Risks: An Australian Perspective', *Sociology of Health and Illness*, vol. 27, no. 4, pp. 448–67.

Lupton, D. & McLean, J. 1998, 'Representing Doctors: Discourses and Images in the Australian Press', *Social Science and Medicine*, vol. 46, no. 8, pp. 947–58.

Marjoribanks, T. 2007, 'Media and Popular Culture', in J. Germov & M. Poole (eds), *Public Sociology: An Introduction to Australian Society*, Allen & Unwin, Sydney, pp. 389-405.

McKinlay, J. 1979, 'Epidemiological and Political Determinants of Social Policies Regarding the Public Health', *Social Science and Medicine*, vol. 13A, no. 5, pp. 541–58.

Media Watch 2008a, 'Gilding the Lily', ABC TV. Available online: <http://www.abc.net. au/mediawatch/transcripts/s2249537.htm>

Media Watch 2008b, 'Bitter Pill', ABC TV. Available online: <http://www.abc.net.au/ mediawatch/transcripts/s2297042.htm>

Moynihan, R. & Cassels, A. 2005, *Selling Sickness: How the World's Biggest Pharmaceutical Companies are Turning us all into Patients*, Allen & Unwin, Sydney.

Moynihan, R. & Henry, D. 2006, 'The Fight against Disease Mongering: Generating Knowledge for Action', *PLoS Medicine*, vol. 3, no. 4, pp. 1–4. Available online: <http:// www.plosmedicine.org>

Moynihan, R., Health, I. & Henry, D. 2002, 'Selling Sickness: The Pharmaceutical Industry and Disease Mongering', *British Medical Journal*, vol. 324, pp. 886–91.

Payer, L. 1992, *Disease-mongers: How Doctors, Drug Companies, and Insurers are Making you Feel Sick*, Wiley & Sons, New York.

Petersen, A. 2001, 'Biofantasies: Genetics and Medicine in the Print News Media', *Social Science & Medicine*, 52, pp. 1255–68.

Petersen, A. 2002, 'Replicating Our Bodies, Losing Our Selves: News Media Portrayals of Human Cloning in the Wake of Dolly', *Body & Society*, vol. 8(4), pp. 71–90.

Seale, C. 2002, *Media and Health*, Sage, London.

Seale, C., Cavers, D. & Dixon-Woods, M. 2006, 'Commodification of Body Parts: By Medicine or by Media?', *Body & Society*, vol. 12, no. 1, pp. 25–42.

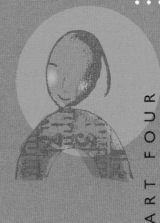

The Social Organisation of Health Care: Professions, Politics, and Policies

The chapters in this part of the book are concerned with the social organisation of health care: the role of health policy, political ideology, and the health professions in shaping the institutional features of the Australian health care system. A common theme among the chapters is an analysis of the medical profession's influence on health policy, on other health professions, and on the delivery of health services. The chapters examine the key features of the health system—its history, its structure, and the changes under way—to understand why the health system is organised the way that it is and how it could be otherwise.

Part 4 is divided into seven chapters:

That any sane nation, having observed that you could provide for the supply of bread by giving bakers a pecuniary interest in baking for you, should go on to give a surgeon a pecuniary interest in cutting off your leg, is enough to make one despair of political humanity.

GEORGE BERNARD SHAW
1908, *The Doctor's Dilemma*, preface

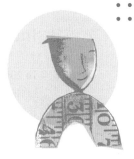

CHAPTER 18

Power, Politics, and Health Care

HELEN
BELCHER

Overview

- What is the nature of the Australian health care system?
- What role do ideology, politics, power, and interests play in shaping Australian health insurance arrangements?
- How have history, culture, and social structure influenced health insurance?

THE POLITICS OF MEDICARE

The first Rudd Labor Government budget increased the Medicare Levy Surcharge thresholds for singles from $50,000 to $70,000 and for families from $100,000 to $140,000. Treasurer Wayne Swan argued the increase was warranted as the previous government's failure to adjust the threshold had unfairly burdened families on modest incomes. It was welcomed as long overdue by the Secretary of the Health Service Union of Australia who had previously supported the scrapping of the 30 per cent Private Health Insurance Rebate. In her opinion the rebate diverted funds from the public sys-tem to 'prop up' the private health system. The Australian Medical Association, the private health insurance sector, and the Federal Liberal–National Party Opposition argued the increase in the threshold would see many younger high-income earners give up private health insurance, that it would force hundreds of thousands of mainly frail and elderly patients onto public hospital waiting lists, place an extra burden on the ailing public system, and put insurers and private hospitals in jeopardy (*Canberra Times*, 11 May 2008). How can these differ-ences be explained?

Introduction

In 2000, the Senate Community Affairs References Committee observed that 'much of the debate and commentary (on Australian health policy) often seems to focus on the requirements of funding agencies such as governments and the needs of practitioners' (2000, p. 3). Earlier, Sidney Sax had argued that the Australian health care system responds to vested interests and influences—'a strife of interests' (Sax 1984)—many of which are seemingly unrelated to health (1990). Gwendolyn Gray extended this argument by claiming that 'the competing ideological perspectives of Australia's major parties are the principal reasons for the frequent and major changes in policy direction' (1991, p. 184).

The financing and organisation of private health insurance reflects a clash of **ideology**, not so much over the need for insurance but over the issue of compulsion or freedom of choice and over who should be responsible. In Sax's opinion there are two major players: politicians and doctors—with hospitals and the insurance industry playing supporting roles (Sax 1984). Specifically they compete over the role of the **state**, the role of the individual/community and the role of the **market**. Importantly, the strength of the differences can be overstated. In fact, there has been a tendency to strike compromises and over time these have been embedded into health care arrangements; nevertheless, Australian health insurance reflects an ideological struggle between social and economic **liberalism**, which has found political expression in the two major political parties: the Australian Labor Party (ALP) and the Liberal–National Party Coalition. Generally speaking, the working class, through the trade unions, has aligned itself with the ALP, whereas doctors, private hospitals, and the insurance industry have supported the Coalition. After an overview of the Australian health care system, this chapter analyses the influence of ideology, politics, and vested interest on health-insurance policy.

The Australian health care system

There are two key characteristics of the Australian health care system: its federal structure and a public/private division of responsibilities. These characteristics provide a backdrop for the organisation of the Australian health care system, and ultimately health policy.

Federal structure

In 1901, the colonies of New South Wales, Victoria, South Australia, Queensland, Tasmania, and Western Australia agreed to the establishment of the Commonwealth of Australia; however, the 'founding fathers' were anxious to balance the needs

ideology
In a political context, ideology refers to those beliefs and values that relate to the way in which society should be organised, including the appropriate role of the state.

state
A term used to describe a collection of institutions, including the parliament (government and opposition political parties), the public-sector bureaucracy, the judiciary, the military, and the police.

market
Any institutional arrangement for the exchange of goods according to economic demand and supply. This term is often used to describe the basic principle underlying the capitalist economy.

liberalism
An ideology that regards the interests of individuals and their position in the market-place as being of primary importance.

of the Australian people as a whole against the **rights** of individual states. Hence they adopted a federal structure, which provided for the operation of a national government (the Commonwealth) in parallel with six state governments. A third tier of government, local government, was not included in the Constitution, relying for its existence on its respective state (for a fuller discussion of the Australian political system, see Singleton et al. 2008).

Section 51 of the Constitution divides responsibilities between the Commonwealth and state governments but, as Dean Jaensch notes, 'the division of powers was more complex' (1984, p. 30). Some areas, such as defence, customs, and excise were granted to the Commonwealth as exclusive powers whilst others were allocated as shared powers. Thus, Federal and state governments share responsibility for such things as taxation, marriage and divorce, and conciliation and arbitration. If there is conflict Section 109 stipulates that federal legislation should prevail, although either may appeal to the High Court of Australia. All other powers, known as residual powers, remain with the states (Singleton et al. 2008, p. 29). Although designed to protect the interests of the states, this arrangement has created problems for the adequate management of health services, particularly due to overlapping responsibilities.

Shared government responsibilities

The Commonwealth Government plays a leadership role in national health matters but also exercises a significant financial role. In 2005–06 it funded 43 per cent of total health expenditure (see Figure 18.1). While the Commonwealth's share has fallen since 2000–01—down from 44.3 per cent (AIHW 2008, p. 400)—it is still the major source of funds. These are delivered via the Pharmaceutical Benefits Scheme (PBS) and Repatriation Pharmaceutical Benefits Scheme (RPBS); Specific Purpose Payments (SPPs) to the states/territories including payments specified by the Australian Health Care Agreements and Public Health Outcomes Funding Agreements; and Medicare (AIHW 2008, pp. 398–9). The latter provides 'free or subsidised treatment by medical practitioners, participating optometrists, services delivered by a practice nurse on behalf of a general practitioner (GP)', along with a limited range of services provided by dentists and allied health practitioners (AIHW 2008, p. 316). It also provides free public hospital care for patients who elect to be treated as 'public hospital' patients. The Medicare levy, which is calculated on the basis of 1.5 per cent of taxable income plus a surcharge of 1 per cent for high income earners who do not have private health insurance, supports Medicare. Despite the inference, though, the levy is not a 'hypothecated' tax, that is, the money raised by the levy is not specifically allocated to health. Nor does the levy cover the full cost of the Commonwealth's expenditure on health. Indeed in 2005–06 the levy provided only 18 per cent of Commonwealth funds with the remainder coming from general revenue (Duckett 2007, pp. 41–50; AIHW 2008, p. 316).

rights
Socially prescribed privileges and entitlements for individuals and social groups.

State government expenditure inclusive of local government contributed 25 per cent of the funds for total health expenditure in 2005–06 (see Figure 18.1). This was up from 23 per cent in 2001–02, which is partly explained by the decrease in the Commonwealth's share of expenditure (AIHW 2008, p. 400). The states and territories deliver and manage public acute and psychiatric hospital services and a wide range of community and public health services including school health, dental health, maternal and child health, and environmental health programs (Bloom 2000; AIHW 2008). They are also responsible for the regulation of health professionals.

Local government funds are drawn from the respective state/territory government, and local taxes and charges. It is a minor, but nevertheless important, player being responsible for aspects of environmental control, some personal preventive services, and home care services (Bloom 2000, p. 25; AIHW 2008, p. 401).

The federal division of responsibilities, which arises out of the Constitutional definition of powers, has implications for health policy and thus the quality of care. Indeed, the National Health and Hospital Reform Commission (NHHRC 2008, p. 20) note: '[l]ack of clarity of accountability and definition of responsibilities creates the environment for a blame game, as each government is able to blame the other for shortcomings attributed to each other's programs. The losers are the public who wait longer for care or don't have their service needs met'.

Public/private division of responsibilities

In addition to the federal division of responsibility there is a public/private division. In 2005–06, private sources such as health insurance funds, out-of-pocket payments, and compulsory third party motor vehicle and workers' compensation insurers, funded 32 per cent of total health expenditure (see Figure 18.1). Amongst other things, private sources provided 59 per cent for private hospitals (AIHW 2008, p. 399). It is worth noting, that private hospitals benefited indirectly from the Commonwealth's payment of the private health insurance rebate. In 2005–06 it amounted to 34 per cent of the gross funding provided by private health insurers to private hospitals (AIHW 2008, pp. 398–9).

The importance of the public/private division is highlighted by the influence exerted by private providers—most notably doctors—upon the organisation and financing of health care services (Thame 1974; Sax 1984; Crichton 1990; Gillespie 1991; Richardson 1998; Scotton 1998; Gray 2004). For example, the lifting of thresholds described in the vignette was opposed by the Australian Medical Association (AMA) on the grounds that 'it will cause people to drop out of private health insurance' (Capolingua 2008). Politicians, too, exert considerable influence. Throughout the term of its government (1996–2007) the Liberal–National Party tinkered with Medicare in favour of private health insurance arrangements. It introduced measures that reflected its ideological position, especially the privatisation

Figure 18.1 Percentage of health expenditure according to source of funds, 2005–06

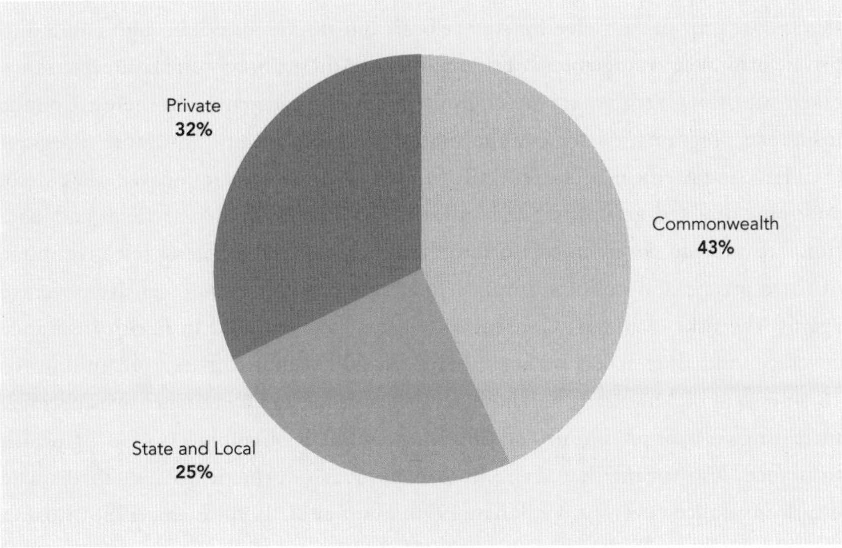

Source: Adapted from AIHW 2008, Table 3, p. 400

agenda of the then Prime Minister, John Howard (Gray 2004. p. 90–1). Consequently, the Coalition Government introduced the non-means tested 30 per cent rebate, the Medicare levy surcharge and the targeted eligibility based 'Medicare Safety Net'. The nature and language of each helps to redefine publicly provided health care as a welfare measure, not a shared system; they suggest that cover should be limited to those unable to provide for themselves, a residual rather than universal, or institutional, approach to health (McAuley & Menadue 2007).

International comparisons

The Australian health care system can best be described as 'mixed'. The public and private sector are responsible to varying degrees for the financing, organisation, and provision of health services. Most notably private practitioners provide health services in public institutions for which they are reimbursed on the basis of a fee-for-service or sessional payment financed by a combination of Medicare payments, private health insurance, and payments by individuals. The American system, by way of contrast, is largely dependent on the private sector, while the British system is largely public in character.

The United States' system of health insurance, a 'proxy measure of access to health care' (National Center for Health Statistics [NCHS] 2007, p. 56), is largely the result of a movement sponsored by the providers of health care services (Bates

Helen Belcher

1983). The need for hospitals, combined with a political philosophy that emphasised individual responsibility, resulted in a largely private health care system. Almost all services are provided on a fee-for-service basis and are supported through public and private insurance arrangements. The majority of Americans rely on private insurance taken out through employers under group policy arrangements, but there are public insurance programs: Medicare, the State Children's Health Insurance Program (SCHIP), and Medicaid. The federally funded Medicare program covers the elderly and some disabled groups, while Medicaid and SCHIP draw on federal and state funds to provide cover for low-income families. As well as being selective, none of these private and public insurance programs provides comprehensive coverage against the risks of illness. Consequently, gaps have emerged in health insurance coverage, and thus access to health care. In 2005, approximately 42 million or 16.4 per cent of Americans had no insurance. The lack of comprehensive coverage, increasing costs of premiums and falls in the number of employers offering health insurance, also meant that an unknown number of Americans had inadequate health insurance coverage (Callahan 1990; Ham et al. 1990; Hehir 1996; Ross et al. 1999; DeNavas-Walt et al. 2004; NCHS 2007).

British health insurance began as 'a movement run by consumers for their mutual benefit' (Bates 1983, p. 104). The fact that this movement was backed by a strong working class helps explain the British adoption of a more collectivist, and hence public, approach. The government, through the National Health Service (NHS), provides comprehensive free health care for everyone, funded by all taxpayers (Ham 1992; Ross et al. 1999). Reforms introduced by the Conservative Government in 1989, however, opened up health care provision to market forces, moves that have not been reversed by the New Labour Governments of Tony Blair, and now Gordon Brown. It was argued that these changes would promote competition, increase consumer choice, and devolve decision-making and accountability to the local level (Ross et al. 1999). In addition, the Thatcher Conservative Government of the 1970s encouraged the development of private insurance, which now stands at approximately 11 per cent of the population. A significant proportion of these policies are paid for by employers. Whilst the British health care system retains its public nature, the private sector has emerged as a relatively small but important player, a role seemingly supported by New Labour (Wallis 2004).

gross domestic product (GDP)
The market value of all goods and services that have been sold during a year.

In 2005, Australian health expenditure, as a percentage of the **gross domestic product (GDP)** was 8.8 per cent, compared with 15.3 per cent for the USA and 8.3 per cent for the United Kingdom (see Figure 18.2). Higher expenditure has, however, not resulted in better health (see Tables 18.1 and 18.2). In fact, when compared with Australia and the United Kingdom, Americans have poorer health and limited access prompting the observation that universal, comprehensive health coverage leads to better health outcomes.

Figure 18.2 Health expenditure for Australia and selected Organization for Economic Co-operation and Development (OECD) countries as a percentage of GDP, 1976–2005

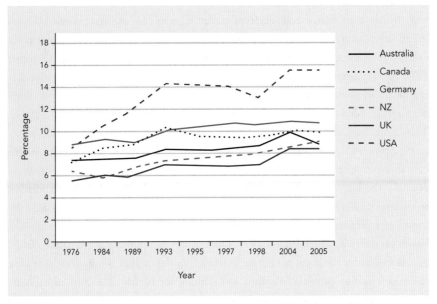

Source: Adapted from AIHW 2008, Table S8.4, p. 403

Table 18.1 Neonatal and infant mortality rates* for Australia, the United Kingdom, and the USA, latest available year per 1000 live births

Country	Neonatal	Infant
Australia (2005)	3.6	5.0
United Kingdom (2004)	3.5	5.1
USA (2004)	4.5	6.8

* Neonatal: less than 28 days of birth; Infant: less than one year.

Source: Adapted from AIHW 2008, Table S8, p. 485

Table 18.2 Life expectancy at selected ages for Australia, the United Kingdom, and the USA, 2005

Country	Life expectancy (years of age)					
	At birth		At age 25–29		At age 65–69	
	Males	*Females*	*Males*	*Females*	*Males*	*Females*
Australia	79.0	83.7	55.0	59.4	18.6	21.7
UK	76.6	81.1	52.6	56.8	16.7	19.6
USA	75.3	80.4	51.7	56.3	17.1	19.9

Source: Adapted from AIHW 2008, Table S11, p. 487

Helen Belcher

Health insurance

The purpose of insurance is to provide protection against loss. This involves 'a contract whereby, for a stipulated consideration, called a premium, one party undertakes to indemnify or guarantee another against loss by a certain specified contingency or peril, called a risk, the contract being set forth in a document called a policy' (Titmuss 1974, p. 90). Generally, it is a market commodity, but 'insurance, by its very nature, is a means of buying out of the discipline of market forces ... the tendency to over-use a service because it is covered by insurance' (McAuley & Menadue 2007, p. 14). This 'moral hazard' is not such a problem in some areas of insurance such as home and car insurance, but health is unlike other goods and services. The need for health care is largely uncertain; the costs of health care are high, and most consumers do not have the knowledge that enables them to make an informed choice in relation to treatment. What is more, illness can restrict others, either through the risk of the spread of infection, through emotional and psychological suffering, or through the loss of productivity (McClelland 1991; Duckett 2007; McAuley & Menadue 2007). Access to health care, then, cannot be simply left to the market as not all citizens have the means to buy protection against loss. Paying for health care must incorporate measures that provide both access and equity (Scotton & Macdonald 1993). In other words, health insurance requires some level of collective responsibility. 'Community rating', the cross-subsidisation of sicker and poorer members of society by the healthier and wealthier members through the payment of set premiums, is Australia's acknowledgment of that responsibility (Scotton & Macdonald 1993). Determining the degree of collective responsibility is informed by ideology.

Ideology

The meaning of 'ideology' is contentious (Abercrombie et al. 1988), but it generally refers to 'a set of beliefs and values which express the interests of a particular social group' (Haralambos & Holborn 1991, p. 21). Ideology shapes judgments about fairness and justice, often characterised as contests between freedom and equality— between the right to 'do as I choose' and the need to ensure that societal benefits are fairly distributed.

The concept of 'liberty' or 'freedom' refers to the ability of the individual to make choices independently of outside interference. It assumes individual responsibility. The concept of equality relates to equality of outcome and, as such, implies some level of collective responsibility. Conflict emerges over the question of fairness or equity. In cases in which liberty assumes importance, questions of fairness are decided on the basis of merit. Access to goods and services must be 'earned'. When this system fails, targeted welfare services may be provided. These services are linked to demonstrations of willingness to work. Welfare provision is residual—available only as a last resort. If equality is perceived to be more important, then it is more likely that fairness will be determined on the basis of need. Satisfaction of that need is more likely to be seen in terms of a collective responsibility requiring public and universal provision: an institutional approach. Rather than holding the individuals responsible for their predicament, this approach acknowledges structured inequality and opts for institutional provision in order to ensure equality of outcome (Gardner 1995; Dalton et al. 1996). Both responses are legitimate and even defensible when viewed from their ideological basis; however, adoption of either must consider the questions of access and equity.

From Left to Right

Traditional understandings of freedom and equality stretch along a political continuum from Left to Right, from **socialism** to liberalism. Equality is generally associated with the socialist end of the continuum, and freedom with the liberal end. While this understanding is too simplistic (see Kymlicka 1990), it provides a useful guide to understanding health insurance policy. It is worth noting that Australian history has tended to be a history of liberalism rather than of socialism. 'The classic values of **individualism**, competition, individual freedoms, and inequality, have combined with an acceptance of a minor role for government in protection for the "really needy"' (Tulloch 1983, p. 255). Consequently, the dominant view of welfare is residual (Beilharz et al. 1992).

Social and economic liberalism

Understandings of liberty range from 'freedom from' coercion to 'freedom to' benefit. Both understandings acknowledge the concept of rights, but the former views these rights as negative—freedom from interference—whereas the latter sees rights as positive—the right to services and benefits that enable participation in society.

One person's 'right' entails another's obligation. It also creates expectations. In the case of health, a negative right entails an obligation not to interfere in the actions of another. A positive right entails an obligation to provide appropriate care and an expectation that such care will be forthcoming (Beauchamp & Faden 1979). The splitting of rights into negative and positive types is simplistic, as rights are 'complex, containing both negative rights and positive rights' (Beauchamp & Faden 1979, p. 120). There is, for example, a tension between the right not to insure and the right of the community not to have to support the non-insured in times of adversity. Simplistic as it is, the division into negative and positive broadly defines two types of liberalism.

Proponents of negative rights generally argue for non-interference, which is linked to their advocacy of the libertarian variety of liberty—freedom from coercion.

socialism
A political ideology with numerous variations, but with a core belief in the creation of societies in which private property and wealth accumulation are replaced by state ownership and distribution of economic resources.

individualism/ individualisation
A belief or process supporting the primacy of individual choice, freedom, and self-responsibility.

Helen Belcher

The state may only intervene to limit the liberty of an individual when and if the exercise of that liberty will harm others. This justification is a feature of narrow and conservative social health programs. Rights and expectations are framed within an individualistic perspective, which argues for the satisfaction of health access through private provision. Public provision should be limited to cases in which harm may flow from the actions of others, such as quarantine of contagious diseases, or to the provision of those public goods for which individuals are unlikely to pay. Rather than the public provision of goods and services, preference is given to the operation of the market. Unfortunately, some will fail, but eventually the rewards will 'trickle down' and people will receive some benefit. Failing that, they can turn to charity. The moral justification of this outlook lies in the proposal that libertarianism is grounded in free choice. Libertarianism extends its defence of individual freedom to the assertion that taxation is inherently wrong because it violates people's rights to dispose of their wealth as they see fit (Kymlicka 1990). When all is said and done, individuals 'earn' access to goods and services.

Such a belief underpins the concept of **economic rationalism** (also known as economic liberalism or neo-liberalism), which refers to the capacity of the market to allocate resources efficiently (Beilharz et al. 1992). Economic efficiency drives not only economic policy but also health and social policy. It requires the cutting back of government responsibilities, the introduction of private sector competition, and the promotion of independence, all in the name of economic efficiency (Rees & Rodley 1995). The privatisation of government functions is necessary in order to return responsibility to the individual, thereby ending the culture of dependency. People should be free to make their own choices and their own mistakes. In the case of health, this idea finds expression in the call for individuals to finance their own health care needs through the purchase of private health insurance, thereby leaving the public health care system to care only for those who cannot afford private health care.

Social liberalism, by way of contrast, views rights as positive: liberty means 'freedom to' benefit. This ideology acknowledges that compensation is needed to counteract the excesses of the marketplace. This is done by assuming some degree of collective responsibility for improving access to health care services, which in turn enables individuals to participate fully in society. State intervention, through either the levying of taxes, legislation, or public provision, is expected even if not always welcome (Beilharz et al. 1992). The influence of socialism, with its emphasis on equality, is evident in social liberalism. Equality extends beyond equality of opportunity to equality of conditions and outcomes. Hence the emphasis is not on 'the abstract individual' who exists before his or her social situation (Forder et al. 1984, p. 16), but upon the **social structure** that either limits or enhances the conditions of individuals and hence their **life chances**. Resources are allocated according to need, not merit. Moreover it holds that reliance on the idea of individual, negative

economic rationalism/economic liberalism
Terms used to describe a political philosophy based on small-government and market-oriented policies, such as deregulation, privatisation, reduced government spending, and lower taxation.

social liberalism
An ideology that is based on individual freedom but acknowledges the need for state intervention to overcome the inadequacies of the market, which can act to limit the freedom of individuals fully to participate in society.

social structure
The recurring patterns of social interaction through which people are related to each other, such as social institutions, and social groups.

life chances
Derived from Max Weber, the term refers to people's opportunity to realise their lifestyle choices, which are often assumed to differ according to their social class.

rights is insufficient. These must be supplemented by positive rights, which allow for the 'freedom to' benefit. The state needs to be involved so that those obstacles that hinder individual development can be addressed (Beilharz et al. 1992). Universal health insurance enables access to health care services and benefits, and so enables individuals to participate in society. By definition, it impinges on personal liberty in the interest of equality.

Politics and power

Politics is the process of resolving conflict between rival understandings and interests over the allocation of scarce resources. Politics is about power. While there are several definitions of power, ranging from elitist through pluralist to radical theories (see Gardner 1995), **pluralism** is dominant. The pluralist view maintains that health policy outcomes are a consequence of compromise between the interests of government and various interest groups, the most significant of which are those groups representing doctors. This is a legitimate exercise of power.

A contrasting view is provided by Stephen Lukes (1974), who identifies three dimensions of power. The first is equivalent to pluralism and is evident in issues over which there is observable conflict. The second refers to those occasions where decision-making is confined to safe issues through the process of non-decision-making. The use of power suppresses conflicts so its use is covert. Issues are kept out of the political or decision-making process by removing them. Tactics used include transferring a contentious issue to a committee for examination and co-opting opponents to the committee, knowing full well that nothing will happen or that the dissenting voices will be neutralised (Lukes 1974). The third dimension offers a radical critique of power by highlighting the actual shaping of interests and preferences, usually without individuals being aware that they are being shaped. Lukes maintains that people's expressed preferences and interests are shaped by **socialisation**, education, and the media, thereby creating a system of dominant values and beliefs: ideology. Conflict is latent—sleeping until woken—because people are unaware of their real preferences and interests. This enables those who exercise power to protect their interests at the expense of the powerless.

Lukes' theory of power can be combined with the 'structural interest perspective' developed by Richard Alford (1975). He maintains that health policy and the organisation of health care are the products of the social, political, and economic forces that exist at a particular time. Vested or structural interests are formed. These may be classified as dominant (professional monopoly), challenging (corporate rationalism), or repressed (equal health advocacy). Interests are dominant if they have achieved ideological status—that is, they do not have to organise to defend their interests because other institutions do that for them. Challenging interests seek the overthrow or modification of the dominant interests, while repressed interests are kept under

pluralism
A theory whereby state power is shared with a large number of pressure or interest groups.

socialisation
The process of learning the culture of a society (its language and customs), which shows us how to behave and communicate.

Helen Belcher

control by the actions of dominant and challenging interests. To be heard they usually must align themselves with the dominant or challenging interests

Pluralist accounts of health insurance assume too level a playing field. They ignore the role of ideology in shaping the context within which decision-making occurs, as well as the dominance of some interests over others. Pluralism also ignores the unequal distribution of resources, although this inequality impedes the effective mobilisation of competing interests (Gardner 1995). More satisfying explanations are provided by Lukes and Alford.

By far the most powerful group of people within the health care system are doctors—the professional monopolists. **Medical dominance** is derived not through a natural process but, rather, through scientific medical knowledge, which means that 'patients depend on their doctor to define their malady and propose the alternative treatments available. This monopoly of therapeutic knowledge' underpins the profession's dominance (Gillespie 1991, p. 16). Moreover, fee-for-service medicine provides economic autonomy. It allows doctors to set their own fees albeit modified by the operation of government fee schedules. Maintenance of this arrangement is supported by private health insurance. Hence doctors have a strong incentive to support its retention. Whilst fee-for-service medicine appears secure in Australia, support for private health insurance is fluid. This chapter now turns to an examination of that situation.

Health insurance arrangements in Australia

There are various health insurance models, which range across two continuums: selective–universal coverage and public–private provision.

Selective coverage, influenced by economic liberalism, is targeted, usually by means testing, so that only those considered unable to provide for themselves receive benefits and/or services. It assumes that most people will be responsible for their own health care needs and hence favours private provision purchased in the market. Private health insurance then is a residual measure.

Universal coverage, a product of social liberalism, provides benefits and/or services for the whole population. It assumes collective responsibility that is delivered by the state and financed through taxation. Attitudes to health insurance in Australia have oscillated between these two broad approaches.

Organisation of health care in Australia has its origins in colonial settlement. At that time, the colony's administration was the only source of health care. This was partly attributable to the government's responsibility for the needs of the convicts and their gaolers, but is also explained by the absence of two traditional sources of support: families and the Church (see Sax 1984). Throughout the nineteenth century, the emphasis was on self-help, an ideal embodied in the **Friendly Societies**. In exchange for the payment of regular amounts, members and their families were

---

medical dominance
A general term used to describe the power of the medical profession in terms of its control over its own work, over the work of other health workers, and over health resource allocation, health policy, and the way that hospitals are run.

Friendly Societies
An organisation based on membership fees that serves the collective interests of its members, offering health insurance and welfare services, and sometimes social club activities such as dances and sports teams.

entitled to the services of a 'lodge doctor', who entered into contracts with the Societies in exchange for a capitation fee (Green & Cromwell 1984; Gillespie 1991).

Throughout the nineteenth century, growth in medical knowledge and medical status led to increased demand for medical and hospital care, not only among the poor but also among those considered able to pay. Government, however, opted for a 'hands-off' policy, leaving hospital funding to voluntary charitable organisations. This resulted in a three-tiered system:

1   The better-off in the community sought private medical services. They were also expected to contribute to charities for the support of the poor (Crichton 1990).
2   Friendly Societies catered for the working man and his dependants (Green & Cromwell 1984; Gillespie 1991).
3   Those who could not afford private medical services or Friendly Society contributions either went without or attended public hospital out-patient clinics. The poor depended on charity (Sax 1984; Crichton 1990; Daniel 1995).

The question of who could be treated free of charge created a dilemma for medical professionals and for the state, reaching crisis points between the two World Wars. James Gillespie argues that this dilemma provided the climate for the development of hospital insurance schemes that 'epitomised the two major tendencies of the organisation of interwar medical practice—the move towards collective responsibility for the costs of health care and the hegemony of the hospital' (1991, p. 27).

By 1949, a clear division had developed between conservative and labour forces over health insurance arrangements. Many doctors, who were aligned with the newly formed conservative Liberal Party, pushed for fee-for-service medicine financed by private contribution, and subsidies for those unable to provide for themselves or their families (Crichton 1990). Working-class leaders, aware of the strain placed on the Friendly Societies by the economic depressions of the 1890s and the 1930s, identified with the Australian Labor Party and its push for universal, non-contributory health care schemes.

Tensions between the two major political parties and their supporters were evident in the debates over Labor's attempts to introduce a comprehensive 'free' national health scheme (Dewdney 1972). Doctors—partly influenced by the experience of their British colleagues with National Health Insurance and their fear of loss of autonomy (Gillespie 1991)—combined with conservative politicians. Together they depicted Labor's attempts as a communist threat. The failure of the Chifley Government adequately to counter medical and opposition tactics thwarted any changes that would threaten doctors' control of the health care system (Crichton 1990). In fact, doctors' influence was extended, most notably through the addition of Paragraph xxiii (A) to section 51 of the Constitution.

In 1945, the Victorian Attorney-General, acting on behalf of the Victorian branch of the British Medical Association (BMA), challenged the *Pharmaceutical*

Benefits Act 1945 (Cwlth) in the High Court. This Act allowed patients to receive pharmaceutical benefits only if the doctor's prescription was written on a government-supplied form. The Court ruled the Commonwealth did not have the power to provide or finance health services. Therefore, the government's request that doctors use a prescribed form was unconstitutional (Gillespie 1991). Alarmed by this ruling, the government sought to amend Section 51 of the Constitution by referendum. Robert Menzies, the leader of the Liberal Party, agreed to the change but insisted on the inclusion of the phrase 'but not so as to authorise any form of civil conscription'. It had been suggested by the BMA president who was concerned the amendment as proposed would allow for the nationalisation of medical and dental services (Dewdney 1972; Sax 1984; Gillespie 1991). The government agreed to the addition, finally putting to the people an amendment that would allow for a wide range of welfare services, such as the widows' pensions, family allowances, pharmaceutical, hospital, medical and dental benefits (though civil conscription of doctors was specifically barred). The success of the referendum enabled government to provide a wide range of welfare services (Bloom 2000), but it also provided doctors with a mechanism to forestall attempts that might subject them to non-medical control (Sax 1984).

Following the defeat of the Chifley Government in 1949, the new Conservative Menzies Government introduced a voluntary health insurance scheme known as the Page Plan. It replaced Labor's universal and compulsory scheme with a subsidised voluntary insurance scheme that required a 'co-payment'. Voluntary insurance was 'the Christian idea of mutual assistance' (Fadden cited in Gillespie 1991, p. 253), and as such would be 'Australia's answer to socialized medicine' (Page cited in Gillespie 1991, p. 254). Existing voluntary insurance organisations, including Friendly Societies, served as the administrative vehicles, a move that accelerated implementation, but also ensured market involvement. The Plan did not remove state intervention. Universal fee-for-service benefits originally gazetted by the Chifley Government were enshrined 'as the central principle of medical remuneration, but only at the expense of handsome subsidization by the taxpayer' (Gillespie 1991, p. 280). Finally, the Plan preserved the existing doctor–patient relationship. All Australians would receive good medical treatment 'regardless of ability to pay the full price ... without destroying or damaging beyond repair the freedom of the medical profession and the vital relationship between doctor and patient' (Page cited in Fox 1963, p. 876). Voluntary subsidised insurance, then, reflected the government's concern with individual initiative, market involvement, and limited state intervention (Dewdney 1972; Sax 1984; Gray 1991; Scotton & Macdonald 1993, pp. 9–11).

By the end of the 1960s it was clear that there were problems with the Page Plan, not the least being rising contribution rates and gaps in coverage that meant patients were liable for one third instead of one tenth of doctor's fees (Sax 1984; Scotton &

Macdonald 1993). As Sax explained, approximately 17 per cent of the population had no insurance and an unspecified number were underinsured. While they were not turned away from hospitals 'they deprived themselves of other goods and services in order to discharge their debts or the hospitals had to write off bad debts. Because insured benefits were roughly proportional to fees, high use contributors accumulated big out-of-pocket expenses' (1984, p. 78). Clearly the biggest impact fell on those least able to fend for themselves—the chronically ill, the aged, and poor. Moreover there were rumblings about the rapid growth in public expenditure, much of which was generated by suppliers, with little evidence of improved health outcomes (Dewdney 1972; Crichton 1990).

The election of a Labor Government in December 1972 offered an opportunity to address growing levels of dissatisfaction. Labor argued voluntary health insurance had failed, that the playing field was not level, and therefore that as a matter of justice the community as a whole should bear the responsibility for the health of its citizens. Access was not a privilege, but a right, and this was best achieved by a compulsory scheme (Sax 1984). Consequently it introduced Medibank, which provided universal cover for free public hospital accommodation and treatment, and 85 per cent of the schedule fee for medical services, with a maximum $5 gap payment (Willcox 1991). Its introduction was strongly resisted by doctors, private hospitals, and private health insurance providers. They argued that the scheme amounted to unwarranted interference in the market and in the relations between doctor and patient (Sax 1984).

The Coalition's return to power in December 1975, only months after the introduction of Medibank, marked a gradual move away from universality and a return to selectivity, all in the name of choice and competition. Over a period of several years, Medibank was slowly dismantled culminating in the Fraser Government's 1981 abandonment of the goal of universal coverage and the re-establishment of a private insurance system. Financial insecurity and the debt collector again became features of the Australian health care system (Scotton & Macdonald 1993; Gray 2004).

The reintroduction of universal health insurance, renamed Medicare, followed the ALP's win in the 1983 election. Old animosities between the medical profession and the ALP re-emerged, finding expression in the New South Wales specialists' strikes of 1983 and 1985. Ostensibly these strikes were over Section 17 of the *Health Insurance Act 1983* (Cwlth), which sought 'to safeguard the balance between the private and public sectors within public hospitals, to restrain the rates of growth of diagnostic services, and to protect the interests of patients by ensuring the appropriateness of fees charged where publicly funded facilities were used to provide services' (Committee of Inquiry into Rights of Private Practice, as cited in Sax 1990, p. 75). Doctors, on the other hand, perceived Section 17 as unnecessary interference in their right to practise and as an attempt to nationalise the health care system (Crichton 1990; Sax 1990). An ideological clash between doctors and politicians erupted, with the doctors arguing for freedom of choice and the government arguing for the right to control practice in the interest of economic stability. The Federal Government eventually backed down, but Medicare survived and grew in popularity. Private health insurance declined—down from 50 per cent in June 1984 to 34.3 per cent in December 1995 (AIHW 1996)—prompting grim predictions that the public hospital system would collapse under the weight of public admissions. Doctors and conservative politicians argued this could only be avoided by increasing the numbers of privately insured individuals and/or the dismantling of Medicare, which they argued promoted over-servicing and inefficiency.

The election of the Coalition in March 1996 again shifted the focus of the health insurance debate. Defeat in the 1993 election—partly attributed to the Liberal–National Party's promise to replace Medicare with a private system—prompted a Coalition change of heart. Consequently, the Howard Government retained Medicare, but set about increasing the attractiveness of private health insurance. In the 1996 Budget, two moves were announced to encourage the purchase of private health insurance. The first entitled those with private health insurance to an annual tax rebate worth $450 for families and $125 for individuals. The second added a 1 per cent surcharge to the Medicare levy for individuals/families with no health insurance. These incentives were justified by recourse to the argument that they supported the right of individuals to choose, and they would reduce the pressure on public hospitals (Gray 2004; Foster & Fleming 2008).

The level of private insurance did not increase, but rather continued to fall reaching its lowest level in December 1998. In an effort to redress this fall, the Coalition replaced its 1996 initiative with the non-means tested 30 per cent tax rebate, an initiative that met with only limited success. Further measures were required; hence the Coalition Government announced a modification of the community rating system and introduced 'Lifetime Health Cover'. As of July 2000, private health insurers were permitted to set a different premium for different people depending on the age that they first took out private health insurance cover. The government argued this would 'stabilise the private health sector, it will take the pressure off Medicare, and give Australians a real choice in their health care' (Wooldridge 1999). In the 12 months leading up to its introduction, Australians were bombarded with an advertising campaign that critics argue implied Medicare was in crisis (Gray 2004). Regardless, the introduction of 'Lifetime Health Cover' is credited with a reversal with coverage increasing from 32.2 per cent in the quarter prior to its introduction to 45.7 per cent in the September 2000 quarter (Duckett 2007, p. 56; PHIAC 2008).

The introduction of Medibank in 1975 and Medicare in 1984 was strongly resisted by doctors, who clung to the old bogey that it would mark the fall of medicine to a socialist scheme. In particular, they raised concerns related to 'fees, conditions of service in public hospitals, a perceived threat to private hospitals and the pernicious threat that could be exerted by a single government-directed paymaster' (Sax 1984, pp. 109–10). Health insurance funds, drawing on the ideology of economic liberalism, argued for 'the virtues of freedom of choice through subsidised insurance and the retention of an element of market activity' (Sax 1984, p. 112). Dilution of either would compromise the quality of care, a view that also accorded with that of the Coalition (Sax 1984; Gray 2004). While the medical pressure of doctors, supported by the insurers and the Coalition, did result in some modification of both schemes, their influence was moderated by the efforts of the corporate rationalisers and equal health advocates (Duckett 1984). Doctors and their allies still retain a large measure of professional and economic control, which finds expression in continued support for private health insurance. During its term, the Howard Government, mindful of the popularity of Medicare, vowed it would retain the scheme in its entirety. At the same time it introduced measures that accorded with its ideological commitment to freedom of choice and individual responsibility, views that accorded with those of the medical profession (Gray 2004).

In November 2007, the Coalition was defeated and the ALP assumed power. During the course of the election it promised to retain key aspects of the Coalition's private health arrangements, including the retention of the 30 per cent rebate and 'Lifetime Health Cover'. It also retained the Medicare surcharge, but in line with its commitment to middle- and low-income earners it announced it would raise the income threshold that triggered its activation.

BOX 18.1 Doing health sociology: unpacking health insurance debates

Private health insurance is generally perceived as a legitimate and preferable means of funding access to health care in Australia, partly because it provides choice and takes the pressure off Medicare and the public system (Australian Health Insurance Association 2005). There are nevertheless concerns that it is administratively expensive, removes the brake on provider costs, acts as a disincentive to provide public goods, and compromises the achievement of equity (McAuley 2008). Health sociology acts as a lens through which we can examine the social patterns and interactions that constitute health insurance arrangements. Historical, cultural, and structural factors highlight the influence of our personal views on arrangements that facilitate access to health care. A critical eye suggests alternative ways of providing access. Use of the sociological imagination then helps us to understand the links between personal troubles, such as illness, and public issues, such as access to health care services.

Helen Belcher

Beyond Left and Right: the pragmatics of health policy

Critics argue improving the attractiveness of private health insurance increases the pressure to introduce 'opting out' provisions similar to those that marked the end of Medibank. Indeed, they argue that support for private health insurance reflects an ideological position that downplays government involvement and supports the operation of the market for those who can afford to pay and charity for those unable to pay. This ideological nature is reflected in the cost of the 30 per cent health insurance rebate, which amounted to $3.2 billion in 2005–06 (AIHW 2008, p. 401 and 427), money which would best be directed towards increasing investment in public hospitals and the public health care system. The Coalition's support for private health insurance and moves to privatise health are consistent with a legitimate view of the world, but questions remain as to its desirability. Certainly, support for the 30 per cent rebate encourages individual responsibility, but it also distorts health care arrangements in that it impinges on the access of others, most notably the poorer and sicker members of society who cannot afford health insurance premiums. Private health insurance not only allows individuals to 'jump the queue' but also denies access to doctors who cannot be in two places at the same time.

> There is, therefore, a head-on-head conflict between the liberal–libertarian 'right' of individuals to spend their income on health care and the communitarian–solidarity 'right' of individuals in a community to have equal access to high-quality medical care. The latter goal must necessarily be achieved by imposing some constraint upon income-based preferential care to a particular group in the community. In Australia, this 'penalty' has taken the form of requiring full taxation and payment of the Medicare levy by those who are likely to use Medicare services less because they have purchased private health insurance, and consequently, are more likely to use private services (Richardson 2003, p. 13).

It is generally agreed that medical care should be available to all those who need it, but differences emerge over how this is best achieved. While no party can claim a monopoly on any one view, doctors and conservative politicians—influenced by economic liberalism's emphasis on self-help and individual responsibility—have generally opted for restricted state intervention when the market and the family break down. The ALP and its supporters—influenced by social liberalism—have tended to opt for the expansion of state intervention in the belief that this will allow citizens not only to enjoy the fruits that society can offer but also to participate in the shaping of society (Sax 1984). Each government has tended to keep key aspects of the previous government's policies whilst also tinkering with those policies so that they reflect their own ideological position. 'The result is a set of programs, some "socialist", some "market", and many lacking any ideological basis other than a wish to serve the needs of privileged interest groups' (McAuley & Menadue 2007, p. 10).

Conclusion

The value of the sociological imagination applied to health policy is that it reveals its complexity. At the same time it enables analysts to identify the impediments to change and may assist in the identification of solutions. This chapter has outlined the historical and cultural influences upon the development of health policy, in this case health insurance. Australia's penal origins, her smallness, and isolation, produced a citizenry that unlike her American counterparts looks to the state for some measure of collective responsibility for the welfare of her population. At the same time she has been suspicious of 'big brother', a fact also attributable to our origins, our size, and isolation.

Structural factors that have shaped the way health policy and more particularly health insurance have been organised include the federal organisation of the Australian health care system, the role of ideology, and the relationship between, and power exercised by, the various structural interests, namely the professional monopolists, the corporate rationalisers, and equal health advocates. The present health insurance arrangements are not a 'natural' part of Australian health policy. Rather, they are a consequence of historical, social, political, economic, ideological, and cultural factors, which together with vested interests have produced the current health insurance arrangements.

Understanding the role of the first three blocks of the sociological imagination is important for any decision on how things might be improved for the benefit of all Australians. The history of Australian health care financing reveals that government involvement is a contested issue, especially as it relates to the question of compulsion versus freedom of choice (Sax 1984; Crichton 1990; Duckett 1995; Gray 2004). It also reveals a strong pragmatic streak. The Coalition retained Medicare—a consequence of strong community support (Medicare Australia 2007)—but introduced measures that assist private health insurance. Similarly, the ALP retained the privatisation measures but moulded them to reflect its preferred shape. For that reason it opted for changes to the income thresholds described in the vignette. As already noted, Australians tend to look to government for solutions, but at the same time retain a suspicion of too much interference. Solutions that fail to take account of these tendencies will either falter or face a stormy passage, which may explain the contrary political positions. Perhaps, then, it would be preferable to argue that health insurance policy in Australia reflects the influence of ideology, politics, and vested interest tempered by pragmatism. Any alternative policy, then, must accept the role of both public and private providers and acknowledge the need to maintain choice whilst also insisting on the need to ensure access for all in need, regardless of income.

Helen Belcher

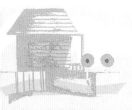

Summary of main points

» Health policy concerns the role of the state, the individual, the community, and the market.

» Key players include doctors, health insurers, private hospitals, and politicians.

» Government involvement is a contested issue.

» Health insurance policy reflects an ideological struggle between economic and social liberalism, which finds expression in the two major political parties: the Australian Labor Party and the Liberal–National Party Coalition.

» Australian health insurance arrangements are marked by pragmatism.

» History, culture, and structure have all contributed to current health insurance arrangements.

Sociological reflection: Medicare reforms

Using the four features of the sociological imagination, analyse the responses to the Rudd Government's proposal to raise the income threshold at which the Medicare surcharge is activated.

Discussion questions

1 Given that both major federal political parties have maintained key aspects of each other's health insurance measures when in government, is it reasonable to argue that health policy reflects the relationship between politics, power, ideology, and structural interests?

2 Reflect on your attitude to health insurance. Should individuals remain free to spend their own money in whatever way they choose?

3 The cost of the private health insurance rebate amounted to $3.2 billion in 2005–06. Would this money be better directed to the support of the public health system?

4 Is it possible to have public and private provision of health care services without having a two-tier health system?

5 Thirty-eight private insurers operate in Australia. What problems does this create? Would these problems be removed if the thirty-eight insurers were replaced with a single national insurer?

6 Identify and explain the case for and against health care co-payments.

Further investigation

1 Proponents of private health insurance argue it increases choice and removes pressure from the public system while others argue the case for a single national insurer. Discuss.

2 The National Health and Hospitals Reform Commission (2008) argues that Medicare is focused on access to doctors and hospitals and not the whole person. Explain and analyse this concern.

Further reading

Beilharz, P., Considine, M. & Watts, R. 1992, *Arguing about the Welfare State: The Australian Experience*, Allen & Unwin, Sydney.

Duckett, S. J. 2007, *The Australian Health Care System*, 3rd edn, Oxford University Press, Melbourne.

Foster, M. & Fleming, J. 2008, 'The Health Care System in Australia' in S. Taylor, M. Foster & J. Fleming (eds), *Health Care Practice in Australia*, Oxford University Press, Melbourne, pp. 46–73.

Gillespie, J. A. 1991, *The Price of Health: Australian Governments and Medical Politics 1910–1960*, Cambridge University Press, Melbourne.

Gray, G. 2004, *The Politics of Medicare: Who Gets What, When and How*, UNSW Press, Sydney.

Hindle, D. & McAuley, I. 2004, 'The Effects of Increased Private Health Insurance: A Review of the Evidence', *Australian Health Review*, vol. 28. no. 1, pp. 119–38.

McAuley, I. & Menadue, J. 2007, *A Health Policy for Australia: Reclaiming Universal Health Care*, Centre for Policy Development, Sydney. Available online: <http://cpd.org.au>

National Health and Hospitals Reform Commission 2008, *Beyond the Blame Game: Accountability and Performance Benchmarks for the Next Australian Health Care Agreements*, NHHRC, Woden.

Web resources

Australian Department of Health and Ageing: <http://www.health.gov.au/>
Australian Institute of Health and Welfare (AIHW): <http://www.aihw.gov.au/>
Australian Labor Party (ALP): <http://www.alp.org.au/>
Australian Medical Association (AMA): <http://www.ama.com.au/>
Centre for Policy Development (CPD): <http://www.cpd.org.au/>
Doctors Reform Society of Australia: <http://www.drs.org.au/index.html>

Helen Belcher

• • **Online case study**
Visit the Second Opinion
website to access
relevant case studies.

Liberal Party of Australia (LPA): <http://www.liberal.org.au/>

National Health and Hospitals Reform Commission (NHHRC): <http://www.nhhrc.org.au/>

Private Health Insurance Administration Council (PHIAC): <http://www.phiac.gov.au>

Documentaries/films

Difference of Opinion (2007): 50 minutes, SBS TV. 'Do either of the main political parties have the right plan for our health system?' This episode of the current affairs program explores the major issues facing the Australian health system and the differences and similarities between the major political parties. Available online: <http://www.abc.net.au/tv/differenceofopinion/content/archives/doo_20071011.htm>

Hospital: An Unhealthy Business (1997): 57 minutes, Film Australia/ ABC TV. Based at St Vincent's Hospital, Melbourne, the documentary shows the daily problems faced in treating patients amid severe financial constraints.

References

Abercrombie, N., Hill, S. & Turner, B. 1988, *Dictionary of Sociology*, Penguin, London.

Alford, R. R. 1975, *Health Care Politics: Ideological and Interest Group Barriers to Reform*, University of Chicago Press, Chicago.

Anonymous 2008, 'Hands Off Health Rebates, Critics Say', *The Canberra Times*.

Australian Health Insurance Association 2005, 'Beyond the Hospital Gate: A New Province for Private Health Insurance AHIA Submission House of Representatives Standing Committee on Health: Inquiry into Health Funding'. Available online: <http://www.ahia.org.au/documents/AHIA%20Submission,%20House%20of%20Representatives%20-%20Inquiry%20into%20Health%20Funding%202005.pdf>

Australian Institute of Health and Welfare 1996, *Australia's Health 1996*, AGPS, Canberra.

Australian Institute of Health and Welfare 2008, *Australia's Health 2008*, AIHW, Canberra.

Bates, E. 1983, *Health Systems and Public Scrutiny: Australia, Britain and the United States*, Croom Helm, London.

Beauchamp, T. L. & Faden, R. R. 1979, 'The Right to Health and the Right to Health Care', *The Journal of Medicine and Philosophy*, vol. 4, no. 2, pp. 118–31.

Beilharz, P., Considine, M. & Watts, R. 1992, *Arguing about the Welfare State: The Australian Experience*, Allen & Unwin, Sydney.

Bloom, A. L. 2000, *Health Reform in Australia and New Zealand*, Oxford University Press, Melbourne.

Callahan, D. 1990, *What Kind of Life: The Limits of Medical Progress*, Simon & Schuster, New York.

Capolingua, R. 2008, 'Dr Rosanna Capolingua Discusses Private Health Insurance Figures and Increasing the Income Threshold on ABC 720 Perth—Mornings', in *AMA Media Transcripts*. Available online: <http://www.ama.com.au/web.nsf/doc/WEEN-7GK6DB>

Commonwealth of Australia, Senate Community Affairs References Committee 2000, *First Report—Public Hospital Funding and Options for Reform*, Commonwealth of Australia, Canberra. Available online: <http://www.aph.gov.au/senate/Committee/clac_ctte/completed_inquiries/1999-02/phealth_first/report/index.htm>

Crichton, A. 1990, *Slowly Taking Control? Australian Governments and Health Care Provision 1788–1988*, Allen & Unwin, Sydney.

Dalton, T., Draper, M., Weeks, W. & Wiseman, J. 1996, *Making Social Policy in Australia: An Introduction*, Allen & Unwin, Sydney.

Daniel, A. 1995, 'The Politics of Health: Medicine Versus the State', in G. M. Lupton & J. M. Najman (eds), *Sociology of Health and Illness: Australian Readings*, 2nd edn, Macmillan, Melbourne, pp. 57–76.

DeNavas-Walt, C., Proctor, B. D. & Mills, R. J. 2004, *Income, Poverty, and Health Insurance Coverage in the United States: 2003*, US Government Printing Office, Washington, DC.

Dewdney, J. C. H. 1972, *Australian Health Services*, John Wiley & Sons, Sydney.

Duckett, S. J. 1984, 'Structural Interests and Australian Health Policy', *Social Science & Medicine*, vol. 18, no. 11, pp. 959–66.

Duckett, S. J. 1995, 'The Australian Health Care System: An Overview', in G. M. Lupton & J. M. Najman (eds), *Sociology of Health and Illness: Australian Readings*, 2nd edn, Macmillan, Melbourne.

Duckett, S. J. 2007, *The Australian Health Care System*, 3rd edn, Oxford University Press, Melbourne.

Forder, A., Caslin, T., Ponton, G. & Walklate, S. 1984, *Theories of Welfare*, Routledge & Kegan Paul, London.

Foster, M. & Fleming, J. 2008, 'The Policy Context of Health Care Practice' in S. Taylor, M. Foster & J. Fleming (eds), *Health Care Practice in Australia*, Oxford University Press, Melbourne, pp. 131–60.

Fox, T. 1963, 'The Antipodes: Private Practice Publicly Supported', *Lancet*, vol. 20, 4 May, pp. 988–94.

Gardner, H. (ed.) 1995, *The Politics of Health: The Australian Experience*, 2nd edn, Churchill Livingstone, Melbourne.

Gillespie, J. A. 1991, *The Price of Health: Australian Governments and Medical Politics 1910–1960*, Cambridge University Press, Melbourne.

Gray, G. 1991, *Federalism and Health Policy: The Development of Health Systems in Canada and Australia*, University of Toronto Press, Toronto.

Gray, G. 2004, *The Politics of Medicare: Who Gets What, When and How*, UNSW Press, Sydney.

Green, D. G. & Cromwell, L. G. 1984, *Mutual Aid or Welfare State: Australia's Friendly Societies*, Allen & Unwin, Sydney.

Ham, C. 1992, *Health Policy in Britain: The Policies and Organisation of the National Health Service*, 3rd edn, Macmillan, London.

Ham, C., Robinson, R. & Benzeval, M. 1990, *Health Check: Health Care Reforms in an International Context*, King's Fund, London.

Haralambos, M. & Holborn, M. 1991, *Sociology: Themes and Perspectives*, 3rd edn, Collins Educational, London.

Hehir, J. B. 1996, 'Justice and Healthcare', *Chicago Studies*, vol. 35, no. 3, pp. 238–48.

Jaensch, D. 1984, *An Introduction to Australian Politics*, 2nd edn, Longman Cheshire, Melbourne.

Kymlicka, W. 1990, *Contemporary Political Philosophy: An Introduction*, The Clarendon Press, Oxford.

Lukes, S. 1974, *Power: A Radical View*, Macmillan, London.

McAuley, I. 2008, *More Than One Health Insurer is Too Many: The Case for a Single Insurer*. Available online: <http://cpd.org.au/paper/the-case-a-single-insurer>

McAuley, I. & Menadue, J. 2007, *A Health Policy for Australia: Reclaiming Universal Health Care*, Centre for Policy Development, Sydney. Available online: <http://cpd.org.au>

McClelland, A. 1991, *In Fair Health? Equity and the Health System*, Background Paper no. 3, AGPS, Canberra.

Medicare Australia 2007, *Medicare Australia 2006–07 Annual Report*. Available online: <http://www.medicareaustralia.gov.au/about/governance/reports/06-07/index.jsp>

National Center for Health Statistics, 2007, *Health, United States, 2007, With Chartbook on Trends in the Health of Americans*, Hyattsville, MD.

National Health and Hospitals Reform Commission (NHHRC) 2008, *Beyond the Blame Game: Accountability and Performance Benchmarks for the Next Australian Health Care Agreements*, NHHRC, Woden.

Private Health Insurance Administration Council 2008, Membership Statistics. Available online: <http://www.phiac.gov.au/statistics/membershipcoverage/table1.htm>

Rees, S. & Rodley, G. (eds) 1995, *The Human Costs of Managerialism: Advocating the Recovery of Humanity*, Pluto Press, Sydney.

Richardson, J. 1998, 'The Health Care Financing Debate', in G. Mooney & R. Scotton (eds), *Economics and Australian Health Policy*, Allen & Unwin, Sydney, pp. 192–213.

Richardson, J. 2003, 'Priorities of Health Policy: Cost Shifting or Population Health', Paper presented to the Australian Health Care Summit, Health Economics Unit, Monash University, Melbourne.

Ross, B., Nixon, J., Snasdell-Taylor, J. & Delaney, K. 1999, 'International Approaches to Funding Health Care', *Occasional Papers: Health Financing Series*, vol. 2, Commonwealth of Australia, Canberra. Available online: <http://www.health.gov.au/internet/main/publishing.nsf/Content/health-historicpubs-hfsocc-occpahsfv2.htm>

Sax, S. 1984, *A Strife of Interests: Politics and Policies in Australian Health Services*, Allen & Unwin, Sydney.

Sax, S. 1990, *Health Care Choices and the Public Purse*, Allen & Unwin, Sydney.

Scotton, R. B. 1998, 'The Doctor Business', in G. Mooney & R. Scotton (eds), *Economics and Australian Health Policy*, Allen & Unwin, Sydney, pp. 72–92.

Scotton, R. B. & Macdonald, C. R. 1993, *The Making of Medibank,* School of Health Services Management, University of New South Wales, Sydney.

Singleton, G., Aitkin, D., Jinks, B. & Warhurst, J. 2008, *Australian Political Institutions*, Election Update Edition, Pearson Education Australia, Frenchs Forest.

Thame, C. 1974, 'Health and the State: The Development of Collective Responsibility for Health Care in Australia in the First Half of the Twentieth Century', PhD thesis, 'The Doctors versus the Nurses' 1962, *Nursing Times*, 15 June, pp. 783–4.

Titmuss, R. M. 1974, *Social Policy: An Introduction*, Allen & Unwin, London.

Tulloch, P. 1983, 'The Welfare State and Social Policy', in B. Head (ed.), *State and Economy in Australia*, Oxford University Press, Melbourne, pp. 252–71.

Wallis, G. 2004, 'The Demand for Private Medical Insurance' in *Economic Trends*, no. 606, pp. 46–56.

Willcox, S. 1991, *A Health Risk? Use of Private Insurance*, Background Paper no. 4, AGPS, Canberra.

Wooldridge, M. 1999, 'Lifetime Cover now a Reality', Press Release 28 September 1999. Available online: <http://www.health.gov.au/internet/main/publishing.nsf/Content/health-mediarel-yr1999-mw-mw99088.htm>

Helen Belcher

CHAPTER 19

Challenges to Medical Dominance

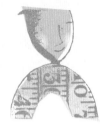

JOHN
GERMOV

Overview

- What is medical dominance?
- How did medicine become the dominant health care profession?
- In what ways are challenges to medical dominance affecting the medical profession and the organisation, delivery, and use of health services?

AUSTRALIA'S DR DEATH

In 2005, events at Bundaberg Base Hospital made media headlines worldwide due to the actions of general surgeon Dr Jayant Patel, often referred to as 'Dr Death' in the media. He has been linked to eighty-seven deaths of patients under his care, and many more cases of patient mistreatment and negligence; though these allegations are the subject of legal proceedings (Dunbar et al. 2007; Thomas 2007). While the Patel case represents an extreme example of the failure of professional peer review and hospital management to ensure patient safety, it exposes the systemic problem of medical dominance and the difficulty in challenging the clinical autonomy of doctors. Of particular concern, was the fact that whistleblowers failed to get hospital managements and fellow doctors to act in response to their claims, and ultimately turned to politicians and the media to have matters addressed.

Introduction

There would never be any public agreement among doctors if they did not agree to agree on the main point of the doctor being always in the right.

George Bernard Shaw (1908), *The Doctor's Dilemma*, preface

The term **medical dominance** refers to the fact that medicine is clearly the most powerful profession in the health system, despite comprising only 13 per cent of the total health professional workforce (ABS 2006). This chapter briefly explains what medical dominance is, how it was established, and the problems it poses to the delivery of optimal health care. The chapter then focuses on the various challenges to medical dominance that are said to be undermining medicine's influence over health care delivery, other health professions, and patients. It then examines the effectiveness of various challenges to the medical profession, showing that medical dominance has never gone unchallenged, and has often been resisted in formal and informal ways.

medical dominance
A general term used to describe the power of the medical profession in terms of its control over its own work, over the work of other health workers, and over health resource allocation, health policy, and the way that hospitals are run.

What is medical dominance?

According to Eliot Freidson (1970), a key author in the field, the professional dominance of medicine is due to doctors' clinical role of diagnosis and treatment; the ability of doctors to exert control over the knowledge base and occupational territory of other health professions; the requirement that doctors request and supervise the work of other health practitioners; and the unequal public status of medicine compared to other health professions. Furthermore, Henry Mintzberg states: '[t]he professional's power derives from the fact that not only is his [*sic*] work too complex to be supervised by managers or standardized by analysts, but also that his services are typically in great demand ... which enables him to insist on considerable autonomy in his work' (1979, p. 357).

The medical profession dominates every aspect of health care delivery, particularly other health professions such as nursing and allied health, in the following ways:

- Only doctors can formally diagnose disease and sign birth and death certificates, and they have significant control over access to non-medical benefits, such as sick leave, workers' compensation, and early retirement due to health reasons.
- Doctors' control of diagnosis and treatment means that they effectively have administrative and financial authority over other health professions. The decisions of doctors set in train the work of nursing and allied health professionals who are either directly or indirectly responsible to doctors' authority, particularly

John Germov

within the hospital system. This means that doctors can control access to a range of therapies through the requirement of a doctor's referral before other health professions can treat a patient.

- Doctors are over-represented on hospital management boards, the registration boards of most other health professions, health policy advisory bodies, and the bodies that fund health research. Such a situation limits the ability of alternative, nursing, and allied health practitioners to produce evidence to support their work and expand their occupational roles, which could potentially challenge the legitimacy of medical expertise if their treatments are proven to be particularly effective.

As Freidson points out, the key feature of medical dominance is autonomy, which he defines as the 'authority to direct and evaluate the work of others without in turn being subject to formal direction and evaluation by them' (Freidson 1970, p. 135). Mary Elston (1991) makes a useful distinction between three forms of medical autonomy that highlights the basis of medicine's dominance:

1   *economic autonomy*: the right of doctors to determine their pay rates (fee-for-service)
2   *political autonomy*: the right to make policy decisions as the legitimate experts on health matters
3   *clinical autonomy*: the right to set professional standards about treatment, which dictate hospital expenditure and the work of other health care workers (this right is enacted through licensing laws, which protect medicine from occupational encroachment).

The notion of autonomy helps to explain why many other occupational groups have achieved limited success in attempting to mimic medicine's attributes by adopting a strategy of **professionalisation**. Professionalisation assumes that professional status can be gained by simply meeting a set of criteria or traits which, once acquired, function collectively to transform an occupation into a profession. Such a **trait approach** to professionalisation reflects functionalist theory, which views professions as performing essential 'functions' for society by possessing certain attributes from which they derive their high status and rewards. The assumption behind such an understanding is that, if any occupation acquires similar attributes or traits (such as university qualifications, highly specialised knowledge and skills, or a code of ethics) it can become a profession. Despite their professional projects, nursing and allied health professions have not achieved the same level of power or status as medicine because they have been unable to acquire the essential characteristic of autonomy. They have also been deprived of the special historical and political advantages that provided the medical profession with its exclusive professional status, as the following section describes.

professionalisation
The process of becoming a profession, whereby an occupational group attains publicly recognised and government-legitimated monopoly and autonomy over its area of work.

trait approach
A functionalist theory of professions that assumes professional status can be achieved by meeting a set of criteria (usually defined as specialised expertise and training, and self-regulation through a code of ethics).

• • • **TheoryLink**
• • • Chapter 2 discusses
• • • functionalism in more
• • • detail

Medical dominance: a brief history

A number of significant works have examined the issue of professions, particularly the rise of the medical profession (see Freidson 1970, 1994; Johnson 1972; Larson 1977; Starr 1982; Larkin 1983; Abbott 1988; Gillespie 1991; see also Porter 1997; Duffin 1999; and Le Fanu 1999 for general histories of medicine). In Australia, the landmark text on the rise of the medical profession remains Evan Willis's *Medical Dominance* (1983, 1989), on which much of this section's content is based.

Medical dominance is less than a century old. During most of the nineteenth century and even in the early twentieth century, most people did not consult a doctor when they were sick, but rather visited the more affordable and accessible homeopaths, chemists, Chinese herbalists, and midwives. In the early nineteenth century, doctors had few cures and little scientific understanding of disease. Most doctors serviced the wealthy who resided in the major cities and could afford their fees. The general population was highly sceptical of medicine, particularly of surgeons, because of the high death rate from post-operative infection, particularly due to the lack of antiseptic procedures that only came into use in the 1880s (Porter 1997).

Doctor numbers in Australia were also small, with only 18 doctors for Melbourne's 20,000 residents in 1841, rising to more than 500 by 1863 (Willis 1989). As their numbers increased, mostly because of an oversupply in the United Kingdom, doctors used two political strategies to gain a competitive advantage over unqualified practitioners (the 'quacks', as some doctors refer to them) (Willis 1989). The main way to achieve this advantage was for doctors to expand their client base by establishing a health care monopoly. First, medical associations were formed to unify doctors against their competition, and second, the associations lobbied the **state** to ban 'quacks'. In 1862, the Victorian Government (with other colonies to follow) became the first to pass legislation giving doctors significant advantages, such as the exclusive use of medical titles, and the right to sign death certificates, hold government appointments, and sue for non-payment of fees. Because of the dominance of a laissez-faire ideology (minimal state intervention in economic matters), most governments were unwilling to ban 'quacks', viewing this as a curtailment of people's freedom of choice.

The major legal development that firmly entrenched medical dominance was an amendment to the Australian Constitution. Doctors have traditionally been aligned with conservative political forces that favour free enterprise and private health insurance arrangements and support the development of medical dominance. In 1946 it was the federal Labor Government that secured medical dominance by allowing a minor constitutional amendment of section 51, paragraph xxiiiA, by referendum. The primary purpose of the referendum was to enable the federal government to make laws on a range of welfare services such as maternity allowances, pensions, unemployment benefits, and medical services. The Australian branch of the British

state
A term used to describe a collection of institutions, including the parliament (government and opposition political parties), the public sector bureaucracy, the judiciary, the military, and the police.

Medical Association (BMA)—a separate Australian Medical Association (AMA) did not form until 1962—believed that the wording of the referendum would result in the nationalisation of medicine (as had occurred in the United Kingdom). On behalf of the BMA, Robert Menzies (the leader of the Opposition at the time) introduced an additional phrase, which forbade any form of civil conscription of medicine (Gillespie 1991). The Labor Government agreed to this request to lessen opposition to the referendum, which was passed by popular vote (this was one of only eight successful referenda in Australia to date). The constitutional amendment allowed federal governments to provide a wide range of welfare services, but it effectively enshrined medical autonomy in the constitution—medicine was now the only profession to be granted freedom from civil conscription. It is worth mentioning that the exact meaning of the amendment with respect to medicine has never been challenged or clarified; rather, it has been accepted as the hallmark of medical dominance in Australia and is now regarded as a naïve slip on the part of the then Labor Government.

Decades later, it was again the federal Labor Government that further entrenched medical dominance. In an effort to gain the medical profession's support in establishing Medicare in 1984, the government allowed doctors a specific 'job perk': the right to treat private patients in public hospitals. In effect, Medicare subsidises the fee-for-service system. It sets a schedule fee, which doctors and hospitals can charge for public patients, but the schedule is not compulsory for private patients since most doctors are private contractors to the public system. The system provides an incentive for doctors and hospitals to treat private patients because of the greater revenue private patients provide. Such an open-ended system—ensuring little accountability with regard to doctor and hospital practice—has sustained doctors' economic autonomy under Medicare.

As Willis (1989), among others, argues, the development of the medical profession's monopoly was guaranteed by the state through the support of fee-for-service, self-regulation, medical education (particularly the independent specialist colleges), and the suppression of competition from other health practitioners. State support was partly achieved through **class** allegiances between the profession and conservative political forces (Connell 1988). This has resulted in a commonality of lifestyles and interests between doctors and the upper class to the extent that 'doctors as a group, and medical organisations as institutions, have particular political and economic interests they do not share with most of their patients: interests in maintaining a sharp division of labour in health care, in a substantial amount of public ignorance about health, and in seeing that self-help arrangements for health care remain marginal or ineffective' (Connell 1988, p. 214). It is indeed ironic that while the state helped to establish medical dominance, a large segment of the medical profession opposes significant forms of public health care, as shown by the AMA's continued opposition to **Medicare**.

class (or social class)
A position in a system of structured inequality based on the unequal distribution of power, wealth, income, and status. People who share a class position typically share similar life chances.

Medicare
The publicly funded Australian federal government scheme that provides access to free health care in public hospitals and free or subsidised treatment by general practitioners and some specialist services.

Maintaining dominance

Willis (1989) describes four methods by which medicine has exerted control over its competition in an attempt to maintain its dominance:

1 *subordination*: ensuring that some health workers, such as nurses, midwives, and allied health practitioners, all work under the direct authority of doctors, especially within the hospital system

2 *limitation*: legally restricting the occupational territory of other health workers, such as physiotherapists, dentists, and optometrists, particularly through doctor representation on registration boards

3 *exclusion*: denying legitimacy to alternative health practitioners, such as acupuncturists, chiropractors, and homeopaths, by excluding them from registration, state-supported education, research, and public health insurance (Medicare) coverage

4 *incorporation*: the absorption of occupational territory into medical practice, such as doctors practising 'spinal manipulation'.

Despite using incorporation, subordination, limitation, and exclusionary practices, medicine has never completely dominated health care. In fact, other health professions have resisted medical dominance, with varying degrees of success. The introduction of Medibank and then Medicare (see Chapter 18) is evidence that governments can introduce policies to which many doctors are opposed. Medicine's dominance over other health therapies has also been incomplete (see Chapters 20–23).

In 1978, after a long struggle against medicine, chiropractors were able to gain formal recognition as a profession by the state through registration and funding of a university degree course (Willis 1989). Willis argues that the success of chiropractors in challenging medical dominance resulted from public support and a record of successful treatment. Chiropractors are still unable to hold positions in public hospitals and are not covered by Medicare, even though all workers' compensation schemes recognise chiropractors as primary practitioners (that is, patients do not need a doctor's referral to see them). Therefore, it is important to note that the achievement and maintenance of medical dominance does not mean that doctors have total control, and there have been, and continues to be, effective forms of resistance to the power held by this profession.

Problems with medical dominance

Medicine has often been criticised for being self-serving—placing self-interest over patient or public interest—in the delivery of health services and the treatment of disease. The profession has been accused of not being open to self-criticism, with self-regulation unable effectively to address issues of fraud, negligence, misconduct, or incompetence among its members. Media exposés of medical fraud and negligence have made the public increasingly aware of the potentially damaging effects of medical treatment and of some practitioners' exploitation of patients, which Ivan Illich (1977) termed **iatrogenesis** (see also Germov 1993, 1994). Various forms of fraud have been exposed over the years—particularly scientific fraud in the form of biased medical research (La Follette 1992), pharmaceutical fraud such as the promotion of thalidomide (Braithwaite 1984), and medical technology fraud such as the marketing of the Dalkon Shield (Cashman 1989). The patient deaths and abuses at Chelmsford Hospital and the Auckland Women's Hospital further demonstrate that self-regulation can result in the unwillingness of health professionals to engage in 'whistle-blowing' (see Daniel 1998) even in the face of allegations of gross negligence (see Coney 1988; Bromberger & Fife-Yeomans 1991).

The problems of self-regulation have often been linked with the issue of fee-for-service and the pursuit of profit, which have raised concerns over whether clinical or financial concerns determine appropriate courses of treatment (Navarro 1976, 1986, 1992). Doctors' clinical autonomy means that their decisions significantly shape resource usage in the health system, making it difficult for hospital administrations and governments to control health expenditure or evaluate the effectiveness and quality of the health care provided. Claims of overservicing and quality problems are given credence by studies showing significant variations in surgery rates between practitioners, hospitals, and regions within a country (Renwick & Sadkowsky 1991), as well differences in the diagnosis rates of certain mental health conditions, which can vary substantially between countries (Turner 1995). Medicine's monopoly over clinical decision-making in terms of the diagnosis and treatment of disease has marginalised the role of other health therapies, to the possible detriment of providing optimal health care. Moreover, the **biomedical model** displaced a concern with the social origins of disease and led to the **medicalisation** of social problems and some social groups.

Medicine's monopoly has often been considered **patriarchal** for much of the last century, with many writers accusing the profession of sexism in the research, diagnosis, and treatment of disease, and in terms of discrimination against female doctors (see Broom 1991; Fee & Krieger 1994; Pringle 1998; Annandale & Hunt 2000; Annandale 2004). Barbara Ehrenreich and Deidre English (1973) highlight the oppressive role of medicine in the persecution of women healers, who were often accused of being witches in medieval Europe. The medical profession initially denied women access to medical education to become doctors. It also opposed the professionalisation of female-dominated occupations such as nursing by lobbying against the establishment of state-supported nurse registration, university education, and nurse practitioner autonomy.

Although women were initially not allowed to study medicine at university, there was a gradual entry of women into universities and thus into the profession during

iatrogenesis/ iatrogenic

A concept popularised by Ivan Illich that refers to any adverse outcome or harm as a result of medical treatment.

biomedicine/ biomedical model

The conventional approach to medicine in Western societies, based on the diagnosis and explanation of illness as a malfunction of the body's biological mechanisms. This approach underpins most health professions and health services, which focus on treating individuals, and generally ignores the social origins of illness and its prevention.

medicalisation

The process by which non-medical problems become defined and treated as medical issues, usually in terms of illnesses, disorders, or syndromes.

patriarchy

A system of power through which males dominate households. It is used more broadly by feminists to refer to society's domination by patriarchal power, which functions to subordinate women and children.

the second half of the twentieth century. Women now make up around 50 per cent of medical school enrolments in Australia, but still comprise only 26 per cent of medical practitioners, with the number of female practitioners expected to rise to 42 per cent by the year 2025 (AIHW 1996). The **women's health movement** and the increasing numbers of female doctors provide circumstantial evidence to show that medical dominance can be effectively challenged in this domain (see Chapter 7; Broom 1991; Pringle 1998).

Challenges to medical dominance: countervailing powers

It is important to point out that medical dominance has never been absolute and has also been the subject of resistance and contestation. Donald Light's (1993, 2000) concept of countervailing powers attempts to convey this situation, noting that 'the state, patient groups, the medical–industrial complex, alternative therapies ... pursue their interests resulting in power struggles' (2000, p. 203). Most doctors work in some form of **professional bureaucracy** (Mintzberg 1979) and have always been subject to bureaucratic and budgetary constraints (Abbott 1988; Light 1993, 2000; Barnett et al. 1998). For example, a number of authors have written about how the organisation of hospitals reflects a constant tension between the power structures of bureaucratic authority and medical autonomy (Turner 1995). Therefore, while the medical profession has considerable power over the provision of health care, there are countervailing powers that constrain and even oppose medical influence.

Many authors have highlighted a range of factors that imply that medical dominance is in decline, such as the professionalisation strategies of allied health practitioners (see Chapter 22); new models of health that focus on prevention, social factors, and community care (see Chapter 24); and the increasing popularity of alternative therapies (see Chapter 21). In the remainder of this chapter we will discuss three broad social trends that represent the major challenges to medical dominance: **deprofessionalisation**, **corporatisation**, and **McDonaldisation**.

Deprofessionalisation

Deprofessionalisation is the process by which medicine's monopoly over knowledge, and its authority over the patient, is reduced as a result of increased public knowledge and influence over the health system (Haug 1973, 1988). According to Marie Haug, increasing rates of education and the emphasis on health promotion have produced a vast health literature as well as increased awareness of health issues, meaning that the power and mystique of medical practice is in decline. The media has contributed

women's health movement
A term used broadly to describe attempts to address sexism in medicine by highlighting the importance of gender in health research and treatment. Achievements include women's health centres and the National Women's Health Policy.

professional bureaucracy
Henry Mintzberg's (1979) term for an organisation that relies on staff with specialised knowledge and expertise to deliver complex services that require decision-making autonomy at the point of service delivery.

deprofessionalisation
A general theory predicting the decline of medical status and power due to the public's increased education about health issues and diminishing trust in medical practice as a result of media exposés of medical fraud and negligence.

corporatisation
A process referring to the decline of medical power as a result of the salaried employment of doctors in private sector health organisations, whereby corporate managers impose controls over medical practice.

McDonaldisation
A term coined by George Ritzer to expand Weber's notion of rationalisation; defined as the standardisation of social life by rules and regulations, such as increased monitoring and evaluation of individual performance, akin to the uniformity and control measures used by fast-food chains.

further to the demystification of medicine through exposures of medical fraud and medical negligence, leading to a decline of medical status.

The extent of medical fraud has been estimated at 7 per cent of health expenditure (Germov 1995). Medi-fraud can take a number of forms, such as:

- charging for work never done or for services more extensive than those provided
- overservicing (unnecessary treatment, testing, and hospitalisation)
- unnecessary referrals to other specialists as a result of fee-splitting arrangements
- treating so many patients per day that adequate treatment is rendered impossible
- unfairly giving private patients priority over public patients in public hospitals because of the increased revenue they provide.

Overservicing may not only result from conscious attempts to defraud, but may also be the consequence of improper clinical practices, negligence (see Box 19.1), or the lack of alternative forms of treatment. Where overservicing results in direct financial gain to the practitioner, it is a form of fraud (Auditor-General 1992; Health Insurance Commission 1993). While attempts to explain medi-fraud can easily lead to the demonisation of doctors, the key issue is that the structure of the health system allows self-regulation, which provides an incentive for some doctors to pursue profit at patient and public expense.

BOX 19.1 Medical negligence and adverse events

In 1996, *The Quality in Australian Health Care Study* found that 16 per cent of hospital patients experienced an 'adverse event', 50 per cent of which were preventable, and 10 per cent of which resulted in disability or death (TQAHC 1996; see also Wilson et al. 1999). More recent estimates suggest the cost to the health system of medical errors in Australia is between $1 and 2 billion each year (Armstrong et al. 2007). While this is an alarming figure, the numbers partly reflect the known risks and chance of human error that can occur when people undergo some medical procedures. The figures for adverse events are significantly higher than those reported in the USA. Despite the conclusions of the 1996 Report, the Federal Government never endorsed or systematically

acted on its findings (Wilson et al. 1999), and thus there are insufficient data to determine whether any improvements have occurred. A study of Victorian hospitals in 2003–04 is suggestive of little improvement, finding that adverse events cost the state health system around $460 million, representing 16 per cent of total hospital expenditure (Ehsani et al. 2006). A review of so-called 'sentinel events'— medical accidents involving operations on the wrong patient or body part, or leaving medical instruments in a patient's body leading to the need for another operation—found 130 reported events in 2004–05, with 41 per cent of cases concerning operating on the wrong patient or body part (AIHW 2007).

The deprofessionalisation trend is also reflected in the organised efforts of the women's health movement and the consumer health movement (these include carers, and disability and illness-specific interest groups, for example), which have emphasised patient rights of choice of treatment, access to information, and informed consent (including informed financial consent). The acknowledgment of patient rights represents a clear displacement of medical autonomy in favour of patient autonomy, and they are increasingly being recognised by the courts and governments. Moreover, the introduction of the *Australian Charter of Healthcare Rights* on 22 July 2008 (see: <http://www.safetyandquality.gov.au>) and the establishment of health care complaints commissions by state governments are further evidence of a shifting balance of power between doctors and patients.

The focus on patient rights can often involve a conception of an 'ideal' health consumer who is assertive, knowledgeable, critical, and prepared to shop around for the best deal. Treating patients as consumers tends to replace concerns about access and equity with a more individualistic model, in which the emphasis on meeting consumer demands ignores all those 'consumers' who find it difficult to make demands, such as the elderly, the chronically sick, and the disabled (Hindess 1987). The assumption of the 'ideal consumer' pervades the discussion of patient rights, according to which decisions and actions are based on maximising the satisfaction of individual wants and desires, ignoring the possibility that choices may be manipulated or determined by an individual's social location or by inequalities in **social structure**, particularly in the case of marginalised groups (Stretton & Orchard 1994). There is little evidence that doctor–patient interaction has moved away from the traditional relationship of trust and dependence: most patients continue not to invoke their rights as 'active' consumers, rarely question doctors even when they have not understood what they have been told, and are generally unable to evaluate whether medical services are good or bad (Lloyd et al. 1991). Such findings dampen the enthusiasm surrounding patient rights and highlight the limits of the deprofessionalisation challenge to medical dominance.

The deprofessionalisation thesis also predicted that medicine's monopoly over health care delivery would be undermined by competition from alternative practitioners. Some authors suggest that a new form of **medical pluralism** is emerging whereby people are increasingly using a range of traditional, orthodox, and alternative health therapies to maintain health and address illness, similar to what existed in the era before medical dominance (see Cant & Sharma 1999). The popularity of alternative health care is increasingly challenging medicine, leading some doctors to incorporate alternative therapies such as acupuncture and spinal manipulation into their own practice. Such a development means that doctors can practise alternative therapies with minimal training and receive Medicare payments (with no cost to the patient) under the pretence of a normal consultation, giving them an unfair advantage over alternative practitioners (who are not covered by Medicare). In this

social structure
The recurring patterns of social interaction through which people are related to each other, such as social institutions and social groups.

medical pluralism
A general term that refers to the vast array of healing modalities across the globe, in particular to the increasing popularity of alternative therapies and their coexistence with biomedicine in Westernised societies.

way, medical dominance is actually reasserted as alternative therapists suffer a market disadvantage by having to charge patients full fees for service or primarily rely on patients who have private health insurance which may cover some of the costs of alternative therapies.

From proletarianisation to corporatisation

John McKinlay and John Stoeckle (1988) proposed a neo-Marxist proletarianisation thesis to explain developments in the United States' health system, in which profit-motivated health companies had transformed the way medical services were delivered (McKinlay & Arches 1985; McKinlay & Stoeckle 1988; Salmon 1990, 1994). According to this view, corporations are increasingly controlling the provision of health care, with doctors employed on salaries and thus subject to corporate goals and organisational regulations that serve to diminish their clinical and economic autonomy. The proletarianisation thesis always encountered **empirical** problems when applied to countries such as the United Kingdom and Australia with predominantly public health systems. In both countries, medicine has retained self-regulation and has maintained substantial influence over the use of health resources through clinical and political autonomy. Most commentators have ceased using the term proletarianisation and replaced it with corporatisation, as a more accurate depiction of the trend towards corporate control of health care delivery.

In recent years there has been a growing trend towards the corporatisation of general practice in Australia, which may lend further weight to the corporatisation thesis. A number of large companies have expanded their presence in the field of general practice by taking over the ownership and management of existing clinics (see White 2000; Travaglia & Braithwaite 2007). Corporate ownership is likely to place constraints on doctors' clinical autonomy through restrictive work practices and revenue quotas as corporations seek to increase shareholder value through significant yearly returns on investment (Starr 1982; Saks 2003; Cockerham 2004). Not only may this have negative implications for the quality of patient care, but 'corporatised doctors' would be required to use company specialists and diagnostic services (pathology and radiology clinics), intensifying the **medical–industrial complex** and potentially providing an incentive for overservicing.

The term 'medical–industrial complex', originally coined by Vicente Navarro and colleagues in the late 1960s (see Navarro 1998) and popularised by Arnold Relman (1980), describes the role of large profit-oriented corporations in health care. It highlights the **commodification of health care** (Connell 1988) and the often stark contradiction between earning profits and meeting the health needs of the community. This has been an especially important insight in the USA, which has a significantly underfunded public health system, whereby more than 47 million Americans have no public or private health cover (National Coalition on Health Care 2008).

empirical
Describes observations or research that is based on evidence drawn from experience. It is therefore distinguished from something based only on theoretical knowledge or on some other kind of abstract thinking process.

medical–industrial complex
The growth of profit-oriented medical companies and industries, whereby one company may own a chain of health services, such as hospitals, clinics, and radiology and pathology services.

commodification of health care
Treating health care as a commodity to be bought and sold in the pursuit of profit maximisation.

McDonaldisation

A neo-Weberian perspective on challenges to medical dominance highlights the increasing bureaucratic and managerial control of doctors' work, in which new managerial strategies have been introduced to constrain doctors' clinical autonomy. George Ritzer (1993) conceptualises these attempts as part of a wider social trend towards the McDonaldisation of society—in which the characteristic features that govern the work organisation of fast-food restaurants are coming to dominate increasing areas of society. Ritzer uses the example of 'McDoctors', who work in 24-hour fast-food-type clinics that are 'based on rules, regulations, and controls so that what physicians do in them will be highly predictable' (1993, p. 97). McDoctors have limited autonomy as a result of increased monitoring and evaluation of their daily work performance. In Australia such private chains have had a limited impact to date. A more substantial development has been the rise of **managerialism** in the public health sector.

Managerialism and clinical governance

Since the 1990s, successive waves of managerial strategies have been introduced into public health sectors, such as 'best practice' and Total Quality Management (TQM), to name only a couple. Such strategies have involved highly specified performance criteria, sometimes in the form of contractual relations, performance targets and measures, and work-specific protocols, which have attempted to rein in doctors' clinical autonomy.

An extensive literature has examined the impact of managerialism in the health sector, with a particular emphasis on its impact on medicine (see Coburn 1988, 2006; Clarke & Newman 1997; Exworthy & Halford 1999; Clarke et al. 2000; Harrison & Ahmad 2000; Hughes & Light 2002; Allsop 2006; Dent 2006; Hunter 2006; Kelleher et al. 2006). To varying degrees, there is an emerging consensus in the literature that managerial strategies are making inroads into constraining medical autonomy. The success of the new public sector managers cannot be judged by the profits they earn (as with their private sector counterparts); rather, they are judged by the 'savings' they can accrue. The focus on management is to 'do more with less'; but as numerous critics point out, the danger is that in doing so concerns with quality service delivery become marginalised. Nonetheless, managerialism has been one of the key trends affecting the work of all health professionals, particularly doctors.

One of the first applications of managerialism in the health sector in Australia involved the introduction of 'casemix' and Diagnosis Related Groups (DRGs). Casemix is a funding system that relates hospital resource use to specific treatments given to patients and makes possible the comparison of hospital performance. DRGs are a casemix classification system based on the grouping of patients of similar

TheoryLink
Chapter 2 discusses Weberianism in more detail.

managerialism
The introduction of private sector management techniques into the public sector.

clinical conditions to determine treatment costs. Concerns have been raised that such funding models lead to the premature release of patients to keep costs down (discharging patients 'quicker and sicker'), with hospitals shifting responsibility for continued care onto the community (Draper 1992; Braithwaite & Hindle 1998).

Clinical governance is a term that has gained currency in the United Kingdom as part of the Labour Government's reforms of the health system. It is often used as an umbrella term to describe a range of quality assurance measures at the clinical level, but its exact meaning and the measures it refers to remain the subject of some debate (Flynn 2002). Liam Donaldson (1998, 2000), one of the original architects of clinical governance measures in the United Kingdom, views them as a means to address variations in medical practice, prevent unnecessary errors and ensure that clinical practice reflects state-of-the-art **evidence-based medicine (EBM)**. Clinical governance essentially refers to attempts to control doctors' clinical autonomy through the standardisation of their clinical practices using various types of performance measurement, work protocols, and benchmarking. It involves the measurement, comparison, and standardisation of medical practitioners' individual and team performance in hospital settings, and represents the extension of the rationalisation process to clinical activity. For example, 'critical pathways' (also known as clinical pathways) are commonly being developed to direct medical treatment decisions. A critical pathway is a set of clinical practice guidelines that map the provision of services in a chronological manner in terms of diagnosis and treatment for a specific condition. The pathway also serves to identify and remove variance in patient treatment and aims to achieve optimal patient care.

Clinical governance essentially involves an attempt to micro-manage the daily clinical decisions and work practices of health professionals. In this sense it is a direct response to the issues of rising health care costs, fraud, negligence, and error, as well as an attempt to address patient rights in terms of public accountability. Clinical governance heralds an era where the performance of individual doctors and hospitals can be publicly comparable in terms of cost, timeliness, and clinical standards of effective treatment outcomes. It is an attempt by the state to exercise control over the medical profession at the clinical level—the last bastion of medical dominance. Since the establishment of clinical protocols require the cooperation of clinicians, it remains to be seen how effective a challenge they will be to medical dominance.

Managerialism in its general and clinical modes may represent the most effective challenge to medical dominance to date. In particular, the move towards clinical governance has been cushioned from severe medical resistance because it is difficult to object to the pursuit of accountability and comparability of performance, although they ultimately represent a significant threat to the clinical and economic autonomy of medicine. As with all predictions of the imminent demise of medical dominance, caution should be adopted, as the medical profession has proven itself to be highly adaptable and resilient.

clinical governance
A term to describe a range of quality assurance measures that control doctors' clinical decision-making through standardised work protocols and performance measurement at the clinical level.

evidence-based medicine (EBM)
An approach to medicine that maintains that all clinical practice should be based on evidence from randomised control trials (RCTs) to ensure treatment effectiveness and efficacy.

BOX 19.2 Doing health sociology: negotiating managerialism

An Australian study examined the impact of managerialism on a broad range of nursing, allied health, and medical practitioners (Germov 2005). The study found that health professionals were able to exercise considerable agency to influence the way in which managerial strategies were implemented at the clinical level. Due to the complexity of clinical work, the imposition of clinical governance cannot take place without the explicit involvement and at least tacit agreement of health professionals themselves. According to the study findings, managerial strategies at the clinical level, while designed and implemented by health professionals, had the effect of standardising professional practice through clinical protocols, critical pathways, and contractual relations. Such managerial strategies were incorporated into professional practice as a 'survival strategy' in the context of cost and staffing pressures (Germov 2005).

Future directions: continuing challenges to medical dominance

Despite predictions of the decline of medical dominance in the context of increasing bureaucratic and corporate constraints, Freidson (1994) maintains that the medical profession has been able to respond to changing social circumstances and to stave off the major threats to its power. He acknowledges that individual doctor autonomy is increasingly constrained by consumer, bureaucratic, and corporate requirements, but discounts these developments and maintains that the collective autonomy of the medical profession remains relatively intact (Freidson 1986, 1994). He argues that the medical profession has been able to maintain its power by becoming internally stratified between 'rank-and-file professionals', who continue to deliver clinical services to patients, and 'supervisory professionals' who 'are accountable for the aggregate performances of the workers ... [and who] tend to have an organizational perspective' (Freidson 1994, p. 142). Mike Dent (1998, p. 221) comes to a similar conclusion, arguing that '[m]edical autonomy can be seen to be under revision and the *individual* autonomy of the physician is giving way to a *group* version'. According to this view, the medical profession is going through a process of re-stratification (Riska 1993). Others argue that the re-stratification thesis underestimates the extent to which the extension of state control, through various managerial and financial measures, is constraining medical autonomy (Coburn et al. 1997), yet it has long been observed that the complex and indeterminate nature of medical work means that it is not easily subjected to control (Mintzberg 1979; Freidson 1994). As Dent

John Germov

● ● **TheoryLink**
● ● See Chapter 2 for an
● ● overview of symbolic
● ● interactionism.

negotiated order
A symbolic interactionist concept that refers to any form of social organisation in which the exercise of authority and the formation of rules are outcomes of human interaction and negotiation.

agency
The ability of people, individually and collectively, to influence their own lives and the society in which they live.

symbolic interactionism
This theory focuses on the micro-worlds of people as these are constructed by individuals themselves. It positions individuals, including those with mental illness, as social actors who draw from wider cultural meanings to describe their lives and circumstances.

nurse practitioner
The title given to nurses with an enhanced and extended role, such as the ability to prescribe certain drugs and undertake procedures such as Pap smears and minor surgery. In some countries (such as the USA) it may also refer to the nurse's ability to charge a fee for service.

notes, 'clinical decision-making is a complex process which cannot be standardised because patients are not standard and disease processes are themselves highly variable' (1998, p. 207).

The indeterminacy of much health care work along with the contributions of nursing and allied health professionals has always meant that medical dominance has been the product of a **negotiated order** (Strauss et al. 1963; Strauss 1978; Fine 1984). While this perspective has been criticised for implying that everything is 'open to negotiation' and thus downplaying the unequal distribution of power within an organisation such as a hospital (Day & Day 1977), it exposes the need to take into account the **agency** that nursing and allied health professionals do exert in their experience of medical dominance; something that Marxist and Weberian accounts have tended to neglect.

The concept of a negotiated order stems from the **symbolic interactionist** perspective and highlights the importance of understanding the daily interaction between health professionals, whereby nurses and allied health professionals regularly challenge and undermine medical dominance in direct and indirect ways. Furthermore, the introduction of **nurse practitioners** in Australia and elsewhere may pose a significant threat to medical practice. Moreover, the introduction of Enhanced Primary Care (EPC) to facilitate (and fund) collaboration among medical and allied health professionals heralds the opening-up of Medicare funding for allied and preventive services (see chapter 22).

David Coburn and Evan Willis (2000) point out that it is now difficult to write about the medical profession as a single group because it is increasingly fragmented into diverse and sometimes competing factions, such as the various specialities, GPs, and salaried doctors, meaning that the medical profession no longer speaks in a unified voice and that disunity among doctor ranks is not uncommon. For example, the two most active medical representative bodies—the AMA and the DRS (Doctors Reform Society)—are diametrically opposed on many key issues such as Medicare and private health insurance reform.

Conclusion

Challenges to medical dominance such as deprofessionalisation, corporatisation, and McDonaldisation, and the medical profession's responses to such challenges, reflect the dynamic nature of the health system. Medical dominance will continue to be the subject of formal and informal challenge, and it remains to be seen how long-lasting these trends will be in eroding the professional autonomy of medicine. What appears certain is that at all three levels—political, economic, and clinical autonomy—medical dominance is being challenged and steadily undermined. The recent development of clinical governance, though still in its infancy in Australia, may prove to be the most significant challenge yet. It has always been the case that the clinical decisions of doctors determine, to a large extent, health expenditure and the work of other health practitioners. While the McDonaldisation of medical practice represents new forms of accountability and constraint over the medical profession, it is not without inherent problems and may undermine the flexibility and quality of health care provided if the primary concern becomes one of cost-cutting and rule-following. With increasing pressure on governments to find innovative ways to control rising health expenditure, the future of medical dominance will continue to be contested. Freidson (1994) asks what the alternative to medical dominance might be. His answer is that medicine needs to be 'liberated' from 'material self-interest'; only in this way will the negative aspects of medical dominance be quashed.

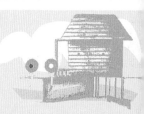

Summary of main points

» Medicine monopolises health care delivery, health policy, and the nature of health practice.

» Medical dominance was achieved through political means and was granted and guaranteed by the state through legislation and constitutional amendment in Australia.

» Medical dominance has always been the subject of resistance and challenge, but recent challenges may result in the most significant curtailment of medical autonomy to date.

» The main challenges to medical dominance are deprofessionalisation, corporatisation, and McDonaldisation.

Sociological reflection: medical dominance methods

The key aspect of medical dominance is professional autonomy, which is evidenced in three main ways:

» economic autonomy
» political autonomy
» clinical autonomy.

Define each form of medical autonomy and identify at least one challenge to it. How effective do you think the challenges you have identified have been?

John Germov

Discussion questions

1 How would you define medical dominance?

2 How was medical dominance achieved?

3 What are some examples of deprofessionalisation? To what extent does it represent a challenge to medical dominance?

4 What are some examples of corporatisation in the health sector? To what extent do they represent a challenge to medical dominance?

5 What might be some of the positive and negative outcomes of McDonaldisation in the health sector?

6 What could be done to address the problems related to medical dominance further?

Further investigation

1 There is considerable debate over whether the power of the medical profession is being undermined by the trends of deprofessionalisation, corporatisation, and McDonaldisation. What do these trends involve and to what extent have they curtailed the political, economic, and clinical autonomy of the medical profession?

2 Examine the impact of medical dominance on one other health profession such as nursing or an allied health profession (e.g. dietetics, occupational therapy, physiotherapy, pharmacy, and so on). How is the profession you have chosen challenging medical dominance and to what extent has it been effective?

3 Discuss the challenge that managerialism poses to medical dominance in Australia.

Further reading

Commonwealth of Australia 2006, *The Blame Game: Report on the Inquiry into Health Funding*, House of Representatives Standing Committee on Health and Ageing, Canberra. Available online: <http://www.aph.gov.au/house/committee/haa/healthfunding/report.htm>

Freidson, E. 2001, *Professionalism: The Third Logic*, Polity Press, Cambridge.

Kelleher, D., Gabe, J. & Williams, G. (eds) 2006, *Challenging Medicine*, 2nd edn, Routledge, London.

'Medical Dominance Revisited' 2006, Special Issue of *Health Sociology Review*, vol. 15, no. 5, pp. 421–534.

Pringle, R. 1998, *Sex and Medicine: Gender, Power and Authority in the Medical Profession*, Cambridge University Press, Cambridge.

Productivity Commission 2005, *Australia's Health Workforce*, Productivity Commission, Canberra. Available online: <http://www.pc.gov.au/projects/study/healthworkforce/docs/finalreport>

Riska, E. 2001, *Medical Careers and Feminist Agendas: American, Scandinavian, and Russian Women Physicians*, Aldine de Gruyter, New York.

Saks, M. 2003, *Orthodox and Alternative Medicine: Politics, Professionalization and Health Care*, Sage, London.

Waitzkin, H. 2000, *The Second Sickness: Contradictions of Capitalist Health Care*, 2nd edn, Rowman & Littlefield, Lanham.

Willis, E. 1989, *Medical Dominance*, revised edn, Allen & Unwin, Sydney.

Web resources

Australian Commission on Safety and Quality in Health Care: <http://www.safetyandquality.gov.au/>

Australian General Practice Network: <http://www.adgp.com.au/site/index.cfm>

Australian Medical Association (AMA): <http://www.ama.com.au>

Centre for Clinical Governance Research in Health: <http://www.med.unsw.edu.au/medweb.nsf/page/ClinGov_About>

Consumers' Health Forum of Australia: <http://www.chf.org.au>

Doctors Reform Society of Australia (DRS): <http//www.drs.org.au/index.html>

Health Issues Centre (HIC): <http://www.healthissuescentre.org.au/>

Public Health Association of Australia (PHAA): <http://www.phaa.net.au>

Online case study • • •
Visit the Second Opinion website to access relevant case studies.

Documentaries/films

The Doctor (1991): 125 minutes, starring William Hurt and directed by Randa Haines. A film about an arrogant doctor who becomes a patient and deals with issues of doctor-patient interaction.

First do no Harm (2007): 50 minutes, Four Corners, ABC TV. Examines hospital scandals and the problems of a self-regulating medical profession. Available online: <http://www.abc.net.au/4corners/content/2007/s2013033.htm>

Patch Adams (1998): 125 minutes. Starring Robin Williams. Produced by Universal Pictures, directed by Tom Shadyac, USA. A sentimental film about a doctor who 'treats the patient, not the disease'.

Paying the Price (2001): 45 minutes, Four Corners, ABC TV. Investigates the pharmaceutical industry and its attempts to undermine Australia's Pharmaceutical Benefits Scheme, which subsidises many medicines.

Patients Held Hostage (1992): 43 minutes, Yorkshire Television/Four Corners, ABC TV. Examines medical fraud in US psychiatric hospitals operated by National Medical Enterprises and Psychiatric Institutes of America, which illegally abducted and abused patients in the pursuit of profit.

Sicko (2007): 110 minutes. A Michael Moore documentary on the problems of profit-oriented health care in the USA compared to free public health systems in Canada, the UK, and France.

The Trouble with Medicine (1993): 6 part documentary series (each around 55 minutes) dealing with various challenges and limitations relating to biomedicine, ABC TV, BBC TV & Thirteen-WNET.

References

Abbott, A. 1988, *The System of Professions: An Essay on the Division of Expert Labor*, University of Chicago Press, Chicago.

Allsop, J. 2006, 'Medical Dominance in a Changing World: The UK Case', *Health Sociology Review*, vol. 15, no. 5, pp. 444–57.

Annandale, E. 2004, *Feminist Theory and the Sociology of Health and Illness*, Routledge, London.

Annandale, E. & Hunt, K. (eds) 2000, *Gender Inequalities and Health*, Open University Press, Buckingham.

Armstrong, B. K., Gillespie, J. A., Leeder, S. A., Rubin, G. L. & Russell, L. M. 2007, 'Challenges in Health and Health Care for Australia', *Medical Journal of Australia*, vol. 187, no. 9, pp. 485–9.

Auditor-General 1992, *Medifraud and Excessive Servicing*, Audit Report no. 17, Health Insurance Commission, Canberra.

Australian Bureau of Statistics 2006, *Australia (Australia), Occupation (a) (UNIT GROUPS) by sex*, Cat. no. 2068.0, ABS, Canberra.

Australian Institute of Health and Welfare 2007, *Sentinel Events in Australian Public Hospitals 2004–2005*, AIHW Cat. no. HSE 51, AIHW, Canberra.

Australian Institute of Health and Welfare 1996, *Female Participation in the Australian Medical Workforce*, AIHW, Canberra.

Barnett, J. R., Barnett, P. & Kearns, R. A. 1998, 'Declining Professional Dominance? Trends in the Proletarianisation of Primary Care in New Zealand', *Social Science & Medicine*, vol. 46, no. 2, pp. 193–207.

Braithwaite, J. 1984, *Corporate Crime in the Pharmaceutical Industry*, Routledge & Kegan Paul, London.

Braithwaite, J. & Hindle, D. 1998, 'Casemix Funding in Australia: Time for a Rethink, *Medical Journal of Australia*, vol. 168, pp. 558–60.

Bromberger, B. & Fife-Yeomans, J. 1991, *Deep Sleep: Harry Bailey and the Scandal of Chelmsford*, Simon & Schuster, Sydney.

Broom, D. 1991, *Damned if We Do: Contradictions in Women's Health Care*, Allen & Unwin, Sydney.

Cant, S. L. & Sharma, U. 1999, *A New Medical Pluralism? Alternative Medicine, Doctors, Patients and the State*, Routledge, London.

Cashman, P. 1989, 'The Dalkon Shield', in P. Grabosky & A. Sutton (eds), *Stains on a White Collar*, Hutchinson, Sydney.

Clarke, J. & Newman, J. 1997, *The Managerial State: Power, Politics and Ideology in the Remaking of Social Welfare*, Sage, London.

Clarke, J., Gewirtz, S., & McLaughlin. E. (eds) 2000, *New Managerialism, New Welfare?*, The Open University and Sage, London.

Coburn, D. 1988, 'Canadian Medicine: Dominance or Proletarianization?', *The Milbank Quarterly*, vol. 62, no. 2, pp. 92–116.

Coburn, D. 2006, 'Medical Dominance Then and Now: Critical Reflections', *Health Sociology Review*, vol. 15, no. 5, pp. 432–43.

Coburn, D., Rappolt, S. & Bourgeault, I. 1997, 'Decline vs. Retention of Medical Power Through Restratification: An Examination of the Ontario Case', *Sociology of Health & Illness*, vol. 19, no. 1, pp. 1–22.

Coburn, D. & Willis, E. 2000, 'The Medical Profession: Knowledge, Power, and Autonomy', in G. L. Albrecht, R. Fitzpatrick, & S. C. Scrimshaw (eds), *Handbook of Social Studies in Health and Medicine*, Sage, London, pp. 377–93.

Cockerham, W. C. 2004, *Medical Sociology*, 9th edn, Prentice Hall, Englewood Cliffs, NJ.

Coney, S. 1988, *The Unfortunate Experiment*, Penguin, Melbourne.

Connell, R. W. 1988, 'Class Inequalities and "Just Health"', *Community Health Studies*, vol. 12, no. 2, pp. 212–17.

Daniel, A. 1998, *Scapegoats for a Profession: Uncovering Procedural Injustice*, Harwood Academic, Amsterdam.

Day, R. & Day, J. V. 1977, 'A Review of the Current State of Negotiated Order Theory: An Appreciation and a Critique', *The Sociological Quarterly*, vol. 18, Winter, pp. 126–42.

Dent, M. 1998, 'Hospitals and New Ways of Organisation of Medical Work in Europe: Standardisation of Medicine in the Public Sector and the Future of Medical Autonomy', in P. Thompson & C. Warhurst (eds), *Workplaces of the Future*, Macmillan, London.

Dent, M. 2006, 'Disciplining the Medical Profession? Implications of Patient Choice for Medical Dominance', *Health Sociology Review*, vol. 15, no. 5, pp. 458–68.

Donaldson, L. J. 1998, 'Clinical Governance and Service Failure in the NHS', *Public Money and Management*, vol. 18, no. 4, pp. 10–11.

Donaldson, L. J. 2000, 'Clinical Governance—a Mission to Improve', *British Journal of Clinical Governance*, vol. 5, no. 1, pp. 1–8.

Draper, M. 1992, *Casemix, Quality and Consumers*, Health Issues Centre, Melbourne.

Duffin, J. 1999, *History of Medicine*, University of Toronto Press, Toronto.

Dunbar, J. A., Reddy, P., Beresford, B., Ramsey, W. P & Lord, R. S. A. 2007, 'In the Wake of Hospital Inquiries: Impact on Staff and Safety', *Medical Journal of Australia*, vol. 186, no. 2, pp. 80–3.

Ehrenreich, B. & English, D. 1973, *Witches, Midwives and Nurses*, Old Westbury Feminist Press, New York.

Ehsani, J. P., Jackson, T. & Duckett, S. J. 2006, 'The Incidence and Cost of Adverse Events in Victorian Hospitals 2003–04', *Medical Journal of Australia*, vol. 184, no. 11, pp. 551–5.

Elston, M. A. 1991, 'The Politics of Professional Power: Medicine in a Changing Health Service', in J. Gabe, M. Calnan & M. Bury (eds), *The Sociology of the Health Service*, Routledge, London, pp. 58–88.

Exworthy, M. & Halford, S. (eds) 1999, *Professionals and the New Managerialism in the Public Sector*, Open University Press, Buckingham.

Fee, E. & Krieger, N. (eds) 1994, *Women's Health, Politics, and Power: Essays on Sex/Gender, Medicine, and Public Health*, Baywood, New York.

Fine, G. A. 1984, 'Negotiated Orders and Organizational Cultures', *Annual Review of Sociology*, vol. 10, pp. 239–62.

Flynn, R. 2002, 'Clinical Governance and Governmentality', *Health, Risk & Society*, vol. 4, no. 2, pp. 155–73.

Freidson, E. 1970, *Profession of Medicine*, Harper & Row, New York.

Freidson, E. 1986, *Professional Powers: A Study of the Institutionalisation of Formal Knowledge*, University of Chicago Press, Chicago.

Freidson, E. 1994, *Professionalism Reborn: Theory, Prophecy and Policy*, Polity Press, Cambridge.

Germov, J. 1993, 'The Waiting List Bypass', *Health Forum*, vol. 27, October, pp. 23–4.

Germov, J. 1994, 'Medi-fraud: The Systemic Infection', *Australian Journal of Social Issues*, vol. 28, no. 3, pp. 301–4.

Germov, J. 1995, 'Medifraud, Managerialism and the Decline of Medical Autonomy: Proletarianisation and Deprofessionalisation Reconsidered', *Australian and New Zealand Journal of Sociology*, vol. 31, no. 3, pp. 51–66.

Germov, J. 2005, 'Managerialism in the Australian Public Health Sector: Towards the Hyper-rationalisation of Professional Bureaucracies', *Sociology of Health & Illness*, vol. 27, no. 6, pp. 738–58.

Gillespie, J. A. 1991, *The Price of Health: Australian Governments and Medical Politics 1910–1960*, Cambridge University Press, Melbourne.

Harrison, S. & Ahmad, W. I. 2000, 'Medical Autonomy and the UK State 1975 to 2025', *Sociology*, vol. 34, no. 1, pp. 129–46.

Haug, M. 1973, 'Deprofessionalisation: An Alternative Hypothesis for the Future', *Sociological Review Monograph*, vol. 20, pp. 195–211.

Haug, M. 1988, 'A Re-examination of the Hypothesis of Deprofessionalisation', *Milbank Quarterly*, vol. 2 (supp.), pp. 58–66.

Health Insurance Commission 1993, 'Medicare Fraud and Over-Servicing: What the Health Insurance Commission Proposes', *Health Issues*, vol. 36, September, p. 20.

Hindess, B. 1987, *Freedom, Equality, and the Market: Arguments on Social Policy*, Tavistock, London.

Hughes, D. & Light, D. W. (eds) 2002, *Rationing: Constructed Realities and Professional Practices*, Blackwell, Oxford.

Hunter, D. J. 2006, 'From Tribalism to Corporatism: The Continuing Managerial Challenge to Medical Dominance', in D. Kelleher, J. Gabe & G. Williams (eds), *Challenging Medicine*, 2nd edn, Routledge, London, pp. 1–23.

Illich, I. 1977, *Limits to Medicine, Medical Nemesis: The Exploration of Health*, Penguin, Harmondsworth.

Johnson, T. 1972, *Professions and Power*, Macmillan, London.

Kelleher, D., Gabe, J. & Williams, G. (eds) 2006, *Challenging Medicine*, 2nd edn, Routledge, London.

La Follette, M. C. 1992, *Stealing into Print: Fraud, Plagiarism and Misconduct in Scientific Publishing*, University of California Press, Berkeley, CA.

Larkin, G. 1983, *Occupational Monopoly and Modern Medicine*, Tavistock, London.

Larson, M. S. 1977, *The Rise of Professionalism: A Sociological Analysis*, University of California Press, Berkeley, CA.

Le Fanu, J. 1999, *The Rise and Fall of Modern Medicine*, Abacus, London.

Light, D. W. 1993, 'Countervailing Power: The Changing Character of the Medical Profession in the United States', in F. W. Hafferty & J. B. McKinlay (eds), *The Changing Medical Profession: An International Perspective*, Oxford University Press, New York.

Light, D. W. 2000, 'The Medical Profession and Organizational Change: From Professional Dominance to Countervailing Power', in C. Bird, P. Conrad & A. M. Fremont (eds), *Handbook of Medical Sociology*, 5th edn, Prentice Hall, Englewood Cliffs, NJ.

Lloyd, P., Lupton, D. & Donaldson, C. 1991, 'Consumerism in the Health Care Setting: An Exploratory Study of Factors Underlying the Selection and Evaluation of Primary Medical Services', *Australian Journal of Public Health*, vol. 15, pp. 194–201.

McKinlay, J. B. & Arches, J. 1985, 'Towards the Proletarianization of Physicians, *International Journal of Health Services*, vol. 15, no. 2, pp. 161–95.

McKinlay, J. B. & Stoeckle, J. D. 1988, 'Corporatization and the Social Transformation of Doctoring', *International Journal of Health Services*, vol. 18, no. 2, pp. 191–205.

Mintzberg, H. 1979, *The Structuring of Organizations*, Prentice Hall, Englewood Cliffs, NJ.

National Coalition on Health Care 2008, 'Health Insurance Coverage', *National Coalition on Health Care*. Available online: <http://www.nchc.org/facts/coverage.shtml>

Navarro, V. 1976, *Medicine Under Capitalism*, Prodist, New York.

Navarro, V. 1986, *Crisis, Health and Medicine: A Social Critique*, Tavistock, London.

Navarro, V. 1992, *Why the United States Does Not Have a National Health Program*, Baywood Publishing, New York.

Navarro, V. 1998, 'Book Review of Private Medicine and Public Health: Profits, Politics and Prejudice in the American Health Care Enterprise by Lawrence D. Weiss', *Contemporary Sociology*, vol. 27, no. 4, pp. 419–20.

Porter, R. 1997, *The Greatest Benefit to Mankind: A Medical History of Humanity from Antiquity to the Present*, HarperCollins, London.

Pringle, R. 1998, *Sex and Medicine: Gender, Power and Authority in the Medical Profession*, Cambridge University Press, Cambridge.

Relman, A. S. 1980, 'The New Medical-Industrial Complex', *New England Journal of Medicine*, vol. 303, no. 2, pp. 963–70.

Renwick, M. & Sadkowsky, K. 1991, *Variations in Surgery Rates*, AGPS, Canberra.

Riska, E. 1993, 'Introduction', in E. Riska & K. Wegar (eds), *Gender, Women and Medicine: Women and the Medical Division of Labour*, Sage, London.

Ritzer, G. 1993, *The McDonaldization of Society*, Pine Forge Press, Thousand Oaks, CA.

Saks, M. 2003, *Orthodox and Alternative Medicine: Politics, Professionalization and Health Care*, Sage, London.

Salmon, J. W. (ed.) 1990, *The Corporate Transformation of Health Care: Issues and Directions*, vol. 1, Baywood, New York.

Salmon, J. W. (ed.) 1994, *The Corporate Transformation of Health Care: Perspectives and Implications*, vol. 2, Baywood, New York.

Starr, P. 1982, *The Social Transformation of American Medicine: The Rise of a Sovereign Profession and the Making of a Vast Industry*, Basic Books, New York.

Strauss, A. 1978, *Negotiations: Varieties, Contexts, Processes, and Social Order*, Jossey-Bass, San Francisco.

Strauss, A., Schatzman, L., Ehrlich, D., Bucher, R. & Sabshin, M. 1963, 'The Hospital and its Negotiated Order', in E. Freidson (ed.), *The Hospital in Modern Society*, Free Press, New York.

Stretton, H. & Orchard, L. 1994, *Public Goods, Public Enterprise, Public Choice*, Macmillan, London.

Taskforce on Quality in Australian Health Care 1996, *The Final Report of the Taskforce on Quality in Australian Health Care*, Australian Health Ministers' Advisory Council, Canberra.

Thomas, H. 2007, *Sick to Death*, Allen & Unwin, Sydney.

Travaglia, J. & Braithwaite, J. 2007, *The Privatisation and Corporatisation of Hospitals: A Review of the Citations and Abstracts in the Literature*, Centre for Clinical Governance Research, Sydney.

Turner, B. S. with Samson, C. 1995, *Medical Power and Social Knowledge*, 2nd edn, Sage, London.

White, K. 2000, 'The State, the Market, and General Practice: The Australian Case', *International Journal of Health Services*, vol. 30, no. 2, pp. 285–308.

Willis, E. 1983, *Medical Dominance*, Allen & Unwin, Sydney.

Willis, E. 1989, *Medical Dominance*, revised edn, Allen & Unwin, Sydney.

Wilson, R. M., Gibberd, R., Hamilton, B. & Harrison, B. 1999, 'Safety of Healthcare in Australia: Adverse Events to Hospitalised Patients', in M. M. Rosenthal, L. Mulcahy, & S. Lloyd-Bostock (eds), *Medical Mishaps: Pieces of the Puzzle*, Open University Press, Buckingham, pp. 95–106.

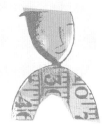

CHAPTER 20

Sociology of Nursing

HELEN
KELEHER

Overview

- Why is it important to understand nursing's history in order to comprehend the contemporary health system?
- To what extent is Australian nursing focused on illness care compared to health promotion and primary health care?
- What are some of the challenges and opportunities for the role of nurses in Australia?

NURSES AND THE HEALTH PROMOTING HOSPITAL

For as long as she could remember, Catherine had wanted to be a nurse. She gained good grades that allowed her to enter a Bachelor of Nursing degree at university. Catherine studied hard for the 3 years of the course and gained registration as a nurse at the end of those 3 years. She was then offered a graduate year with a large public hospital but felt that the pressure of technological demands, insufficient time to deliver patient-centred care, and the busy wards meant a lack of personal support for new graduates. Catherine completed the graduate year but she did not enjoy it. Her doubts were rising about whether she really did want to be a nurse. She was always dealing with sickness, crisis, and pressure.

She decided to take a working holiday in Scotland. As soon as she arrived, Catherine was offered a job as a nurse in a cardiac ward in a major hospital. There she became involved in the development of health promotion roles for hospital nurses. In Catherine's undergraduate course in Australia, there had very little content about health promotion and health education, and she found that she really loved the principles and concepts of health promotion. She became involved in the implementation of the 'health promoting hospital' concept. She loved the idea of helping people to learn about staying well through health education. The hospital had developed training and materials for staff members to enable them to work in health-

promoting practices. Catherine found
the team approach to this work to be very
supportive and much preferred it to the
hierarchical structures she had experienced
in her first hospital. Moreover, she gained a
great deal of satisfaction knowing that she
was doing more than just fixing illness. After
2 years of working in Scotland, Catherine

decided to return home to study a Master of
Public Health so she could work in a range
of settings and use her expanded skills and
knowledge. For her next job, perhaps she
would seek work in remote Australia or a
developing country where health promotion
and public health nurses are in much
demand.

Introduction

Nursing is regarded as the predominant caring profession, one that is multiskilled
and has varied career paths. The common image of a nurse is of one who works in
a hospital but nursing work varies widely; nurses work in many different types of
settings including primary care clinics, general practice, community and **primary
health care** services, women's health services, maternal and child health, schools,
aged-care facilities, rural and remote outreach areas, mental health, district nursing
services, academia, and government departments. The roles of the nursing profession include 'the promotion of health, prevention of illness, and the care of ill,
disabled and dying people. Advocacy, promotion of a safe environment, research,
participation in shaping health policy and inpatient and health systems management, and education are also key nursing roles' (ICN 2008).

> **primary health care (PHC)**
> Both the point of first contact with the health care system and a philosophy for delivery of that care.

Directions of development in nursing change over time, usually in response
to policy directions of governments, and demand pressures for nursing services
by employers. This chapter will begin with a brief history of the development of
nursing in Australia—with an emphasis on nursing's professionalising strategies
and the directions taken by nursing through its history—before turning to new
directions and the opportunities and challenges which lie ahead for nursing. Themes
that emerge are the changing relationships between nursing and other medical
professions, and advances in nurses' professional status.

Development of nursing

Florence Nightingale's nineteenth century writings on nursing were full of high
moral tone and missionary zeal about women's roles in the care of the sick. Her views
reflected Victorian values about women's duties and responsibilities, views which

Helen Keleher

were embraced in Australia. Nursing services in Australia developed in the late nineteenth century from grassroots services provided by charity organisations to the poor members of society, providing a combination of sick-care and welfare. District Nursing Associations, established from 1895, expected nurses to be Christian and to spread the 'gospel' of hygiene and moral influence (*ANJ* 1903). The nurse was to be 'rewarded by the material and visible results of her ministrations' (*ANJ* 1908, p. 97) rather than a decent wage.

Hospitals had been established since the mid-1800s, primarily by charities and churches. Prior to the arrival in 1868 of the first Nightingale-trained nurses, nursing training was unsystematic and localised (Ehrenreich & English 1973). Efforts of senior nurses to set up systems for nurses learning on and off the wards were not always supported by hospital management beyond that which was aimed at the indoctrination of nurses with moral values of hygiene, order, and discipline. Many powerful doctors failed to see the need for nurses to learn and expected them to perform well at 'sweating', which included menial work and hygiene, as well as patient care. As a result, senior nurses became locked in power struggles with doctors and hospital management for control over nursing. Menial work was whatever a hospital wanted it to be such as cooking, serving meals, or the washing of ward linen, while hygiene involved lots of scrubbing. Change was very slow, but from the early 1900s nurses started to become more organised.

Early professionalising strategies

Nurses understood that they needed to work collectively for change. The first Australian nursing organisation was the Victorian Trained Nurses' Association (VTNA), formed in 1902, with a register for nurses and the first nursing journal, *UNA* (United Nurses Association). By 1907, five states had established similar organisations with membership lists and central management of examinations which nurses had to pass to be entered on the membership list of that state. The exclusion of untrained workers from practising as nurses was one of the earliest professionalising strategies. In **professionalisation** theory, this strategy is known as closure, which is a necessary step for a group of workers to become a profession. Nursing achieved closure through registration while other professionalising strategies included increasing nurses' knowledge base through education, identifying nurses' scope of practice, and the development of career pathways as well as improvements to pay and work conditions. Theories about professionalisation in nursing are much debated from a range of positions which are outlined in Box 20.1.

A characteristic of early nursing organisations was the lay membership category that was taken up by many doctors, who for many years held the positions of chairman and often treasurer of those nursing organisations, as well as editorship of *UNA* and the *Australasian Nurses' Journal* (*ANJ*). As editors, they could control the publication of articles. Medical bias dominated the editorial content. For example,

professionalisation/ professional project
The process of becoming a profession, whereby an occupational group attains publicly recognised and government-legitimated monopoly and autonomy over its area of work.

class (or social class)
A position in a system of structured inequality based on the unequal distribution of power, wealth, income, and status. People who share a class position typically share similar life chances.

state
A term used to describe a collection of institutions, including the parliament (government and opposition political parties), the public-sector bureaucracy, the judiciary, the military, and the police.

medical dominance
A general term used to describe the power of the medical profession in terms of its control over its own work, over the work of other health workers, and over health resource allocation, health policy, and the way that hospitals are run.

BOX 20.1 Doing health sociology: theories of professions and gender in nursing

The normative trait theory was an influential theory in the sociology of professions (Greenwood 1957). Trait theory was essentially a prescription of qualities and attributes that described and justified hierarchies in the labour market. In this theory, a profession is regarded as having core characteristics including an abstract body of knowledge acquired during a prolonged period of training and education, and a science orientation (Hearn 1982). Other characteristics include the mastery of techniques, self-regulation, autonomy, social status, and prestige. This theory puts forward an ideal type that ignores conceptual accounts of **class**, power, monopoly, divisions of labour, and relations between professionals and the **state**.

Professions operate within social structures wherein power is a central dynamic. All professions aim to create restrictive practices to control their market of professional services. In doing so they have created both mystique and self-serving social status. Eliot Freidson (1970), another classic analyst of the sociology of professions, argues that the professions have acquired distinctive places in the occupational hierarchy by engaging in political processes to gain full control over their work, and legitimated authority which is dependent on support from the state. Evan Willis (1989) took these theories further by demonstrating how **medical dominance** of the health system was created through its achievement of occupational autonomy and control over practice to limit other occupational groups, and either exclude or subordinate others. He analyses medicine in relation to midwifery and nursing to illustrate the processes involved in exclusion, limitation, and subordination.

Feminist theorists analyse the patriarchal foundations of theories of the professions arguing that professionalisation is a divisive, elitist model.

Eva Gamarnikow (1978) and Jeff Hearn (1982) argue that the suppression of female nurses by a predominantly male medical profession is based on a sexual division of labour in health care. Others (Fee 1983; Doyal 1997) demonstrate the gendered social processes involved in the physical and emotional work of caring. Jane Salvage (1985), Sandra Speedy (1991) and Celia Davies (1995) reject the masculine foundations of professionalisation theories which they see as unsuitable for the nursing profession. They argue that the professionalising strategies of the medical profession have produced oppressive power relations within nursing that are counter-productive and draw attention to the needs of the profession rather than the needs of the people for whom the health system is established. Further, they see that the construction of caring as a deeply gendered form of women's work is also counter-productive because they exclude men from nursing.

Gender is a social construct that demonstrates systems of social relations and how those relations are constrained by norms, values, and perceptions of the roles of men and women in society. Gendered norms and attitudes are present in all parts of social life which are fundamentally constructed by gender divisions and stereotypes and shape organisational structures, institutions, and the labour market. In health care, one of the historical functions of gender was to exclude women from medicine using the power derived from male, class-privileged power (Witz 1992). These exclusionary practices were based on beliefs about the second-class status of women, beliefs about what it is to be a woman, and women's suitability for science versus caring roles. Of course, many of these social practices have steadily been broken down since the mid to late twentieth century both in medicine and nursing.

Helen Keleher

gender/sex
This pair of terms refers to the socially constructed categories of feminine and masculine (the cultural identities and values that prescribe how men and women should behave), and the social power relations based on those categories, as distinct from the categories of biological sex (female or male).

public health/public health infrastructure
Public policies and infrastructure to prevent the onset and transmission of disease among the population, with a particular focus on sanitation and hygiene such as clean air, water, and food, and immunisation. Public health infrastructure refers specifically to the buildings, installations, and equipment necessary to ensure healthy living conditions for the population.

nurses' agitation for improved pay and conditions was roundly condemned as disregarding women's duties and responsibilities (Keleher 2000).

The journal was a key player in what one historian described as a 'prolonged and determined battle' (Russell 1990, pp. 23–4) over efforts to establish state-run nursing registration boards. Up until about 1920, most states (with the exception of Queensland, which established a board in 1912) showed no interest in the quality of nurses training or subsequent learning opportunities, preferring to delegate responsibility for the conditions of registration to hospitals and state-based organisations. Political support for state nursing registration boards was gradually achieved in all states: South Australia (1920), Western Australia (1921), Victoria (1923), New South Wales (1924), and Tasmania (1927) (Bowe 1960). It is interesting to note that medical practitioners in Australia did not achieve full state-run registration boards until 1936, long after the *Australian Medical Journal* (later the *MJA*) was established in 1857 and the Melbourne Medical School in 1862 (Keleher 2000).

Certainly, nursing was socially constructed as women's work that involved gendered social processes. These social relations were instrumental in securing the dominant position of the emerging medical profession in the health and social structures of Australia. Doctors were also working on professionalising strategies that included limiting the practices of various health workers including midwives and nurses (Willis 1989). The medical profession had to manage nursing in order to control it. Nonetheless, as a profession, nursing has never seemed to pose any threat to the power of medicine in Australia. Indeed, the loyalties of nursing to hospitals and the illness model were captured very early, while nursing organisations narrowed the vision for nursing in Australia because they failed to see the value of nursing beyond the hospital walls.

Early public health nursing

During the late 1800s, a **public health** movement gained momentum in Australia and internationally, eventually providing new opportunities for nursing. The public health movement was led by champions who could see how the health of the public could be improved by safe water supplies, sanitation systems, safe food supplies, breastfeeding of infants, better working conditions in factories, and widespread education about hygiene. Public health services were spearheaded by local governments which had employed male sanitary inspectors since about 1860 for the 'safeguarding of home life, safeguarding of industrial life and for the prevention of the transmission of disease' (*ANJ* 1921, p. 344). From 1900, local government authorities started to appoint Medical Officers of Health and soon after, the first women health visitors or 'nurse inspectors' were employed. They undertook home visits for hygiene monitoring and the provision of advice to mothers of new infants in efforts to reduce what were alarming infant mortality (death) rates (IMR) among the poor. Infant mortality rates in Sydney peaked at 194 per 1000 in 1875, which was higher than rates in London. Public health reforms gradually made a difference to these rates of tragic loss of infant life. By 1900, the IMR ranged from 126.1 per 1000 live births in Western Australia to 95.2 in Victoria. School medical services began employing school nurses around 1902. Infant welfare clinics were established by local government in poor suburbs first, but by the 1930s, most mothers had access to a nurse whether in a city suburb, or a rural town, or via a visiting baby-health van in remote areas. At first, the baby-health clinics employed midwives (registered nurses with an obstetrics certificate) but they were soon required to carry an extra certificate in Infant Welfare Nursing in order to work in baby health clinics (Keleher 2000).

Still, public health nurses in Australia were marginalised by the dominance of the hospital nurse culture. Nurses who sought careers in district or public health nursing were regarded as entering a different culture from what was seen as 'real nursing'. There was no representation of public health or district nurses on registration boards, nor were they identified in nurses' awards. Indeed, it wasn't until 1943 that the Victorian Government granted the request of infant-welfare nurses to be brought under the nurses' wages board. Public health nursing was effectively marginalised by these processes despite international directions to ensure that nurses in community settings and within government agencies were properly educated and supported (Keleher 2000).

Power in nursing

Historically, nursing in Australia has been extremely hospital-centric and nurses' learning was effectively subjugated to the needs of hospital medicine. Hospital matrons eventually established their power over nursing organisations and nurses' registration boards although members of the medical profession often held the balance of power—an important plank in medicine's determined intentions to limit and control nursing practice (see Box 20.1).

Hierarchical class divisions between ward nurses and administrative nurses were evident. Most of nursing's early leaders were 'lady nurses' who were drawn from the middle classes because they could afford to pay the premiums for entry to the lady nurse ranks. They were not aligned with the rank and file of the labour movement from where most of the ward nurses were recruited and they were ambivalent about their role in acting for those staff on matters of pay and conditions (Bessant & Bessant 1991, pp. 11–12). Nursing organisations were also reluctant to engage in industrial issues, undoubtedly because they were dominated by matrons and the medical profession.

Hospital matrons derived their power from their alignment with hospital medicine and the powerful position of the medical profession. In turn, hospital nurses

Helen Keleher

perceived that they acquired a degree of status from their close working relationship with the medical profession. This not only made nurses reluctant to be militant about their training and working conditions, but it gave them a sense of security from the approval they received from the medical profession as well as reflected status which was a trade-off for nursing's archaic conditions of employment. Hospital nursing, which controlled nurses' training and learning, had acquired power within the Australian health care system and its policies that neglected broader learning by nurses and suppressed the development of other types of nursing.

Nursing organisations

The VTNA became the Royal Victorian College of Nurses (RVCN) which was the only college in Australia that could offer award-bearing courses until the late 1940s. The medical profession provided many of the lectures to nurses in the sister–tutor and nursing administration courses that were designed to meet the needs of the hospital system. There were attempts in the 1920s and again in the 1930s to have postgraduate nursing courses provided in conjunction with the University of Melbourne. The RVCN Committee established to negotiate this development ran aground amid factional disputes over professional control over the courses, so these efforts came to nothing and the Committee was disbanded. University education for Australian nurses did not become a reality until the late 1980s, unlike in many other countries which were much more progressive than Australia. For example, from the 1920s, every university and medical school in Brazil was required to establish a school of nursing providing public health nursing as well as hospital nursing. By 1923, postgraduate courses in public health nursing were available in twenty universities in the USA including the prestigious campuses of Michigan (Ann Arbor), Yale, Columbia (New York City), Berkeley, and Cleveland, all of which also provided pre-registration nursing degrees on campus and in association with university-affiliated hospitals, community health centres, and other appropriate settings (Keleher 2000). Eventually, the College of Nursing Australia (now the Royal College of Nursing Australia) was established in 1949 with branches in each state, with a brief to provide what was called 'post-basic' education, and their courses played an important role in enabling nurses to advance their careers. Still, they remained very hospital-centric and they were not affiliated with any universities.

Winds of change

A landmark report on Australian nursing was prepared in 1968 by Rae Chittick, Emeritus Professor of the prestigious Canadian McGill University, in her capacity as a consultant to the World Health Organization. Chittick found 'a deeply troubled profession [in which] the self-sacrificing and somewhat self-righteous nurse [had] became a way of life' (Chittick 1968, p. 58). She saw that the educational programs available in hospital-based schools of nursing were narrow and provided almost no preparation for practice outside the walls of the hospital, nor did they make student nurses aware of the social, political, or cultural problems they must face as citizens: 'perhaps no other group of young people in modern society receives such a narrow, restricted and unimaginative type of education' (Chittick 1968, p. 213). Any community-service ideal that did exist among nurses was eclipsed by the dominance of the hospital model and its leaders' adherence to traditional values about service to hospital medicine. She noted that many nurses 'harbour bitter memories of the attitude of the medical profession towards change in the nursing profession and their great indifference to our hopes and aspirations' (Chittick 1969, p. 63). She was very clear about the necessity of setting up university programs for nurses, noting that the lack of suitable educational programs had been a significant impediment to the development of public health nursing and primary health and community nursing. On the basis of a report such as that, nursing's status as a profession seemed somewhat in doubt but it was one of the winds blowing change through Australian nursing. There were numerous inquiries and many reports into the problems and possible solutions to nursing education and the issues were hotly debated (Smith 1999); it seemed that reform was inevitable.

Another breath of fresh air came from the launch of Australia's Community Health Program (CHP) in the early 1970s by the Whitlam Labor Government. The CHP attempted to develop more comprehensive health services than hospitals and general practice could provide. The reforms were based on a **social model of health** and aimed to increase access to services in community settings. The CHP embraced broader concepts of health, based on the World Health Organization's understandings that health is not merely the absence of disease but the ability to function effectively within one's environment. This was the era of the new public health which was given further impetus by the Alma-Ata Charter for Primary Health Care (WHO 1978) and the Ottawa Charter for Health Promotion (WHO 1986; see also Chapters 23 & 24). These developments provided new opportunities for nursing particularly for generalist community nurses who worked in the newly established community health services (Keleher 2000).

During the 1970s and 1980s, nurses and nursing organisations kept up pressure on governments to act on the findings of inquiries and reports to advance the education of nurses. These were difficult years. Nursing education had become a sensitive political issue and nurses were becoming militant, using strike action to press their case. With the election of a new Hawke Labor Government in 1983, nurses were successful in securing a commitment to transfer nursing education to the higher education sector, a decision that was announced by Dr Neal Blewett, the (then) Minister for Health (Smith 1999, pp. 234–5). The implementation of the decision was complex, requiring substantial legislative and administrative changes to be made in both hospitals and universities, but nursing in Australia has never looked

social model of health
Focuses on social determinants of health such as the social production, distribution, and construction of health and illness, and the social organisation of health care. It directs attention to the prevention of illness through community participation and social reforms that address living and working conditions.

Helen Keleher

back. In a speech made by Dr Blewett in 1993, he said, '[t]he nurses were successful in securing greater recognition of their professional status, in gaining new career structures, and in winning better pay and improved working conditions' (Blewett 1993 cited in Smith 1999, p. 237).

As nursing transferred from the apprentice-style system of training to university education, there was a strong emphasis in the new curriculum on primary health care practice underpinned by philosophies based on the World Health Alma-Ata Charter for Primary Health Care (WHO 1978) which was regarded as the key to achieving the goal of *Health For All by the Year 2000*. In the early twenty-first century, nursing's focus is firmly on the education of a workforce for the acute-care sector albeit driven by workforce shortages and increased demands on hospitals from increased patient acuity, with public and community/primary health given no more than a token place in nursing curriculum. Indeed, even today, while many nursing students find a great deal of attraction in the affinity with hospital medicine and its technological challenges, many do not, and end up leaving the profession. Nursing is failing to provide sufficient curriculum to ensure that nurses find it easy to find alternative career paths in community and primary nursing. The retention of nurses in the profession is an issue of national concern (Johnstone and Stewart 2002; Productivity Commission 2005) both for new graduates, who are inducted into the hospital sector, and more experienced nurses who leave the profession for various reasons such as burn-out and a lack of family-friendly workplaces.

Contemporary challenges for nursing

Career pathways

Australia is experiencing a generalised shortage of nurses (Productivity Commission 2005). Simultaneously, national health care policy is firmly embracing a prevention and promotion agenda that is directed at cultural change about keeping people out of hospital care. These policy directions follow international trends because many countries are finding the costs of hospital care to be rising towards unsustainable levels (see Chapter 18).

Care is being focused on community-based services and settings with improved coordination of services and integration of multidisciplinary care, which has too often been fragmented and poorly coordinated, especially at the interface between hospital and community. Further, social and demographic changes are driving health care reforms including ageing, rising levels and complexity of chronic conditions, and health care workforce shortages especially of general practitioners. The increasing level of health inequalities demands improvements in access to primary care by underserved groups and communities. There are high-level considerations of reforms to the scope of practice and job redesign of health professionals (Keleher et al. 2007). These are circumstances that require a considered response from nursing and a cultural shift that demonstrates its capacity to meet these challenges, given commonly held opinions among the nursing faculty that some types of nursing practice are more legitimate than others (Happell 2002).

Other challenges include confusion about generalist and specialist roles, and a lack of learning framework or career structure for nurses working in settings other than hospitals, with little transferability between settings. Nursing registers show the somewhat restricted nature of nursing. Those registers, held by nurses' boards, identify registered general nurses, mental health nurses, midwives, and nurse practitioners. By comparison, the United Kingdom holds registers for nurses, midwives, and specialist community public health nurses. This latter category signifies a much stronger value placed on nurses who work outside hospitals in the United Kingdom.

The place of nurses in public and community health in the United Kingdom is on the agenda of health policy reforms. In 2002, the United Kingdom set out a health policy for prevention and **health promotion** with a series of government papers, one of which was *Liberating the Talents: Helping Primary Care Trusts and Nurses to Deliver the NHS Plan* (Department of Health 2002). This paper described the main activities of community nurses under the headings of first-contact care, management of long-term conditions and public health, but 5 years later, there were concerns that despite a positive reception, the approach had not impacted on education or workforce planning (Department of Health 2007). To progress reforms in nursing career pathways to better meet the needs of the population, the Department of Health issued a discussion paper proposing a new framework for nursing careers. Box 20.2 sets out the five care pathways on which reforms to nursing careers in the United Kingdom will be based.

health promotion
Any combination of education and related organisational, economic, and political interventions designed to promote behavioural and environmental changes conducive to good health, including legislation, community development, and advocacy.

BOX 20.2	Nursing careers in the five care pathways proposed for the United Kingdom

The Children, Public and Family Health Pathway will help build dedicated public health capacity and capability into the system. The emphasis will be on intervening at a population level and in working in partnership to address the determinants of health. Health-needs assessment for populations, communities, groups, families, and individuals will be a key component and will provide the basis for intervention to improve health, reduce health inequalities, and increase support for vulnerable families and individuals. This pathway will also encompass the maintenance and improvement of the health of children and young people within a philosophy of family-centred care in a range of settings.

The First Contact, Access and Urgent Care Pathway will develop nurses who can respond to

... »

a variety of undifferentiated needs, supporting children, families, and adults to manage their own health care through advice, information, or treatment of minor injury or illness or disturbances in mental health and well-being.

The Long-Term Care Pathway takes account of the increased number of people living with long-term (chronic) health conditions because of demographic changes and improved living conditions. The nursing contribution will focus on supporting self-care, independent living, personalised care, case management of complex conditions, and end-of-life care. It will span the full range of long-term conditions, covering all ages, including mental health and learning disabilities. It will see nurses working across organisational boundaries in partnership with patients and carers.

The Acute and Critical Care Pathway will ensure nurses are able to offer scheduled or unscheduled care for people needing continuous clinical, technical, and nursing support, often in potentially life-threatening situations, following elective surgery, or acute psychotic episodes. The pathway covers patients of all ages and backgrounds and in various settings, such as community outreach and tertiary settings.

The Mental Health and Psychosocial Care Pathway will build the capacity of nurses to work with mental health service users and other clients requiring psychosocial care. It will encourage a holistic approach and help nurses work across a range of settings—including acute and community care settings as well as clients' own homes—in order to build strengths and optimise health and well-being.

Source: Department of Health 2007

What the framework in Box 20.2 shows is that working in hospital wards is only one of many career options open to nurses in the United Kingdom, but is Australian nursing ready for such reforms? Nursing is undoubtedly a versatile workforce, and with general practitioners, is well placed to meet population health challenges that need enhanced primary and community health care service delivery. Another challenge for nursing is to overcome the institutionalisation of the illness paradigm in Australia's nursing registers and nurse education. Community and primary care nursing lacks a national policy, and nursing provides limited education opportunities for careers in primary and community nursing. Yet, 'it is in general practice and community settings that increasingly complex health care conditions are managed, with rapidly emerging needs for appropriately prepared case managers/coordinators of care' (Keleher et al. 2007, p. 2).

Practice nursing

Practice nurses are employed by general medical practices with a scope of practice defined by the needs of the practice:

> Practice nurses can be either registered nurses or enrolled nurses, but there are no
> formal post registration/enrolment educational requirements or professional regula-
> tions associated with practice nursing, as there are with nurse practitioners. (National
> Nursing and Nursing Education Taskforce 2006, p. 4)

Practice nursing is a large and growing area of practice in the United Kingdom,
Canada, and New Zealand, and more recently in Australia. Certainly, nursing as a
profession has been ambivalent about nurses working alongside medical practitioners in general practice settings, perhaps because of concerns about loss of
professional autonomy and limitations on nurses' scope of practice (Bonawit &
Watson 1996); however, the support by governments for practice nursing (PN) has
required nursing organisations and university nursing schools to become more
engaged with research, policy, and education for PNs. A lack of career development
in non-acute and community-based contexts of practice has limited the attractiveness of employment in these settings (Brookes et al. 2004). Certainly, practice
nursing in Australia is an area of somewhat casualised or sessional employment
without a career pathway although there is recognition that a career pathway needs
to be developed (Pascoe et al. 2006). Further, practice nurses' skill levels and scope
of practice are not linked to the needs of patients, but to the needs of the practice
(Keleher et al. 2007). There is a sense that practice nursing poses a threat to nursing's hard-won gains in professionalism, working conditions, and autonomy, but
just as members of the medical profession felt that to control nursing they had to
manage it, so it is for practice nursing. Rather than keeping practice nursing at arm's
length, the profession of nursing must engage with and manage the developments in
practice nursing if it is to steer the future of practice nursing into the pathway of
nursing's standards of professional status.

Nurse practitioners

The introduction of nurse practitioners in Australia since the early 1990s has been
a divisive issue between some parts of the medical profession and nursing, but it has
been an important professional step forward for nurses. In the early days of nurse
practitioners, the Australian Medical Association (AMA) objected vigorously to
nurse practitioners amid threats felt by some medical practitioners that nurse practitioners might compete for doctor's jobs or undermine their authority; objections
to nurse practitioners have subsided and they are now an integral, and small but
increasing, part of the overall nursing workforce. Nurse practitioners have advanced
qualifications, extensive nursing experience and are governed by registration requirements. They are:

> authorised to practise in an expanded nursing role in clinical settings as diverse as
> hospitals and aged care facilities, as well as in the community ... [and] have developed
> the skills and knowledge to expand their role to include ... prescribing medications

and ordering diagnostic tests. (National Nursing and Nursing Education Taskforce 2006, p. 2)

In Australia, the title of 'nurse practitioner' is protected by legislation administered by nurses' registration boards. While there remain some restrictions on nurse-practitioner practice compared to the advanced scope of practice that has been developed in the United Kingdom and Canada, it is likely that nurse practitioners, with their advanced practice capacity, will increasingly find their place in addressing workforce shortages in many parts of Australia's health system.

Conclusion

An understanding of the history of nursing allows us to appreciate the contested and gendered nature of nursing's struggle for professional status and control. Traditionally, nursing in Australia has been hospital-centred and illness-focused, though gradually changing as university nursing curricula address health promotion and the social model of health. In recent years, professional opportunities for nurses have expanded both within and outside the hospital system, through the introduction of nurse practitioners and the expansion of community and practice nursing.

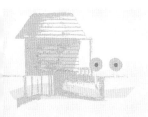

Summary of main points

» History has shown that nursing's professional status is tied to control over the education of nurses, their registration requirements, and their scope of practice.
» Nursing registers that are confined to nurses who work in acute care are restricting the attractiveness of nursing work beyond the walls of hospitals.
» There is no requirement for specific skills or knowledge about community, primary, or public health nursing, so the curriculum in nursing schools is not directed towards a workforce for those sectors despite the increasing national agenda for prevention and community and primary care.
» An expanding scope of practice for experienced and appropriately qualified nurses is the next step in the moving forward of nursing's professional status.

Sociological reflection: vested interests

The health system is driven by powerful interests that are imposed by dominant groups that have a vested interest in maintaining medical dominance and current funding systems that support the treatment of illness.

» What might roles for nurses look like in a health promoting health system?

» How can sociological analysis inform our understandings of the power relationships that maintain a focus on cure and illness, and how do those power relationships affect the profession of nursing?

Discussion questions

1 What were some of the key factors in the early development of nursing?

2 How is nursing's history important for understanding current challenges?

3 How have theories of professionalism been used by nursing to construct its own agenda of professionalisation?

4 What are some of the career options and challenges for nurses?

5 Why is the role and title of nurse practitioner a professional advance for nursing?

6 In what ways would a stronger undergraduate nursing curriculum about health promotion and public health be of benefit to graduate nurses?

Further investigation

1 Compare and contrast theories of professionalism and their influence on nursing.

2 Nursing in Australia has neglected both public health and primary care career pathways. Discuss, using the Further Readings to inform your response.

3 Nurse practitioners represent a fundamental challenge to medical dominance in Australia. Discuss.

Further reading

Hart, C. 2004, *Nurses and Politics: The Impact of Power and Practice*, Palgrave Macmillan, Basingstoke.

Liimatainen, L., Poskiparta, M. & Sjögren, A. 1999, 'Student Nurses and Reflective Health Promotion Learning in Hospital', Paper Presented at the European Conference on Educational Research, Lahti, Finland, 22–25 September 1999. Available online: <http://www.leeds.ac.uk/educol/documents/000001151.htm>

Sourtzi, P., Nolan, P. & Andrews, R. 1996, 'Evaluation of Health Promotion Activities in Community Nursing Practice', *Journal of Advanced Nursing*, vol. 24, no. 6, pp. 1214–23.

Thompson, P. & Kohli, H. 1997, 'Health Promotion Training Needs Analysis: An Integral Role for Clinical Nurses in Lanarkshire, Scotland', *Journal of Advanced Nursing*, vol. 26, no. 3, pp. 507–14.

Helen Keleher

Toffoli, L. & Henderson, J. 2007, 'Progress in Nursing: Multidisciplinary and Shared Care', in Willis, E., Reynolds, L. and Keleher, H. (eds), *Understanding the Australian Health Care System*, Sydney, Elsevier, pp. 179–88.

Wicks, D. 1999, *Nurses and Doctors at Work: Rethinking Professional Boundaries*, Allen & Unwin, Sydney.

Web resources

Australian Nursing Federation (ANF): <http://www.anf.org.au>

International Council of Nurses: <http://www.icn.ch>

National Nursing and Nursing Education Taskforce, Australian Health Ministers' Advisory Council: <http://www.nnnet.gov.au/index.htm>

New South Wales Nurse Practitioners: <http://www.health.nsw.gov.au/nursing/practitioner/nurse_practitioner.asp>

Documentaries/films

The Burning Times (1990): 56 minutes, National Film Board of Canada, Canada. Documents how female healers were persecuted as witches.

The Doctor (1991): 125 minutes, produced by Buena Vista, directed by Randa Haines, USA. Starring William Hurt, this is a film about an arrogant doctor who becomes a patient and deals with issues of doctor–patient interaction.

Handmaidens and Battleaxes (1989): 55 minutes, Silver Films. Examines the changing role of nursing in Australia.

References

Australasian Nurses' Journal 1903, 'Notes', July, p. 37.

Australasian Nurses' Journal 1908, 'District Nursing Associations', October, p. 97.

Australasian Nurses' Journal 1921, 'Training School for Infant Welfare: First under Karitane in Australia', 15 October, p. 344.

Bessant, J. & Bessant, B. 1991, *The Growth of a Profession: Nursing in Victoria 1930s–1980s*, La Trobe University Press, Bundoora.

Bonawit V. & Watson L. 1996, 'Nurses Who Work in General Medical Practices: A Victorian Survey', *Australian Journal of Advanced Nursing*, vol. 13, no. 4, pp. 28–34.

Bowe, E.J. 1960, 'The Story of Nursing in Australia since Foundation Day', New South Wales College of Nursing, Eighth Annual Oration, Sydney.

Brookes K., Davidson P., Daly J. & Hancock K. 2004, 'Community Health Nursing in Australia: a Critical Literature Review and Implications for Professional Development', *Contemporary Nurse*, April–June, vol. 3, no. 16, pp. 195–207.

Chittick, R. 1968, *Assignment Report for Western Pacific Regional Office of the World Health Organization*, WHO, Manila.

Chittick, R. 1969, 'Our Anabasis', *Australasian Nurses' Journal*, March, pp. 58–60.

Davies, C. 1995, *Gender and the Professional Predicament in Nursing*, Open University Press, Buckingham.

Department of Health, 2002, *Liberating the Talents: Helping Primary Care Trusts and Nurses to Deliver the NHS Plan*, Department of Health, London.

Department of Health, CNO Directorate, 2007, *Towards a Framework for Post-registration Nursing Careers*, Department of Health, London.

Doyal, L. 1997, *What Makes Women Sick: Gender and the Political Economy of Health*, Macmillan, London.

Ehrenreich, B. & English, D. 1973, *Witches, Midwives and Nurses*, Old Westbury Feminist Press, New York.

Fee, E. (ed.) 1983, *Women and Health: The Politics of Sex in Medicine,* Baywood Publishing Company, New York.

Freidson, E. 1970, *Profession of Medicine*, Dodd Mead, New York.

Gamarnikow, E. 1978, 'Sexual Division of Labour: The Case of Nursing', in A. Kuhn & A. Wolpe (eds), *Feminism and Materialism*, Routledge & Kegan Paul, London.

Greenwood, E. 1957, 'The Attributes of a Profession', *Social Work*, vol. 2, pp. 44–55.

Happell, B. 2002, 'The Role of Nursing Education in the Perpetuation of Inequality', *Nurse Education Today*, vol. 22, no. 8, pp. 632–40.

Hearn, J. 1982, 'Notes on Patriarchy, Professionalization and the Semi-professions', *Sociology*, vol. 16, no. 2, pp. 184–201.

International Council of Nurses (ICN) 2008, Definition of Nursing. Available online: <http://www.icn.ch/definition.htm>

Johnstone, M. J. & Stewart, M. 2002, 'Ethical Issues in the Recruitment and Retention of Graduate Nurses: A National Concern', *Contemporary Nurse*, vol. 14, issue 3, pp 240–7.

Keleher, H. 2000, 'Australian Nursing: For the Health of Medicine or the Health of the Public?', PhD thesis, La Trobe University, Bundoora.

Keleher H., Parker R., Abdulwadud O., Francis K., Segal L. & Dalziel K. 2007, *Systematic Review of Primary and Community-Based Nursing*, Department of Health Science, Monash University, Melbourne.

National Nursing and Nursing Education Taskforce 2006, 'Myth Busters', Australian Health Ministers' Advisory Council. Available online: <http://www.nnnet.gov.au/downloads/mythbusters_np.pdf>

Helen Keleher

Pascoe T., Hutchinson R., Foley E., Watts I., Whitecross L. & Snowdon T. 2006, 'General Practice Nursing Education in Australia', *Collegian*, vol. 13, no. 2, pp. 22–5.

Productivity Commission 2005, *Australia's Health Workforce, Research Report.* Productivity Commission, Canberra.

Russell, L. 1990, *From Nightingale to Now: Nursing Education in Australia,* Harcourt Brace Jovanovich, Sydney.

Salvage, J. 1985, *Politics of Nursing,* Heinemann, London.

Smith, R. 1999, *In Pursuit of Nursing Excellence: A History of the Royal College of Nursing,* Australia, 1949–1999, Oxford University Press, Melbourne.

Speedy, S. 1991, 'The Contribution of Feminist Research', in G. Gray & R. Pratt (eds), *Towards a Discipline of Nursing,* Churchill Livingstone, Melbourne.

World Health Organization 1978, *Primary Health Care: Report of the International Conference on Primary Health Care,* WHO, Alma-Ata, USSR.

World Health Organization 1986, *Ottawa Charter for Health Promotion,* WHO, Geneva.

Willis, E. 1989, *Medical Dominance,* Allen & Unwin, Sydney.

Witz, E. 1992, *Professions and Patriarchy,* Routledge, London.

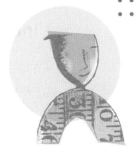

CHAPTER 21

The Sociology of Complementary and Alternative Medicine

ALEX
BROOM

Overview

- What is complementary and alternative medicine (CAM)?
- Why is CAM increasingly popular?
- What are some of the benefits and limitations of CAM?

THE HUNT FOR LIAM

On 28 November 1998, 3-year-old Liam Williams-Holloway was taken into hospital by his parents with what was initially thought to be the mumps. It took ten days to confirm that Liam had neuroblastoma, a rare form of childhood cancer. Given a fifty-fifty chance of survival with chemotherapy, and none without, Liam received two courses but, on 5 January 1999, oncologists were told that Liam's parents wanted no further chemotherapy treatment for Liam. The state responded to this by making Liam a 'ward of court' (i.e. custody is handed over to the state) in an effort to ensure that he received chemo-therapy, with police and social services involved in the 'hunt for Liam'. Aided by public donations, and in hiding, the family pursued alternative cancer treatments, eventually travelling to Mexico and Germany. This sparked a heated public debate over the right to live versus the right to choose, and the role of the state in deciding for individuals what constitutes an 'effective' treatment. Liam died in late October 2000, within 2 years of his initial diagnosis, but also living significantly longer than his oncologists expected he would without chemotherapy.

Introduction

The above vignette provides a vivid illustration of the complex issues emerging in an increasingly pluralistic therapeutic landscape, highlighting tensions between the right to choose (from the parents' perspective) and the right to live (from the child's perspective), within the context of a **biomedical** monopoly over **state**-provided cancer treatment. While not all decisions about health are this complex or serious, Australians increasingly have to weigh up a range of perspectives on health and illness, and competing claims to expertise, such as those between naturopaths and general practitioners (GPs). **Complementary and alternative medicine (CAM)** has become increasingly popular, with a conservative estimate finding that Australians spend around $1.8 billion of their own money each year on CAM and CAM therapists (MacLennan et al. 2006). Despite high levels of public support and recent political pressure, currently there is no formal health policy in Australia addressing CAM-related issues. Furthermore, the relationship between various CAM and biomedical organisations remains tense, a situation acknowledged in a recent senate inquiry (NHMRC 2005; Senate Community Affairs References Committee 2005). As examined in this chapter, sociologists have done a lot of work examining the reasons why people are using CAM and the nature of the divisions between CAM and biomedicine in Australia and internationally. The focus of this body of work has been on the ideological differences and organisational structures limiting CAM legitimation and integration. Furthermore, there has been interest in disentangling what additional benefits CAM may provide for individuals, who are currently provided biomedical care. In order to provide some context to the sociological work done on CAM, it is useful to provide some reflection on issues of definition and the historical trajectories of CAM and biomedicine.

What is CAM?

What actually constitutes a complementary or alternative medicine is a question that continues to cause researchers considerable problems in terms of how to measure levels of usage in the wider population. CAM is now largely accepted as a broad descriptor, though other labels are frequently used including 'alternative', 'natural', 'folk', 'holistic', and 'complementary' (see Broom 2002). Such terms are ideologically loaded in their own unique way and each holds certain qualities that neither CAM practitioners nor biomedical practitioners have accepted. For example, the term *complementary* is, for many CAM practitioners, considered to mean 'non-essential'. Moreover, *alternative* is equally problematic for some CAM practitioners because it implies an incompatibility with biomedicine. For some medical practitioners, 'alternative' denotes legitimacy in terms of being considered an effective 'alternative' to biomedical treatment. As a result there is still ongoing debate over what CAM actually is, what characterises CAM practices, and thus, what to call its practitioners.

**biomedicine/
biomedical model**

The conventional approach to medicine in Western societies, based on the diagnosis and explanation of illness as a malfunction of the body's biological mechanisms. This approach underpins most health professions and health services, which focus on treating individuals, and generally ignores the social origins of illness and its prevention.

state

A term used to describe a collection of institutions, including the parliament (government and opposition political parties), the public-sector bureaucracy, the judiciary, the military, and the police.

complementary and alternative medicine (CAM)

A broad term to describe both alternative medical practitioners and practices that may stand in opposition to orthodox medicine and also those who may collaborate with, and thus complement, orthodox practice (are also referred to as integrative medicine).

Sociologists tend to take a different approach to issues of terminology by exploring the common sense assumptions underlying terms, such as 'scientific', 'evidence-based', 'natural', 'holistic', and 'invasive'. Rather than trying to secure a concrete definition, what is important is the purpose, impact, and durability of certain categories. From a sociological perspective, CAM is ultimately a **socially constructed** and dynamic entity that is historically and culturally variable. Moreover, it contains concrete or 'harder' elements (basic artefacts such as acupuncture needles or crystals) and 'softer' elements (health ideology or approaches to the therapeutic relationship) which are represented in certain ways and categorised to be certain things. CAM does not exist *per se*; it has no identifiable, concrete boundaries or borders outside of the sense-making practices that we all utilise. Rather, the term is a somewhat clumsy, but nevertheless useful, over-arching category that helps us ascribe meanings to practices that are hugely diverse.

At various points in time there have been attempts to establish a lasting definition of CAM, to make a durable list of which modalities are essentially CAM or bio-medical. As could be predicted, such a list invariably fails the test of time; 'what is CAM' is variable over time and space. The socially and culturally mobile nature of CAM plagues base-line survey research (Zollman & Vickers 1999) and there is a lack of consistency in definitions of CAM between studies with significant implications on the results. For example, the inclusion of spiritual practices as CAM—which can be anything from praying for healing to consulting a spiritual healer—greatly increases the reported percentage of CAM users in a population (see Richardson et al. 2000). Moreover, a flat percentage of CAM users provides little information regarding the usage of particular modalities (e.g. chiropractic versus psychic surgery). Thus, statistics tend to tell us little about which alternative modalities are most frequently used and tend to promote an image of the ascendance of all CAMs, which may be inaccurate.

While it is important to emphasise the socially and culturally relative nature of CAM, as presented in Table 21.1, we can also say certain things about the general features of many CAM modalities, including broad distinctions between the principles of health espoused by CAM practitioners versus those generally promoted by the medical profession.

> **social construction/ constructionism**
> Refers to the socially created characteristics of human life based on the idea that people actively construct reality, meaning it is neither 'natural' nor inevitable. Therefore, notions of normality/ abnormality, right/ wrong, and health/ illness are subjective human creations that should not be taken for granted.

Table 21.1 The complementary and alternative medicine (CAM) model

Key features	Description
Self-healing	The body has a 'natural' ability to heal itself and maintain homeostasis
Holism	A person is a subtle and complex blend of body, mind, and spirit
Patient-centred	Treating root causes is more important than just managing symptoms—each person is unique
Self-help	The patient must take responsibility for his or her own wellness
Intimacy	The client/practitioner relationship is seen to aid healing through intimacy, intentionality, and awareness of multiple variables in illness

Source: Broom & Tovey 2008

Alex Broom

Broadly, the category CAM is used to refer to a wide range of therapeutic practices including aromatherapy, naturopathy, herbalism, homeopathy, reiki, acupuncture, and spiritual healing. Moreover, there are certain parallels we can draw between CAMs. What largely characterises CAMs is, first, a lack of integration into Western health care systems and, second, their tendency to espouse models of care that incorporate physical and metaphysical elements in treatment processes. There is also some merit in distinguishing between 'whole systems' approaches like naturopathy or homeopathy and the less ideologically driven healing approaches such as reiki, aromatherapy massage, or healing touch. Even though these categories are disputed, and should not be viewed as in any way static, the following table from the National Centre for Complementary and Alternative Medicine in the US provides one (albeit limited) schema for differentiating between different CAMs.

Table 21.2 Categories of CAM

CAM type	Description
Alternative medical systems	Alternative medical systems are built upon complete systems of theory and practice. Often, these systems have evolved apart from and earlier than the conventional medical approach used in the United States. Examples of alternative medical systems that have developed in Western cultures include homeopathic medicine and naturopathic medicine. Examples of systems that have developed in non-Western cultures include traditional Chinese medicine and ayurveda
Mind–body interventions	Mind–body medicine uses a variety of techniques designed to enhance the mind's capacity to affect bodily function and symptoms, including meditation, prayer, mental healing, and therapies that use creative outlets such as art, music, or dance
Biologically based therapies	Biologically based therapies in CAM use substances found in nature, such as herbs, foods, and vitamins. Some examples include dietary supplements, herbal products, and the use of other so-called natural therapies (for example, using shark cartilage to treat cancer)
Manipulative and body-based methods	Manipulative and body-based methods in CAM are based on manipulation and/or movement of one or more parts of the body. Some examples include chiropractic or osteopathic manipulation, and massage
Energy therapies	Energy therapies involve the use of energy fields. They are of two types: 1 Biofield therapies are intended to affect energy fields that purportedly surround and penetrate the human body. The existence of such fields has not yet been scientifically proven. Some forms of energy therapy manipulate biofields by applying pressure and/or manipulating the body by placing the hands in, or through, these fields. Examples include qigong, reiki, and therapeutic touch. 2 Bioelectromagnetic-based therapies involve the unconventional use of electromagnetic fields, such as pulsed fields, magnetic fields, or alternating-current or direct-current fields

Source: National Center for Complementary and Alternative Medicine 2008

There are similar definitional issues with terms such as 'Western' or 'modern' medicine. Historically, Western medicine has been referred to as 'modern', 'conventional', or 'orthodox'. Yet, these categories have obvious limitations. For example, some biomedical techniques and practices developed from what we may consider premodern times, and in non-Western regions (Tovey et al. 2007). Thus this chapter refers to 'modern medicine' as biomedicine. Biomedicine refers to the scientific basis of the practices generally recognised as modern medicine, such as biology and biochemistry, rather than suggesting its progressiveness (i.e. modern) or geographical roots (i.e. Western). The next section briefly overviews how biomedicine came to be (for further detail see Chapters 1 and 19).

Biomedicine in social and historical contexts

Biomedicine is often represented as having always been 'conventional', even though in actuality, it came into being through a relatively recent process of securing state validation, professional autonomy, and self-regulation (Willis 1989). Through the implementation of various policies, Acts, regulations and laws, biomedicine, to a large extent, ensured the exclusion of certain other practices from receiving state legitimation (see Willis 1989). Biomedicine is, ultimately, the product of historical struggles over access to resources, rights to practise, state validation, and occupational territories. Throughout these struggles, biomedicine has been relatively successful in establishing a monopoly over the delivery of primary (e.g. general practitioners) and secondary health care (e.g. hospitals). As such, the dominance of biomedicine has been as much about political manoeuvring, and achievement of self-regulation, as it has been about effectiveness. Of course, one cannot separate effectiveness from access to resources. Alliances, state funding, and the flow-on effect of political power all contribute to claims about the legitimacy of the biomedical model, with resources spent on furthering the biomedical approach, thus boosting the performance of biomedicine over other therapeutic modalities (Broom & Tovey 2008).

Medical dominance is a relatively recent phenomenon. In Europe, before the widespread emergence of the medical profession, a range of modalities were available including astrology, herbalism, and healing (Larner 1992). The pattern until the nineteenth century was for different modalities to wax and wane in popularity, but, in the mid-nineteenth century, one of these modalities, **allopathy** (what has now evolved into what we call biomedicine), began to rise into a position of dominance (Willis 1989). The initial development of the medical profession in England in the nineteenth century came about through the merging of apothecaries, surgeons, and physicians (Abbott 1988). In 1815, the General Pharmaceutical Association initiated the *Apothecaries Act*, looking to the government to raise the standard of entry into the profession and to prohibit 'unqualified persons' from practising. The Act was the outcome of an ongoing struggle to create defined occupational boundaries between

medical dominance
A general term used to describe the power of the medical profession in terms of its control over its own work, over the work of other health workers, and over health resource allocation, health policy, and the way that hospitals are run.

allopathy
A descriptive name often given to orthodox medicine. Allopathy is the treatment of symptoms by opposites.

the apothecaries, druggists and chemists, physicians and surgeons (Dew 1998). The Act introduced the concept of a qualified or registered practitioner into English law, which gave the General Medical Council powers of control over who could practise medicine (Waddington 1973).

With medical dominance came a specific set of understandings about the body, the nature of disease, and the patient/provider relationship; what we generally refer to as the biomedical model (Samson 1999). This model of therapeutic practice espoused ideas that would dramatically alter the treatment of illness and disease in the twentieth and twenty-first centuries. Importantly, these biomedical assumptions, and now entrenched treatment practices, are crucially relevant to the reasons why individuals may utilise CAM, their experiences of biomedical care, and paradigmatic conflict between CAM and biomedicine.

The biomedical model and the embodiment of its assumptions within pharmaceutical and technological advances are self-perpetuating. If it is accepted that disease is reducible to the organ, cellular, or genetic levels (i.e. not connected to such things as the mind, spirit, or social environment), then more is spent on technologies that focus on organ, cell, and gene-specific problems. Thus, medical technologies, interventions, and practices significantly frame how we make sense of illness—they effectively render some things treatable and others untreatable. The result is an increasing reliance on the ability of biomedical experts to discover new and better ways of fixing us—that is, to produce new technologies that can discover (diagnosis), predict (prognosis), and cure—in accordance with the tenets of the biomedical approach.

The **reductionist** approach of biomedicine stresses the central role of the clinician in the healing process. The intervention of the clinician is active, and, in general, downplays the role of any social, psychological, or emotional factors that may cause the disease or play a role in its natural evolution or treatment. It is important at this point to stress that this is a model of health care prominent within biomedicine, not a description of the approach generally taken by medical practitioners, though it strongly influences how they approach treatment processes (Broom & Tovey 2008). Furthermore, the biomedical model still dominates public health provision in Australia and internationally (Turner & Samson 1995), even though CAM increasingly competes for legitimacy among the public. The failure of biomedicine to cure (or even decrease the prevalence of) common conditions including many cancers, chronic illnesses, and even the common cold, has led to a reduction in public deference to biomedical expertise and increased support for CAM.

Theoretical approaches to CAM: conceptualising patient engagement

Over the last two decades, sociologists have been attempting to understand the changes occurring in health care consumption (i.e. what people are using) and the

reductionism
The belief that all illnesses can be explained and treated by reducing them to biological and pathological factors.

consumerism
The processes and institutions by which individuals satisfy their needs by purchasing goods and services in a market. Mass consumerism refers to post-Second World War consumer practices, whereby the reduction of the cost of goods and the extensive use of advertising and new credit arrangements created a mass market. It is often argued that consumerism has less to do with the satisfaction of wants than with the desire to be different and distinctive.

relationships between professional groups and organisations (e.g. doctors and CAM practitioners). In terms of changing patient preferences, sociologists have developed a range of theoretical ideas to conceptualise CAM popularity among the wider population, including arguments about:

- a postmodernisation of social life
- processes of reflexive modernisation
- the emergence of new forms of selfhood and 'well-being'.

Some sociologists view the increased presence of CAM as reflecting wider patterns related to the so-called postmodernisation of social life (e.g. Bakx 1991; Siahpush 1998; Eastwood 2000; Rayner & Easthope 2001). Postmodernisation is broadly seen to denote an increased fragmentation of people's experience, **consumerism**, **individualisation**, and aestheticisation (judgments of taste or sensory value) of social life. Within this social context, the biomedical model is viewed as being subsumed by subjective individualised knowledges (people's own world views and perspectives) that inform how health and illness occur. CAM use, within this approach, is viewed as a rejection of medical dominance and the biomedical model in favour of individualised understandings of disease and treatment regimens. Implicit in such arguments is the increased prioritisation of **lay concepts of health and illness**, and importantly, the rejection of the superiority of scientific knowledge and expertise. While this theoretical stance has been widely drawn on, its applicability has been seriously questioned and has rarely been subject to empirical investigation (Broom & Tovey 2007b).

There have also been attempts to link CAM consumption to a wider cultural transition to **reflexive modernity**. Less suggestive of a complete cultural shift away from **modernity**, this period is characterised by individuals becoming more sceptical of the judgments or advice of scientific 'experts' (Lupton & Tulloch 2002) and actively assessing the merits of particular claims rather than merely accepting the status quo (Tovey et al. 2001; Low 2004). Moving beyond the rather over-simplistic 'fragmentation of social life' and 'individualisation' themes implicit in the postmodernisation thesis, one focus of the reflexive modernity thesis is on the increased tendency of people to be more critical of expert knowledge (Giddens 1991; Beck 1992). In this light the increased popularity of CAM could be explained as a backlash against the perceived failings of science and biomedical interventions (Tovey et al. 2001).

There have also been attempts to theorise use of CAM at the level of the individual, with well-being (as opposed to 'health' or 'disease prevention') as the new focus in contemporary health care (see Doel & Segrott 2003; Sointu 2006). Departing from biomedical notions of being 'cured', 'healthy', or 'disease-free', the notion of achieving well-being has emerged as a potentially useful concept for characterising what CAM offers to those who use it. Well-being encapsulates notions of:

- authenticity (i.e. being true to one's own spirit or being, regardless of external influences)

TheoryLink

See Chapter 2 for an overview of postmodernism and reflexive modernity.

individualism/ individualisation

A belief or process supporting the primacy of individual choice, freedom, and self-responsibility.

lay concepts of health and illness

Refers to personal and non-expert explanations of health attainment and illness causation and treatment.

reflexive modernity

A term coined by Ulrich Beck and Anthony Giddens to refer to the present social era in developed societies, in which social practices are open to reflection, questioning, and change, and therefore in which social traditions no longer dictate people's lifestyles.

modernity/ modernism

A view of social life that is founded upon rational thought and a belief that truth and morality exist as objective realities that can be discovered and understood through scientific means.

Alex Broom

- recognition (i.e. external acknowledgment of the validity of subjective experience)
- **agency** (i.e. the individual is central and powerful in the healing process).

agency
The ability of people, individually and collectively, to influence their own lives and the society in which they live.

Essentially, this involves the conceptualisation of 'health' as a subjective and individualised process (Bishop & Yardley 2004; Sointu 2006). CAM use, in this light, becomes a project of the self—part of the creation of an individual's identity.

Empirical research has, however, illustrated the limitations of these theoretical ideas for understanding people's use of CAM. For example, drawing on interviews with 80 British cancer patients, Alex Broom and Philip Tovey (2007b) argue that these notions of a wider cultural shift (postmodernisation) or rejection of 'objective' scientific expertise (reflexive modernisation) do not reflect grassroots patient experiences. Rather, what characterises individuals' engagement with CAM is a tension between the appeal of individualisation (a focus on the subjective self) and depersonalisation (the appeal of knowledge gained from scientific expertise). Furthermore, in this same study it was found that CAMs were valued because they allow for and promote agency and self-determination, particularly the reclaiming of hope, subjective experience and personal control. These were viewed as elements that were neglected in biomedical cancer care (Broom & Tovey 2007b). Yet there is also emerging evidence that highlights significant limitations to many CAM practices (and models of care), which can be hugely problematic for patients.

Theorising the limitations of complementary and alternative medicines

While there has been significant attention paid to the benefits of CAM and the problems with biomedicine, there is emerging concern regarding the potentially restrictive and controlling aspects of some CAM practices. Specifically, permeating some CAM practices are strong discourses of 'positivity' and self-responsibility, often linked to notions of self-actualisation and self-healing (see Gray & Doan 1990; Rittenberg 1995; De Raeve 1997; Bolletino 2001; Goldstein 2003; Broom & Tovey 2008; Broom forthcoming). What is interesting for sociologists is the degree to which CAM ideologies and practitioners encourage potentially restrictive, or even spurious, models of healing. An example, is the view, evident in some CAM practices, that one can actively shape or change one's reality (Bolletino 2001), and that to heal oneself necessarily involves an active reconstructing of one's worldview (Hay 1999). Such ideological frameworks ultimately denote a degree of self-responsibility for disease, and place the burden squarely on the individual patient (see Gray & Doan 1990; Rittenberg 1995; De Raeve 1997). It is not suggested here that such ideas are purely negative for patients, but it does point to a repositioning of responsibility, and potential guilt, for being ill (see also Frankl 1992). In the context of cancer and end-of-life care, for example, people may feel as if they 'failed' in healing themselves, adding an extra burden to an already difficult time.

This emerging problem of self-responsibility in CAM is illustrated in Broom's recent study of Australian cancer patients who use CAM (Broom forthcoming). The findings of this work suggest that CAM can act in such a way as to have liberating effects, including patient empowerment and promoting self-determination. It was also shown that there are normative and coercive facets to certain CAM modalities popular with cancer patients in Australia (e.g. strict naturopathic, dietary, or self-help programs). Interviews with cancer patients revealed the difficulties of 'maintaining positivity' and 'self-healing' in everyday contexts of having cancer. CAMs, it would seem, can act as disciplinary, controlling devices (Foucault 1991; Petersen 1997; Rose 1999), and carers and family members can unwittingly encourage this through wanting the person to 'be strong' and 'remain positive' (see also Brownlie 2004). Common statements from CAM practitioners like 'you must be positive' and 'you can heal yourself' might be deployed to suit the needs of those in supportive or caring roles (and those of CAM practitioners), rather than those of the individual patient (see Broom forthcoming).

In another study, Broom and Tovey (2008) found that the notions espoused by many CAM practitioners (i.e. self-healing, self-help, well-being, and self-awareness) may actually make the transition to death quite difficult for some individuals. The notion of 'healing oneself' through diet, meditation, and self-discipline may in fact be hard to let go of as the cancer progresses and the more rigorous CAM therapies become unrealistic. Moreover, there is concern regarding how patients reconcile 'success' when they get to an advanced stage of disease (i.e. 'have I done enough?'; 'maybe I wasn't positive enough') in the context of discourses around self-healing and self-responsibility (see Broom & Tovey 2008). Thus, it remains critical that in seeking to understand CAM sociologically, we acknowledge both the liberating and constraining elements of different therapeutic modalities.

Theorising the relationship of CAM to biomedicine: inter- and intra-profession issues

While sociologists have been particularly interested in the experiences of people who use CAM, there has also been a lot of work done on the disputes between CAM and biomedicine (Willis 1989; Tovey & Adams 2001; Kelner et al. 2004; Hirschkorn & Bourgeault 2005; Mizrachi et al. 2005). Within this literature, among other things, it has been argued that increases in public support for CAM represent a potential challenge to the power and structure of biomedicine. The increasing provision of CAM by general practitioners and private health funds, for example, can be seen as potentially challenging the current biomedical monopoly over primary and secondary health care. As such, the increased role of CAM in Australian health care could be seen as contributing, among other factors, to the **deprofessionalisation** of biomedicine (Haug 1973, 1988). Deprofessionalisation in this context denotes a demystification of medical expertise—making it more accessible to lay people—and increasing lay scepticism about biomedical health professionals (Broom 2005; Tovey & Broom 2007). This process of deprofessionalisation is seen to result from reductions in the monopolisation of medical knowledge, autonomy in work performance, and authority over clients (Haug 1988; Gray 2002; Lewis et al. 2003).

Arguments about CAM as challenging or potentially diminishing biomedical power are being problematised by research done in grassroots clinical contexts. Recent work suggests a view of the waning power or influence of the medical profession/al is oversimplified, if not erroneous (Broom 2006; Broom & Tovey 2007a). For example, key factors viewed as impacting on medical practice, such as CAM, the internet, or medical managerialism, may in fact be resulting in a series of adjustments to the current social context rather than a breakdown in professional control (Germov 1995; Lewis et al. 2003; Broom 2005).

Research by Broom indicates the emergence of complex strategies on the part of medical professionals to maintain their position of authority and monopoly over patient care (Broom 2005; Tovey & Broom 2007). In one study involving doctors working in the cancer wards of two Australian hospitals, it was found that, in medical consultations with patients, medical specialists frequently utilise unsubstantiated notions of 'risk'—'CAM will interfere with your chemotherapy' or 'CAM will harm you'—as a key strategy to stop their patients from using CAM (Broom & Adams forthcoming). Even though we may view CAM popularity as problematising medical dominance, research is also showing how grassroots interactions, such as medical consultations, can involve communication strategies that reassert biomedical models of care and expertise that undermine patient use of CAM.

deprofessionalisation
A general theory predicting the decline of medical status and power due to the public's increased education about health issues and diminishing trust in medical practice as a result of media exposés of medical fraud and negligence.

BOX 21.1 Doing health sociology: doctors and CAM

In their study, Tovey and Broom (2007) found three main types of reactions by doctors to their cancer patients' use of CAM:

1 explicit or implicit negativity
2 supportive ambivalence
3 pragmatic acceptance.

Findings illustrated that if doctors were negative or ambivalent toward their patients' interest in CAM, they risked alienating them and concealment of future CAM use. While historically doctors have focused heavily on warning against CAM use, this study found that a focus on understanding subjective benefits of CAM and patients' individual experiences would actually enhance doctor–patient communication, facilitate discussion of risks, and thus improve the quality of care provided.

Over the last few decades there have been numerous struggles between biomedicine and CAM modalities seeking state legitimacy and community recognition. Seen by many as the success stories of complementary and alternative medicine, chiropractic and acupuncture embarked on a long struggle for recognition in Australia (Willis 1989), and in doing so, some argue, have submitted to the hegemonic influences of biomedicine, dropping their mesmeric origins in exchange for access to the hospital and insurance industries. Kevin Dew (1998) reiterates this, stating that by moving towards the core of biomedicine to seek validation, chiropractic and acupuncture potentially compromised their ideological roots.

In health care contexts such as **primary health care**, there has been an increase in the adoption or 'integration' of specific CAM practices (e.g. acupuncture). In the USA, the notion of integrative medicine is particularly popular with the privatisation of health care facilitating the consumer-driven provision of CAM in conjunction with conventional medical treatments. Yet, as sociologists have noted, integration may in fact be more about strategic co-option of certain CAM procedures and technologies than the coming together of CAM and biomedicine (Broom & Tovey 2007a). Again, the provision of acupuncture and other CAM practices in biomedical settings has arguably resulted in a muting of their metaphysical overtones (i.e. notions of energy fields, qi, or chakras) in an attempt to increase their compatibility with the biomedical model. It is argued that this process of assimilation has been exacerbated by processes of professionalisation and in particular the establishment of qualifications, licensing, and regulatory bodies (Saks 1998).

> **primary health care (PHC)**
> Both the point of first contact with the health care system and a philosophy for delivery of that care.

Nursing and CAM

Historically, the relationship between CAM and the nursing profession has been quite different to that of the medical profession. Nursing has frequently presented itself as patient-centred rather than disease-centred and holistic rather than mechanistic in approach. This, it could be argued, gives nursing practice something of a 'natural' affinity to some CAM approaches (Light 1997), but also reflects some important differences between the trajectory of nursing and medicine (Boschma 1994). CAM therapies like reiki, spiritual healing, reflexology, meditation, or massage may be seen on one level to have broadly compatible objectives in terms of patient outcomes to that of nursing practice (reducing anxiety, stress, pain, and discomfort). The vast popularity of CAM is thus potentially less challenging to the nursing profession than it is to certain elements of the medical profession. This is perhaps best reflected in the increased levels of CAM advocacy within the nursing literature. There is significantly more support for integration and more research into the potential benefits of utilising CAM in conjunction with biomedicine (Chong 2006; Lengacher et al. 2006). Moreover, at least within some facets of nursing, knowledge of, and the ability to offer advice on, CAM is represented as a valuable element to the nurse's role in patient care (Lee 2005).

Alex Broom

On another level, certain sub-groups within nursing, it would seem, have begun to present the incorporation of CAM as a means of establishing inter- and intra-professional distinction (Tovey & Adams 2003). CAM, in part, has emerged as a means of differentiating nursing from medicine and also within nursing itself, such as 'holistic' or 'CAM nurse' specialists versus purely 'biomedical' nurses. Studies also show the ways in which nurses are selecting and giving advice about CAM, and thus acting as gatekeepers (excluding certain practices and promoting others) (Tovey & Broom 2007). Thus, it would seem nursing is both involved in CAM advocacy, to a degree, but is also contributing to the delimiting of CAM provision according to their own professional goals and belief systems. Nurses, as gatekeepers and legitimisers of CAM, thus play an important role in shaping what patients want from CAM, what they use it for, and how they view it in relation to biomedicine. This places nurses in a potentially powerful position in shaping the form of CAM integration into mainstream health services (Broom & Adams forthcoming).

Conclusion

Complementary and alternative medicine represents a fascinating site of tension, conflict, and change for health sociologists. Early work in the sociology of CAM focused primarily on the professions (Willis 1989), but increasingly sociologists have been exploring the lived experiences of CAM users and the complexities of what CAM may achieve for different individuals in a range of disease contexts. There is still a need for more research examining the role of gender, class, and ethnicity in shaping experiences of CAM, but it seems clear that CAM achieves certain things often not 'done well' in biomedicine. This includes recognising the subjectivity of health and illness, the importance of the therapeutic relationship, and the utility of allowing people to have a sense of agency and control over their illness. As illustrated in this chapter, it is critical that we also acknowledge and interrogate the limitations of CAM rather than idealising practices as 'liberating' and 'empowering' merely because they are excluded from mainstream health care delivery. Emphasising the disciplinary and digressive aspects of some CAM practices and practitioners would not denigrate the value of CAM. Rather, critical analysis of this kind would facilitate progress by reflecting a more accurate and nuanced picture of what actually occurs when people engage with non-biomedical options.

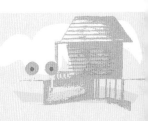

Summary of main points

» From a sociological perspective, CAM is a constructed and dynamic entity that is historically and culturally variable.

» The value of CAM seems to be embedded to the tendency of CAM modalities to promote agency and self-determination, and to acknowledge and promote subjectivity.

» Some CAM modalities and practitioners promote strong discourses of hyper-positivity and self-responsibility that can be problematic for some patients, particularly those with cancer.

» Even though CAM is often presented as a potential challenge to the biomedical organisational culture, biomedical professionals are utilising complex interpersonal strategies to reinforce their position of authority and monopoly over health care provision.

» For certain elements of the nursing community, CAM has emerged as a means of differentiation from the medical community and support for CAM can be linked to broader processes of distinction and professionalisation within nursing.

Sociological reflection: using CAM

» Do you use CAM? Think about some of the reasons why you do or do not.
» Are there some CAM therapies you would never consider using? Why?
» Which CAM therapies are most likely to be integrated with biomedicine? Why?
» To what extent do CAM therapies individualise notions of health and illness by promoting self-responsibility and self-healing? Is this a good or bad thing?

Discussion questions

1 What are some of the reasons people use CAM therapies?

2 What would be the benefits and the limitations of the increased regulation of complementary and alternative medicines like naturopathy or herbal medicine?

3 What might the implications be if CAM therapies like acupuncture or homeopathy were delivered by general practitioners?

4 Should treatments only be provided to patients if there is evidence to back them up? What constitutes 'evidence' and who should decide this?

5 People are increasingly making use of CAM; should the Australian Government provide CAM as well as biomedical health care if the population views it as useful?

Alex Broom

6 If you could decide on one CAM being integrated into mainstream health care which one would it be and why?

7 What is more important: the right to live or the right to choose? Should parents be allowed to choose alternative treatments for their children over conventional care?

Further investigation

1 CAM is contributing to a reduction in the power of biomedicine and its practitioners. Discuss.

2 The increasing popularity of CAM therapies result from the processes of reflexive modernity. Discuss.

3 Choose an example of CAM (such as homeopathy, acupuncture...) and examine:
   a The historical background to the development of the therapy and its practice.
   b The implicit and explicit cultural values underpinning the particular therapeutic approach to diagnosis and treatment.
   c The way it is regulated and the institutions in which it is practised.
   d The critical challenge it presents to orthodox approaches to health.

Further reading

Adams, J. (ed.) 2007, *Researching Complementary and Alternative Medicine*, Routledge, London.

Barry, A. 2006, 'The Role of Evidence in Alternative Medicine: Contrasting Biomedical and Anthropological Approaches', *Social Science and Medicine,* vol. 62, no. 11, pp. 2646–57.

Cant, S. & Calnan, M. 1991, 'On the Margins of the Medical Marketplace? An Exploratory Study of Alternative Practitioners' Perceptions', *Sociology of Health and Illness,* vol. 13, no. 1, pp. 39–57.

Cant, S. L. & Sharma, U. 1999, *A New Medical Pluralism? Alternative Medicine, Doctors, Patients and the State*, Routledge, London.

Dew, K. 2000, 'Deviant Insiders: Medical Acupuncturists in New Zealand', *Social Science and Medicine,* vol. 50, no. 12, pp. 1785–95.

Jackson, S. & Scambler, G. 2007, 'Perceptions of Evidence-based Medicine: Traditional Acupuncturists in the UK and Resistance to Biomedical Modes of Evaluation', *Sociology of Health and Illness,* vol. 29, no. 3, pp. 412–29.

Sointu, E. 2006, 'The Search for Well-being in Alternative and Complementary Health Practices', *Sociology of Health and Illness,* vol. 28, no. 3, pp. 330–49.

Tovey, P., Easthope, G. & Adams, J. (eds), 2004, *The Mainstreaming of Complementary Medicine*, Routledge, London.

Willis, E. & Coulter, I. 2004, 'The Rise and Rise of Complementary and Alternative Medicine: A Sociological Perspective', *Medical Journal of Australia*, vol. 180, no. 11, pp. 587–9.

Web resources

Australian Traditional Medicine Society: <http://www.atms.com.au/>

Canadian Interdisciplinary Network for Complementary and Alternative Medicine Research: <http://www.incamresearch.ca/index.php?home&lng=en>

Complementary and Integrated Medicine Research Unit (UK): <http://www.cam-research-group.co.uk/>

International Society for Complementary Medicine Research: <http://www.iscmr.org/>

Journal of Complementary and Integrative Medicine: <http://www.bepress.com/jcim>

National Center for Complementary and Alternative Medicine (NCCAM): <http://nccam.nih.gov/>

Documentaries/films

Lorenzo's Oil (1992): 129 minutes. Directed by George Miller and starring Susan Sarandon and Nick Nolte, the film traces the plight of a family attempting to save their young son from a rare brain disease for which medicine has no cure.

Second Opinion (2005): ABC TV series with a focus on alternative therapies (30 minute episodes). Available online: <http://www.abc.net.au/tv/secondopinion/>

The Trouble with Medicine (1993): 6 part documentary series (each around 55 minutes) dealing with various challenges and limitations relating to biomedicine, ABC TV, BBC TV & Thirteen-WNET.

References

Abbott, A. 1988, *The System of Professions: An Essay on the Division of Expert Labor*, University of Chicago Press, Chicago.

Bakx, K. 1991, 'The "Eclipse" of Folk Medicine in Western Society', *Sociology of Health and Illness*, vol. 13, pp. 20–38.

Beck, U. 1992, *Risk Society: Towards a New Modernity*, Sage, London.

Bishop, F. & Yardley, L. 2004, 'Constructing Agency in Treatment Decisions: Negotiating Responsibility in Cancer', *Health*, vol. 8, no. 4, pp. 465–82.

Reader bonus

Available on the Second Opinion website: Easthope, G. 2005, 'Alternative Medicine', in J. Germov (ed.), *Second Opinion: An Introduction to Health Sociology*, 3rd edition, Oxford University Press, Melbourne.

Online case study

Visit the Second Opinion website to access relevant case studies.

Alex Broom

Bolletino, R. 2001, 'A Model of Spirituality for Psychotherapy and Other Fields of Mind–Body Medicine', *Advances in Mind–Body Medicine,* vol. 17, pp. 90–107.

Boschma, G. 1994, 'The Meaning of Holism in Nursing: Historical Shifts in Holistic Nursing Ideas', *Public Health Nursing,* vol. 11, no. 5, pp. 324–30.

Broom, A. 2002, 'Contested Territories: The Construction of Boundaries Between "Alternative" and "Conventional" Cancer Treatments', *New Zealand Journal of Sociology,* vol. 17, no. 2, pp. 215–34.

Broom, A. 2005, 'Medical Specialists' Accounts of the Impact of the Internet on the Doctor/Patient Relationship', *Health,* vol. 9, no. 3, pp. 319–38.

Broom, A. 2006, 'Reflections on the Centrality of Power in Medical Sociology: An Empirical Test and Theoretical Elaboration', *Health Sociology Review,* vol. 15, no. 5, pp. 55–70.

Broom, A. forthcoming, '"I'd Forgotten about Me in All of This": Discourses of Self-healing, Positivity and Vulnerability in Cancer Patients' Experiences of Complementary and Alternative Medicine', *Journal of Sociology.*

Broom, A. & Adams, J. forthcoming, 'Oncology Clinicians' Accounts of Discussing Complementary and Alternative Medicine with their Patients', *Health: An Inter-disciplinary Journal for the Social Study of Health, Illness and Medicine.*

Broom, A. & Tovey, P. 2007a, 'Therapeutic Pluralism? Evidence, Power and Legitimacy in UK Cancer Services, *Sociology of Health and Illness,* vol. 29, no. 3, pp. 551–69.

Broom, A. & Tovey, P. 2007b, 'The Dialectical Tension Between Individuation and Depersonalisation in Cancer Patients' Mediation of Complementary, Alternative and Biomedical Cancer Treatments', *Sociology,* vol. 41, no. 6, pp. 1021–39.

Broom, A. & Tovey, P. 2008, *Therapeutic Pluralism: Exploring the Experiences of Cancer Patients and Professionals,* Routledge, London and New York.

Brownlie, J. 2004, 'Tasting the Witches' Brew: Foucault and Therapeutic Practices', *Sociology,* vol. 38, no. 3, pp. 515–32.

Chong, O. 2006, 'An Integrative Approach to Addressing Clinical Issues in Complementary and Alternative Medicine in an Outpatient Oncology Center', *Clinical Journal of Oncology Nursing,* vol. 10, no. 1, pp. 83–8.

De Raeve, L. 1997, 'Positive Thinking and Moral Oppression in Cancer Care', *European Journal of Cancer Care,* vol. 6, no. 4, pp. 249–56.

Dew, K. 1998. *Borderland Practices: Validating and Regulating Alternative Therapies in New Zealand,* Victoria University of Wellington, Wellington.

Doel, M. & J. Segrott 2003, 'Self, Health, and Gender: Complementary and Alternative Medicine in the British Mass Media', *Gender, Place and Culture,* vol. 10, no. 2, pp. 131–44.

Eastwood, H. 2000, 'Postmodernisation, Consumerism and the Shift Towards Holistic Health', *Journal of Sociology,* vol. 36, pp. 133–55.

Foucault. M. 1991, 'Governmentality', in G. Burchell et al. (eds), *The Foucault Effect: Studies in Governmentality,* Harvester Wheatsheaf, Hempstead, pp. 87–104.

Frankl, V. 1992, *Man's Search for Meaning*, Deakin, Boston.

Germov, J. 1995, 'Medifraud, Managerialism and the Decline of Medical Autonomy', *Journal of Sociology*, vol. 31, no. 3, pp. 51–66.

Giddens, A. 1991, *Modernity and Self-identity: Self and Society in the Late Modern Age*, California, Stanford University Press, Stanford, CA.

Goldstein, M. 2003, 'Complementary and Alternative Medicine: Its Emerging Role in Oncology', *Journal of Psychosocial Oncology*, vol. 21, no. 2, pp. 1–21.

Gray, D. 2002, 'Deprofessionalising Doctors? The Independence of the British Medical Profession is Under Unprecedented Attack', *British Medical Journal*, vol. 324, no. 7338, pp. 627–9.

Gray, R. & B. Doan 1990, 'Heroic Self-healing and Cancer', *Journal of Palliative Care*, vol. 6, no. 1, pp. 32–41.

Haug, M. 1973, 'Deprofessionalisation: An Alternative Hypothesis for the Future', *Sociological Review Monograph*, vol. 20, pp. 195–211.

Haug, M. 1988, 'A Re-examination of the Hypothesis of Deprofessionalisation', *Milbank Quarterly*, vol. 2, (supp.), pp. 58–6.

Hay, L. 1999, *You Can Heal Your Life*, Hay House, Carlsbad, CA.

Hirschkorn, K. & I. Bourgeault 2005, 'Conceptualising Mainstream Health Care Providers' Behaviours in Relation to Complementary and Alternative Medicine', *Social Science and Medicine*, vol. 61, pp. 157–70.

Kelner, M., Wellman, B., Boon, H. & Welsh, S. 2004, 'Responses of Established Healthcare to the Professionalization of Complementary and Alternative Medicine in Ontario', *Social Science and Medicine*, vol. 59, pp. 915–30.

Larner, C. 1992, 'Healing in Pre-industrial Britain', in M. Saks (ed.), *Alternative Medicine in Britain*, Clarendon Press, Oxford.

Lee, C. 2005, 'Communicating Facts and Knowledge in Cancer Complementary and Alternative Medicine', *Seminars in Oncology Nursing*, vol. 21, no. 3, 201–14.

Lengacher, C., Bennett, M., Kip, K., Gonzalez, L., Jacobsen, P. & Cox, C. 2006, 'Relief of Symptoms, Side Effects, and Psychological Distress Through Use of Complementary and Alternative Medicine in Women with Breast Cancer', *Oncology Nursing Forum*, vol. 33, no. 1, pp. 97–104.

Lewis, J., Marjoribanks, T. & Pirotta, M. 2003, 'Changing Professions: General Practitioners' Perceptions of Autonomy at the Front Line', *Journal of Sociology*, vol. 39, no. 1, pp. 44–61.

Light, K. 1997, 'Florence Nightingale and Holistic Philosophy', *Journal of Holistic Nursing*, vol. 15, no. 1, pp. 25–40.

Low, J. 2004, 'Managing Safety and Risk: The Experiences of People with Parkinson's Disease Who Use Alternative and Complementary Therapies', *Health*, vol. 8, no. 4, pp. 445–63.

Lupton, D. & Tulloch J. 2002, 'Risk is Part of Your Life: Risk Epistemologies among a Group of Australians', *Sociology*, vol. 36, no. 2, pp. 317–35.

MacLennan, A., Myers, S. & Taylor, A. 2006, 'The Continuing Use of Complementary and Alternative Medicine in South Australia: Costs and Beliefs in 2004', *Medical Journal of Australia*, vol. 184, no. 1, pp. 27–31.

Mizrachi, N., Shuval, J. & Gross, S. 2005, 'Boundary at Work: Alternative Medicine in Biomedical Settings', *Sociology of Health and Illness*, vol. 27, no. 1, pp. 20–43.

National Center for Complementary and Alternative Medicine 2008, *What is CAM?*. Available online: <http://nccam.nih.gov/health/whatiscam/>

National Health and Medical Research Council 2005, *NHMRC Response to Senate Community Affairs References Committee Report: The Cancer Journey: Informing Choice*, National Health and Medical Research Council, Canberra. Available online: <http://www.aph.gov.au/Senate/committee/clac_ctte/completed_inquiries/2004-07/cancer/response.pdf >

Petersen, A. 1997, *Foucault, Health and Medicine,* Routledge, London.

Rayner, L. & Easthope, G. 2001, 'Postmodern Consumption and Alternative Medications', *Journal of Sociology*, vol. 37, no. 2, pp. 157–76.

Richardson, M. A., Sanders, T., Palmer, J. L., Greisinger, A. & Singletary, S. E. 2000, 'Complementary/alternative Medicine use in a Comprehensive Cancer Center and the Implications for Oncology', *Journal of Clinical Oncology*, vol. 18, pp. 2505–14.

Rittenberg, C. 1995, 'Positive Thinking: An Unfair Burden for Cancer Patients?', *Supportive Care in Cancer*, vol. 3, no. 1, pp. 37–9.

Rose, N. 1999, *Governing the Soul,* 2nd edn, Free Association Books, London.

Saks, M. 1998, 'Medicine and Complementary Medicine: Challenge and Change' in Scambler, G. & Higgs, P. (eds), *Modernity, Medicine and Health,* Routledge, London.

Samson, C. 1999, 'Biomedicine and the Body', in C. Samson (ed.), *Health Studies: A Critical and Cross-Cultural Reader,* Blackwell Publishers, Oxford.

Senate Community Affairs References Committee (SCARC) 2005, *The Cancer Journey: Informing Choice*, Commonwealth of Australia, Canberra.

Siahpush, M. 1998, 'Postmodern Values, Dissatisfaction with Conventional Medicine and Popularity of Alternative Therapies', *Journal of Sociology*, vol. 34, no. 1, pp. 58–70.

Sointu, E. 2006, 'Recognition and the Creation of Well-being', *Sociology*, vol. 40, no. 3, pp. 493–510.

Tovey, P. & Adams, J. 2001, 'Primary Care as Intersecting Social Worlds', *Social Science and Medicine*, vol. 52, pp. 695–706.

Tovey, P. & Adams, J. 2003, 'Nostalgic and Nostophobic Referencing and the Authentication of Nurses' Use of Complementary Therapies', *Social Science & Medicine*, vol. 56, 1469–80.

Tovey, P. & Broom, A. 2007, 'Oncologists' and Specialist Cancer Nurses' Approaches to Complementary and Alternative Medicine Use and Their Impact on Patient Action', *Social Science and Medicine*, vol. 64, pp. 2550–64.

Tovey, P., Atkin, K. & Milewa, T. 2001, 'The Individual and Primary Care: Service User, Reflexive Choice Maker and Collective Actor', *Critical Public Health*, vol. 11, no. 2, pp. 153–66.

Tovey, P., Chatwin, J. & Broom, A. 2007, *Traditional, Complementary and Alternative Medicine and Cancer Care: An International Analysis of Grassroots Integration*, Routledge, London and New York.

Turner, B. S. & Samson, C. 1995, *Medical Power and Social Knowledge*, 2nd edn, Sage Publications, London.

Waddington, I. 1973, 'The Struggle to Reform the Royal College of Physicians 1767–1771: A Sociological Analysis', *Medical History*, vol. 17, pp. 107–26.

Willis, E. 1989, *Medical Dominance: The Division of Labour in Australian Health Care*, Allen & Unwin, Sydney.

Zollman, C. & Vickers, A. 1999, 'Complementary Medicine and the Doctor', *British Medical Journal*, vol. 319, pp. 1558–61.

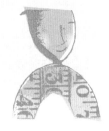

CHAPTER 22

Jostling for Position:
A Sociology of Allied Health

LAUREN
WILLIAMS

Overview

- What role does allied health play in the delivery of health care to Australians and to what extent is its role affected by medical dominance?
- What strategies have allied health practitioners used to seek professional status, and how successful have they been?
- What are the current threats and opportunities for allied health as a grouping in the health system?

STROKE AND ALLIED HEALTH

A 69-year-old man, John, was admitted to hospital following a cerebrovascular accident. The stroke caused some damage in the right side of the brain that resulted in paralysis down the left hand side of the body, and slightly slurred speech. John was admitted to the stroke ward where he was cared for by a team including doctors, nurses, and allied health staff (medical radiation scientists, speech pathologists, dietitians, physiotherapists, occupational therapists, and social workers). All played their distinctive roles in his treatment and recovery. After a week, John was discharged and went home, having received care and education from professionals who worked together as a team.

Jill, a 57-year-old woman, was admitted to the same hospital with renal (kidney) failure, which made her extremely unwell. She was seen by doctors, who were trying to diagnose why her kidneys failed, and provided with routine care by nurses. Renal failure requires dietary modification by a dietitian, but a dietitian consult was not requested and Jill was receiving a high protein diet, which would exacerbate kidney failure. After several days of lying in bed she had fluid in her lungs. A physiotherapist could have cleared her lungs or mobilised her, but no physiotherapist was requested. Three weeks later, Jill's kidney failure was resolved and the doctors said she could be discharged, but the relatives refused as she was so weak she could not even sit up. Jill was not assessed by an occupational therapist for her ability to care for herself at home.

Instead she was sent to an outlying hospital to further recuperate, prolonging the cost to the public health system. She left feeling sick and confused, having had a very negative experience because the doctors only focused on the medical nature of her disease, and there was no team to manage other aspects of her care.

Introduction

Allied health professionals provide specialised services directly to patients, as distinct from services provided by doctors or nurses. The range of services provided by allied health is broad, addressing the physical, psychological, social, functional, nutritional, pharmaceutical, and informational needs of patients. The aim of this chapter is to describe, and then analyse from a sociological perspective, the role of allied health practitioners, focusing on their development into professions in a health system characterised by **medical dominance**. To study the division of labour in what Evan Willis (1989) calls the **social structure** of health care delivery, we must look at how the various professions operate within the system. Much has been written from a sociological or political perspective about medicine and, increasingly, nursing. The critical perspective offered by sociology will uncover barriers to success and thereby inform the future direction of the allied health professions. It is the purpose of this chapter to provide such a perspective. We will see how members of the allied health professions seek to position themselves within the health system in order to be able to deliver effective patient care.

Description of the allied health professions

First, let us examine the term 'allied health professions'. 'Allied' means 'related to' or 'connected with', which was traditionally taken to mean 'allied to medicine'. 'Health' refers to the type of care delivered by these workers and to the system within which this care is delivered. The term 'professions' connotes a specific level of occupation: one that confers a high status. Some authors argue that this group would more correctly be called para- or semi-professionals, but use of the term 'profession' by allied health occupations indicates that these groups individually and collectively regard themselves as meeting the criteria for professional status. The previous labels

medical dominance
A general term used to describe the power of the medical profession in terms of its control over its own work, over the work of other health workers, and over health resource allocation, health policy, and the way that hospitals are run.

social structure
The recurring patterns of social interaction through which people are related to each other, such as social institutions and social groups.

Lauren Williams

for this group were 'ancillary' and 'paramedical'. Paramedical literally means 'beside medicine' and is defined as 'supplementing and supporting medical work' (*Australian Oxford Dictionary* 2004).

The Australian Bureau of Statistics (ABS) groups allied health practitioners into two categories: the health occupations (those with a diagnostic and treatment role, such as physiotherapists, occupational therapists, speech pathologists, and dietitians); and the health-related occupations (including psychologists, social workers, and counsellors) (AIHW 2004). Allied health professions, as defined above, made up 13 per cent of the total number of the health occupations at the 2006 census (see Table 22.1). The table shows that the number of allied health workers is increasing, as for other health occupations. It also shows the female proportion of the profession.

Table 22.1 Health personnel in Australia, by occupation, from the 2006 and 2001 census

	2006 (% female)[1]	2001[2]	Percentage change
Allied health practitioners			
Audiologists	1 080 (76.5)	801	35
Dietitians	2 584 (92.2)	2 001	29
Medical radiation scientists*	7 791 (67.6)	8 325	–6
Occupational therapists	6 835 (93.1)	5 343	28
Orthoptists	526 (86.3)	438	20
Orthotists and prosthetists	345 (33.0)	372	–7
Pharmacists	14 717 (56.1)	12 600	17
Physiotherapists	12 277 (71.0)	11 500	7
Psychologists	11 622 (78.2)	11 100	5
Social workers	12 420 (82.8)	9 124	36
Speech pathologists	3 871 (97.1)	2 997	29
Podiatrists	2 096 (61.5)	1 763	19
Total allied health practitioners	76 184	66 364	15
Total health occupations	592 848	391 328	5

* Previously listed as radiography (2006 number includes medical diagnostic radiographer and medical radiation therapists).

Source: 1. ABS 2006; 2. DOHA 2004a

Allied health workers form a homogeneous group in the sense that, broadly, they have a common role within the health system: supporting patient care. The fact that Australia has national, state, and special-purpose organisations of allied health professions—the work of which includes annual conferences and developmental projects—reflects this commonality. In addition, allied health professions previously operated under the same or similar management structures within the health system, although as we will see later, restructuring over the past decade has created other organisational models. University programs educating individual professions are also usually grouped together in schools or departments of 'allied health' or 'health sciences'.

A closer analysis of the functions of the individual professions illustrates their heterogeneity, and most have their own professional associations, fostering a specific professional identity. This chapter does not attempt to explore the diversity of the various allied health groups; it is more important for a sociological analysis to focus on the features common to the group as a whole.

Nature of the work of allied health professionals

Table 22.2 lists some key hospital-based allied health professions in Australia and describes important features of each. These professions predominantly work in multidisciplinary teams in public or private health settings. The role of an allied health professional within the acute care setting involves the following steps:

1 Individual needs of the patient are assessed to determine the extent of a problem, taking the present and past physical condition and lifestyle of the patient into consideration.
2 Treatment goals are decided upon, in consultation with the patient, and treatment is provided while the patient is in the acute care setting.
3 Records are kept and patient progress is communicated to other members of the health care team.
4 If patients need to continue treatment they are educated in the hospital and/or follow-up is organised to be provided in an out-patient setting.

Table 22.2 Characteristics of a sample of allied health professions in Australia

Role in health care delivery	Main place of work	Origins[1]
Physiotherapy The use of physical and manual methods in the treatment and prevention of injury and disease, with the aim of maximising normal movement	Mainly private practice, also hospital, and out-patient setting	Massage therapy in the early twentieth century, and university degree training since the 1970s
Occupational therapy Aims to maximise the quality of life of people affected by developmental delay, ageing, physical illness or injury, or psychological or social disability	Hospital, or community health settings, with increasing numbers in private practice	Workers in care of mentally ill in late eighteenth century. Established in Australia after the Second World War. University-based training established in 1945 at the University of Queensland

Table 22.2 (continued)

Role in health care delivery	Main place of work	Origins[1]
Speech pathology The diagnosis and treatment of problems with communication and with higher brain function involving speech and language	Community health, rehabilitation, hospitals, and increasing numbers in private practice	Developed as a result of the two World Wars and was firmly established in Australia by the end of the Second World War
Dietetics The application of nutritional knowledge in the dietary treatment of disease. Dietitians also advise on dietary changes to prevent illness in groups, communities, and populations	Half employed in the public hospital system, others in private practice, the food industry, and public health	Pre-1930s, dietitians were from the USA (home economics based), or nurses studied dietetics in the United Kingdom. University-based training established at the University of Melbourne in 1938
Medical radiation science Covers four distinct professional streams that produce images to assist diagnosis and to treat disease: medical imaging; ultrasonography; radiation therapy and non-ionising radiation; and radioactive and stable nuclides	Predominantly private practice, also in public hospitals	Arose from male-dominated science and technical background, but feminised in the 1930s as nurses gained necessary qualifications
Podiatry Previously known as chiropody, podiatry deals with prevention, diagnosis, treatment, and rehabilitation of medical and surgical problems concerning feet and lower legs	Majority in private practice, some in community health	This male-dominated profession arose in the early twentieth century to treat returned soldiers; 12-month courses by private colleges were replaced by tertiary degrees in the 1970s

1 This table gives only a brief overview, and each profession has its own complex history of development: see Phillipa Martyr (1994) for a history of the rehabilitation professions in Australia: physiotherapy, occupational therapy, and speech pathology; Heather Nash (1989) for the dietetic profession in Australia; Anne Witz (1992) for the feminisation of radiography.

Historical, cultural, and structural analysis of the allied health professions

In examining the issues facing allied health professions today, it is important to be aware of the history of their development. This section also examines issues relating to the culture of the allied health professions and/or their location within the health system's division of labour. These topics have been placed together since some issues, such as medical dominance, cross both cultural and structural perspectives.

Allied health professions arose as part of a trend towards increasing specialisation by encroaching on tasks that were previously performed by doctors or nurses. In the development phase of allied health in Australia, these new occupations were mostly staffed by nurses who underwent further specialised training (du Toit 1995), with fully specialised training established in the 1940s (see Table 22.2).

Working within a medically dominated public health system: 'it is always the doctor's patient'

Cultural and structural issues, for the allied health professions, are largely defined by the existence of medical dominance, which is outlined in Chapter 19. In this discussion, we will examine what impact this dominance has on the allied health professions.

Eliot Freidson (1970) has defined four key dimensions of medical dominance that impact on allied health:

1   control over the work and knowledge base of other health professions
2   the physician role of diagnosis and treatment
3   the need for the work of others to be requested and supervised by medicine
4   the unequal status of medicine and other health professions.

Evan Willis (1989) notes that, in Australia, medicine has used strategies of subordination, limitation, exclusion, and incorporation to produce and reproduce medical dominance of the health system. The strategy that has most characterised the relationship between medicine and the allied health professionals within the hospital system is subordination. Willis (1989) defines this as a mode of domination in which the occupations work under the direct control of doctors. This is reflected in the American Medical Association (AMA) 1981 definition of allied health personnel as using 'independent judgement, within their areas of competence *as approved by the supervising physician*' (my italics) (Donini-Lenhoff 2008, p. 49). These non-medical occupations are usually predominantly female, thereby creating a relationship between the **sexual division of labour** and the occupational division of labour.

The medical dominance strategy of subordination has affected allied health professionals in several ways:

1   doctors having positions of authority within the hospital and health system, and therefore administrative and financial control over allied health
2   doctors possessing absolute autonomy over their work, and controlling the amount of autonomy available to allied health professionals
3   doctors having direct or indirect control of **state** recognition of some allied health professions through representation on registration boards.

First, subordination is implemented by doctors having traditionally dominated the structure of the health system's division of labour, including having power over allocation of funding and resources. Although this situation is gradually changing with the increasing bureaucratisation and structural reorganisation of the hospital

sexual division of labour
Refers to the nature of work performed as a result of gender roles. In contemporary English-speaking societies, the stereotype is that of the male breadwinner and the female homemaker, even though this pattern is far from an accurate description of most people's lives.

state
A term used to describe a collection of institutions, including the parliament (government and opposition political parties), the public-sector bureaucracy, the judiciary, the military, and the police.

system, medicine continues to receive significantly more funding for practice and research than do other health areas. This situation is reinforced by medical representation on committees that control the allocation of funds.

Second, subordination affects the autonomy of the allied health professions. Autonomy is defined as control over one's own work, and has been identified by Freidson (1970) as the most important feature of **professionalisation**. An important question is that of the extent to which allied health professionals have autonomy in delivering clinical care. An Australian study looked at issues of dominance, autonomy, and authority for nursing and for four allied health professions (physiotherapy, occupational therapy, speech pathology, and psychology) within the hospital setting (Kenny & Adamson 1992). It found that allied health professionals, on average, believe that they have professional autonomy, but that this was truer for practitioners with more years of experience. A staggering 20 per cent of health workers in their first year of practice felt unable to make recommendations on patient care to referring doctors. While allied health may be gaining more power as a group within an organised system, doctors have not relinquished control of the patient in the hospital setting, and the responsibility for the care of the patient lies with the doctor.

To increase autonomy within the public hospital system would require significant changes in current policy on the delivery of patient care within hospitals, since most allied health professionals operate on medical request or referral. While allied health professionals can subvert this system by finding alternative means of seeing patients or by receiving referral from nurses or other allied health professionals, the doctor retains the power to ignore their recommendations or to cease contact between the patient and the allied health professional.

Allied health practitioners have greater autonomy within the private practice setting, with the right to consult patients without medical referral. The changes to Medicare, introduced with the Enhanced Primary Care (EPC) system in 2004, threaten this autonomy to some extent, since the ability of patients to obtain a rebate for allied health services depends on medical referral (see the section on working within Medicare p. 464). Allied health professional associations have begun to lobby for this requirement to be removed.

Finally, subordination is implemented through medical representation on registration boards for allied health, which is ironic, since many of the professions (for example, occupational therapy and physiotherapy) invited medicine to play this role. In the USA, allied health professions were accredited by the American Medical Association (AMA), a relationship which began in the early 1930s and did not cease until 1994 (Donini-Lenhoff 2008).

The question of profession

Authors have referred to the need for allied health occupations to achieve professional status as a struggle for survival (Willis 1989; Gardner & McCoppin 1995). Some

professionalisation
The process of becoming a profession, whereby an occupational group attains publicly recognised and government-legitimated monopoly and autonomy over its area of work.

authors have argued that allied health professionals would be more correctly called 'semi-professionals', since they lack the autonomy, power, status, and economic remuneration of traditional professions such as medicine (Willis 1989).

Allied health professionals, on the other hand, would argue that they meet the criteria for professional status by possessing an independent body of knowledge and expertise, by having university degrees as a minimum requirement, by achieving recognition of professional status by the state, and through ethical decision-making (which are all characteristic of the medical profession). Arguments such as these are based on the **trait approach** to professions, which in turn reflects functionalist theory. The assumption is that professions perform necessary functions for society, and hence the criteria that define a profession represent essential characteristics. This reasoning fails to explain why allied health occupations, if they are professions according to these criteria, are still poorly paid, have low status, and are subordinated to medicine.

Not surprisingly, then, trait theory has itself come under criticism for obscuring the historical and political conditions under which occupations professionalise. In a review of the professionalisation of occupational therapy, Rob Irvine and Jenny Graham (1994) found that trait theory was still accepted, relatively uncritically, by occupational therapy. They argued that occupational therapists have limited themselves by defining their professional role according to this trait approach and advocated a critical approach as a more useful framework. This model emphasises social power, control, and monopoly of markets, and the authors conclude by suggesting that power is the only logical basis upon which to distinguish between dominant professions and other occupations. Anne Witz (1992) also rejected a trait approach, but noted that those taking a critical approach have neglected to recognise the relationship between **gender** and professionalisation.

Gender and profession in the case of allied health

Feminist theory describes how the production of labour by women can reduce economic costs. Just as women reduce the cost of domestic labour by performing household chores without financial remuneration, allied health professionals, who are predominantly female, cheapen the cost of labour in the acute care setting by being paid significantly less than doctors (Turner 1995). Marjorie De Vault (1995) asserts that the type of work done by predominantly female allied health professions is 'women's work' in that it consists of 'devalued tasks that connect the actualities of people's lives with more abstract, "governing" bodies of knowledge, in this case, the practical application of medical knowledge'.

Witz (1992) applies a feminist analysis of gender to the division of labour in the health system by viewing it within the context of **patriarchy**—the society-wide system of male dominance. Medical dominance, then, is also male dominance, since the majority of doctors are male and most allied health professionals are female. This

---

TheoryLink

Chapter 2 discusses functionalism in more detail.

trait approach

A functionalist theory of professions that assumes professional status can be achieved by meeting a set of criteria (usually defined as specialised expertise and training, and self-regulation through a code of ethics).

gender/sex

This pair of terms refers to the socially constructed categories of feminine and masculine (the cultural identities and values that prescribe how men and women should behave), and the social power relations based on those categories, as distinct from the categories of biological sex (female or male).

feminism/feminist

A broad social and political movement based on a belief in equality of the sexes and the removal of all forms of discrimination against women. A feminist is one who makes use of, and may act upon, a body of theory that seeks to explain the subordinate position of women in society.

TheoryLink

Chapter 2 discusses feminist theory in more detail.

patriarchy
A system of power through which males dominate households. It is used more broadly by feminists to refer to society's domination by patriarchal power, which functions to subordinate women and children.

social closure
A term first used by Max Weber to describe the way that power is exercised to exclude outsiders from the privileges of social membership (in social classes, professions, or status groups).

norms
Expectations about how people ought to act or behave.

class (or social class)
A position in a system of structured inequality based on the unequal distribution of power, wealth, income, and status. People who share a class position typically share similar life chances.

trend seems set to continue, with 78 per cent of 2006 enrolments in undergraduate health courses being female (AIHW 2008). The proportion of each profession that is female is shown in Table 22.1.

Research on the career aspirations of health profession graduates by Lena Nordholm and Mary Westbrook (1981) found that female graduates were more likely to aspire to intermediate supervisory positions, while males aspired to leadership positions. Thus, as these professions masculinise, gender will increasingly play a role in determining the nature of work, with males having increasingly greater structural input into organisation within the health setting (Turner 1987, 1995). These males take the 'glass escalator' within a male-managed system. A US study of registered dietitians conducted by Prudence Pollard and colleagues (2007) found females experienced negative wage discrimination, with a median wage gap of nearly US$5000 between males and females.

Professionalising strategies

Witz (1992) has conceptualised the search for professional recognition of specific occupations as the professionalising project of the group. Witz defines the professionalising projects as 'strategies of occupational closure, which aim for occupational monopoly over the provision of certain skills and competencies in a market for services' (1992, p. 5). The setting of boundaries around specified professional domains is known as **social closure**.

Allied health professions and nursing have tended to adopt the professionalising project of medicine. Susan Roberts (1983) identifies this strategy as being typical of the behaviour of oppressed groups and describes how the subordinate group internalises the **norms** of the dominant group. The subordinate group believes that if it can just be more like the dominant group it will achieve the same level of power and control. Professionalisation strategies that have been adopted by the subordinate allied health professions include:

- adopting a scientific body of knowledge and a code of professional conduct
- developing professional associations and accreditation of members
- establishing a university degree as the entry-level qualification.

These traits are all typical of the dominant group: medicine. While medicine has achieved a high degree of autonomy and professional closure within its domain, sanctioned and maintained by the state, the same strategies will not work for the allied health professions. This is, first, because power that already existed within a privileged social **class** was used politically to achieve the professional status of medicine, rather than that power being conferred as a result of possessing the above-mentioned traits. Second, no government is likely ever again to deliver as much power to one profession as it did to medicine; indeed, the state is presently working to try to limit medicine's power (see Chapter 19).

Given that allied health professions are likely to remain subordinate to medicine, within the hospital system at least, there are few groups left within the health system over which allied health can exert power and control. This leads to conflicts between the constituent professions of the allied health grouping, and between allied health and nursing. These groups jostle each other for power and position since they cannot successfully challenge medicine.

Threats to professional domains

Willis conceptualises the division of labour in health care as 'a continuing struggle over appropriate occupational territories' (1989, p. 4). Threats to the current boundaries of practice within allied health may come from three directions:

1 **vertical encroachment** from above
2 vertical encroachment from below
3 **horizontal encroachment**.

Vertical encroachment from above

This term refers to the possibility that the work of allied health professionals will be taken over by doctors. Physiotherapy may be at risk from doctors' use of electrotherapy or manipulative therapy (du Toit 1995), but otherwise, as long as allied health professionals continue to do the work that doctors are not interested in doing, doctors are unlikely to encroach upon their role. While allied health professionals see their work as a specialised role that doctors are untrained to perform, doctors largely perceive these tasks to be unchallenging or too time consuming. If allied health professionals encroached upon the work of doctors, though, the latter group would act quickly either to exclude the allied health professionals from performing that role or to claim a superior skill in the task (Gardner & McCoppin 1995). For example, proposals for physiotherapists to have referral rights to specialists or limited prescription rights have so far been quashed by the medical profession.

Vertical encroachment from below

The threat that is probably most underestimated by allied health professions is that of encroachment from below. Multiskilling of generic health workers has been proposed (e.g. in New South Wales in 1992 (Gardner & McCoppin, 1995)). Generic health workers would undertake less specialised tasks after one to two years of training and be paid substantially less than allied health professionals. The allied

encroachment (vertical and horizontal)
The threat to professionals' occupational territory. Vertical encroachment can be from above (from medicine, for instance) or from below, whereby less qualified workers do some of the tasks previously done by a professional. Horizontal encroachment refers to the occupational takeover of one profession by another, where both have similar status and power.

health professions and nursing react strongly against such proposals at professional association and union levels. While such proposals have not been implemented, the threat has not disappeared. Other examples of encroachment from below are the encroachment of diversional therapists on occupational therapists (especially in the USA where they do not require registration) and of physiotherapist aides on physiotherapists (du Toit 1995).

Horizontal encroachment

Allied health professionals also encroach on each other's territory as they vie for a better position within the system. For example, occupational therapy has expanded its role by encroaching on the work of physiotherapists in what is now a recognised speciality of occupational therapy. Complementary practitioner groups, while not usually employed in hospitals, have the potential to encroach on the traditional territory of allied health professionals in the private practice setting. These professions are increasingly being legitimised by Medicare and health insurers who provide rebates for their services. In the three months April–June 2008, Medicare rebated 30,204 occasions of service by chiropractors and osteopaths for patients referred by their general practitioner (Medicare Australia 2008). These people might otherwise have consulted a physiotherapist.

Recognising allied health as professions: the role of the state and professional associations

In Australia, the state formally recognises allied health occupations as professions. There are three types of agencies that are responsible for this task:

1 Commonwealth government authorities;
2 state and territory government authorities;
3 professional associations.

Commonwealth and state governments control the qualifications that practitioners require in order to practise in Australia, through legislation. Thus, the state legitimates the production and reproduction of professional status for these occupations (Willis 1989).

In some cases, the government has devolved this responsibility to the professional associations in a system known as 'self-regulation'. This is consistent with a national move to establish self-regulation for professions that were previously registered in only one or two of the states and territories. Both dietetics and speech pathology were deregistered in this way during the 1990s (Gardner & McCoppin 1995). In some self-regulating professions, practitioners are recognised through association membership, whereas others have developed further systems of differentiation that involve compliance with continuing education requirements. Table 22.3 lists the allied health professions that required registration or were self-regulating at the end of 2008.

Setting and examining the criteria for Australian recognition of overseas qualifications was previously the responsibility of the state, but this role has been devolved to professional associations. This provides the professional associations with more scope to practise exclusionary tactics, with the risk that the access to job opportunities of practitioners trained overseas will be limited in a strictly controlled job market. Changes to Medicare have provided further opportunity for professional associations to exert control over practice. The Dietitians Association of Australia (DAA), for example, ensured that the government would only register dietitians for Medicare rebates if they participated in the self-regulation scheme (for which practitioners must be members of DAA and meet minimum educational and documentation requirements).

In 2008, the new Rudd Government proposed a move to national, rather than state-based, registration. The initiative arose in response to several high-profile media cases for medical malpractice, where it was found that doctors deregistered in one state merely set up practice in another. The proposal included nine health professions: medical practitioners, nurses and midwives, pharmacists, physiotherapists, psychologists, osteopaths, chiropractors, optometrists, and dentists (including dental hygienists, dental prosthetists and dental therapists) (Health Workforce Australia 2008), presumably with others to follow. This is the first step toward eliminating the states and territories from the professional recognition process.

Table 22.3 Registration and self-regulation of health professions

Type of regulation	Occupation
State-based registration	Medical radiation scientists (except ACT)
	Occupational therapists (except Tas, ACT, NSW, and Vic)
	Optometrists
	Pharmacists
	Physiotherapists
	Podiatrists (except NT)
	Psychologists
Self-regulation (managed by professional associations)	Dietitians
	Medical scientists (registration required in ACT only)
	Social workers
	Speech pathologists (registration required in Queensland only)
	Welfare workers

Source: Australian Skills Recognition Information (ASRI), 2006

Lauren Williams

Working within Medicare: how the state supports medical dominance in the private practice setting

One means of threatening the medical workforce is by granting non-physician health providers the right to independent practice. While Australian allied health practitioners have legally held that right for decades, health funds colluded with medicine to keep allied health professionals subordinate, by specifying the need for a doctor's referral before reimbursing a consultation with an allied health professional. This practice is now almost non-existent among health funds, allowing allied health professionals to consult without referral with the notable exception of the AMA Health Fund Limited (the fund of the Australian Medical Association). The ability of patients to self-refer has increased the viability of private practice for the allied health professions but a recent government initiative is challenging the independent base of private practitioners.

Changes to Medicare have meant that the state has reintroduced the need for a doctor's referral to allied health professionals. Medicare Plus, also known as the Enhanced Primary Care scheme (EPC), was introduced by the Howard Government in the lead-up to the 2004 federal election. Patients with chronic health conditions and complex care needs became entitled to Medicare rebate for services by Aboriginal health workers, audiologists, chiropodists, chiropractors, dietitians, mental health workers, osteopaths, physiotherapists, podiatrists, psychologists, occupational therapists, and speech pathologists (DOHA 2004b). These practitioners were invited to register with the Health Insurance Commission, provided they met the specified requirements (registration or participation in the self-regulation system of professional associations). Allied health organisations that had lobbied the federal government for years to be eligible for Medicare rebates celebrated this initiative, hoping it would improve the access of people on low incomes to their services.

Despite having the potential to make private practice more lucrative for allied health professionals by increasing their client base, Medicare Plus is much more lucrative for general practitioners (GPs) (Foster et al. 2008). The GPs receive Medicare rebates for preparing their management plan and for coordinating team arrangements. The GP then refers the patient to the allied health practitioner. The scheduled fee for allied health services in 2008 was $56.25 (of which the patient can claim 85 per cent), which is likely to be less than the usual fee for many practitioners. Any difference in price needs to be met either by the practitioner (compromising business growth), or the patient (counter to improving equity of access to allied health services). Strenuous reporting requirements are placed on the allied health practitioners, who are not remunerated for their administration, providing a further disincentive to practitioners.

The system also reinforces medical dominance through the referral process, where the GP determines not only which individual practitioner the patient must see, but how many times they may see them (up to a maximum of five visits in a 12-month period). The number of visits specified may well be insufficient for best practice, putting a metaphorical band-aid on patients rather than providing them with effective treatment.

Despite the reinforcement of medical dominance by the EPC system, federal funding has increased the occasions of service by allied health professionals outside the hospital and community health sectors. The three most commonly claimed allied health services in Australia in April-June 2008 were physiotherapy (155,267 services), podiatry (139,714 services), and dietetics (36,055 services) (Medicare Australia 2008). The extension of Medicare rebates to services by allied health professions may be susceptible to political whim and a change of government, although thus far the Rudd Labor Government has made no changes to the system.

Alternatives to Medicare

People ineligible to obtain allied health services under Medicare can still access practitioners by either bearing the full cost of the consultation or paying part of the cost with rebates from private health insurers. Around 45 per cent of Australians had some form of private health insurance by June 2008 (PHIAC 2008); however, only those who had some type of 'extras cover' were able to claim for a rebate for so-called 'ancillary services'. As at June 2006, 42 per cent of the population had some ancillary cover (PHIAC 2006). The average amount of benefits paid for some ancillary services was $26.00 for physiotherapy and $31.00 for podiatry (PHIAC 2006). Although these amounts had increased by 1.3 per cent and 1.0 per cent respectively from the previous year (PHIAC 2006), the amounts are unlikely to cover the cost of even a single consultation and are less than the Medicare rebate. Thus the 'out-of-pocket' expense for the patient is not significantly reduced by private insurance.

Allied health in the hospital system: restructuring and economic rationalism

As we have seen, allied health practitioners deliver services through the public (state-administered) health care setting, or in private practice. The public and private settings will be treated separately. Traditionally, in Australian hospitals, individual allied health departments were directly responsible to the medical superintendent or director of medical services. For example, an occupational therapist would report to the chief occupational therapist (or occupational therapist in charge), who would in turn report to the medical superintendent (or the medical superintendent's deputy). The medical superintendent would thus be responsible for each individual allied health group, as well as for all the medical services. Nursing services were organised separately under a matron or director of nursing. A difficulty inherent in this system was that medical superintendents were, by definition, doctors, and so had limited understanding of the diverse professional groups in their charge. What they did have a good understanding of was the role of doctors, which had implications for the way in which they directed funding and resource allocation to both groups.

economic rationalism
Terms used to describe a political philosophy based on small-government and market-oriented policies, such as deregulation, privatisation, reduced government spending, and lower taxation.

Hospital restructuring during the 1990s, driven by **economic rationalism**, resulted in changes to this traditional structure. Two main alternatives emerged for allied health in this restructuring:

1   the divisions of allied health model
2   the dispersed unit model (Boyce 1996).

The first model, where various allied health departments are grouped together in a single division, was generally favoured by allied health professions and their unions, and emerged as the main alternative to the traditional model, evident in 37 per cent of Australian hospitals at the turn of the millennium (Boyce 2001); (for a comprehensive review of this shift in the 1980s and 1990s see Boyce 2001). In the era of cost-cutting and justification of service outcomes, allied health professionals found that they had more in common with other allied health professionals than with medicine. As a result, they grouped together to be responsible to hospital administration through an allied health administrator. (Even if the group was not organised in this way in formal lines of responsibility, there was a tendency for the informal grouping of these professions to be recognised by management in lines of communication.) The advantages of the division of the allied health system are that the allied health professions maintain discipline-specific units under the umbrella of allied health, and that they have the potential to achieve representation on the executive of hospital management. The potential disadvantages include the lack of an influential power base for those professions not represented on the executive, and the possibility of internal conflicts over who should manage the group, and which professions should be included in the allied health grouping.

The other possible structure, the dispersed unit model, where allied health professionals are responsible to either medical or nursing clinical units, was less popular with the allied health professions, and was evident in only six per cent of Australian hospitals (Boyce 2001). Resistance to this model was based on concern about the destruction of established allied health career structures, lack of control over distribution of workloads, and lack of a united voice for allied health. As health sector costs continue to rise there will be further pressure to rationalise and reorganise.

Future directions: critical analysis of the allied health professions

Becoming allied with each other

The word 'allied' in the term 'allied health' traditionally meant allied to medicine. However, the term could be reinterpreted to mean that these professions form allegiances with each other as a group. In grouping together for political and special purposes, allied health professions gain sufficient numbers to form an effective power bloc. Rosalie Boyce (1995) suggests that for allied health to survive in the era of economic rationalism, the constituent professions must ally with each other, both inside and outside the health system. There is evidence that this has indeed occurred in Australia over the past decades (Boyce 2006). High-level management positions established within hospitals and state health departments are specifically staffed by allied health practitioners (Law & Boyce 2003). Reorganisation into divisions has brought allied health professionals closer in terms of clinical practice, and has also fostered research alliances, reflected in the papers presented at the annual national conferences of allied health. Allied health groupings in the public health system have forged links with colleagues located in similar groupings at universities. Extending this relationship further, the first Australian Chair in Allied Health was filled in 2004 through collaborative funding of the University of Newcastle and the then Central Coast Area Health Service in New South Wales. This role was primarily established to strengthen links between researchers and practitioners of allied health. Organisations to promote evidence-based practice in allied health have also been formed (see the Centre for Allied Health Evidence at <http://www.unisa.edu.au/cahe>). Universities are further fostering the cooperation of individual allied health professions through a shift to multi-professional undergraduate training (Smith et al. 2005).

In response to the threat of reorganisation into clinical teams (Callan et al. 2007), allied health professionals have formed a variety of national, state, and special purpose bodies of allied health. The Allied Health Professions Australia (AHPA) is regarded by the federal government as the peak allied health group in Australia and it provides representation to national committees and working groups. The AHPA (formerly the HPCA) is essentially a collaboration of individual allied health professional associations under the one umbrella (audiology, dietetics, exercise physiology, occupational therapy, orthoptics, orthotics and prosthetics, pharmacy, podiatry, psychology, radiography, social work, sonography, and speech pathology). This group has previously been criticised for not being a significant lobby group (Gardner & McCoppin 1995). Part of this failure can be attributed to the difficulties experienced by a national association in dealing with health care systems and industrial conditions that are subject to the interests of the individual states, resulting in a growth of state-based organisations. These groups then lobby state health departments for resources, and are currently lobbying universities over their financial contribution to student supervision.

Allied health alliances have been formed for specific purposes—for example, the National Allied Health Casemix Committee, the Allied Health Best Practice Consortium (Boyce 1991) and more recently the National Allied Health Organisational Structures Network (NAHOSN). SARRAH (Services for Australian Rural and Remote Allied Health) is the strongest special purpose group to have emerged in recent years. Although this body was specifically formed with the intention of increasing the allied health services outside metropolitan areas, the group has been effective in lobbying for funds that support the allied health professions more broadly. SARRAH joined with the Australian Rural and Remote Health Taskforce of the HPCA to form the National Rural and Remote Allied Health Advisory Service in 2002 (NRRAHAS), supported by federal funding. These organisations each formed with different purposes and to some extent compete for the same scarce resources.

BOX 22.1 Doing health sociology: the rise of allied health organisations as a power bloc

When the public sector hospital restructuring commenced in the 1990s, it became clear to allied health that the biggest risk to their practice within the health system was organisation into clinical teams. This might mean, for example, that a former department of fifteen physiotherapists would be 'redistributed' across ten different teams, so that some would work in a division of medicine, some in a division of surgery and so on, reporting to a doctor instead of a senior physiotherapist. The NAHOSN was formed to lobby against this change. By forming a special purpose organisation the AHPs have united to use collectivism to increase their power.

Exploring options outside the traditional acute care setting

Medicine clearly dominates its traditional territory of the acute care setting, particularly in metropolitan areas. This is because the majority of doctors prefer to work in these settings with the potential for advancement, academic recognition, and research funding. Allied health therefore has an opportunity in areas outside this domain, such as in the rural health setting, or in the field of community health or **public health**. With the greying of the population profile, as the baby boomers approach old age, there is general recognition that care for complex or chronic problems is a priority and that current resources will not meet the need. Allied health professionals need to seize the opportunity to play a key role in the treatment of chronic problems in delivery of patient care in the community.

Spiralling costs of medical treatment make prevention a more palatable option for decision makers, and an emphasis on prevention has gained a stronger hold in health care (see Chapter 23 for more detail). The World Health Organization (WHO) *Ottawa Charter for Health Promotion 1986* brought about international recognition of the need for a preventive approach to health care. Dianna Kenny and Barbara Adamson (1992) have identified **health promotion** as one of the broader social forces undermining medical power. Although medicine still has a strong input into health

public health/public health infrastructure
Public policies and infrastructure to prevent the onset and transmission of disease among the population, with a particular focus on sanitation and hygiene such as clean air, water and food, and immunisation. Public health infrastructure refers specifically to the buildings, installations, and equipment necessary to ensure healthy living conditions for the population.

promotion and public health, it does not control it to the extent that it controls the hospital or illness system. As such, allied health professionals who work in this area can potentially be freed from the dominance of the medical model. Dietetics is one example of a profession that is expanding in numbers by broadening in focus from acute care to apply its knowledge of nutrition in a preventive setting (Meyer et al. 2002). Other allied health professionals would perhaps do well to strengthen alternative avenues of employment along similar lines.

Refocusing the professionalising projects

In attempting to establish domains of practice, and to obtain power and prestige, many of the allied health professions have tried to model themselves on medicine. The fallacy of this approach is that it involves rejecting the cultural identity of the individual professions. This identity could be used instead to harness a different type of strength, which, as De Vault (1995) points out, is more practical and embodied. For example, most allied health professionals spend significantly longer time in direct contact with patients than do doctors. The increased counselling role could be used to foster a model of patient empowerment, which medicine has failed to develop (despite rhetoric to the contrary).

Rather than trying to adopt the traits of medicine, allied health professionals could change the nature of their professionalising project and focus on challenging medical dominance by seeking to increase professional autonomy. The right to independent practice—that is, the ability to see patients without a doctor's referral—was an important step in seeking this autonomy, and needs to be maintained.

health promotion
Any combination of education and related organisational, economic, and political interventions designed to promote behavioural and environmental changes conducive to good health, including legislation, community development, and advocacy.

Conclusion

Interestingly, the theme for the 2009 biannual National Allied Health conference was 'Allied Health Leading Change', a much more positive title than that used 4 years previously: 'Innovation or Extinction? Adapting Roles and Practice'. While the position of allied health professions has strengthened over recent years, the challenge to obtain sufficient funding and autonomy to continue to perform their specialised roles in patient care remains. Doctors will continue to dominate the hospital system for as long as the bulk of health and research funding goes to acute care. Doctors are happy to coexist with other health professions in a system of medical dominance until that dominance is challenged. It is up to the allied health professions to focus professionalising projects to achieve a status that confers prestige and respect within the health system, and one that results in optimal outcomes for patient care. Allied health professions have an opportunity to work together in hospitals within a division of allied health model and to strengthen their position in the less traditional fields of community and public health, and in the rural setting. Allied health professionals

Lauren Williams

also need to lobby against the medical control of the EPC process in order to prevent erosion of this right. Overcoming the limitation of medical dominance would allow the allied health professions to focus their expertise and efforts on delivery of specialised patient care, which is, after all, the reason for their emergence.

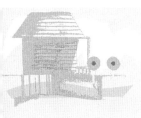

Summary of main points

» The allied health professions arose out of an increasing trend towards specialisation in the delivery of patient care within the health system.

» In working within the health system, allied health professions are subject to the forces that characterise it: the dominance of the medical profession (and consequent subordination of the allied health professions) and the current era of restructuring resulting from economic rationalism.

» While some professions have made more gains than others, allied health remains largely subordinate to medicine. This subordination is gender related, since the predominantly female allied health professionals do 'women's work' within the health system.

» Because they cannot challenge medical dominance, individual allied health professions struggle against encroachment on their territory by nursing, alternative or complementary health, and other allied health professions.

» Many of the allied health professions are following the professionalising project of medicine in trying to establish domains of practice, and obtain power and prestige. They could instead build upon their own distinctive strengths and develop their own professionalising projects.

» The extent to which the allied health professions will be successful in enhancing their status depends upon their ability to redevelop a professional project appropriate to their culture, present an allied front, and embrace continuity of care in the community, and a shift to a preventive (rather than curative) approach to practice.

Sociological reflection: where does medical dominance begin? The structure within the allied health education sector

If you are studying to be an allied health professional, where is your program (e.g. physiotherapy or nutrition and dietetics) located within the university structure? Are your lecturers located in a school or department with other allied health professionals? Does your university have a medical degree? If so, what is the link between your lecturers and the medical lecturers? Are they in the same department? The same faculty? Reflect on what message structural organisation within the university setting sends about the role of allied health professions.

Discussion questions

1 Allied health professionals perform specialised tasks within the hospital system. What would the consequences be for patient care in a hospital setting if such professions were not there to fulfil that role?

2 Why is it that the allied health professions do not have total autonomy within the hospital system?

3 Discuss the role of gender in determining the nature of work done by allied health professionals, and the respect with which that work is regarded within the system.

4 Why is the organisation of allied health within the public hospital system important to the survival of these professions?

5 How do the professions apply trait theory and what are the limitations to this approach? Discuss the alternatives.

6 What factors challenge, threaten, or undermine the role of allied health professions in the health system? What opportunities exist for the allied health professions to strengthen their position?

Further investigation

1 Choose one specific allied health profession. Identify the nature of the professionalising project of that profession by one or all of the following means:
   • Interview a professional currently working in the public or private health sector
   • Search the website of the professional association (or obtain written information from that association)
   • Interview a final-year student of that profession (provided he or she has had significant practical experience).

2 Choose an allied health organisation and critique the strategies it is employing in terms of how successful it will be in improving the position of individual allied health professions within the health sector.

Further reading

Boyce, R. A. 2001, 'Organisational Governance Structures in Allied Health Services: A Decade of Change', *Australian Health Review*, vol. 24, no. 1, pp. 22–36.

Boyce, R. 2006, 'Emerging from the Shadow of Medicine: Allied Health as a "Profession Community" Subculture', *Health Sociology Review*, vol. 15, no. 5, pp. 520–34.

Lauren Williams

Foster, M. M., Mitchell, G., Haines, T., Tweedy, S., Cornwell, P. & Flemming, J. 2008, 'Does Enhanced Primary Care Enhance Primary Care? Policy Induced Dilemmas for Allied Health Professionals', *Medical Journal of Australia*, vol. 188, no. 1, pp. 29–32.

Gardner, H. & McCoppin, B. 1995, 'Struggle for Survival by Health Therapists, Nurses and Medical Scientists', in H. Gardner (ed.), *The Politics of Health*, 2nd edn, Churchill Livingstone, Melbourne.

Kenny, D. & Adamson, B. 1992, 'Medicine and the Health Professions: Issues of Dominance, Autonomy and Authority', *Australian Health Review*, vol. 15, p. 3.

Web resources

6th National Allied Health Conference: <http://www.sapmea.asn.au/conventions/allied health/index.html>

Allied Health Professions Australia (HPCA): < http://www.ahpa.com.au>

Australian Association of Occupational Therapists: <http://www.ausot.com.au/>

Australian Association of Social Workers (AASW): <http://www.aasw.asn.au/>

Australian Education International, National Office of Overseas Skills Recognition <http://aei.dest.gov.au/AEI> and search NOOSR

Australian Institute of Radiography: < http://www.air.asn.au/html/s01_home/home.asp>

Australian Physiotherapy Association (APA): <http://physiotherapy.asn.au>

Australian Podiatry Council <http://www.apodc.com.au>

Australian Psychological Society (APS): <http://www.psychology.org.au/>

Dietitians Association of Australia (DAA): <http://www.daa.asn.au/>

Health Workforce Australia: <http://www.nhwt.gov.au/>

Optometrists Association Australia: <http://www.optometrists.asn.au/>

Private Health Insurance Administration Council: <http://www.phiac.gov.au>

Services for Rural and Remote Allied Health (SARRAH): <http://www.sarrah.org.au>

Speech Pathology Australia: <http://www.speechpathologyaustralia.org.au/>

Online case study

Visit the Second Opinion website to access relevant case studies.

Documentaries/films

The Trouble with Medicine (1993): 6 part documentary series (each around 55 minutes) dealing with various challenges and limitations relating to biomedicine, ABC TV, BBC TV & Thirteen-WNET.

References

Australian Bureau of Statistics 2006, *Australia (Australia), Occupation (a) (UNIT GROUPS) by Sex*, Cat. no. 2068.0, ABS, Canberra.

Australian Government Department of Immigration and Citizenship 2006, *Australian Skills Recognition Information (ASRI)*. Available online: <http://www.immi.gov.au/asri/a-z.htm#s>

Australian Institute of Health and Welfare (2004), *Australia's Health 2004*, AIHW, Canberra.

Australian Institute of Health and Welfare (2008), *Australia's Health 2008*, AIHW, Canberra.

Australian Government Department of Immigration and Citizenship 2006, *Australian Skills Recognition Information (ASRI)*. Available online: <http://www.immi.gov.au/asri/a-z.htm>

The Australian Oxford Dictionary, 2nd edn, Oxford University Press, Melbourne.

Boyce, R. A. 1991, 'Hospital Restructuring: The Implications for Allied Health Professionals', *Australian Health Review*, vol. 14, pp. 147–54.

Boyce, R. A. 1995, 'The Business of Economic Reform in Health: What's Allied Health Got To Do With It?', *Proceedings of the South-West Pacific Regional Dietitians Conference*, 11–13 May 1995, Brisbane, Dietitians Association of Australia, Canberra.

Boyce, R. A. 1996, 'Researching the Organisation of Allied Health Professions: Sorting Fact from Fantasy', Paper Presented at the Second National Allied Health Conference, 15–16 November, Sydney.

Boyce, R. A. 2001, 'Organisational Governance Structures in Allied Health Services: A Decade of Change', *Australian Health Review*, vol. 24, no. 1, pp. 22–36.

Boyce, R. 2006, 'Emerging from the Shadow of Medicine: Allied Health as a "Profession Community" Subculture', *Health Sociology Review*, vol. 15, no. 5, pp. 520–34.

Callan V. J., Gallois C., Mayhew M. G., Grice T. A., Tluchowska M., & Boyce R. 2007, 'Restructuring the Multi-professional Organization: Profession Identity and Adjustment to Change in a Public Hospital', *Journal of Health and Human Service Administration*, vol. 29, no. 4, pp. 448–77.

De Vault, M. L. 1995, 'Between Science and Food: Nutrition Professionals in the Health Care Hierarchy', in J. J. Kronenfeld (ed.), *Research in the Sociology of Health Care: Patients, Consumers, Providers and Caregivers*, vol. 12, JAI Press, Connecticut, pp. 60–75.

Department of Health and Ageing 2004a, *National Allied Health Workforce Report*, June 2004, DOHA, Canberra.

Department of Health and Ageing 2004b, *Medicare Benefit Schedule*, Allied Health and Dental Services, DOHA, Canberra.

Donini-Lenhoff, F. G. 2008, 'Coming Together, Moving Apart: A History of the Term *Allied Health* in Education, Accreditation, and Practice', *Journal of Allied Health*, vol. 37, no. 1, pp. 45–52.

du Toit, D. 1995, 'The Allied Health Professionals in Australia: Physio, Occupational and Speech Therapy Professions', in G. M. Lupton & J. M. Najman (eds), *Sociology of Health and Illness: Australian Readings*, 2nd edn, Macmillan, Melbourne.

Foster, M. M., Mitchell, G., Haines, T., Tweedy, S., Cornwell, P. & Flemming, J. 2008, 'Does Enhanced Primary Care Enhance Primary Care? Policy Induced Dilemmas for Allied Health Professionals', *Medical Journal of Australia*, vol. 188, no. 1, pp. 29–32.

Freidson, E. 1970, *Profession of Medicine*, Harper & Row, New York.

Gardner, H. & McCoppin, B. 1995, 'Struggle for Survival by Health Therapists, Nurses and Medical Scientists', in H. Gardner (ed.), *The Politics of Health*, 2nd edn, Churchill Livingstone, Melbourne, pp. 371–427.

Health Workforce Australia 2008, *National Registration and Accreditation Scheme*. Available online: <http://www.nhwt.gov.au/natreg.asp>

Irvine R. & Graham J. 1994, 'Deconstructing the Concept of Profession: A Prerequisite to Carving a Niche in a Changing World', *Australian Occupational Therapy Journal*, vol. 41, pp. 9–18.

Kenny, D. & Adamson, B. 1992, 'Medicine and the Health Professions: Issues of Dominance, Autonomy and Authority', *Australian Health Review*, vol. 15, no. 1, pp. 3.

Law, D. & Boyce, R. A. 2003, 'Beyond Organisational Design: Moving From Structure to Service Enhancement', *Australian Health Review*, vol. 26, no. 1, pp. 175–85.

Martyr, P. 1994, 'The Professional Development of Rehabilitation in Australia, 1870–1981', PhD thesis, the University of Western Australia and P. Martyr.

Medicare Australia 2008, *Requested Medicare Items Processed from April 2008 to June 2008*. Available online: <https://www.medicareaustralia.gov.au/statistics/mbs_item.shtml>

Meyer, R., Gilroy, R., & Williams, P. 2002, 'Dietitians in New South Wales: Workforce Trends 1984–2000', *Australian Health Review*, vol. 25, no. 3, pp. 122–30.

Nash, H. 1989, *The History of Dietetics in Australia*, Dietitians Association of Australia, Canberra.

Nordholm, L. A. & Westbrook, M. T. 1981, 'Career Selection, Satisfaction and Aspirations among Female Students in Five Health Professions', *Australian Psychologist*, vol. 16, p. 1.

Pollard, P., Taylor, M. & Daher, N. 2007, 'Gender-based Wage Differentials Among Registered Dietitians', *Health Care Management*, vol. 26, no. 1, pp. 52–63.

Private Health Insurance Administration Council 2006, *Operations of the Registered Health Benefits Organisations Annual Report 2005–2006*, PHIAC, Canberra.

Private Health Insurance Administration Council 2008, *General Treatment—Benefits: June 2008*. Available online: <http://www.phiac.gov.au/statistics/trends/index.htm>

Roberts, S. J. 1983, 'Oppressed Group Behaviour: Implications for Nursing', *Advances in Nursing Science*, vol. 5, no. 4, pp. 21–30.

Smith, A., Williams, L., Lyons, M., & Lewis, S. 2005, 'Pilot Testing a Multiprofessional Learning Module: Lessons Learned', *Focus on Health Professional Education*, vol. 6, no. 3.

Turner, B. S. 1987, *Medical Power and Social Knowledge*, Sage, London.

Turner, B. S. with Samson, C. 1995, *Medical Power and Social Knowledge*, 2nd edn, Sage, London.

Willis, E. 1989, *Medical Dominance*, revised edn, Allen & Unwin, Sydney.

Witz, A. 1992, *Professions and Patriarchy*, Routledge, London, pp. 23–45.

World Health Organization 1986, *Ottawa Charter for Health Promotion*, First International Conference on Health Promotion: The Move Towards a New Public Health, 17–21 November, Ottawa, Canada, and WHO, Geneva.

ACKNOWLEDGMENTS

I gratefully acknowledge Lana Hebden for her help with word processing and research assistance on this chapter.

Lauren Williams

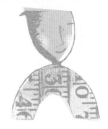

CHAPTER 23

A Sociology of Health Promotion

KATY
RICHMOND
and
JOHN
GERMOV

Overview

- What dilemmas arise in relation to programs that give information about health to individuals and groups?
- What are the differences between individualist and structuralist health promotion programs?
- How can individualist health promotion programs further the medicalisation of everyday life?

UPSTREAM AND DOWNSTREAM

Medical professionals spend their time caring for the sick. The sick can be likened to people near the mouth of a rapidly flowing river, having been thrown into the river from a cliff further upstream. Instead of only rescuing people from drowning, we should focus our efforts upstream to find out who is throwing people into the river in the first place. We might build a few fences. Even better, we might do something about assist-ing people to change direction, helping them to travel towards a tropical paradise or a cool mountain stream, away from the dangerous cliff face. In other words, doing some planning upstream at the cliff face— working towards structural change to promote good health—is, in the end, more effective than saving people from drowning one by one (metaphor adapted from Irving Zola cited in McKinlay 1994, pp. 509–10).

Introduction

Health promotion aims to improve the health of whole populations. Before the 1970s, there was a three-pronged approach to health and illness: providing communities with basic public health facilities (clean water, sewerage); providing doctors and hospitals; and providing 'top-down' health education. The philosophy of health promotion has developed since the 1970s and reflects a **social model of health**, or what has commonly come to be known as the **new public health** approach. This approach was intended to change the health agenda in a modestly radical direction towards community participation and empowerment, and structural and environmental change. However, in Australia and elsewhere, health promotion has essentially remained committed to old-style 'top-down' health education. This chapter provides a critique of this approach and offers some examples and suggestions for the future.

The path through the health promotion story is complex, since health promotion practices range along a broad continuum. These practices can be simplified by categorising them into two polar 'types'. The conservative end of health promotion can be termed **individualist health promotion (IHP)** and the more radical end **structuralist–collectivist health promotion (SCHP)**. IHP is, in essence, health education about lifestyle. SCHP, on the other hand, encompasses participatory health programs at the community level, legislation, and bureaucratic interventions, which range from small local programs such as the provision of needle exchanges to more significant measures such as laws restricting tobacco advertising and the creation of smoke-free environments.

A brief history of health promotion

Concerns about **public health** and disease prevention, as discussed in Chapter 1, date back to the nineteenth century. These concerns dissipated as medical treatments improved and it was not until the 1970s that any significant interest in public health was renewed. As the so-called 'lifestyle diseases' or 'diseases of affluence' (heart disease, cancer, and stroke) became the leading causes of death in developed countries, governments and health professionals turned their attention to disease prevention. Health promotion as a term was popularised through the 1974 report, *A New Perspective on the Health of Canadians* (1974), known as the Lalonde Report, after Marc Lalonde, the then Canadian Minister of Health and Welfare. The report identified four key 'health fields' that influenced the health of individuals:

1   the physical and social environment (over which individuals have little control)
2   human biology (physical and mental health)

health promotion
Any combination of education and related organisational, economic, and political interventions designed to promote behavioural and environmental changes conducive to good health, including legislation, community development, and advocacy.

social model of health
Focuses on social determinants of health such as the social production, distribution, and construction of health and illness, and the social organisation of health care. It directs attention to the prevention of illness through community participation and social reforms that address living and working conditions.

new public health
A social model of health linking 'traditional' public health concerns about physical aspects of the environment (clean air and water, safe food, occupational safety), with concerns about the behavioural, social, and economic factors that affect people's health.

Katy Richmond and John Germov

individualist health promotion (IHP)
IHP is a set of programs that provide health education about health risks to persuade people to change their lifestyles. A wide group of professionals are involved in these programs, including doctors, nurses, allied health professionals, psychologists, educators, and media and marketing experts.

structuralist–collectivist health promotion (SCHP)
SCHP encompasses a wide range of interventions, including participatory community programs, legislation, and bureaucratic interventions. The latter range from needle exchanges to the enactment of laws restricting industrial pollution, fireworks, flammable nightwear, cigarette advertising, and smoking in public places.

public health
Public policies and infrastructure to prevent the onset and transmission of disease among the population, with a particular focus on sanitation and hygiene such as clean air, water, and food, and immunisation. Public health infrastructure refers specifically to the buildings, installations, and equipment necessary to ensure healthy living conditions for the population.

3 lifestyle (over which individuals allegedly have control)
4 the nature and resourcing of health care services.

The Lalonde Report is generally regarded as providing the impetus for global initiatives in health promotion, the major driving force of which has been the World Health Organization (WHO), a United Nations body. WHO has hosted a series of important international health conferences, out of which have emerged a number of highly influential health policy documents. These include the Alma-Ata Declaration of 1978 (WHO 1978), which was released at its International Conference on Primary Health Care held at Alma-Ata in the USSR, the 1981 report entitled *Global Strategy Health for All by the Year 2000*, and the *Ottawa Charter for Health Promotion* of 1986 (WHO 1986). The consistent message of all of these publications is a movement away from a focus on illness towards **positive health**. These documents urge health professionals and policy-makers not only to educate people about health matters, but also to change the environments in which people live and to involve the community in projects to improve health.

The Ottawa Charter was subtitled *The Move towards a New Public Health* and has been the dominant influence over health promotion approaches to this day. The model is a novel attempt to integrate health education and individual behaviour-change strategies, with broader structural strategies that aim fundamentally to reorient health care services and public policies to address the social determinants of health. As Figure 23.1 depicts, the new public health approach is envisaged as five interrelated principles, which highlight the need to:

- *strengthen community action:* through community consultation and participation in priority setting, planning, decision-making, and implementation processes
- *develop personal skills:* through health education to enable behaviour/lifestyle change
- *create supportive environments:* in terms of environmental sustainability and wider support systems that ensure social life is safe and satisfying
- *reorient health services:* towards prevention, holistic and culturally appropriate care, and power-sharing between health professionals, community groups, and individual users of health services
- *build healthy public policy:* by means of interventions beyond the health system that aim to make living and working conditions conducive to health and equity.

Subsequent health promotion declarations (see Box 23.1) in Adelaide, Jakarta, Mexico City, and Bangkok have reiterated the original principles espoused in the Ottawa Charter, adding greater detail and examples of their practical application. In particular, since the 1997 Jakarta Declaration, health promotion activities have focused on 'settings for health' as a practical way to implement the five Ottawa Charter principles—that is, the everyday settings in which health promotion strategies can be enacted, such as the school, the workplace, and the local sports club.

Figure 23.1 Ottawa Charter for Health Promotion

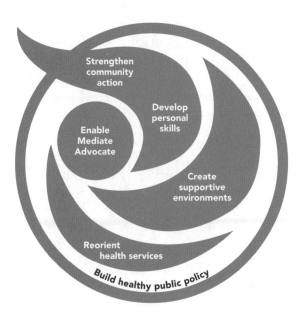

BOX 23.1 Global health promotion declarations to date

1986 Ottawa Charter for Health Promotion

1988 Adelaide Recommendations on Healthy
Public Policy

1991 Sundsvall Statement on Supportive
Environments for Health

1997 Jakarta Declaration on Leading Health
Promotion into the Twenty-first Century

2000 Mexico Ministerial Statement for the
Promotion of Health: From Ideas to
Action; Framework for Countrywide
Plans of Action for Health Promotion

2005 Bangkok Charter for Health Promotion
in a Globalized World

Stimulated by international debate, the Australian Federal Government released an initial report, *Promoting Health: Prospects for Better Health Throughout Australia* (1979), and since then has produced a range of reports (see O'Connor-Fleming & Parker 2007). Despite the developments at the national and international level in support of making social environments conducive to health, most health promotion activity in Western countries such as Australia has continued to be very narrowly focused around educating people to change their lifestyles. Such programs assume that all that is needed is to 'educate' people about the fact that they are putting their health at risk by smoking cigarettes, eating unhealthy food, drinking too much, and not exercising enough. In this approach, the problem of illness is

positive health
A holistic view of health that focuses on wellness, rather than disease, and that it is culturally relative, incorporating notions of spirituality, community, and social support.

Katy Richmond and John Germov

conceptualised in terms of individuals' non-compliance with health advice. Some people are said to have 'failed' to give up full-cream milk or butter, for instance. Smokers are said to have 'failed to understand' that lung cancer and coronary heart disease are major risks of smoking (Borland et al. 1994). In contrast to the focus on individual responsibility of such approaches, sociological contributions to health promotion have focused on the social determinants of health behaviour and the **social construction** of health advice.

Criticisms of individualist health promotion

Individualist health promotion programs of these kinds are difficult to challenge because they are couched in rhetoric that seems so manifestly benevolent (Lupton 1995). They are generally promoted as both successful and cost effective. Adequate evaluations have rarely been attempted because of a variety of methodological weaknesses in the studies themselves and because of the fact that the effect of any particular health message cannot be easily isolated from other social changes occurring in the community (Byde 1995).

Criticisms of IHP start by pointing out that few programs succeed for any length of time (Mechanic 1994). Alan Beattie (1991) goes so far as to claim that on some occasions in the United Kingdom, news of the lack of success of these programs is politically suppressed. Successes are often limited to that segment of the population that is highly motivated to change, and the people who arguably really need to change are often impervious to health messages (Van Beurden et al. 1993). In a Newcastle study of cardiovascular disease, those who did not respond to invitations to be involved were more likely to be overweight or obese (Elliott 1995).

These individualist health programs continue despite their lack of long-term success because they are supported by a range of powerful interest groups, not least a range of medical and allied health professionals. As Alan Petersen argues, 'Health promotion is not a value free enterprise. It is enmeshed in power relations' (1996, p. 56). The IHP model has widespread support because it makes governments look authoritative and active, while at the same time it avoids confrontations that might prove politically costly (Lupton 1995). IHP has the support of the medical profession because it expands medical turf and it provides work for **epidemiologists**, allied health professionals, psychologists, and educationalists, to the extent that the area has become overcrowded (Beattie 1991). Furthermore, IHP meshes well with psychological models of behaviour and is widely supported by media and marketing experts, who circulate its attendant slogans. Drug companies also do well out of some IHP campaigns. For example, in the 1990s, fears about heart disease at the onset of menopause sent thousands of women in their fifties off to pharmacies with doctors' prescriptions to buy packets of oestrogen and progesterone.

---

social construction
Refers to the socially created characteristics of human life based on the idea that people actively construct reality, meaning it is neither 'natural' nor inevitable. Therefore, notions of normality/abnormality, right/wrong, and health/ illness are subjective human creations that should not be taken for granted.

epidemiology
The statistical study of patterns of disease in the population. Originally focused on epidemics, or infectious diseases, it now covers non-infectious conditions such as stroke and cancer. Social epidemiology is a sub-field aligned with sociology that focuses on the social determinants of illness.

risk society
A term coined by Ulrich Beck to describe the centrality of risk calculations in people's lives in Western society, whereby the key social problems today are unanticipated hazards, such as the risks of pollution, food poisoning, and environmental degradation.

Ulrich Beck characterises contemporary life as a **risk society** in which people are regularly concerned about 'preventing the worst' (Beck 1992, p. 49). The study of **risks** has escalated in health journals, and the struggle to reduce or eliminate risk factors has become an activity of considerable importance and prestige within the health professions (Skolbekken 1995). Thus, what was essentially a medical discussion about the probabilities of getting a particular disease has now entered our daily discourse—a striking example of the **medicalisation** of everyday life.

The social construction of risks is not confined to medicine, of course. Governments face economic pressures because of the costs of hospital-based medicine, and thus people are encouraged to take responsibility for their own health and well-being. As part of this process, people are taught how to 'read' symptoms and to watch for changes in bodily behaviour (Pinell 1996). Women, for example, are taught to examine their breasts for symptoms of cancer, and more recently men have been urged to watch for early signs of prostate cancer. Deborah Lupton suggests that the body is now regarded as 'a site of toxicity' that necessitates a high degree of personal surveillance (Lupton 1995, p. 433).

This anxious surveillance of our bodies is paradoxical because our lives are, overall, increasingly under control and our life expectancy has greatly increased. There are, of course, human-made risks such as acid rain, and terrorist acts, but overall the risks from our environment are reducing (Skolbekken 1995). Yet we often regard these risks as overwhelming, and it is as if our anxieties condense around our bodies —almost as if the rest of our problems might become manageable if we could only get our bodies under control (Williams & Calnan 1996). Robert Crawford (1980) describes this as **healthism** and says that this extreme concern with personal health has now become a national preoccupation. In fact, it can be argued that our preoccupation with bodily health is unhealthy. The hazards that we face are often rare, and some say that the risks are so small they should be ignored (Skolbekken 1995).

Healthism has generated a consumer culture in which health has become a market commodity. We are all exhorted to make use of aerobics classes, gymnasiums, exercise bicycles, health food shops, and new diet foods. We watch television programs discussing 'the healthy lifestyle', and we read magazines telling us what to eat (Nettleton 1995). The lifestyle choices that we make are each given a moral value, and how we consume these various commodities helps to constitute our sense of self (Johanson et al. 1996). The sign of being normal is to have a healthy body. So what emerges from such health **consumerism** is a set of status distinctions that become elaborated into a system of **social control** (Crawford 1980).

IHP programs are based on highly simplified psychological models that exaggerate the ease with which behaviour can be changed based on the assumption of a direct connection between health knowledge and behaviour modification (see, for example, Bennett & Hodgson 1992). In fact, little is known about how people choose between various courses of action in relation to their health. No one has ever found

risk/risk discourse
Risk refers to 'danger' and risk discourse is often used in health promotion messages warning people that certain actions involve significant risks to their health.

medicalisation
The process by which non-medical problems become defined and treated as medical issues, usually in terms of illnesses, disorders, or syndromes.

healthism
The extreme preoccupation with personal health that is evident within the general population.

consumerism
The processes and institutions by which individuals satisfy their needs by purchasing goods and services in a market. Mass consumerism refers to post-Second World War consumer practices, whereby the reduction of the cost of commodities and the extensive use of advertising and new credit arrangements created a mass market. It is often argued that consumerism has less to do with the satisfaction of wants than with the desire to be different and distinctive.

social control
Mechanisms that aim to induce conformity, or at least to manage or minimise deviant behaviour.

Katy Richmond and John Germov

clear links between 'knowing' and 'doing', and much ordinary, everyday behaviour is hard to change; this is particularly true for the most disadvantaged (Kaplan 1988; Siskind et al. 1992; Kassulke et al. 1993). As one respondent in a Sydney study said, the healthy choice is 'not that easy to do even if you know it, believe in it and want to do it' (Ritchie et al. 1994, p. 101). David Mechanic is a particularly strident critic. He argues that 'health actions that must depend on persistent conscious motivation' are unlikely to be successful in the long run (1994, p. 487). Weight loss, dietary modification, and quitting smoking are all difficult to achieve. Individual aspects of behaviour are integrated into a person's sense of self and of belonging to a particular social group (Giddens 1991, p. 121). Social isolation is something that people quite reasonably consider when they contemplate making changes in their daily lives. If the people all around them smoke, they would place themselves in a marginal position if they were to stop smoking (Byde 1995).

The limits of epidemiology

It is only recently that the medical approach to health promotion, and in particular epidemiology, has been challenged on its claims to scientific objectivity (Crawford 1980). The job of epidemiologists is to research the statistical risks of acquiring particular diseases, but their language is the language of probability, not certainty. We are a long way from being able to predict illnesses perfectly. Some associations between risks and outcomes are strong and others are weak, yet the community is encouraged to think of risks in all-or-none terms. For example, there is a proven link between smoking and lung cancer (though not all people who smoke get the disease). Yet, the links between fat consumption and heart disease, or between exercise and heart disease, are not of the same order of risk, and it has been argued that it is dishonest and counterproductive to suggest otherwise (Kaplan 1988; Davison et al. 1992; Germov & Williams 1996).

Coronary heart disease, for example, can only be partly explained by orthodox behavioural risk factors. Genetic factors are also significant in explaining why some people get heart disease and others do not (Tannahill 1992; McKinlay 1996). Critics go further than simply maintaining that the messages of the epidemiologists have been misapplied. Critics argue that there should be far more criticism of epidemiological research itself (see Chapter 3). There are two sets of arguments here. First, critics point to methodological flaws in epidemiology where fake risks have been created. These include cases in which epidemiological studies have selectively cited supportive trials and ignored non-supportive data (Skolbekken 1995). The second set of criticisms surround the social construction of the statistical data upon which epidemiology is based. In an important study, John McKinlay (1996) argues that the statistics about women and heart disease are socially constructed, and that a rereading of basic coronary heart disease data indicates that, in each age category, women's risk of heart disease is about the same as, or slightly lower than, men's. Risk does not rise suddenly at the time of menopause. One of the major flaws in the statistical data, so McKinlay argues, is the lack of recognition that a sizeable proportion of women in their fifties arriving at hospital with heart attacks have experienced unrecognised coronary 'incidents' earlier in their lives. McKinlay also points to inaccuracies in cause-of-death attribution, which under-report the number of early coronary heart disease deaths in women before menopause.

The complexities of epidemiological research data are largely ignored by IHP programs, the basic currency of which are simple slogans that frequently go well beyond the evidence (Le Fanu 1986). The lay population experiences illness as sets of events related to people they know or read about. Some smokers they know may live to a ripe old age, and some people who jog regularly drop dead from a heart attack— such examples are referred to as the 'prevention paradox' (Rose 1985; Hunt & Emslie 2001). Simplifying disease prevention messages based on risk factors ignores both the scientific and lay evidence, whereby some people with risk factors never get the actual disease, while others with no risk factors do. Public scepticism is further entrenched when it appears that health scientists change their minds about health risks (Davison et al. 1992; Tannahill 1992). One Sydney study found that their respondents indicated that health messages, especially relating to food, generated confusion: '[o]ne minute red meat is bad for you, chicken is good. The next thing you know chicken is bad and pork's the thing' (Ritchie et al. 1994, p. 100). Admittedly, public confusion over health messages is often fuelled by the marketing efforts of companies, when they exaggerate scientific findings to promote the alleged health benefits of certain products. Yet, the medical scientific community is not without fault either when it comes to exaggerating the links between risk factors derived from population-based studies and the implications these have for an individual's health.

The structuralist approach

Critics writing from the structuralist perspective argue that the ineffectiveness of the lifestyle approach to health promotion wastes community resources. More importantly, they argue that these programs are fundamentally misconceived. The failure of individuals to comply with health warnings is not the problem; the problem is with governments and powerful corporate interests, such as the tobacco lobby, who do not accept responsibility for major diseases in the community. Putting pressure on people to change their lifestyles is, in effect, **victim-blaming**, and does nothing to correct the structural causes of ill health (Waitzkin 1983). Structuralists, often from a neo-Marxist perspective, argue that '[t]o focus on individual life-styles is to assume an independence and freedom of the individual that is an illusion' (Navarro 1986, p. 35). Health promotion policy should instead do something about the social situations that

victim-blaming
The process whereby social inequality is explained in terms of individuals being solely responsible for what happens to them in relation to the choices they make and their assumed psychological, cultural, and/or biological inferiority.

TheoryLink

See Chapter 2 for an overview of Marxism.

frame the decisions that individuals make about their health, especially situations such as inadequate incomes and lack of choice of employment and housing.

In the first place, living in disadvantaged neighbourhoods reduces access to health services, which 'gives rise to physical, service, and social environments that impede residents from finding, travelling to, and affording health care services' (Kirby & Kaneda 2005, p. 28). There are also material impediments to people's ability to put health messages into practice. William Cockerham (2005) argues that IHP approaches are most effective in positive circumstances and least effective under negative conditions. One example comes from a study of food-buying in Canada, which looked at five low-income women and how they budgeted for food for their families (Travers 1996). It was found that they were not adhering to a 'live-for-today' mentality, and what determined their food purchases was their low income, which reduced their capacity to select appropriate foods or to shop at more distant locations, where food was cheaper. Another significant factor was the pressure that the women faced from their children, who saw food advertised on television. Max Travers argues that 'good food' messages are phrased in dogmatic terms and list unfamiliar, often expensive, and not easily available foods. He concludes that teaching someone to budget does not address the structural inequity created by inadequate welfare allowances (Travers 1996). Travers' argument has particular relevance for remotely located Indigenous Australians whose access to modestly priced fruit and vegetables is greatly restricted. In relation to diet, A. J. McMichael concludes that '[h]ealthy choices are not usually easy choices for the socially disadvantaged' (1991, p. 10).

The structuralist perspective provides two sets of arguments about why working-class people suffer more ill health than middle-class people. The first is a **materialist analysis**: working-class people do not have access to the same range of choices as middle-class people (Whitehead 1992). They live in suburbs close to toxic waste; their houses are overcrowded, and in some rural communities sanitation may be poor. Many working-class jobs are associated with health hazards, and generate illnesses and disabilities that only become apparent years or even decades after employment has ceased, such as deafness. There are also a range of occupationally induced cancers, asbestos-related diseases, and respiratory illnesses associated with industrial chemicals. Coal miners' lives, for example, are severely curtailed by the inhaling of coal dust (Cockerham 2004, 2005). Some industrial pollution also affects those who live in suburbs near to industrial areas. Furthermore, industrial chemicals adhering to workers' clothing can cause illnesses among those washing this clothing. People with material wealth, on the other hand, have cars and access to jobs with good working environments, and they live in pleasant suburbs a long distance from industrial pollution (Burdess 1996).

The second set of explanations relates to cultural factors that limit people's ability to purchase appropriate health care, and that promote differences not only in behaviours relating to diet, smoking, alcohol, and exercise, but also in attitudes to

materialist analysis
An analysis that is embedded in the real, actual, material reality of everyday life.

taking risks. These cultural factors often have their basis in material circumstances. There are, for example, important emotional consequences of working in jobs with considerable surveillance, low levels of personal fulfilment and creativity, and the stress that accompanies the constant threat of unemployment (Link & Phelan 1995; Burdess 1996; see Chapter 5 for further detail).

The basic reason for the lack of a connection between 'knowing' and 'doing' lies in the power to choose. The rhetoric of IHP is that, if you know the health risks of a particular form of behaviour, then you have some choice and some power in your life. This vastly exaggerates the options for the poor and economically vulnerable. Individuals in the middle class may well have some control over their lives, and therefore some capacity to care for their own bodies, but such messages often simply create anxiety for those with fewer material resources.

Health promotion practitioners, by definition, see health as a top priority, but some people see health differently. Though this 'difference of opinion' might appear to be a cultural matter, ultimately our views about life's priorities depend on material resources. Living healthily, according to IHP wisdom, means acknowledging risks. Yet, these risks are framed in the way that middle-class people (the health promoters) see the risks (Nettleton 1995). When faced with health promotion relating to lifestyle, people undertake what is essentially a cost–benefit analysis. They look at what they will lose by undertaking healthy lifestyles and think about what the health promoters tell them about their future 'gains' (Tannahill 1992). If they believe that their lives are dominated by things they cannot do anything about, then the pleasures that they gain from the so-called unhealthy aspects of their life are not worth giving up. Most people with little choice about their lives regard their immediate comfort to be of far greater importance than end-stage health (Davison et al. 1992; Ritchie et al. 1994).

A survey of 1000 people in the Hunter Region of New South Wales found that drugs, crime, and road safety were major concerns, and that health was of far less importance. Cancer came sixth on the list of concerns, and fears of heart disease were placed even further down the list. Respondents in this study thought that heart problems were almost inevitable when you got older and could be dealt with appropriately when the time came through drug therapies or surgery (Higginbotham et al. 1993).

The structuralist perspective also criticises IHP programs for targeting their health messages to particular groups in the community. The apparently value-free activity of giving people health messages can become an important form of discrimination (Thorogood 1992). To target the working class, for example, assumes this social category is clearly defined and identifiable. The potential danger of such an approach is that it conveys a patronising and paternalistic message, whereby middle-class 'experts who know best' tell the working class how to live. There is also a strong possibility that **stigmatisation** and a sense of failure will emerge in the targeted

stigma/ stigmatisation
A physical or social trait, such as a disability or a criminal record, that results in negative social reactions such as discrimination and exclusion.

Katy Richmond and John Germov

group. Such stigmatisation will be accentuated in the case of marginalised groups, such as drug-takers or sex workers. For example, the 'Grim Reaper' AIDS campaign in 1986 swamped diagnostic and pathology services with 'worried well' low-risk individuals, and also extended socially divisive attitudes towards homosexuals (Bray & Chapman 1991).

class (or social class)
A position in a system of structured inequality based on the unequal distribution of power, wealth, income, and status. People who share a class position typically share similar life chances.

There is, in fact, a strong **class** dimension to IHP activity. IHP programs work within a set of concepts that are familiar to middle-class people. These include the need to plan for the future, and the importance of self-improvement and self-control (Crawford 1980). In essence, health promotion messages are created by the middle class and visited upon the working class, who are then chastised for their 'failure to listen'. Crawford, for example, suggests that health is a moral discourse that allows middle-class people visibly to demonstrate their capacity for self-discipline—to 'strut the turf' and to display not only their control over themselves, but also their control over others (1984, p. 80). If health promotion messages are perceived as authoritarian and class-biased, then working-class people may resist or ignore them. People do not like being told what to do and such 'advice' can easily be seen as interference or as personally offensive (McMasters 1996).

Moving towards a structuralist–collectivist approach

The SCHP approach involves both small-scale local interventions and broader national or global social change (such as legislative change and humanitarian interventions in developing countries). Australia has been successful in enacting a wide range of health-related legislation. Laws include those outlawing industrial pollution, fireworks, flammable nightwear, cigarette advertising, and smoking in public places; as well as laws requiring water fluoridation, compulsory car seat belts, and the labelling of poisons. Some of these legislative changes have emerged through debate within the major political parties, but others have been the result of pressure from groups of individuals who have worked outside conventional political processes, such as environmental groups and the non-profit health and welfare sectors. Legislation rarely brings about radical change. Some legislation that looks good on the surface may be no more than symbolic because, in the end, 'weak-kneed' politicians compromise with powerful interest groups (Barraclough 1992).

In the 1980s, with the onset of HIV/AIDS and the rise in illicit drug use, an alternative approach of harm minimisation was adopted. For example, needle-exchange programs have been very effective in minimising the spread of HIV/AIDS and Hepatitis C through needle drop-off points in suburban shopping centres, particularly near pharmacies. Australia also has a program providing free needles to drug users through the services of participating pharmacists, but this program is limited by the understandable reluctance of pharmacists to be involved because of the fear of being known in the community as establishments that cater for drug users. More recently, there has been limited acceptance of the inner Sydney Kings Cross Drug-Injecting Room, which provides clean needles and safe, clean cubicles for drug users in that community.

Community-based approaches

The collectivist underpinning of SCHP is based on community participation so that health priorities and interventions reflect the concerns of particular communities. Yet, this makes it difficult to prescribe exactly what SCHP strategies should actually be, and therefore some argue that the approach should be about processes and not about end results (Baum & Sanders 1995). It is conventional to suggest that SCHP should be community based. Much of what has occurred so far in the name of community-based health promotion is not structural change at all, but health education in disguise (Beattie 1991). Where health education has been imposed on communities, there has been some negative reaction, especially with regard to matters such as quitting smoking and controlling alcohol intake (Flaherty et al. 1991; Brown & Redman 1995). This suggests that community-based SCHP programs clearly need to be 'bottom up' rather than 'top down'. Making this a reality is not as easy as it sounds.

There is a great deal of unrecognised hostility within community health promotion programs. Conflict usually emerges when community gatekeepers 'bite the hands that feed them' by challenging the domination of health services and policies by local medical and allied health professionals (Beattie 1991, p. 178). Sometimes this conflict is suppressed, and control stays in the hands of doctors, hospitals, and some special interest groups (Brownlea 1987). Sometimes the hostility is so intense that the community program is denied funding. Since one of the major stumbling blocks in community health promotion programs is professional inflexibility, one of the most obvious concerns of SCHP programs should be the restructuring of professional groups, at least at the local level, so that they are less rigid and more cooperative (Beattie 1991). Some critics doubt that empowerment of community groups is a real possibility given 'the imbalance of participatory capacity between participants' (Kelly & Van Vlaenderen 1996, p. 1245) (see Chapter 24 for more discussion on community health).

Examples of SCHP

The following examples illustrate the differences between the IHP and the SCHP approaches, but do not attempt to be comprehensive of the topics discussed. Several

Katy Richmond and John Germov

of the suggested approaches listed here are already being utilised in some areas of Australia.

Example 1: smoking

Smoking is a major cause of heart disease and lung cancer. While the educative efforts of IHP programs 'advising' people not to smoke have their place, the most effective measures have involved structural change. For example, since the 1990s public health policy has considerably improved this area, with legislation in particular making an impact on smoking rates in the population, which are now down to around a quarter of the population (AIHW 2003). Tobacco advertising has been comprehensively outlawed in Australia and explicit health warnings on cigarette packets are mandatory. In most states, retail outlets are required to limit the display of cigarette packets on stands and store-owners are under considerable surveillance in relation to selling cigarettes to minors. Smoking restrictions in public venues commenced with workplaces, public buildings, and public transport. Such legislation is now being extended to restaurants, pubs, and clubs. Some high-profile public venues remain exempt, such as some casinos and sporting events (Pikora et al. 1999). For example, the Grand Prix held in Melbourne each year is still permitted to advertise cigarettes. Further measures are still needed to prevent the discounting of cigarettes in larger pack sizes (Hill & White 1995; Hill et al. 1995). Given the fact that community hostility towards smoking is increasing, further attempts should be made to increase taxes on smoking, as the cost of cigarettes can be a particularly effective tool to prevent the onset of habitual smoking in teenagers (Crowley et al. 1995).

Example 2: diet

Governments have a great deal of power in relation to food. They can control the ingredients and labelling of processed food and can create incentives for primary producers of meat and grain. They can also ban inappropriate food produce, such as little drink packages that look like orange juice but that, in fact, contain alcohol (McMichael 1991). Rather than trying to change individual behaviour in relation to adding salt to food (the IHP approach), it would be more effective and economical to change food-processing laws to reduce the salt content of tinned and frozen foods (a SCHP approach) (Jamison 1995). Other forms of structural change could include introducing children and parents to good food habits through day care centres, kindergartens, and schools. Measures could include nutrition training for day care centre cooks and specific government legislation concerning standards for the types and amounts of food to be served to the children (Pollard et al. 1999). The state of New South Wales has been the most progressive in this area, with guidelines for school canteens and the *Caring for Children: Food, Nutrition and Fun Activities* program (Bunney & Williams 1999).

Example 3: Aboriginal health

The poor health and life expectancy of Indigenous Australians is well documented and now widely a matter of public concern. One example is the considerably lower birth weight of Aboriginal babies, which is linked to higher rates of neonatal death and early childhood infections (Smith et al. 2000). In many instances such outcomes are preventable if more culturally appropriate antenatal services could be established. In deciding on culturally appropriate services, Aboriginal health workers need to be utilised as community consultants (O'Connor-Fleming & Parker 2007). In addition to the provision of culturally appropriate medical care, structural changes are needed to improve Aboriginal diets and general living conditions because of extreme poverty and limited access to clean water and fresh food in rural and remote communities (Lee et al. 2002). Modest but effective structural interventions in relation to diet could include efforts to improve the stocking of stores where Aboriginal people purchase food (Lee et al. 1994; Scrimgeour et al. 1994; Lee et al. 1996).

Example 4: pollution and workplace health

Structural change to improve public health requires strenuous efforts to limit, or preferably outlaw, industrial pollution. It is difficult to prove concrete links between illness and pollution. Most research of this kind is suggestive rather than definitive, though some geographical areas of Australia are sufficiently isolated to establish reasonably valid linkages. Studies indicate that childhood asthma, for example, has a high prevalence in Victoria's Latrobe Valley, an area where there is large-scale burning of brown coal (Voigt et al. 1998). Health concerns have been expressed about emissions from the aluminium smelter in Portland, Victoria, but this small town also has other potentially polluting industries including fertiliser production (Heyworth et al. 2001). Lead dust is at high levels in many Broken Hill homes, but direct risks to children's health in those homes remain to be ascertained (Boreland et al. 2002).

BOX 23.2 Doing health sociology: health promotion and chronic illness

Promoting good health also means effective management of chronic illness. Diabetes affects 4 per cent of Australians and New Zealanders and complications such as blindness, kidney disease, and limb amputation pose serious problems for the financing of public health. A US report in 2001 concluded that 90 per cent of diabetes-related blindness, 50 per cent of diabetes-related kidney failure, and more than 50 per cent of diabetes-related amputations

. . . »

Katy Richmond and John Germov

could be prevented by better health care systems (Montez & Karner 2005). The IHP approach targets the individual and urges diabetics to monitor their glucose levels, take good care of their feet, and make regular appointments with optometrists. Yet evidence suggests that asymptomatic diabetics often ignore their illness (Lawton et al. 2005) and self-control-based diabetic treatment regimens are in the end largely ineffective (Montez & Karner 2005). The alternative SCHP approach works to limit common complications of diabetes through financial support for improved medical monitoring of glucose levels and cardiovascular and kidney health, provision of diabetic foot care clinics, glucose monitors for home use, and the training of diabetic educators and counsellors.

Conclusion: future directions

A problem facing SCHP is to decide what practical benefits might be provided at the community level by general practitioners (GPs) and allied health professionals (dietitians, psychologists, physiotherapists, occupational therapists, and so on). This not only includes better training of GPs in health promotion, but also health policies that facilitate and reward GPs and allied health professionals for involvement in health promotion. The Federal Government schemes of Enhanced Primary Care (EPC), Coordinated Care Trials (CCTs), and Divisions of General Practice all represent a move in this direction (see Chapters 18, 22, and 24 for further discussion). All of these programs, to greater and lesser degrees, attempt to engage those involved in primary health care in greater collaborative and preventive efforts.

Whatever the structural changes required to improve health, people still need some critically based education about health matters—not information *per se*, but information about how to utilise health services and health resources, and how the social environment impinges on people's health (Beattie 1991, p. 164). People have a right to good health education, and certainly there is evidence that people are anxious to obtain it (Richmond 1995). They do not need lists of the latest epidemiological risk factors for heart disease. Instead they need information about how to evaluate sources of health knowledge. The internet is proving an effective vehicle for improved access to good information. For example, the Federal Government has established *HealthInsite* (see <www.healthinsite.gov.au/>), an online resource of high-quality health information. However, lack of access to the internet for those who cannot afford computers or computer training means that many people are likely to remain 'information poor'.

At the beginning of this chapter, it was noted that health promotion practices range along a broad continuum, but for simplification, they could be categorised into either IHP or SCHP types. The novel feature of the new public health approach, expressed by the Ottawa Charter, is its attempt to bridge the gap between IHP and SCHP approaches by addressing both individual and structural issues. While the argument in this chapter suggests that the new public health has relied primarily on individualistic approaches in practice, such a conclusion must acknowledge the difficulty in overcoming political, economic, and organisational obstacles in attempting to translate the model's rhetoric into reality.

While the philosophies that underpin individualist and structuralist approaches to health promotion cannot always be easily reconciled, there is some ground for convergence. As we have seen in the examples discussed above, health promotion can involve culturally appropriate individualistic methods of health education and lifestyle change, coupled with structural and collective methods aimed at producing wider social change. The future of health promotion clearly needs to head in this direction.

Summary of main points

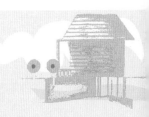

»   Health promotion can be categorised into two types: individualist health promotion (health education about lifestyle change) and structuralist–collectivist health promotion (health programs involving the community, legislation, and bureaucratic interventions).

»   Criticisms of individualist health promotion programs involve their general lack of success in terms of changing behaviour in the long term, and their tendency toward victim-blaming.

»   Much individualist health promotion is based on risk discourse and healthism, and has encouraged such a massive preoccupation with health—often linked to beauty and youth—that health has become a commodity in the marketplace through gyms, health food shops, and diet foods.

»   Examples of structuralist–collectivist health promotion can be found, but much more can be done. It may even be possible for some convergence of IHP and SCHP via the new public health approach.

Katy Richmond and John Germov

Sociological reflection: what's your reaction?

We are constantly bombarded with health education messages. How do you react to such messages? How effective do you think they are? To start with, make a brief list of some of the common messages you are familiar with (for example, 'don't drink and drive', and 'slip, slop, slap'). Then consider the questions below:

» Do you think such messages influence people in general? Why or why not?
» Do such health messages have an impact on you? Have you or would you change your behaviour or lifestyle in response to health education?
» What are some of the underlying assumptions of health education?
» In what ways could health education messages have a negative impact?
» What are some other ways to promote health and prevent illness?

Discussion questions

1   What are the five principles of the Ottawa Charter for Health Promotion? Provide at least one real-life example of a health promotion strategy for each of the five principles.
2   What is healthism? In what ways can healthism have negative implications?
3   What are the major criticisms that can be made of individualist health promotion?
4   What are the major barriers to structuralist–collectivist health promotion?
5   Are individualist health promotion programs easier to implement than structuralist programs?
6   Why might some people be opposed to structuralist–collectivist approaches, and who might these people be?

Further investigation

1   'Public health has, over time, lost its broad gauged approach and moved into a phase of medical dominance and concern for behavioural epidemiology, preventive medicine and health education. It has individualised social and cultural patterns by concentrating on disease categories and risk factor causation principles (heart disease/high blood pressure/less fat/health behaviour change)' (Kickbusch 1989, p. 266). Discuss.
2   What are the differences in how health promotion is understood by the biomedical model compared with the social model of health? Why do these differences exist? Are the limitations of one model addressed by the other? Can the two models be reconciled?

Further reading

Baum, F. 2008, *The New Public Health*, 3rd edn, Oxford University Press, Melbourne.

Bunton, R., Nettleton, S. & Burrows, R. (eds) 1995, *The Sociology of Health Promotion*, Routledge, London.

Cockerham, W. C. 2005, 'Health Lifestyle Theory and the Convergence of Agency and Structure', *Journal of Health and Social Behaviour*, vol. 46, pp. 51–67.

Crawford, R. 1980, 'Healthism and the Medicalization of Everyday Life', *International Journal of Health Services*, vol. 10, pp. 365–88.

Fitzpatrick, M. 2001, *The Tyranny of Health: Doctors and the Regulation of Lifestyle*, Routledge, London.

Hamilton, M., Kellehear, A., & Rumbold, G. (eds) 1998, *Drug Use in Australia: A Harm Minimisation Approach*, Oxford University Press, Melbourne.

Hansen, E. & Easthope, G. 2007, *Lifestyle in Medicine*, Routledge, London.

Keleher, H., MacDougall, C. & Murphy, B. (eds) 2007, *Understanding Health Promotion*, Oxford University Press, Melbourne.

Lupton, D. 1995, *The Imperative of Health: Public Health and the Regulated Body*, Sage, London.

McKinlay, J. 1994, 'A Case for Refocussing Upstream: The Political Economy of Illness', in P. Conrad & R. Kern (eds), *The Sociology of Health and Illness: Critical Perspectives*, 4th edn, St Martin's Press, New York, pp. 509–23.

O'Connor-Fleming, M. E. & Parker, E. 2007, *Health Promotion: Principles and Practice in the Australian Context*, 3rd edn, Allen & Unwin, Sydney.

Petersen, A. & Lupton, D. 1996, *The New Public Health: Health and Self in the Age of Risk*, Allen & Unwin, Sydney.

Web resources

Australian Health Promotion Association: <http://www.healthpromotion.org.au/>

Australian Indigenous Health Promotion Knowledge Network: <http://www.indigenous health.med.usyd.edu.au/>

HealthInsite: <http://www.healthinsite.gov.au/>

Healthy & Active Australia: <http://www.healthyactive.gov.au/>

Primary Health Care Research & Information Service: <http://www.phcris.org.au/>

Public Health Association of Australia (PHAA): <http://www.phaa.net.au>

VicHealth: Victorian Health Promotion Foundation: <http://www.vichealth.vic.gov.au>

World Health Organization, Department of Chronic Diseases and Health Promotion: <http://www.who.int/nmh/about/chp/en/>

World Health Organization, Health Promotion Declarations: <http://www.who.int/health promotion/conferences/en/index.html>

Online case study • • •
Visit the Second Opinion website to access relevant case studies.

Documentaries/films

Sicko (2007): 110 minutes. A Michael Moore documentary on the problems of profit-oriented health care in the USA compared to free public health systems in Canada, the UK, and France.

Strategies to Improve Public Health in Australia (2003): 26 minutes, Video Education Australasia. This short documentary explores the benefits of public health and the key features of the Ottawa Charter in an Australian context.

The Trouble with Medicine (1993): 6 part documentary series (each around 55 minutes). An excellent English–Australian co-production examining a wide range of social and ethical health issues, ABC TV, BBC TV & Thirteen-WNET.

References

Australian Institute of Health and Welfare 2003, *Indicators of Health Risk Factors: The AIHW View*, AIHW Cat. no. PHE 47, AIHW, Canberra.

Barraclough, S. 1992, 'Policy through Legislation: Victoria's Tobacco Act', in H. Gardner (ed.), *Health Policy: Development, Implementation and Evaluation in Australia*, Churchill Livingstone, Melbourne, pp. 183–210.

Baum, F. & Sanders, D. 1995, 'Can Health Promotion and Primary Health Care Achieve Health for All without a Return to their More Radical Agenda?', *Health Promotion International*, vol. 10, no. 2, pp. 149–60.

Beattie, A. 1991, 'Knowledge and Control in Health Promotion: A Test Case for Social Policy and Social Theory', in J. Gabe, M. Calnan & M. Bury (eds), *The Sociology of the Health Service*, Routledge, London, pp. 162–202.

Beck, U. 1992, *Risk Society: Towards a New Modernity*, Sage, London.

Bennett, P. & Hodgson, R. 1992, 'Psychology and Health Promotion', in R. Bunton & G. Macdonald (eds), *Health Promotion: Disciplines and Diversity*, Routledge, London, pp. 23–41.

Boreland, F., Lyle, D., Wodarczyk, J., Balding, W. & Reddan, S. 2002, 'Lead Dust in Broken Hill Homes: A Potential Hazard for Young Children?', *Australian and New Zealand Journal of Public Health*, vol. 26, no. 3, p. 203.

Borland, R., Donaghue, N. & Hill, D. 1994, 'Illnesses that Australians Most Feared in 1986 and 1993', *Australian Journal of Public Health*, vol. 18, pp. 366–9.

Bray, F. & Chapman, S. 1991, 'Community Knowledge, Attitudes and Media Recall about AIDS, Sydney 1988 and 1989', *Australian Journal of Public Health*, vol. 15, pp. 107–13.

Brown, W. & Redman, S. 1995, 'Setting Targets: A Three-stage Model for Determining Priorities for Health Promotion', *Australian Journal of Public Health*, vol. 19, pp. 263–9.

Brownlea, A. 1987, 'Participation, Myth, Realities and Prognosis', *Social Science & Medicine*, vol. 25, pp. 605–14.

Bunney, C. & Williams, L. 1999, *Caring for Children: Food, Nutrition and Fun Activities*, 3rd edn, NSW Department of Health, Sydney.

Burdess, N. 1996, 'Class and Health', in C. Grbich (ed.), *Health in Australia: Sociological Concepts and Issues*, Prentice Hall, Sydney, pp. 163–87.

Byde, P. 1995, 'Contexts and Communication for Health Promotion', in G. M. Lupton & J. Najman (eds), *Sociology of Health and Illness: Australian Readings*, 2nd edn, Macmillan, Melbourne, pp. 301–24.

Cockerham, W. C. 2004, *Medical Sociology*, 9th edn, Prentice Hall, Englewood Cliffs, NJ.

Cockerham, W. C. 2005, 'Health Lifestyle Theory and the Convergence of Agency and Structure', *Journal of Health and Social Behaviour*, vol. 46, pp. 51–67.

Crawford, R. 1980, 'Healthism and the Medicalisation of Everyday Life', *International Journal of Health Services*, vol. 10, no. 3, pp. 365–88.

Crowley, S., Dunt, D. & Day, N. 1995, 'Cost-effectiveness of Alternative Interventions for the Prevention and Treatment of Coronary Heart Disease', *Australian Journal of Public Health*, vol. 19, pp. 336–46.

Davison, C., Finkel, S. & Davey Smith, G. D. 1992, '"To Hell with Tomorrow": Coronary Heart Disease Risk and the Ethnography of Fatalism', in S. Scott, G. Williams, S. Platt & H. Thomas (eds), *Private Risks and Public Dangers*, Ashgate, Aldershot, pp. 95–111.

Elliott, H. 1995, 'Community Nutrition Education for People with Coronary Heart Disease: Who Attends?', *Australian Journal of Public Health*, vol. 19, pp. 205–10.

Flaherty, B., Homel, P. & Hall, W. 1991, 'Public Attitudes Towards Alcohol Policies', *Australian Journal of Public Health*, vol. 15, pp. 301–6.

Germov, J. & Williams, L. 1996, 'The Epidemic of Dieting Women: The Need for a Sociological Approach to Food and Nutrition', *Appetite*, vol. 27, pp. 97–108.

Giddens, A., 1991 *Modernity and Self-identity: Self and Society in the Late Modern Age*, Polity, Cambridge.

Gray, D., Saggers, S., Sputore, B. & Bourbon, D. 2000 'What Works? A Review of Alcohol Misuse Interventions Among Aboriginal Australians', *Addiction*, vol. 95, no. 1, pp. 11–22.

Hart, B. 1989, 'Community Health Promotion Programs', in H. Gardner (ed.), *The Politics of Health: The Australian Experience*, Churchill Livingstone, Melbourne, pp. 414–32.

Heyworth, J., Weller, D., Edwards, J., Guest, C., Smith, P. & Steer, K. 2001, 'A Comparison of the Prevalence of Respiratory Illness and Non-specific Health Symptoms in Two Victorian Cities', *Australian and New Zealand Journal of Public Health*, vol. 25, no. 4, pp. 327–33.

Higginbotham, N., Heading, G., Pont, J., Plotnikoff, R., Dobson, A. J. & Smith, E. 1993, 'Community Worry about Heart Disease: A Needs Survey in the Coalfields and Newcastle Areas of the Hunter Region', *Australian Journal of Public Health*, vol. 17, pp. 314–21.

Hill, D. & White, V. 1995, 'Australian Adult Smoking Prevalence in 1992', *Australian Journal of Public Health*, vol. 19, pp. 305–8.

Hill, D., White, V. & Segan, C. 1995, 'Prevalence of Cigarette Smoking among Australian Secondary School Students in 1993', *Australian Journal of Public Health*, vol. 19, pp. 445–9.

Hunt, K. & Emslie, C. 2001, 'The Prevention Paradox in Lay Epidemiology: Rose Revisited', *International Journal of Epidemiology*, vol. 30, pp. 442–6.

Jamison, J. 1995, 'Australian Dietary Targets in 1995: Their Feasibility and Pertinence to Dietary Goals for 2000', *Australian Journal of Public Health*, vol. 19, pp. 522–4.

Kaplan, R. M. 1988, 'The Value Dimension in Studies of Health Promotion', in S. Spacapan & S. Oskamp (eds), *The Social Psychology of Health*, Sage, Newbury Park, CA, pp. 207–36.

Kassulke, D., Stenner-Day, K., Coory, M. & Ring, I. 1993, 'Information-Seeking Behaviour and Sources of Health Information: Associations with Risk Factor Status in an Analysis of Three Queensland Electorates', *Australian Journal of Public Health*, vol. 17, pp. 51–7.

Kelly, K. & Van Vlaenderen, H. 1996, 'Dynamics of Participation in a Community Health Project', *Social Science & Medicine*, vol. 43, no. 8, pp. 1235–46.

Kickbusch, I. 1989, 'Approaches to an Ecological Base for Public Health', *Health Promotion*, vol. 4, no. 4, pp. 265–8.

Kirby, J. & Kaneda, T. 2005, 'Neighborhood Socioeconomic Disadvantage and Access to Health Care', *Journal of Health and Social Behaviour*, vol. 46, pp. 15–31.

Lawton, J., Peel, E., Parry, P., Gonzalo, A. & Douglas, M. 2005, 'Lay Perceptions of Type 2 Diabetes in Scotland: Bringing Health Services Back In', *Social Science & Medicine*, vol. 60, pp. 1423–35.

Le Fanu, J. 1986, 'Diet and Disease: Nonsense and Non-science', in D. Anderson (ed.), *A Diet of Reason: Sense and Nonsense in the Healthy Eating Debate*, The Social Affairs Unit, London, pp. 109–24.

Lee, A., Bailey, A. P., Yarmirr, D., O'Dea, K. & Mathews, J. D. 1994, 'Survival Tucker: Improved Diet and Health Indicators in an Aboriginal Community', *Australian Journal of Public Health*, vol. 18, pp. 277–85.

Lee, A., Bonson, A. P. V. & Powers, J. R. 1996, 'The Effect of Retail Store Managers on Aboriginal Diet in Remote Communities', *Australian Journal of Public Health*, vol. 20, pp. 212–14.

Lee, A. J., Darcy, A. M., Leonard, D., Groos, A. D., Stubbs, C. O., Lowson, S. K., Dunn, S. M., Coyne, T. & Riley, M. D. 2002, 'Food Availability, Cost Disparity and Improvement in Relation to Accessibility and Remoteness in Queensland', *Australian and New Zealand Journal of Public Health*, vol. 26, no. 3, p. 266.

Link, B. & Phelan, J. 1995, 'Social Conditions as Fundamental Causes of Disease', *Journal of Health and Social Behaviour*, extra issue, pp. 80–94.

Lupton, D. 1995, *The Imperative of Health: Public Health and the Regulated Body*, Sage, London.

McKinlay, J. B. 1994, 'A Case for Refocussing Upstream: The Political Economy of Illness', in P. Conrad & R. Kern (eds), *The Sociology of Health and Illness: Critical Perspectives*, 4th edn, St Martin's Press, New York, pp. 509–23.

McKinlay, J. B. 1996, 'Some Contributions from the Social System to Gender Inequalities in Heart Disease', *Journal of Health and Social Behaviour*, vol. 37, pp. 1–26.

McMasters, A. 1996, 'Research from an Aboriginal Health Worker's Point of View', *Australian Journal of Public Health*, vol. 20, pp. 319–20.

McMichael, A. J. 1991, 'Food, Nutrients, Health and Disease: A Historical Perspective on the Assessment and Management of Risks', *Australian Journal of Public Health*, vol. 15, pp. 7–13.

Mechanic, D. 1994, 'Promoting Health: Implications for Modern and Developing Nations', in L. Chen, A. Kleinman & N. Ware (eds), *Health and Social Change in International Perspective*, Harvard University Press, Cambridge, MA, pp. 471–89.

Montez, J. K. & Karner, T. X. 2005, 'Understanding the Diabetic Body-self', *Qualitative Health Research*, vol. 15, no. 8, pp. 1086–104.

Navarro, V. 1986, *Crisis, Health and Medicine: A Social Critique*, Tavistock, London.

Nettleton, S. 1995, *The Sociology of Health and Illness*, Polity Press, Cambridge.

O'Connor-Fleming, M. E. & Parker, E. 2007, *Health Promotion: Principles and Practice in the Australian Context*, 3rd edn, Allen & Unwin, Sydney.

Johanson, M., Larsson, U. S., Säljö, R. & Svärdsudd, K. 1996, 'Addressing Life Style in Primary Health Care', *Social Science & Medicine*, vol. 43, no. 3, pp. 389–400.

Petersen, A. 1996, 'Risk and the Regulated Self: The Discourse of Health Promotion as Politics of Uncertainty', *Australian and New Zealand Journal of Sociology*, vol. 32, pp. 44–57.

Pikora, T., Phang, J.-W., Karro, J., Corti, B., Clarkson, J., Donovan, R., Frizzell, S. & Wilkinson, A. 1999, 'Are Smoke-free Policies Implemented and Adhered to at Sporting Venues', *Australian and New Zealand Journal of Public Health*, vol. 23, no. 4, pp. 407–9.

Pinell, P. 1996, 'Modern Medicine and the Civilising Process', *Sociology of Health and Illness*, vol. 18, no. 1, pp. 1–16.

Pollard, C., Lewis, J. & Miller, M. 1999, 'Food Service in Long Day Care Centres: An Opportunity for Public Health Intervention', *Australian and New Zealand Journal of Public Health*, vol. 23, no. 6, pp. 606–10.

Richmond, K. 1995, 'Knowledge, Attitudes, Beliefs and Behaviour of Women Factory Workers in Relation to Cardiovascular Disease', in R. Sorger (ed.), *Women Have a Heart Too*, Healthsharing Women's Health Resource Service, Melbourne, pp. 51–5.

Ritchie, J., Herscovitch, F. & Norfor, J. 1994, 'Beliefs of Blue Collar Workers Regarding Coronary Risk Behaviours', *Health Education Research*, vol. 9, pp. 95–103.

Rose, G. 1985, 'Sick Individuals and Sick Populations', *International Journal of Epidemiology*, vol. 14, pp. 32–8.

Scrimgeour, D., Rowse, T. & Knight, S. 1994, 'Food-purchasing in an Aboriginal Community: Evaluation of an Intervention', *Australian Journal of Public Health*, vol. 18, pp. 67–70.

Siskind, V., Najman, J. & Veitch, C. 1992, 'Socioeconomic Status and Mortality Revisited: An Extension of the Brisbane Area Analysis', *Australian Journal of Public Health*, vol. 16, pp. 315–20.

Skolbekken, J. A. 1995, 'The Risk Epidemic in Medical Journals', *Social Science & Medicine*, vol. 40, no. 2, pp. 291–305.

Smith, R., Smith, P., McKinnon, M. & Gracey, M. 2000, 'Birthweights and Growth of Infants in Five Aboriginal Communities', *Australian and New Zealand Journal of Public Health*, vol. 24, no. 2, pp. 124–35.

Tannahill, A. 1992, 'Epidemiology and Health Promotion: A Common Understanding', in R. Bunton & G. Macdonald (eds), *Health Promotion: Disciplines and Diversity*, Routledge, London, pp. 86–107.

Thorogood, N. 1992, 'What is the Relevance of Sociology for Health Promotion', in R. Bunton & G. Macdonald (eds), *Health Promotion: Disciplines and Diversity*, Routledge, London, pp. 42–65.

Travers, K. 1996, 'The Social Organization of Nutritional Inequities', *Social Sciences and Medicine*, vol. 43, pp. 543–53.

Van Beurden, E., James, R., Montague, D., Christian, J. & Dunn, T. 1993, 'Community-based Cholesterol Screening and Education to Prevent Heart Disease: Five Year Results of the North Coast Cholesterol Check Campaign', *Australian Journal of Public Health*, vol. 17, pp. 109–16.

Voigt, T., Bailey, M. & Abramson, M. 1998, 'Air Pollution in the Latrobe Valley and its Impact upon Respiratory Morbidity', *Australian and New Zealand Journal of Public Health*, vol. 22, no. 5, pp. 556–61.

Waitzkin, H. 1983, *The Second Sickness: Contradictions of Capitalist Health Care*, Free Press, New York.

Whitehead, M. 1992, 'The Concepts and Principles of Equity and Health', *International Journal of Health Services*, vol. 22, no. 3, pp. 429–45.

Williams, S. & Calnan, M. 1996, 'The "Limits" of Medicalization? Modern Medicine and the Lay Populace in "Late" Modernity', *Social Science & Medicine*, vol. 42, no. 12, pp. 1609–20.

World Health Organization 1978, *Primary Health Care: Report of the International Conference on Primary Health Care*, Alma-Ata, USSR, 6–12 September, WHO, Geneva.

World Health Organization 1986, *Ottawa Charter for Health Promotion*, First International Conference on Health Promotion: The Move Towards a New Public Health, 17–21 November, Ottawa, Canada, and WHO, Geneva.

CHAPTER 24

Community Health
Services in Australia

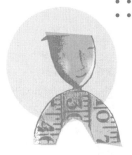

FRAN
BAUM

Overview

- What are community health services and how did their philosophy
  and practice develop in Australia?
- What are some Australian examples of community health services
  in action?
- What are the current policy directions affecting community health
  services in Australia?

COMMUNITY HEALTH:
AN ALTERNATIVE FUTURE

It is 2011 and the Australian Health Ministers are meeting to discuss two key issues: the continued increasing prevalence of chronic disease and associated risk factors in Australia, and the failure of Australia to make progress in reducing the life-expectancy gap between Indigenous and non-Indigenous Australians. For the past few years they have been strongly committed to the idea that improving the management of chronic disease through programs linked to hospitals and general practice working mainly with individuals would solve the problems. Now one of them—a recently appointed health minister in Victoria with a background in

comprehensive community health services and community development—is arguing that the only way to reduce chronic disease and increase Indigenous life expectancy is through a dramatically different approach. She persuades all the health ministers to invest in a big new program that funds a network of healthy and sustainable community programs for 10 years (granted they perform well). These initiatives will link local government with state health departments and will establish community health centres for each 30,000 people living in urban areas and for a size appropriate to the region in rural areas. They will have responsibility for

. . . »

the health and well-being of the population in their area. They will be managed by locally elected boards of management.

In 2021, there is an Australian community health conference which attracts participants from around the world because they want to hear how Australia has turned around the chronic disease epidemic especially in young people and how the Indigenous life expec-

tancy is now 6 years closer to non-Indigenous. This was achieved not through a medical miracle but through giving power and control over health to local communities, taking action on the social determinants of health, and supporting community health with appropriate regulation and legislation to make healthy choices possible and easy.

Introduction:
a history of community health in Australia

Policy frameworks

Australia had a nationally endorsed Community Health Policy for only 3 years: between 1973 and 1976. Initiated by the Whitlam Labor Government, this policy established the framework that led to the expansion of community health in Australia during the 1970s and 1980s. The Community Health Program (CHP) was formed following a recommendation of the Hospitals and Health Services Commission (HHSC). It was established in 1973 as '[a] major community health program to develop facilities and services in a coordinated manner for the provision and planning of prevention, treatment, rehabilitation and related welfare aspects of community health' (HHSC 1973, p. 16).

The chief objective of the national program was 'to encourage the provision of high quality, readily accessible, reasonably comprehensive, coordinated and efficient health and welfare services at local, regional, State and national levels. Such services should be developed in consultation with, and where appropriate, the involvement of, the community to be served' (HHSC 1973, p. 4).

Judith Raftery (1995, pp. 20–1) has summarised the key service components of the CHP as:

1   programs of information and counselling to improve the habits, conditions, and environment that may precede disorders of health
2   direct preventive action
3   disease detection procedures to discover incipient or pre-clinical phases of disease

4 information and counselling programs to motivate individuals to seek care once departure from normal health is perceived

5 specific diagnosis and treatment services

6 rehabilitation and supportive services for those with continuing disease and disability

7 provision of help for those with chronic disability who have to adapt to sheltered living or working conditions.

This program formed the basis for the subsequent development of community health services in Australia. The degree to which the program was radical in intent has been disputed. Alexander (1995) presented it as such and saw it as a forerunner of the Ottawa Charter for Health Promotion and the **new public health**. Raftery (1995, p. 23) interprets the 1973 program as more conservative and says it was unquestioning about certain **biomedical** assumptions: it was 'lacking in ideas about strategies to achieve its objectives; and it was vague and naïve about prevention of illness'. Contrary to Alexander's position, her view is that the 1973 plan was a limited one that did not foreshadow the new public health.

The CHP was reviewed on three occasions, in 1976, 1986, and 1992. Each of these reviews concluded that, while it had not made a significant impact on the nature of the Australian health system, it had allowed some limited experimentation in styles of health care delivery. The main advances were seen in some experimentation with health education and with the provision of community-based services for diagnostic, therapeutic, and rehabilitation services, but each review also noted that there continued to be a strong orientation to service provision and individual treatment, and to tertiary rather than primary or secondary prevention. The 1986 Review, conducted by the Australian Community Health Association (ACHA; formed in 1984), concluded that a community health program with 'some degree of coherence' had been established in all states and territories. It went on to note that the program tended to be a residual and quite conservative service compared to its original intentions, that it had a disease focus, and that it was delivered through secondary and tertiary prevention (ACHA 1986). The reviewers also noted that the CHP had contributed to a broader understanding of health and had made the issue of community involvement more prominent in health debates, but that the CHP had little impact on the overall priorities of the health system. Both Neal Blewett (2000) and Nancy Milio (1983) have noted that the main political champions for more radical change in Australia invested most energy in the establishment of Medicare, Australia's universal health insurance scheme, rather than in the CHP.

The reviews of the CHP did note that its development was patchy across Australia. The Labor Governments in Victoria and South Australia during the 1970s and 1980s did most to establish a network of comprehensive community health services. In contrast, the CHP in Queensland made little progress within a traditional public

new public health
A social model of health linking 'traditional' public health concerns about physical aspects of the environment (clean air and water, safe food, occupational safety), with concerns about the behavioural, social, and economic factors that affect people's health.

biomedicine/ biomedical model
The conventional approach to medicine in Western societies, based on the diagnosis and explanation of illness as a malfunction of the body's biological mechanisms. This approach underpins most health professions and health services, which focus on treating individuals, and generally ignores the social origins of illness and its prevention.

primary health care (PHC)
Both the point of first contact with the health care system and a philosophy for the delivery of that care.

service model characterised by central decision-making, slow responses to local decisions, and no political or bureaucratic commitment to community involvement. In Victoria and South Australia, on the other hand, community health development was at its peak during the 1980s. By this time these states had a network of centres that were developing innovative and creative approaches to comprehensive **primary health care (PHC)**. These states were acknowledged to have made far more significant progress in implementing community health than any of the others.

The 1992 ACHA review analysed the impact of different organisational structures on the ability of community health services to achieve their original aims. The review found that the independently incorporated community health centres, with their own boards of management and control over their own budgets, were the most successful models. South Australia and Victoria also established democratic forms of management for their centres whereby boards of management were elected (Victoria) or appointed (South Australia). These boards were responsible for the overall management and direction-setting for the centres. This form of management is not without problems but during the 1980s and early 1990s the thinking about these challenges showed sophistication and a desire to improve its efficiency (see, for example, Laris 1992, 1995; Legge 1992). David Legge (1992, p. 96) notes:

> The achievements of community health over the last two decades have been huge and in large part are a consequence of the energy and direction gained from real community involvement. Having community members on committees is part of helping staff of the centre to understand the practical health problems that they deal with on a daily basis in the context of the more general concerns of the different communities in the locality.

Since Legge's comment, the policy environment has been less favourable to community health and its development has stagnated and not been encouraged by policy at either federal or state level. Indeed, Legge foreshadowed some of the key reasons for the decline in the fortunes of community health, noting that its underlying principles conflicted with 'new wave managerialism and the underlying ideology of economic rationalism' (Legge 1992, pp. 112).

The period since the early 1990s has seen many changes to community health which has meant that its unique features have been eroded. The election of the Rudd Labor Government with its overt commitment to primary health care might encourage more efforts to strengthen comprehensive community health services based on a social view of health; potentially using them as a basis for reforming mainstream service delivery. This will require significant changes as the direction in most jurisdictions in Australia is towards a system of primary health care, which is about out-of-hospital services, and focuses on chronic disease rather than health promotion, community participation, or the broader promotion of healthy communities.

What are community health services?

There is no simple definition of community health services. They have differed over time and also between states and territories. At neither national nor state level are there any comprehensive databases that describe the activities of community health services. In part this reflects the complexity of community health work, but most significantly it reflects the lack of investment in information systems for community health services. There is also considerable change to the nature and governance of community health services happening at the current time. Nonetheless there are some common features of these services.

Philosophical underpinning

Community health services share a common philosophy with that espoused by the World Health Organization (WHO) in key documents such as the 1978 Alma-Ata *Health for All by the Year 2000* (HFA 2000) Declaration. This document set out a vision for a health system driven by comprehensive primary health care. Grasping the philosophical underpinnings of the HFA 2000 strategy of the WHO is crucial to understanding the sort of comprehensive health service that community health in Australia has always strived for but never achieved. The Alma-Ata Declaration established the following principles:

- Health is a fundamental human right and its achievement would reflect effort in many other social and economic sectors in addition to the health sector.
- Inequities in the health status between people in developed countries and those in developing countries, as well as within countries, are unacceptable, and the key to reducing these inequities and to achieving health for all lies in social and economic development.
- Community participation in planning and implementation of health care is seen as both a right and a duty.

Primary health care is here defined as:

> essential health care based on practical, scientifically sound and socially acceptable methods and technologies made universally accessible to individuals and families in the community through their full participation and at a cost that the community and country can afford to maintain at every stage of their development in the spirit of self-reliance and self-determination. It forms an integral part both of the country's health system, of which it is the central function and main focus, and of the overall social and economic development of the community. It is the first level of contact of individuals, the family and community with the national health system bringing health care as close as possible to where people live and work, and constitutes the first element of a continuing health care process. (WHO 1978)

Fran Baum

The Ottawa Charter for Health Promotion, which in many ways translated the central messages of the HFA 2000 Strategy into a language suitable to developed countries, has also been used extensively by community health services in vision, goal, and planning exercises (see, for example, Sanderson & Alexander 1995). The five strategies of the Ottawa Charter (develop healthy public policy, create supportive environments, encourage community action, develop personal skills, and reorientate health services) provide a fairly accurate description of the work of community health services (as is shown in detail in the section describing their work below).

So the key features of the philosophy behind community health are as follows:

- Multidisciplinary teams are preferable as the basis for community health work.
- Community involvement in the management and running of programs within community health services is an essential part of good practice. The aim of community health is to enable communities to take greater control of the social, economic, and physical environments that influence their health.
- Working in partnership with other sectors is a crucial part of community health work.
- Equity and a **social model of health** are fundamental to the operation and decision-making processes within the services. An understanding of the social and economic determinants of health is fundamental to the logic of the work undertaken in community health services. This legitimacy of this approach has been greatly enhanced in recent years through the work of the Commission on the Social Determinants of Health (CSDH 2008) which argues strongly that health service provision should be underpinned by a detailed understanding of the social determinants of health (CSDH 2008).

The vision of community health as a comprehensive underpinning of the entire health service has unfortunately never been realised. It has always remained marginalised to the mainstream system. While community health has provided a practical example of what could be possible if the model were to be adopted as the basis of the health system, there has never been a political will to implement the community health model in this way.

The main block to this has been the prevalence of fee-for-service general medical practice. This model has precluded the growth of community health because the political will to provide the resources necessary to develop a strong salaried medical workforce within community health centres has been lacking. There are some very real differences between the community health model and the form of health care practised by most general medical practitioners in Australia. The key differences they have identified in services are that whereas a comprehensive model of primary health care stresses **health promotion** and rehabilitation and multidisciplinary team approaches, these are limited in general practice. Rogers and Veale (2000) argue that general practice does not address population-level needs-based planning,

social model of health
Focuses on social determinants of health such as the social production, distribution, and construction of health and illness, and the social organisation of health care. It directs attention to the prevention of illness through community participation and social reforms that address living and working conditions.

health promotion
Any combination of education and related organisational, economic, and political interventions designed to promote behavioural and environmental changes conducive to good health, including legislation, community development, and advocacy.

collaboration across sectors, or education. They also note that general practice does not adopt the philosophy advocated in the World Health Organization's description of primary health care (see above).

Primary medical care is not grounded in a social understanding of health in the way in which community health is. The former is based primarily on the provision of one category of health services to individuals. While general practitioners have begun to do some group and community work through the Divisions of General Practice, this work is limited and is a long way from the vision of comprehensive primary health care offered by the Alma-Ata Declaration. The contrast between a selective model of PHC typically offered in general practice and the more comprehensive model offered in the most progressive community health services is shown in Table 24.1.

Table 24.1 The contrast between comprehensive and selective primary health care

Characteristic	Selective	Comprehensive
Main aim	Reduction/elimination of specific disease	Improvement in overall health of the community and individuals
Strategies	Focus on curative treatment or intervention, with some attention to prevention and promotion	Comprehensive strategy with curative, rehabilitative, and preventive treatment or intervention, and health promotion that seeks to remove root cause of ill health
Planning and strategy development	External, often 'global programs' with little tailoring to local circumstances	Local and reflecting community priorities—professionals 'on tap, not on top'
Participation	Limited engagement in terms of outside experts and tending to be sporadic	Engaged participation that starts with community strengths and their assessment of health issues. Ongoing and aiming for community control
Engagement with politics	Professional and claims to be apolitical	Acknowledges that PHC is inevitably political and engages with local political structures
Forms of evidence	Limited to assessment of disease-prevention strategy based on traditional epidemiological methods usually conducted out of context and extrapolated to the situation	Complex, multiple methods, involving a range of research methods including epidemiology, qualitative, and participatory methodology

Source: Baum 2007

Fran Baum

What do community health services do?

Given the description of the philosophy underpinning community health, it is evident that the activities that these services undertake will be diverse, particularly between services in different states. There are three main areas of activity within community health services: one-to-one services; group programs; and community development and social action. In the early 1990s, community health services that offered this range of programs were still marginal but reasonably widespread. In 2008 there appear to be fewer services that engage in community development and social action. The most comprehensive community health services would normally have some activities in each of these areas. The main service categories in community health have been defined in South Australia and these represent the range of work that might be done within a community health service.

Clinical services

Community health services offer a range of clinical services to individuals. These may include medical services. Other services that may be offered are counselling, podiatry, physiotherapy, speech pathology, dietetics, and nutrition. The emphasis within these services is to encourage rehabilitation and prevent the likelihood of problems recurring in the future. Around Australia there is an increasingly strong focus on chronic disease and counselling of women experiencing domestic violence and/or sexual abuse is a service that is commonly provided.

Medical services offered within community health centres differ from those offered in most private general practitioner services. Studies of the work of medical practitioners within women's and community health centres indicate that the users of the centres identify the following advantages of medical practice within community health centres:

- Patients are able to spend more time with the doctor.
- Patients perceive that they are more likely to be treated as a 'whole' person.
- There is easy access to members of the multidisciplinary teams.
- People feel that they are encouraged to have more control of their own health and be involved in decisions about their health.
- Health promotion activities are easier to gain access to.
- Interpreters are more readily available.
- The atmosphere at the centres is supportive and friendly, and is based on trusting relationships (Warin et al. 1998, pp. 87–9).

The service providers in community health services typically offer a range of services in addition to the clinical ones. This is best illustrated by the role of medical practitioners and the ways in which working within a community health centre enables them to take on broader roles beyond one-to-one work. Table 24.2 uses the Ottawa Charter as a framework to describe the potential roles for doctors within community health. The studies on which this table is based show that doctors within the centres are more likely to take on these wider roles than are doctors in private practice.

Table 24.2 Ottawa Charter planning framework: examples of doctors' roles

Ottawa Charter strategy	Examples of doctors' roles in Ottawa Charter strategies in community health centres (mostly done in collaboration with other workers)
Healthy public policy	Advocacy for change in policies and practices of agencies that have an impact on health, for example, harm minimisation approach to drugs
	Assist in the development of asthma-management procedures in schools
Creating supportive environments	Provision of supportive environment for those dependent on illicit drugs
	Lobbying public housing authority to assist patients to find better housing
	Education of private-practice GPs about domestic violence
	Training of other health professionals
Community action	Supporting environmental action by, for example, providing information of health effects of a particular type of pollution
	Supporting community initiatives such as providing a home-detoxification program
Personal skills	Support and education groups: advice and skill development (e.g. management of arthritis, asthma, diabetes, chronic pain, menopause)
Reorientation of health services	Ensuring sufficient time is given to patients and that health promotion approaches are used whenever possible (e.g. responsible use of drugs, encouraging and supporting lifestyle change)
	Applying personal problems from clinical practice to work for public solutions

Source: Adapted from Baum et al. 1996; Warin et al. 1998; Baum & Lawless 2007

Group programs

Community health services typically offer a range of group programs. The exact mix of groups offered by a particular community health service will depend on the needs of that community. Groups may focus on support for:

- a particular age group (for example, young gay people, older Indigenous women)
- people with the same chronic disease (for example, diabetes, cancer, heart disease)
- people with the same social issue (for example, domestic violence, sexual abuse, teenage parenthood, step-parenthood).

Usually the most important features of the groups are that they offer people new information about their situations and provide them with social support. Often the interaction with the other members of the group is as important as the input from the professional workers. These groups are typically offered on a no-fee or very low fee basis. Groups are an important means by which practitioners within a community health centre can move away from a sole focus, as in one-to-one service provision, and be more creative in their work.

Community participation and social action

In the 1980s and early 1990s, community health, and women's and Indigenous services in South Australia and Victoria became engaged in community development or social action campaigns. By 2008 it has become much harder to find examples of such activity although there are some initiatives such as Healthy Cities in Onkaparinga, South Australia that provide strong examples of how a community health service has been the site of innovation in thinking about health promotion (see Box 24.1).

Community development can lead to the development of many health promoting structures in a community such as social support networks, expanded healthy food choices, action and lobbying on environmental issues, and action against social pathologies such as gambling and the misuse of drugs and alcohol. When community development of social action does occur at its best, the local community in concert with the health service controls these initiatives. Community participation is a complex topic and an area in which there is considerable rhetoric about participation. Community development and social action programs are most likely to flourish in community-controlled or managed community health services.

In practice, examples of participation from within the health sector that are not driven by paid professionals are rare. Fran Baum (2008, p. 483) defines four main types of participation that can be identified within the health sector:

- *Consultation*, which asks people to respond to set plans
- *Participation as a means*, which uses participation in an instrumental way to achieve an outcome defined by the health service
- *Substantive participation*, in which people are actively involved in determining priorities and implementation but the initiative remains externally controlled
- *Structural participation*, which is a fully engaged and developmental process in which the community controls the initial agenda and process.

Doing health sociology: Healthy Cities

Onkaparinga (originally Noarlunga) Healthy Cities is an excellent example of how community health has enabled an innovative health promotion project to take root and flourish (Baum et al. 2006). In the past 2 decades one of the major health promotion initiatives of the World Health Organization (WHO) has been the Healthy Cities movement. Noarlunga Health Services became the coordinating site for the Noarlunga Healthy Cities project in 1987. For the first 3 years, funding was provided by the Federal Government, which enabled the appointment of a project manager, who was skilled at both working with senior agency managers and with community members (Baum et al. 2006). This meant the initiative got off to a very good start. What is remarkable is that this project has proved sustainable since then. A key reason for this must be the consistency with which the community health service has supported the Healthy Cities project. Richard Hicks, a senior health service executive of the Southern Area Health Service was the Chairperson of the Noarlunga Healthy Cities project since the beginning to his retirement in 2007. Achievements have included a community arts project, the establishment of an Environmental Health Plan for the area, the clean-up and establishment of wetlands in the local river (the Onkaparinga), and an injury-prevention project. Other initiatives include the Noarlunga Community Action on Drugs, a cross-sectoral program to reduce the harm from drugs in the community, and the Noarlunga injury-prevention project which has established a direct partnership with an injury-prevention project in Bangladesh. This partnership has mutual benefits and demonstrates the value of a global project such as Healthy Cities which enables people to take local ideas and link them globally. The strategic priorities for 2008–11 have been established as Water Security and Climate Change Transport, Planning for Growth and New Communities, Affordable and Appropriate Housing with community participation, and Aboriginal health and well-being as cross-cutting themes to be addressed across the strategic plan.

Through the history of the Onkaparinga project there has been strong and meaningful community involvement. Onkaparinga Healthy Cities is an incorporated body and its constitution states that there must be a majority of community representatives over organisational representatives. The initiative also has strong political support from local government and local members of parliament.

Community management

Community health services have been the most likely parts of the health sector to engage in substantive or structural participation. Community management is the best example of this. The Aboriginal health movement was the first sector to develop

Fran Baum

Indigenous community-controlled health services Independent local organisations, controlled and managed by Indigenous people, which provide a range of services to meet the needs of their particular communities.

the concept of community control; since 1970, **Indigenous community-controlled health services** have been established across Australia. Victorian community health services had boards of management that were directly elected until the mid-1990s and South Australia also had boards of management with some local people elected until the 1990s. This model of governance has some strong advantages in terms of empowering local populations and helping services meet the needs of the population they service (Legge 1992). The Victorian Department of Human Services has reintroduced the concept of direct election to boards of community health centres and so restored community involvement as central to the governance of community health—a crucial step if these services are to be responsive to their communities.

Despite these pockets of community management and control, the practice is rare. The importance of community control of planning management and delivery of Indigenous primary health care services has been stressed in a recent review (Dwyer et al. 2004). They conclude that investment in comprehensive, community-controlled primary health care services offers the best prospect for health system intervention to overcome Indigenous Australians' health disadvantage. This principle can be extended to the whole population and should be seriously considered by governments wishing to develop services that are accountable and responsive to the community. In addition, community-managed health services can offer a voice in public policy discourses which has the potential to counter-balance professional interests. Effective community management requires investment in capacity building and training—an investment that makes sense in terms of the benefits the community involvement has to offer the health system and the community's health.

Twenty-first century primary health care: what role for community health services?

The policy and practice environment in which community health services exist is complex. A review of key policy directions in each Australian jurisdiction suggests the following dilemmas for community health services:

- Health systems are frequently reviewed and reorganised and most reviews call for more emphasis on, and funding commitment to, community-based health services, but there is little evidence of any significant shift of the balance of funding from institutional based care (Dwyer 2004).
- While there are measures designed to integrate different parts of the PHC system in Australia, the systems are still largely fragmented and focused on care for individuals rather than health for populations.

- Increasing rates of chronic disease concern all Australian governments and most are dealing with this by investing in mechanisms to improve coordination of care rather than through upstream prevention and health promotion (Boxall & Leeder 2006).
- More emphasis is being given to community voices in health systems but professional voices, especially medical professional power, are still far more influential and powerful.
- Behaviour modification still dominates the disease-prevention landscape despite evidence of its lack of effectiveness at promoting population health (Baum 2008).
- Attention to the **social determinants of health** is beginning to receive more recognition (especially in Victoria and South Australia), but these efforts are still marginal despite WHO calling attention to the central role of these determinants through the Commission on the Social Determinants of Health (2008).

social determinants of health
The economic, social, and cultural factors that directly and indirectly influence individual and population health.

Primary health care has assumed a much more central place in government thinking about the organisation and development of health services in the past decade. This was evident under the Howard Coalition Government and under the Rudd Labor Government elected in November 2007. An assessment of state and territory health reviews (Dwyer 2004) demonstrates that those recommending change to health systems consistently recommend that primary health care form the centre of the health system. This will, however, not necessarily mean that the ideology and practice associated with community health will flourish. Primary health care, as shown in Table 24.1, can mean different things to different interest groups. Under the Howard Federal Government, there was a selective view of PHC that stressed medical services and behavioural interventions aimed at changing the lifestyles of people at risk of developing chronic disease. This trend has also been evident in many of the policies of many states where the realisation of the growing burden of chronic disease has led to a focus on community-based services. These have tended to be of the selective kind rather than the comprehensive style associated with the community health approach. Thus, chronic disease is being addressed by improving the coordination of services and preventive campaigns that attempt to change the lifestyles of people at risk of chronic disease. There is much less emphasis on activities that address the underlying causes of illness and seek to develop the strengths of communities through empowerment and community development processes.

Chronic disease: a growing concern

Much of the recent emphasis on PHC has been motivated by an awareness of the growing burden of chronic disease on the Australian population. Disadvantaged populations including those in lower socio-economic groups and Indigenous peoples are more likely to suffer from, and die from, chronic disease (Baum 2008). In the past few years, federal, state, and territory governments have placed more emphasis on chronic disease and the need to coordinate care for people with complex and often multiple conditions. An important innovation in primary health care in the 1990s was a series of federally funded coordinated care trials. Twelve trials were established across Australia and each was evaluated thoroughly (Silagy 2000). These trials aimed to test the proposition that services for people with complex and chronic conditions could be improved for no additional cost by improving the coordination of services. This coordination was to be achieved by pooling funds and having care planners to manage the coordination. From the viewpoint of community health, the trials were disappointing because little attempt was made to incorporate community health services within the trials beyond domiciliary and aged-care services. Most of the care coordination was done by GPs and, while they are well suited to providing primary medical care, they are generally neither trained nor experienced in assisting clients to gain access to a range of community services and supports. By contrast, this is exactly the kind of work in which community health services excel. An explicit attempt to involve community health services in care coordination may have improved the outcomes of the trials.

Current reforms in the states and territories are attempting to improve coordination of GP services (which are federally funded via Medicare) and community health services (state and territory funded and managed). For these attempts to be successful it is likely that some changes are required to the organisation, funding, and management of GP services. Each Australian jurisdiction has made chronic disease a central strategic focus and introduced policies which focus on chronic disease. The aims of these policies are similar and shown by the Queensland Strategy for Chronic Disease 2005–15 (launched in 2005). It aims to prevent chronic diseases and associated risk factors, improve the quality of life for people with chronic diseases, and reduce the level of avoidable hospital admissions. Despite widespread recognition of the need to reduce chronic disease, most Australian jurisdictions are focusing primarily on behaviour change strategies and show little evidence of programs to alter the structural conditions in which people make their lifestyle choices. The Commission on the Social Determinants of Health (CSDH 2008) advocates for far greater attention to be paid to social determinants and argues that the comprehensive PHC of the type done by community health services should be far more prominent. It also argues for action in all sectors to promote health and that the health sector has a responsibility to advocate for such action. Australia would be well placed to implement the CSDH recommendations if its community health sector were strengthened and resourced at a much greater level. A comprehensive approach to community health promotion promises to be the most effective way to reduce long-term rates of chronic disease.

Reforming general practice to strengthen community health

Through the 1990s, instead of establishing a strengthened primary health care sector as a whole, the Federal Government established a General Practice Reform Strategy, which injected considerable resources into one part of the primary health care sector. This may well have been a missed opportunity to establish a stronger and more effective primary health care system that could have had a new public health mandate with an emphasis on community participation, multidisciplinary team work, a focus on communities rather than individuals, work across sectors, and health promotion. The main initiative of the General Practice Reform Strategy was the establishment of Divisions of General Practice and a project grants program to encourage GPs to become involved in cooperative activities and improve their integration with the health system (CDHFS 2001).

The Divisions have given GPs the opportunity to develop a range of preventive programs and to take a more population-based approach in their work. By 1995/96 the budget for the General Practice Reform Strategy was $238 million (CDHFS 2001). The strategy has focused on general practitioners and so does not explicitly encourage the multidisciplinary teamwork which is at the heart of community health work. When resources flow to one profession, the power imbalances created tend to undermine effective multidisciplinary teamwork. Despite this, the General Practice Reform Strategy did bring about some changes. For the first time in Australia, it encouraged GPs to come together and take a population view of the community. This has also opened opportunities for them to integrate more effectively with hospitals and community-based health services. Furthermore, it has offered GPs a chance to move away from an exclusive focus on fee-for-service, if they wish. Both of these features are potentially supportive of a more comprehensive PHC.

A review of general practice and community health concluded that if collaboration is to be encouraged (and the reviewers see this as desirable) then it would be important to fund programs that explicitly encourage multidisciplinary teamwork (Fry & Furler 2000). The collaboration will not happen without such incentives. In Victoria, Primary Care Partnerships (PCPs) aim to improve the health of Victorians by engaging consumers, carers, and communities in the planning and evaluation of services: improving health promotion, early intervention, and continuity of care; reducing the use of hospital services; all underpinned by a social model of health (Department of Human Services, Victoria 2001). These partnerships hold promise because they are bringing together all the key players in primary health care, including general practitioners and community health services, in a manner that does not privilege one group above another. The main means of implementing the strategy is through community health plans. These plans map the partnerships that need to be forged,

Fran Baum

and the service systems and infrastructures that need to be better integrated, and are intended to be based on the needs of the population. The evaluation of the partnerships (Swerissen et al. 2003) found that PCPs have had an important impact on the quality of relationships between agencies for service planning and system improvement and have made significant progress towards implementing integrated health promotion plans across regions. The evaluation also noted the limitations of the PCPs in that they are voluntary and have very limited resources at their disposal. Further, they have no direct influence over agency budgets and expenditure. Nonetheless, PCPs have introduced the idea of a networked form of organisation for primary health care that may offer a way forward for a more coordinated and effective primary health care sector that does emphasise the values embedded in the community health movement. Integrated Chronic Disease Management is a specific 'deliverable' for PCPs between 2006–09. As part of this, PCPs will be expected to increase the participation of general practices, general practice divisions, and providers of acute care in PCP activities. It will be a challenge to maintain the community health model while doing this.

Similar programs to improve coordination of GP and community health services are happening in all jurisdictions of Australia; for instance, New South Wales has an Integrated Primary and Community Health Policy (2007–12) which aims at coordinating the community health, GP, and other community-based services; Tasmania has a Primary Health–GP Work project which aims to develop a closer, more effective, working relationship between primary health services and general practice. South Australia has opened a number of GP Plus Centres which aim to offer community health services in a way that is more integrated with the GP sector than in the past.

The community health sector, because of its philosophy and funding model, has been able to take a broader population view of health and put more emphasis on health promotion and disease prevention that is conducted in a way that either addresses or takes account of the social determinants of health. A policy more favourable to comprehensive PHC, encouraging integration between general practice and community health, would fund multidisciplinary Divisions of Primary Health Care with explicit aims of encouraging close coordination between GP and community health. Such an approach would encourage activity across the community health activities from clinical and therapeutic care (from GPs, nurses, psychologists, speech pathologists, physiotherapists), to groups and to community development and social action.

A further way in which general practice and community health services could be integrated is through a program to fund salaried GPs within community health services. These GPs would then have the experience of working within a multidisciplinary team within a service focusing on a social perspective of health. Such a program could offer significant national benefits by allowing a move away from private practice fee-for-service general practice and encouraging a community model for the provision of general practitioner services. The likelihood of investment in salaried medical practitioners working in community health centres has increased with the GP shortages being experienced acutely from 2003 and with the commitment of the Rudd Labor Government to more comprehensive forms of PHC. The salaried model may prove one way of attracting GPs to practise in underserviced areas. Community health centres can provide a more supportive work environment with the potential for referral to a range of professional colleagues in the same organisation. Doctors could also become involved in work beyond one-to-one encounters.

Promising signs for community health

The Rudd Labor Government made a strong commitment to PHC during the 2007 election at which it came to power. Since taking office it has instituted a series of reviews and initiatives that collectively could lead to a significant reform of Australian health services that could see the development of a more comprehensive PHC system based on the community health model. These reviews and initiatives are:

- The Australia 2020 Summit
- The National Health and Hospitals Reform Commission
- The National Preventative Task Force
- The National Indigenous Health Equity Council.

These reviews and initiatives are in their early stages but they have the potential to make recommendations that will shape Australia's health services to be based on comprehensive PHC and to emphasise health promotion and the pursuit of equity. The Australia 2020 summit recommended a much stronger emphasis on disease prevention and a focus on health equity. In terms of Indigenous health, the Rudd Government has made a commitment to close the life expectancy gap in a generation. This will require strengthening of the community-controlled services and ensuring that all health services are accessible to Indigenous peoples. The health sector will also have to lead and monitor efforts to address the social determinants of ill health. It is very likely that the National Indigenous Health Equity Council will take a broad view of its tasks as its Chairperson, Professor Ian Anderson, has written and researched the importance of the social determinants of health and advocated a 'Beyond Bandaids' approach to promoting the health of Indigenous people (Anderson et al. 2007).

While the National Health and Hospitals Reform Commission is likely to focus on hospital services, it has the potential to make recommendations that could lead to investment in comprehensive PHC. The National Preventative Task Force has been asked to focus on tobacco, alcohol, and obesity as risks for chronic disease; this reflects a risk-factor perspective. It is to be hoped that the Taskforce also looks upstream to the factors that underpin these risks and recommends that health services do likewise. Each of these initiatives will be significant in shaping the community health sector over the coming years and their progress should be watched closely by health science students.

Conclusion

The community health sector in Australia is closer to a comprehensive model of primary health care than any other area of health in Australia. The services are planned according to a population health model and develop interventions provided by multidisciplinary teams that focus on individuals, groups, and populations. The philosophy underpinning the services draws on a comprehensive model of primary health care. Most significantly, the services give emphasis to the importance of achieving health equity and plan their services to do this. The community health model was first supported federally during the 1970s and then continued to be strongly supported only by the Victorian and South Australian Governments during the 1980s and early 1990s. Given this, it is true to say that community health has never received sustained long-term commitment from Australian health systems.

If Australian governments are to fulfil the promise of current reviews of health systems in Australia and make a sustained investment in community health, these services could form the backbone of a more sustainable health system that would be focused on effective coordination of care, health promotion, and disease prevention. This system promises to be cost-effective and to offer considerable benefits in terms of population health, especially for low-income and otherwise disadvantaged communities. A national primary health care policy based on a comprehensive strategy, which both ensures effective clinical and therapeutic multidisciplinary care, and encourages and develops a strong disease prevention and health promotion focus, is urgently required. Such a policy would put community health at the centre of a 'health promoting health system' that gives emphasis to preventing the need for unnecessary hospital care and which understands that promoting health requires attention not just to people who are sick but to the whole population in a way that takes account of the social and economic determinants of health.

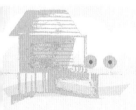

Summary of main points

» Community health services offer the most comprehensive primary health care services in Australia by putting into practice the philosophy of the World Health Organization's 'Health for All' strategy.

» Community health services offer a wide range of services to individuals including medicine, counselling, and a variety of physical therapies. They offer group support to help people to deal with a variety of diseases and social stresses, as well as engaging in social action and community development. Their approach to services is based on the use of multidisciplinary teams.

» Community health services have never been adequately funded and remain marginal to the mainstream health system but current policy changes have the potential to move them to a mainstream position especially as a means of reducing the population burden of chronic disease.

» Community health services can be the basis of a comprehensive PHC system which can ensure high-quality multidisciplinary clinical and therapeutic services and a focus on health promotion and disease prevention in a way that addresses the underlying social determinants of health.

Sociological reflection: the pursuit of wellness

Key features of community health services are the social model of health and the pursuit of wellness, which go beyond physical and psychological considerations by taking into account cultural and spiritual factors, as well as community participation, social support, and the adequacy of material factors such as employment, education, housing, transport, and environmental quality. As a holistic concept, positive health encourages us to consider factors affecting health outside the health system. Community health services also accept that health and wellness are unevenly distributed in our society and so work to redress health inequities.

» Consider the ways in which the organisation of schools, workplaces, local communities, and transport services affect health status.
» What factors affect health equity in Australia?
» What benefits to understanding health and illness can the concept of social determinants bring?

Discussion questions

1 What features of community health services make them different from other parts of the health sector?
2 What are the main differences between medical practice within community health services and within private general practice?
3 What dilemmas do you think community health services encounter when they use community development and social action strategies?

Fran Baum

4   What do you see as the advantages and disadvantages of community manage-
    ment of community health services?
5   What do you think would be the benefits for Australia if its health system were
    based on a network of well-funded community health services?
6   Why do governments seem to prefer to invest in hospitals rather than community
    health services?
7   How can community health services take action on the social determinants of health?

Further investigation

1   The community health services never received a 'sustained long-term commit-
    ment' in the Australian health system. Discuss.
2   Choose a specific area of community health services (for example, Indigenous
    community-controlled health services) and examine its operation in terms of the
    principles of primary health care promoted by the World Health Organization.

Further reading

Baum, F. 2008, *The New Public Health*, 3rd edn, Oxford University Press, Melbourne.

Butler, C., Rissel, C. & Khavarpour, F. 1999, 'The Context for Community Participation
in Health Action in Australia', *Australian Journal of Social Issues*, vol. 34, no. 3,
pp. 253–65.

Commission on the Social Determinants of Health 2008, *Closing the Gap in a Generation:
Health Equity through Action on the Social Determinants of Health*. WHO, Geneva.

Dwyer, J., Silburn, K. & Wilson, G. 2004, National Strategies for Improving Indigenous
Health and Health Care. *Aboriginal and Torres Strait Islander Primary Health Care
Review: Consultants' Report No. 1*, Commonwealth of Australia, Canberra.

Fry, D. & Furler, J. 2000, 'General Practice, Primary Health Care and Population Health
Interface', in Commonwealth Department of Health and Aged Care (ed.), *General
Practice in Australia 2000*, Commonwealth Department of Health and Aged Care,
Canberra, pp. 385–424.

Web resources

Australiahealth.com—Community Health: <http://www.australiahealth.com/>

Carers Australia: <http://www.carersaustralia.com.au/>

Commonwealth Department of Family and Community Services, Community Branch:
<http://www.community.gov.au/>

Human Rights and Equal Opportunities Commission: <http://www.hreoc.gov.au/>

South Australian Community Health Research Unit (SACHRU): <http://www.sachru.sa.gov.au/default.htm>

Victorian Government Health Information—Primary and Community Health: <http://www.health.vic.gov.au/pchtopics/>

Online case study • • •

Visit the Second Opinion website to access relevant case studies.

References

Alexander, K. 1995, 'Community Participation in Hospitals', in F. Baum (ed.), *Health for All: The South Australian Experience*, Wakefield Press, Adelaide.

Anderson, I., Baum, F. & Bentley, M. (eds) 2007, *Beyond Bandaids: Exploring the Underlying Social Determinants of Health*, Co-operative Research Centre in Aboriginal Health (Research Monograph), Darwin.

Australian Community Health Association (ACHA) 1986, *Review of the Community Health Program*, ACHA, Sydney.

Baum, F. 2007, Commentary on the Alma-Ata Declaration, *Social Medicine*, vol. 2, no. 1, pp. 34–41.

Baum, F. 2008, *The New Public Health*, 3rd edn, Oxford, Melbourne.

Baum, F. & Lawless, A. 2007, 'Opposing the Motion that "Family Medicine Should Emphasise Personal Care"', in T. Kenealy & S. Buetow (eds), *Ideological Debates in Family Medicine*, Nova Publishers, New York.

Baum, F., Jolley, G., Hicks, R., Saint, K. & Parker S. 2006, 'What Makes for Sustainable Healthy Cities Initiatives? A Review of the Evidence From Noarlunga after 18 Years', *Health Promotion International*, vol. 21, no. 4, pp. 259–65.

Baum, F., Kalucy, E., Lawless, A., Barton, S. & Steven, I. 1996, *Medical Practice and Women's and Community Health Centres in South Australia*, SACHRU, Adelaide.

Blewett, N. 2000, 'Community Health Services', Speech Given at Annual Public Health Association Conference, Canberra, December.

Boxall, A. & Leeder, S. 2006, 'The Health System: What Should Be Our Priorities?', *Health Promotion Journal of Australia*, vol. 17, no. 3, pp. 200–5.

Commonwealth Department of Health and Family Services (CDHFS) 2001, *General Practice in Australia: 1996*, General Practice Branch, Commonwealth Department of Health and Family Services, Canberra.

Commission on the Social Determinants of Health 2008, *Closing the Gap in a Generation: Health Equity through Action on the Social Determinants of Health*, WHO, Geneva.

Department of Human Services (DHS), Victoria 2001, *A Guide to General Practice Engagement in Primary Care Partnerships*, Aged, Community and Mental Health, Division of the Victorian Government Department of Human Services, Melbourne.

Dwyer, J. 2004, 'Australian Health System Restructuring: What Problem is Being Solved?', *Australia and New Zealand Health Policy*, vol. 1, no. 6, pp. 1–6. Available online:<http://www.anzhealthpolicy.com/home/>

Dwyer, J., Silburn, K. & Wilson, G. 2004, *National Strategies for Improving Indigenous Health and Health Care*, Aboriginal and Torres Strait Islander Primary Health Care Review, Consultant Report no. 1, Department of Health and Ageing, Canberra.

Fry, D. & Furler, J. 2000, 'General Practice, Primary Health Care and Population Health Interface', in Commonwealth Department of Health and Aged Care (ed.), *General Practice in Australia 2000*, Commonwealth Department of Health and Aged Care, Canberra, pp. 385–424.

Hospital and Health Services Commission 1973, *A Community Health Program for Australia*, AGPS, Canberra.

Laris, P. 1992, 'The Way of the Manager: The Context and Roles of Community Health Management', in F. Baum, D. Fry & I. Lennie (eds), *Community Health: Policy and Practice in Australia*, Pluto Press in association with the Australian Community Health Association, Sydney, pp. 64–76.

Laris, P. 1995, 'Boards of Directors of Community Health Services', in F. Baum (ed.), *Health For All: The South Australian Experience*, Wakefield Press, Adelaide, ch. 5, pp. 82–93.

Legge, D. 1992, 'Community Management: Open Letter to a New Committee Member', in F. Baum, D. Fry & I. Lennie (eds), *Community Health: Policy and Practice in Australia*, Pluto Press in association with the Australian Community Health Association, Sydney, pp. 95–114.

McCalman, J., Baird, B. & Tsey, K. 2007, 'Indigenous Men Taking Their Rightful Place—How One Aboriginal Community is Achieving Results', *Aboriginal and Islander Health Worker Journal*, vol. 31, no. 4, 8–9 July/Aug. Available online: <http://search.informit.com.au/documentSummary;dn=955963997149455;res=E-LIBRARY> ISSN: 1037-3403>

Milio, N. 1983, 'Next Steps in Community Health Policy: Matching Rhetoric with Reality', *Community Health Studies*, vol. 2, no. 2, pp. 185–92.

Raftery, J. 1995, 'The Social and Historical Context', in F. Baum (ed.), *Health for All: The South Australian Experience*, Wakefield Press, Adelaide, ch. 1, pp. 19–37.

Rogers, W. & Veale, B. 2000, *Primary Health Care and General Practice: A Scoping Report*, National Information Service, Department of General Practice, Flinders University, Adelaide.

Sanderson, C. & Alexander, K. 1995, 'Community Health Services Planning for Health', in F. Baum (ed.), *Health For All: The South Australian Experience*, Wakefield Press, Adelaide, ch. 10, pp. 161–71.

Silagy, C. 2000, 'Co-ordinated Care Trials', in Commonwealth Department of Health and Aged Care (ed.), *General Practice in Australia 2000*, Commonwealth Department of Health and Aged Care, Canberra, pp. 471–92.

Swerissen, H., Wilson, G., Lewis, H. et al. 2003, *An Evaluation of the Primary Care Partnership Strategy*, Report 3, Australian Institute of Primary Care, La Trobe University, Melbourne.

Warin, M., Baum, F., Kalucy, L., Murray, C. & Veale, B. 1998, *Not Just a Doctor: Community Perspective on Medical Services in Women's and Community Health Centres*, SACHRU, Adelaide.

World Health Organization 1978, 'Declaration of Alma-Ata', International Conference on Primary Health Care, Alma-Ata, USSR, 6–12 September 1978, WHO, Geneva.

ACKNOWLEDGMENT

Thanks to Elsa Barton for researching policy developments that have affected community health in Australian jurisdictions between 2004–07.

Fran Baum

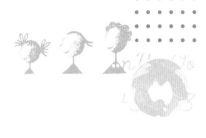

Appendix:
Tips on Planning, Writing, and Referencing Health Sociology Essays

This Appendix provides some handy tips on how to plan, write, and reference an essay, including how to critically assess and reference web-based information, as well as how to correctly reference chapters and information from this book. Much of the information is drawn from Williams, L. & Germov, J. (2001) *Surviving First Year Uni*, Allen & Unwin, Sydney and Germov, J. (2000) *Get Great Marks for Your Essays*, 2nd edn, Allen & Unwin, Sydney. Consult these books for more information on essay writing, referencing, and general academic skills.

Where to start first: don't Google!

When interpreting an essay question, avoid the temptation to Google. You will only end up getting hundreds of dubious 'hits'. Instead, you need to ensure you find credible academic sources and the only way to do this is to stick with university-based library resources. Before jumping deep into library research, you first need to interpret the essay topic and do some preliminary research—that is, a little basic reading on the topic—by doing the following:

• Check the textbook or course readings.
• Check your course guide for any relevant references.
• Check your notes from any relevant lectures.
• Consult some introductory sociological texts found in the library.
• Make use of a sociological dictionary.

By doing this preliminary reading, you will be able to gain a good understanding of the topic and identify key concepts, key authors, and the major sociological debates and theories. You can then use the library databases to find further relevant references (including journal articles).

Essay structure

The basic structure of an essay involves three parts:

- Introduction: clarifies an essay topic for the reader. It should include what your essay will cover, the stance or argument you will take, and briefly define any key terms where necessary.
- Body: a series of logically connected paragraphs where you describe and analyse material relevant to the topic by providing supporting evidence and explanations based on your reading of the literature.
- Conclusion: a short summary, usually in one paragraph, of the evidence and argument presented to answer the essay question. New information should not be included in the conclusion.

Note: unless otherwise stated, the use of subheadings in essays is optional. However, if you use them, be careful to maintain a logical flow in your essay content from one section to the next—that is, what comes before and after a heading should still have a logical connection.

In writing a university-level essay you should:

- Use formal expression and avoid emotive phrases such as slang, clichés, and stereotypes.
- Critically analyse (evaluate strengths and weaknesses) the relevant literature on a topic by taking into account opposing viewpoints.
- Always make use of supporting evidence drawn from authoritative and verifiable sources. Unless you are requested to do so, avoid anecdotal, hypothetical, and personal examples.
- Acknowledge the sources of information used by an accepted system of referencing. This way you avoid plagiarism (theft of another author's work). It also allows readers (including markers) to confirm and follow up on material you present.

What about my opinion? Making your argument, theme, or thesis

Your opinion, preferred explanation, or answer to a topic (sometimes called argument, theme, or thesis) can only be persuasive if it is based on authoritative sources of information (that is, academic books and journals that are related to the discipline you are studying). You should aim to form your opinion about a topic only after you have read the relevant literature and become aware of differing viewpoints. The argument you present in your essay is your considered opinion about a topic, supported with detailed evidence and references.

Writing your essay

- Drafts: writing is a time-consuming process. Once you have completed your notes, you should allow yourself enough time to produce at least two or three drafts before submitting your work.
- Word limits as word targets: aim to write as close to the word limit as possible: 10 per cent above or below the limit is generally acceptable.
- Proof reading: always carefully check your final draft for any spelling, grammatical, or referencing mistakes as marks will be deducted for such errors.

Note-taking and referencing

When you use information from books and journal articles in assignments, you will generally be required to acknowledge your information sources—this is known as referencing. You should reference research findings, statistics, concepts, and theories. You must always provide a reference for direct quotes and paraphrased information (material put into your own words but derived from another source). This may mean that every paragraph in your essay has at least one reference. Therefore, when you make notes of your reading, make sure that you record the bibliographic details (author(s), date of publication, title, page numbers, and so on); this will help you to reference your essay correctly and help you to compile your reference list.

Don't reference lecture notes in your essay

Do not reference or re-use lecture notes in your essays. If you want to use information used in a lecture, you will need to find the original source by conducting your own library research. This is because lecture notes are not publicly available or verifiable documents, and in any case, you are being assessed on your ability to research and synthesise information, not on whether you can copy and repeat lecture notes in essay form.

How to use the Harvard in-text referencing system

There are many types of referencing systems. The preferred one in the social sciences is known as the Harvard in-text referencing system, which is very similar to the APA system used by psychologists. The Harvard system includes references in the text of the essay—for example (Williams & Germov 2001: 5)—this reference tells the reader that information presented in the sentence or paragraph came from a source written by Williams and Germov (surnames only) that was published in 2001 and is found on page 5. All the other details about the information source such as the title, publisher, and place of publication (known as bibliographical information) appear in a list of references at the end of your essay. Here are two examples of what in-text references can look like:

- Germov (2005: 26) states that …

Here the author's name is part of the sentence. Notice the space between the author and the bracket. You may see some variations such as (2005, p. 26) or (2005, 26) —choose one and be consistent unless you have been given specific guidelines to follow.

- It can be argued that … (Germov 2005: 10–16).

If the author is not mentioned in the sentence, then the full reference comes at the end, all in brackets, with the full stop after the bracket.

When one author quotes another, and you want to use the same direct quote

When one author quotes another and you want to use the same direct quote, there is a simple rule to follow. For example, Germov is the author of the book you are using and he has used a direct quote from Mills, which you also want to use. The rule to follow is always reference where you got the information, that is, from Germov. The example below shows you how to reference when one author quotes another:

> Mills (quoted in Germov 2005: 12) states that the sociological imagination is 'a quality of mind that seems most dramatically to promise an understanding of the intimate realities of ourselves in connection with larger social realities'.

Direct quotes and paraphrased material

- In general, aim to paraphrase (put in your own words) the information you gather from other sources. You must still provide a reference for paraphrased information.
- Keep direct quotes to a minimum; they should be no more than 10 per cent of the word count. Copying slabs of information word for word is unacceptable as it is impossible to assess your understanding of the material.
- When using a direct quote, always keep the exact wording and spelling of the original source. Include page number/s with the reference.
- For direct quotes greater than thirty words: do not use quotation marks, but instead indent the quote from the left margin.

Bibliographic details and formatting your reference list

Your reference list is attached to the end of your essay and includes all the bibliographic details of the information sources referenced in your essay. It is only necessary to include the information sources that you referenced in your essay. Do not include other sources that you might have looked at, but not referenced. A reference list should be formatted consistently and organised in alphabetical order (by author surname). The reference list template in Box A2.1 includes examples of the information you need to record and include in your reference list.

BOX A2.1   A reference list template

For a book, provide:

» all author surnames and initials of first names
» date of publication
» book title (italicised or underlined)
» edition (where relevant)
» publisher
» place of publication.

EXAMPLE

Nilan, P., Julian, R. & Germov, J. 2007, *Australian Youth: Social and Cultural Issues*, Pearson Education, Melbourne.

For a chapter in an edited book, provide:

» all author surnames and initials of first names
» date of publication of the book in which the chapter is contained
» chapter title in inverted commas
» initials and surnames of editors, including the abbreviation 'ed.' or 'eds'
» book title (italicised or underlined)
» edition (where relevant)
» publisher
» place of publication.

EXAMPLE

Williams, L. & Germov, J. 2008, 'Constructing the Female Body: Dieting, The Thin Ideal, and Body Acceptance', in J. Germov & L. Williams (eds.), *A Sociology of Food and Nutrition: The Social Appetite*, 3rd edn, Oxford University Press, Melbourne.

For a journal article, provide:

» all author surnames and initials of first names
» date of publication of the journal in which the article is contained
» article title in inverted commas
» journal title (italicised or underlined)
» volume and issue numbers (where relevant)
» first and last page numbers of the article.

EXAMPLE

Skrbis, Z. & Germov, J. 2004, 'The Most Influential Books in Australian Sociology, 1963–2003', *Journal of Sociology*, vol. 40, no. 3, pp. 283–302.

For an online-only journal article, provide:

Same as above, but also include the web address of the online journal (URL) and the date you accessed the website. The inclusion of the URL and date accessed is only necessary if the journal is solely an online journal. If you merely access a hard copy journal via an online database (and download a pdf of an article), then there's no need to include the URL details because the pdf availability means it is exactly the same as the printed version.

EXAMPLE

McClimens, A. & Gordon, F. 2008, 'Presentation of Self in Everyday Life: How People Labelled with Intellectual Disability Manage Identity as they Engage the Blogosphere', *Sociological Research Online*, vol. 13, no. 4, <http://www.socresonline.org.uk/13/4/1.html>, date accessed: 14 September 2008.

For a web source, provide:

» author surnames and initials of first names where available (sometimes the author is an organisation)
» date of publication or last revision/ modification (often included at the bottom of a website)
» title of the publication and/or particular section of a website (italicised or underlined)
» title of the website and the web address (URL)
» date you accessed the website (because web information is often subject to change).

EXAMPLE

Commonwealth of Australia 2008, *Australian Social Trends*, Australian Bureau of Statistics [web site], <http://www.abs.gov.au/>, date accessed: 20 January 2009.

Note: in the text of an essay, you reference web sources in the usual way, noting the author and date. If no author is given, then the title of the website can be used instead (avoid including the URL as this is included in the details you provide in your reference list at the end of the essay). Note also that date accessed details are often not given, as is the case in this book.

How to evaluate the credibility of websites: not all websites are created equal

Because anyone can publish what they like on the web, it is important to exercise caution when obtaining information from a website. You need to evaluate the credibility of a website, before using it as a source of information for assignments. Ask yourself the following questions to help evaluate the credibility of the information contained on a website:

- Can an author be identified?
- Are date and title supplied?
- Are contact details for the author or publisher provided?
- How objective is the information provided? Does it represent the interests of a particular organisation, political party, or pressure group? How might this bias the information presented?
- If the source is an academic one, is it properly referenced and is the material self-published or has it been peer reviewed, such as articles published in online academic journals?

The general point to remember is not to take anything on the web at face value and to ensure that the source is credible. Often the easiest way to judge credibility is to ask yourself whether you would use the source if you had found it in hard copy form on your library shelves.

How to reference this book

A common mistake in referencing an edited book is to reference the editor rather than the chapter author. The first rule to remember when referencing content from an edited book such as *Second Opinion* is to reference the author of the chapter from which you obtained information. For example, let us say you need to reference information in your assignment that you found in the chapter by Lauren Williams, entitled 'Jostling for Position: A Sociology of Allied Health'. In the text of your assignment, you would reference the chapter author, that is, you would reference Williams, so that in your assignment it might appear as:

> Williams (2009) argues that allied health professions are subordinate to the medical profession …

Note that the year is obtained from the date of publication of the book in which the chapter appears. In your reference list at the end of your assignment, the complete reference would appear as:

Williams, L. 2009, 'Jostling for Position: A Sociology of Allied Health', in J. Germov (ed.), *Second Opinion: An Introduction to Health Sociology*, 4th edn, Oxford University Press, Melbourne.

The above entry provides the reader with specific details about where you got your information from, by identifying the chapter author and chapter title, as well as the book it appeared in. Some referencing systems may require you to include the first and last page numbers of the chapter in your reference list, which are usually placed at the end of the reference. While the formatting of your references will depend on which system you employ, you will generally need to include the above information.

Even when the chapter author and the editor are the same person, the same rules apply, so that a chapter by Germov in a book by Germov would appear in your reference list as:

Germov, J. 2009, 'Challenges to Medical Dominance', in J. Germov (ed.), *Second Opinion: An Introduction to Health Sociology*, 4th edn, Oxford University Press, Melbourne.

If you need to reference a section of the book, such as the glossary, you can do so in the following way:

Germov, J. 2009, 'Glossary', in J. Germov (ed.), *Second Opinion: An Introduction to Health Sociology*, 4th edn, Oxford University Press, Melbourne.

Glossary

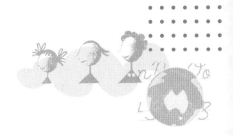

accident proneness
A term invented by industrial psychologists to 'explain' workplace injury and illness. It is based on the false and unproven assumption that workers are careless and malingering, and are therefore solely responsible for accidents.

acute illness
Illness with a rapid onset, short duration, and needing urgent attention.

affect
The expression of feeling or emotion as it influences a person's behaviour; in psychiatric terminology a person suffering from depression may present as 'restricted' or 'flat' in affect.

ageism
A term that denotes discrimination based on age.

agency
The ability of people, individually and collectively, to influence their own lives and the society in which they live.

agribusiness
The complete operations performed in producing agricultural commodities, including farming, manufacture, handling, storage, processing, and distribution.

alcohol misuse
Excessive consumption of alcohol leading to health and/or social problems.

allopathy
A descriptive name often given to orthodox medicine. Allopathy is the treatment of symptoms by opposites.

Alzheimer's disease
An incurable and terminal type of dementia indicated by significant memory loss and degenerative mental and physical abilities, resulting in confusion, language decline, loss of bodily functions, and ultimately, in death.

assimilation/assimilationism

A policy term referring to the expectation that Indigenous people and migrants will 'shed' their culture and become indistinguishable from the Anglo-Australian majority.

autoethnography

An ethnography that focuses on the experience of the researcher.

biobank

The organised collection of biological samples including DNA. It can range in scope from small collections of samples in academic or hospital settings to large-scale national repositories.

biographical disruption

Refers to the effect of chronic illness on a person's self-identity, such as loss of control and certainty, that influences how the person deals with the illness experience.

biological determinism

An unproven belief that individual and group behaviour and social status are an inevitable result of biology.

biomedicine/biomedical model

The conventional approach to medicine in Western societies, based on the diagnosis and explanation of illness as a malfunction of the body's biological mechanisms. This approach underpins most health professions and health services, which focus on treating individuals, and generally ignores the social origins of illness and its prevention.

biopsychosocial model

This model is an extension of the biomedical model. It is a multifactorial model of illness that takes into account the biological, psychological, and social factors implicated in a patient's condition. As with the biomedical model, it focuses on the individual patient for diagnosis, explanation, and treatment.

biotechnology

The use of molecular biology and genetic engineering to modify plants and animals, including humans, at the molecular level.

capitalism

An economic and social system based on the private accumulation of wealth.

Cartesian dualism

Also called mind/body dualism and named after the philosopher René Descartes, it refers to a belief that the mind and body are separate entities. This assumption underpins medical approaches that view disease in physical terms and thus ignore the psychological and subjective aspects of illness.

chronic illness

A long-term or permanent illness condition that has no known cure (for example, diabetes).

citizenship

A collection of social rights and obligations that determine legal identity and membership of a nation state, and function to control access to scarce resources.

civilising process

The 'civilising process' is a concept coined by Norbert Elias to refer to the never-ending social process by which external forms of social control of people's behaviour are replaced by internalised forms of moral self-control.

class (or social class)

A position in a system of structured inequality based on the unequal distribution of power, wealth, income, and status. People who share a class position typically share similar life chances.

clinical governance

A term to describe a range of quality assurance measures that control doctors' clinical decision-making through standardised work protocols and performance measurement at the clinical level.

collective conscience

A term used to describe shared moral beliefs that act to unify society.

colonisation/colonialism

A process by which one nation imposes itself economically, politically, and socially upon another.

commodification of health care

Treating health care as a commodity to be bought and sold in the pursuit of profit maximisation.

commodity culture

The world of advertising and commercial marketing.

communism

A utopian vision of society based on communal ownership of resources, cooperation, and altruism to the extent that social inequality and the state no longer exist. Sometimes used interchangeably with socialism to refer to societies ruled by a communist party. See also *socialism*.

community

A society where people's relations with each other are direct and personal and where a complex web of ties links people in mutual bonds of emotion and obligation.

Community Treatment Order

A legal order made on behalf of individuals by their psychiatrists to enforce treatment outside the confines of the hospital. Conditions of an Order include regular attendance at a nominated public community mental health centre, and adherence to a prescribed medication regimen. Failure to comply with such conditions results in involuntary admission to a psychiatric inpatient unit.

complementary and alternative medicine (CAM)

A broad term to describe both alternative medical practitioners and practices that may stand in opposition to orthodox medicine and also those who may collaborate with, and thus complement, orthodox practice (also referred to as integrative medicine).

consumerism

The processes and institutions by which individuals satisfy their needs by purchasing goods and services in a market. Mass consumerism refers to post-Second World War consumer practices, whereby the reduction of the cost of goods and the extensive use of advertising and new credit arrangements created a mass market. It is often argued that consumerism has less to do with the satisfaction of wants than with the desire to be different and distinctive.

convergence

The process, which may or may not be occurring, whereby orthodox medicine adopts many of the practices of alternative medicine, and alternative medicine acts to become more orthodox by, for example, seeking to license practitioners and make them subject to training.

corporatisation

A process referring to the decline of medical power as a result of the salaried employment of doctors in private sector health organisations, whereby corporate managers impose controls over medical practice.

cultural competence

A set of behaviours, attitudes, policies, and structures that enables the health care system to deliver the highest quality care to patients regardless of race, ethnicity, culture, or language proficiency.

cultural diversity

A term used to refer to the existence of a range of different cultures in a single society. In popular usage, it typically refers to ethnic diversity, but sociologically the term can equally refer to differences based on gender, social class, age, disability, and so on.

cultural stereotypes

Shared images of the members of an ethnic group that are often negative and are based on a simplistic, overgeneralised, and homogeneous view of an 'ethnic' culture.

deinstitutionalisation

A trend in mental health treatment whereby individuals are admitted for short periods of time, rather than undergoing lifetime hospitalisation. In theory, such policies are meant to be supported by extensive community resources, to 'break down the barriers' and integrate the mentally ill into the community. However, in practice, this has not occurred on a wide scale because of the lack of funding of community services.

delusion

A persistent, idiosyncratic belief, unusual in the person's cultural context and which is held on to despite arguments and evidence to the contrary. In psychiatric terminology, delusions may be described as 'grandiose', 'paranoid', 'persecutory', 'hypochondriacal', and 'nihilistic'.

demography/demographic

The statistical study of populations (demography) that identifies selected character- istics of a population (demographics), such as age profile, sex, income, education, and employment.

deprofessionalisation

A general theory predicting the decline of medical status and power due to the public's increased education about health issues and diminishing trust in medical practice as a result of media exposés of medical fraud and negligence.

deviance

Behaviour or activities that violate social expectations about what is normal.

disability

A socially constructed and contested term (for which the definition has varied over time and between cultures) that broadly refers to physical and/or mental limitations, restrictions, or impairments that can be chronic or last for a sustained period of time.

discourse

A domain of language use that is characterised by common ways of talking and think- ing about an issue (for example, the discourses of medicine, madness, or sexuality).

dispossession

The removal of people from land they regard as their own.

dual relationship

Refers to two distinct kinds of relationship with the same person (referred to as 'mul- tiple relationship' when more than two aspects are involved).

dual diagnosis

The presence of a mental health disorder and substance abuse in the same person. Treatment is often problematic as services tend to cater to one diagnostic group, and the symptoms of one disorder may intensify the effects and experiences of the other.

ecological model
Derived from the field of human ecology, and when applied to public health, suggests that an understanding of health determinants must consider the interaction of social, economic, geographic, and environmental factors.

economic rationalism/economic liberalism
Terms used to describe a political philosophy based on small government and market-oriented policies, such as deregulation, privatisation, reduced government spending, and lower taxation.

embodiment
The lived experience of both being a body and having a body.

emotional labour
Refers to the use of feelings by employees as part of their paid work. In health care, a key part of nursing work is caring for patients, often by providing emotional support.

empirical
Describes observations or research that is based on evidence drawn from experience. It is therefore distinguished from something based only on theoretical knowledge or on some other kind of abstract thinking process.

encroachment (vertical and horizontal)
The threat to professionals' occupational territory. Vertical encroachment can be from above (from medicine, for instance) or from below, whereby less qualified workers do some of the tasks previously done by a professional. Horizontal encroachment refers to the occupational takeover of one profession by another, where both have similar status and power.

epidemiology/social epidemiology
The statistical study of patterns of disease in the population. Originally focused on epidemics, or infectious diseases, it now covers non-infectious conditions such as stroke and cancer. Social epidemiology is a sub-field aligned with sociology that focuses on the social determinants of illness.

ethnic communities
Those ethnic groups that have established a large number of ethnic organisations, thus providing a shared context for interaction between members. Only some ethnic groups develop the institutional structure that enables them to become ethnic communities.

ethnicity

Sociologically, the term refers to a shared cultural background, which is a characteristic of all groups in society. As a policy term, it is used to identify migrants who share a culture that is markedly different from that of Anglo-Australians. In practice, it often refers only to migrants from non-English-speaking backgrounds (NESB migrants).

ethnic minorities

Ethnic groups that are not the dominant ethnic group in a society. Unlike the term 'ethnic group', it highlights the power differences between different ethnic groups in society.

ethnocentric

Viewing others from one's own cultural perspective, with an implied sense of cultural superiority based on an inability to understand or accept the practices and beliefs of other cultures.

ethnography

A research method that is based on direct observation of a particular social group's social life and culture—of what people actually do.

ethnospecific services

Services established to meet the needs of specific ethnic groups or a number of ethnic groups. Members of the ethnic group(s) are the targeted clientele, so that these services are distinct from, and often run parallel with, mainstream services.

eugenics

The study of human heredity based on the unproven assumption that selective breeding could improve the intellectual, physical, and cultural traits of a population.

euthanasia

Meaning 'gentle death', the term is used to describe voluntary death, often medically assisted, as a result of incurable and painful disease.

evidence-based medicine (EBM)

An approach to medicine that maintains that all clinical practice should be based on evidence from randomised control trials (RCTs) to ensure treatment effectiveness and efficacy.

feminisation

A shift in the gender base of a group from being predominantly male to being increasingly female.

feminism/feminist

A broad social and political movement based on a belief in equality of the sexes and the removal of all forms of discrimination against women. A feminist is one who makes use of, and may act upon, a body of theory that seeks to explain the subordinate position of women in society.

figurations

A concept developed by Norbert Elias as an alternative to structure and agency. Figurations represent the nexus of structure and agency, and can be conceived of as networks of people in interdependent relationships. They are the product of individuals but beyond the control of any single individual or group. Elias suggested that figurations could best be imagined as a game in which people must depend on one another within the confines of the rules. Social conflict or competition may result in the rules being changed or may cause new forms of figurations to develop.

food security/insecurity

Food security refers to the availability of affordable, nutritious, and culturally acceptable food. Food insecurity is a state of regular hunger and fear of starvation.

Friendly Societies

An organisation based on membership fees that serves the collective interests of its members, offering health insurance and welfare services, and sometimes social club activities such as dances and sports teams.

functional prerequisites

A debated concept based on the assumption that all societies require certain functions to be performed for them to survive and maintain social order. Also known as functional imperatives.

Gemeinschaft

A German term referring to a traditional society in which social relationships are based on personal bonds of friendship and kinship and on intergenerational stability.

gender/sex

This pair of terms refers to the socially constructed categories of feminine and masculine (the cultural identities and values that prescribe how men and women should behave), and the social power relations based on those categories, as distinct from the categories of biological sex (female or male).

gendered health

A term used to acknowledge the different experiences and exposures to health and illness that result from gender.

geneism

A form of discrimination—such as racism, sexism, and ageism—in which people are judged on their ascribed, rather than achieved, status. In this case, their genetic make-up is used as the basis for determining access to social rewards such as employment or health insurance.

genetic manipulation
Alteration of the genetic material of living cells to perform new functions (by rearranging or deleting existing genes), including the transferral of genetic information from one species to another.

genetic reductionism
An assumption that people are simply the sum of their individual genes, so that the causes of disease are reduced to an individual's genes rather than the social, economic, and political context in which people live. See *biological determinism*.

Gesellschaft
A German term referring to an urban society, in which social bonds are based on impersonal and specialised relationships, with little long-term commitment to the group or consensus on values.

globalisation
Political, social, economic, and cultural developments—such as the spread of multi-national companies, information technology, and the role of international agencies—that result in people's lives being increasingly influenced by global, rather than national or local, factors.

gross domestic product (GDP)
The market value of all goods and services that have been sold during a year.

grounded theory
Usually associated with qualitative methods, it refers to any social theory that is derived from (or grounded in) empirical research of social phenomena.

habitus
An expanded notion of habit, 'habitus' refers to the internalised and taken-for-granted personal dispositions we all possess, such as our accent, gestures, and preferences in food, fashion, and entertainment.

health discourses
A domain of language-use that is characterised by common ways of talking and thinking about health.

health promotion
Any combination of education and related organisational, economic, and political interventions designed to promote behavioural and environmental changes conducive to good health, including legislation, community development, and advocacy. See also *primary health care* and *public health*.

healthism
The extreme preoccupation with personal health that is evident within the general population.

hermeneutics
Study of the interpretation and understanding of texts.

high prevalence disorders
This term refers to the most commonly diagnosed mental disorders of anxiety, depression, and substance abuse.

iatrogenesis/iatrogenic
A concept popularised by Ivan Illich that refers to any adverse outcome or harm as a result of medical treatment.

ideal type
A concept originally devised by Max Weber to refer to the abstract or pure features of any social phenomenon.

ideology
In a political context, ideology refers to those beliefs and values that relate to the way in which society should be organised, including the appropriate role of the state.

illness trajectory
Refers to the changing nature of a person's experience of illness over time and how this is influenced by the actions of the patients and their interactions with health professionals, family, and friends.

immigrants
A term for those in the population who were born in another country, which is sometimes extended to the descendants of immigrants through the terms 'second-generation' and 'third-generation' immigrants. However, this usage confuses the term and obscures the key fact that those born overseas have a set of immigrant experiences that their descendants do not have.

Indigenous community-controlled health services
Independent local organisations, controlled and managed by Indigenous people, which provide a range of services to meet the needs of their particular communities.

individualism/individualisation
A belief or process supporting the primacy of individual choice, freedom, and self-responsibility.

individualist health promotion (IHP)
IHP is a set of programs that provide health education about health risks to persuade people to change their lifestyles. A wide group of professionals are involved in these programs, including doctors, nurses, allied health professionals, psychologists, educators, and media and marketing experts.

industrial citizenship

The right of workers to unionise and take collective action such as strikes, protests, and negotiation over improved pay and working conditions.

institutionalisation

A process by which the lives of individuals are regulated in every way, and which creates dependent relationships between the institutionalised person and authority figures.

labelling theory

Focuses on the effect that social institutions and health professions (such as the police, the courts, and psychiatry) have in labelling (defining and socially constructing) what is deviant.

lay concepts of health and illness

Refers to personal and non-expert explanations of health attainment and illness causation and treatment.

lay epidemiology

Refers to people's everyday understanding of health risks, which may or may not be supported by the research evidence.

liberalism

An ideology that regards the interests of individuals and their position in the marketplace as being of primary importance.

life chances

Derived from Max Weber, the term refers to people's opportunity to realise their lifestyle choices, which are often assumed to differ according to their social class.

lifestyle choices/factors

The decisions people make that are likely to impact on their health, such as diet, exercise, smoking, alcohol, and other drugs. The term implies that people are solely responsible for choosing and changing their lifestyle.

low prevalence disorders

This term refers to psychotic disorders, including schizophrenia, which occur significantly less frequently in the population than 'high prevalence' mental disorders.

McDonaldisation

A term coined by George Ritzer to expand Max Weber's notion of rationalisation; defined as the standardisation of social life by rules and regulations, such as increased monitoring and evaluation of individual performance, akin to the uniformity and control measures used by fast food chains.

mainstreaming

A policy term that refers to the provision of services to all members of the community through the same institutional structure. In Australia, it refers to a structure of service provision that is contrasted with that of ethnospecific services.

managerialism

The introduction of private sector management techniques into the public sector.

market

Any institutional arrangement for the exchange of goods according to economic demand and supply. This term is often used to describe the basic principle underlying the capitalist economy.

materialist analysis

An analysis that is embedded in the real, actual, material reality of everyday life.

medical dominance

A general term used to describe the power of the medical profession in terms of its control over its own work, over the work of other health workers, and over health resource allocation, health policy, and the way that hospitals are run.

medical–industrial complex

The growth of profit-oriented medical companies and industries, whereby one company may own a chain of health services, such as hospitals, clinics, and radiology and pathology services.

medical pluralism

A general term that refers to the vast array of healing modalities across the globe, in particular to the increasing popularity of alternative therapies and their coexistence with biomedicine in Westernised societies.

medicalisation

The process by which non-medical problems become defined and treated as medical issues, usually in terms of illnesses, disorders, or syndromes.

Medicare

The publicly funded Australian federal government scheme that provides access to free health care in public hospitals and free or subsidised treatment by general practitioners and some specialist services.

men's health

Running parallel to women's health initiatives, the men's health movement recognises that certain elements of masculine identity and behaviour can be hazardous to health.

mental health

Allows individuals to make sense of the world around them, and their inner experiences. Mentally healthy individuals are able appropriately to fulfil their social roles, conduct relationships with others, and attend to their own basic bodily and psychological needs.

mental illness

Definitions of mental illness differ over time and across cultures. In contemporary Western societies mental illness is formally defined via an elaborate system known as the *DSM-IV-TR*, which describes 374 categories of illness.

meta-analysis and meta-narratives

The 'big picture' analysis that frames and organises observations and research on a particular topic.

modernity/modernism

A view of social life that is founded upon rational thought and a belief that truth and morality exist as objective realities that can be discovered and understood through scientific means. See *reflexive modernity* and *postmodernism*.

moral panic

An exaggerated reaction by the mass media, politicians, and community leaders to the actions and beliefs of certain social groups or individuals, concerns which are often minor and inconsequential, but are sensationally represented to create anxiety and outrage among the general public.

multiculturalism

A policy term referring to the expectation that all members of society have the right to equal access to services, regardless of 'race', ethnicity, culture, or religion. It is based on the recognition that all people have the right to maintain their cultural beliefs and identity while adhering to the laws of the nation state.

muscular ideal

The social construction of the male body that reinforces the desirability of a large, muscular body as epitomising masculinity.

narrative reconstruction

Refers to individuals' beliefs about the causes and implications of their illness and how this shapes a redeveloped sense of self-identity.

negotiated order

A symbolic interactionist concept that refers to any form of social organisation in which the exercise of authority and the formation of rules are outcomes of human interaction and negotiation.

neo-liberalism

A philosophy based on the primacy of individual rights and minimal state intervention. Sometimes used interchangeably with *economic rationalism/economic liberalism.*

new public health

A social model of health linking 'traditional' public health concerns about physical aspects of the environment (clean air and water, safe food, occupational safety) with concerns about the behavioural, social, and economic factors that affect people's health.

norms

Expectations about how people ought to act or behave.

nurse practitioner

The title given to nurses with an enhanced and extended role, such as the ability to prescribe certain drugs and undertake procedures such as Pap smears and minor surgery. In some countries (such as the USA) it may also refer to the nurse's ability to charge a fee for service.

obesity

A socially constructed term that refers to the condition of having a high level of stored body fat, usually defined by body mass index.

orthodox medicine

The medical practices and institutions developed in Europe during the nineteenth and twentieth centuries that are legally recognised by the state. Central to these practices is the teaching hospital, where all new doctors are inducted into laboratory science, clinical practice, and allopathic biomedicine. These practices and institutions are now dominant in all parts of the world.

pandemic

A worldwide epidemic.

patriarchy

A system of power through which males dominate households. It is used more broadly by feminists to refer to society's domination by patriarchal power, which functions to subordinate women and children.

peer group

A group of people who are linked by common interests, equal social position, and (usually) similar age.

Pharmaceutical Benefits Scheme (PBS)

The publicly funded federal government scheme that subsidises the cost of prescribed medicines in Australia.

placebo/placebo effect

Any therapeutic practice that has no clear clinical effect. In practice it usually means giving patients an inert substance to take as a medication. When a patient reacts to a placebo in a way that is not clinically explicable, this is called the 'placebo effect'.

pluralism

A theory whereby state power is shared with a large number of pressure or interest groups.

population health

The collective health status of a specified population.

positive health

A holistic view of health that focuses on wellness, rather than disease, and that is culturally relative, incorporating notions of spirituality, community, and social support.

positivism

Research methods that attempt to study people in the same way that physical scientists study the natural world by focusing on quantifiable and directly observable events.

post-structuralism/postmodernism

Often used interchangeably, these terms refer to a broad perspective that is opposed to the view that social structure determines human action, and instead emphasises a pluralistic world view that explores the local, the specific, and the contingent in social life.

prevalence

The rate at which a particular condition occurs in a population.

primary health care (PHC)

Both the point of first contact with the health care system and a philosophy for delivery of that care.

professional bureaucracy

Henry Mintzberg's (1979) term for an organisation that relies on staff with specialised knowledge and expertise to deliver complex services that require decision-making autonomy at the point of service delivery.

professionalisation/professional project

The process of becoming a profession, whereby an occupational group attains publicly recognised and government-legitimated monopoly and autonomy over its area of work. See *trait approach*.

psychosis

A group of symptoms characterised by gross impairment of perception and thought, which manifests in misapprehension and misinterpretation of the nature of reality, but which is not caused by a physical illness. Hallucinations and delusions are often central to a diagnosis of psychosis.

public health/public health infrastructure

Public policies and infrastructure to prevent the onset and transmission of disease among the population, with a particular focus on sanitation and hygiene such as clean air, water and food, and immunisation. Public health infrastructure refers specifically to the buildings, installations, and equipment necessary to ensure healthy living conditions for the population.

purposive sampling

Refers to the selection of units of analysis to ensure that the processes involved are adequately studied, and where statistical representativeness is not required.

qualitative research

Research that focuses on the personal experiences and beliefs, subjective meanings and interpretations, of the participants being studied.

quantitative research

Research that focuses on the collection of statistical data.

'race'

A term without scientific basis that uses skin colour and facial features to describe what are alleged to be biologically distinct groups of humans. Race is actually a social construction used to categorise groups of people and sometimes implies assumed (and unproven) intellectual superiority or inferiority.

racism

Beliefs and actions used to discriminate against a group of people because of their physical and cultural characteristics.

randomised control trials (RCTs)

A biomedical research procedure used to evaluate the effectiveness of particular medications and therapeutic interventions. 'Random' refers to the equal chance of participants being in the experimental or control group (the group which receives a placebo or no treatment at all and is used for comparison), and 'trial' refers to the experimental nature of the method. RCTs are often mistakenly viewed as the best way to demonstrate causal links between factors under investigation, but tend to privilege biomedical over social responses to illness.

rationalisation

The standardisation of social life through rules and regulations. See *McDonaldisation*.

reductionism

The belief that all illnesses can be explained and treated by reducing them to biological and pathological factors.

reflexive modernity

A term coined by Ulrich Beck and Anthony Giddens to refer to the present social era in developed societies, in which social practices are open to reflection, questioning, and change, and therefore in which social traditions no longer dictate people's lifestyles. See *modernity*.

research methods

Procedures used by researchers to collect and investigate data.

rights

Socially prescribed privileges and entitlements for individuals and social groups.

rigour

A term used by qualitative researchers to describe trustworthy research that carefully scrutinises and describes the meanings and interpretations given by participants.

risk/risk discourse

Risk refers to 'danger' and risk discourse is often used in health promotion messages warning people that certain actions involve significant risks to their health.

risk factors

Conditions, such as alcohol misuse, smoking, and poor diet, that are thought to increase an individual's susceptibility to illness or disease.

risk society

A term coined by Ulrich Beck to describe the centrality of risk calculations in people's lives in Western society, whereby the key social problems today are unanticipated hazards, such as the risks of pollution, food poisoning, and environmental degradation.

ruling class

This is a hotly debated term used to highlight the point that the upper class in society has political power as a result of its economic wealth. The term is often used interchangeably with 'upper class'.

schizophrenia

A long-term mental disorder characterised by a breakdown in the relation between thought, feeling, and behaviour, which results in impaired perception, socially inappropriate behaviours and feelings, and social withdrawal. Both the subjective experiences and observable behaviours involved in this illness are highly variable. In acute stages, delusions and hallucinations are often experienced, whilst chronic symptoms often manifest as lethargy, apathy, and loss of motivation and drive.

self-determination

A government policy designed to ensure that Indigenous communities decide the pace and nature of their future development.

sexism in medicine
Refers to doctors' discriminatory and harmful treatment of women by ignoring women's health concerns in medical research and intervention, not informing women of the availability of other treatments or the side effects of drugs/therapies, and labelling of women's problems as 'psychosomatic' rather than 'real'.

sexual division of labour
Refers to the nature of work performed as a result of gender roles. In contemporary English-speaking societies, the stereotype is that of the male breadwinner and the female homemaker, even though this pattern is far from an accurate description of most people's lives.

sick role
A concept used by Talcott Parsons to describe the social expectations of how sick people are expected to act and of how they are meant to be treated.

social appetite
A term used by John Germov and Lauren Williams to refer to the social patterns of food production, distribution, and consumption.

social capital
A term used to refer to social relations, networks, norms, trust, and reciprocity between individuals that facilitate cooperation for mutual benefit.

social closure
A term first used by Max Weber to describe the way that power is exercised to exclude outsiders from the privileges of social membership (in social classes, professions, or status groups).

social cohesion
A term used to refer to the social ties that are the basis for group behaviour and integration. See *social capital*.

social construction/constructionism
Refers to the socially created characteristics of human life based on the idea that people actively construct reality, meaning it is neither 'natural' nor inevitable. Therefore, notions of normality/abnormality, right/wrong, and health/illness are subjective human creations that should not be taken for granted.

social control
Mechanisms that aim to induce conformity, or at least to manage or minimise deviant behaviour.

social Darwinism
The incorrect application of Charles Darwin's theory of animal evolution to explain social inequality by transferring his idea of 'survival of the fittest' among animals to 'explain' human inequality.

social death

The marginalisation and exclusion of elderly people from everyday life, resulting in social isolation.

social determinants of health

The economic, social, and cultural factors that directly and indirectly influence individual and population health.

social differentiation

A trend toward social diversity based on the creation of social distinction and self-identity through particular consumption choices and through group membership.

social epidemiology

See *epidemiology*.

social exclusion

A broad term used to encompass individuals and groups who experience persistent social disadvantage from a range of causes (poverty, unemployment, poor housing, social isolation etc.), preventing participation in social institutions and political processes.

social institutions

Formal structures within society—such as health care, government, education, religion, and the media—that are organised to address identified social needs.

socialism

A political ideology with numerous variations, but with a core belief in the creation of societies in which private property and wealth accumulation are replaced by state ownership and distribution of economic resources. See also *communism*.

social justice

A belief system that gives high priority to the interests of the least advantaged.

social liberalism

An ideology that is based on individual freedom but acknowledges the need for state intervention to overcome the inadequacies of the market, which can act to limit the freedom of individuals fully to participate in society.

social model of disability

An approach that views society as 'disabling' and thus focuses on the rights of disabled people so as to address cultural and structural discrimination and ensure similar treatment and opportunities afforded to able-bodied people.

social model of health

Focuses on social determinants of health such as the social production, distribution, and construction of health and illness, and the social organisation of health care. It directs attention to the prevention of illness through community participation and social reforms that address living and working conditions.

social structure

The recurring patterns of social interaction through which people are related to each other, such as social institutions and social groups.

social support

The support provided to an individual by being part of a network of kin, friends, or colleagues.

social wage

Government spending on health, social security, education, and housing (often referred to as welfare spending).

socialisation

The process of learning the culture of a society (its language and customs), which shows us how to behave and communicate.

sociobiology

A theory of evolutionary biology, associated with Edward O. Wilson, that seeks to explain the evolution of social organisation and social behaviour in terms of biological characteristics.

sociological imagination

A term coined by Charles Wright Mills to describe the sociological approach to analysing issues. We see the world through a sociological imagination, or think sociologically, when we make a link between personal troubles and public issues.

specialist mental health services

These services, located in both public and private sectors, focus on providing mental health care. They employ professionals who specialise in assessing and treating mental health problems—psychiatrists, psychiatric nurses, and allied health professionals. The specialist sector tends to treat the individuals with the most severe mental health problems, and is usually accessed via a primary care practitioner.

state

A term used to describe a collection of institutions, including the parliament (government and opposition political parties), the public-sector bureaucracy, the judiciary, the military, and the police.

stigma/stigmatisation

A physical or social trait, such as a disability or a criminal record, that results in negative social reactions such as discrimination and exclusion.

'stolen children'

Indigenous children who were forcibly removed from their families during the nineteenth and twentieth centuries by the agents of government in order to assimilate them into mainstream Australia.

structuration
A concept developed by Anthony Giddens to indicate the interrelationship between *structure* and *agency*.

structuralist explanations
Explanations that locate causality outside of the individual. For instance, these may include one's social class position, age, or gender.

structuralist-collectivist health promotion (SCHP)
SCHP encompasses a wide range of interventions, including participatory community programs, legislation, and bureaucratic interventions. The latter range from needle exchanges to the enactment of laws restricting industrial pollution, fireworks, flammable nightwear, cigarette advertising, and smoking in public places.

structure–agency debate
A key debate in sociology over the extent to which human behaviour is determined by social structure.

symbolic interactionism
This theory focuses on the micro-worlds of people as these are constructed by individuals themselves. It positions individuals, including those with mental illness, as social actors who draw from wider cultural meanings to describe their lives and circumstances.

terra nullius
A Latin term used by the British legally to define Australia as an unoccupied land belonging to no one and therefore open to colonisation.

theory
A system of ideas that uses researched evidence to explain certain events and to show why certain facts are related.

therapeutic justice
Specialised courts (such as drug courts) based on a philosophy that some crimes are the result of illness and require a focus on the rehabilitation of offenders.

thin ideal
The dominant aesthetic ideal of female beauty in Western societies, which refers to the social desirability of a thin body shape.

total institutions
A term used by Erving Goffman to refer to institutions such as prisons and asylums in which life is highly regulated and subjected to authoritarian control to induce conformity.

traditional medical system
Indigenous beliefs and practices about health and illness.

trait approach

A functionalist theory of professions that assumes professional status can be achieved by meeting a set of criteria (usually defined as specialised expertise and training, and self-regulation through a code of ethics).

victim-blaming

The process whereby social inequality is explained in terms of individuals being solely responsible for what happens to them in relation to the choices they make and their assumed psychological, cultural, and/or biological inferiority.

women's health movement

A term broadly used to describe attempts to address sexism in medicine by highlighting the importance of gender in health research and services. Achievements include women's community health centres and Australia's 1989 National Women's Health Policy.

Index

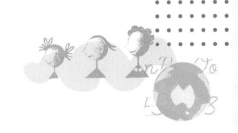